MANUAL OF GASTROENTEROLOGY: DIAGNOSIS AND THERAPY

Fourth Edition

MANUAL OF GASTROENTEROLOGY: DIAGNOSIS AND THERAPY
Fourth Edition

Canan Avunduk, M.D., Ph.D.
Bay State Gastroenterology
Melrose, Massachusetts;
Clinical Associate Professor of Medicine
Tufts University Medical School
Boston, Massachusetts

 Wolters Kluwer | Lippincott Williams & Wilkins
Health

Philadelphia · Baltimore · New York · London
Buenos Aires · Hong Kong · Sydney · Tokyo

Acquisitions Editor: Charles W. Mitchell
Managing Editor: Sirkka Howes
Project Manager: Nicole Walz
Manufacturing Coordinator: Kathleen Brown
Marketing Manager: Angela Panetta
Design Coordinator: Terry Mallon
Cover Designer: Becky Baxendell
Production Services: GGS Book Services

Printed in the USA

Library of Congress Cataloging-in-Publication Data
Avunduk, Canan.
Manual of gastroenterology: diagnosis and therapy/Canan Avunduk.—4th ed.
   p. ; cm.
  Includes bibliographical references and index.
  ISBN-13: 978-0-7817-6974-7 (pbk. : alk. Paper) 1. Gastrointestinal system—
  ISBN-10: 0-7817-6974-4
Diseases—Handbooks, manuals, etc. I. Title.
  [DNLM: 1. Gastrointestinal Diseases—diagnosis—Handbooks. 2. Gastrointestinal
Diseases—therapy—Handbooks. WI 39 A963m 2008]
  RC801.E26 2008
  616.3'3—dc22

                                                2007028861

To all my teachers and students.

CONTENTS

V. SPECIFIC COMPLAINTS AND DISORDERS

The first, second, and third editions of *Manual of Gastroenterology* were well received, both in the United States and abroad. This edition continues the intentions of its predecessors: to be a concise, practical, up-to-date reference for the clinical diagnosis and management of diseases and disorders of the digestive system. The content of all the existing chapters has been carefully reviewed, updated, and supplemented to provide current treatment information for a wide variety of gastrointestinal disorders. References have also been updated for each chapter.

As in the first three editions, the manual is divided into five parts: I. Approach to the Patient with a Gastroenterologic Disorder; II. Diagnostic and Therapeutic Procedures; III. Nutritional Assessment and Management; IV. Gastroenterologic Emergencies; and V. Specific Complaints and Disorders. In most chapters, a brief review of background information or pathophysiology precedes the discussion of diagnosis and treatment.

I believe this book will be particularly useful to primary care physicians, internists, gastroenterologists, medical students, and resident physicians. We also anticipate that other physicians and health care professionals will value *Manual of Gastroenterology* as a guide to gastroenterologic problems that lie beyond their everyday experiences.

Special thanks to Rana H. Bonnice for typing and organizing the manuscript of this book.

Special thanks to Carol Plasse for typing the manuscript for the second, third and fourth editions.

Special thanks to Bill Whall for his unyielding support.

Canan Avunduk, M.D., Ph.D.

Approach to the Patient with a Gastroenterologic Disorder

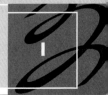

Nearly everyone has experienced a digestive illness. Perhaps it was a self-limiting bout of "intestinal flu" or heartburn or a more serious condition such as chronic ulcerative colitis, Crohn's disease, or carcinoma of the colon. Nevertheless, the social impact of digestive diseases is probably underappreciated.

Cardiovascular disease and cancer are dramatic illnesses that command a great deal of public attention. These disorders are associated with a high mortality and generally affect the older segment of the population. On the other hand, digestive disorders afflict a large number of people in all age groups and are associated with considerable pain, disability, and time lost from school, work, and other activities and considerable health care costs.

In a typical year, digestive disorders affect about 40 million people in the United States. The illnesses are responsible for the long-term inability to pursue ordinary activities, such as school or work, in about a million people, and exact an enormous toll in diminished productivity: more than 150 million days with some restriction in activity, nearly 70 million bed-days, and more than 20 million days lost from work per year. These conditions also result in 40 million annual physician contacts outside the hospital. The illnesses predominantly affect the young and middle-aged, with 70% occurring between the ages of 15 and 64 years. In addition to the losses caused by these predominantly chronic conditions, acute digestive disorders annually affect more than 11 million people and result in 48 million days of restricted activity, 27 million bed-days, and 9 million days lost from work.

Considering all digestive diseases, there are more than 4 million hospitalizations per year, resulting in 28 million hospital days and accounting for 13% of all hospitalizations. Moreover, many digestive diseases are fatal, causing about 9% of all deaths in the United States, or about 220,000 deaths per year, of which 61% are caused by malignancies and 16% by chronic liver disease and cirrhosis. A conservative estimate of the economic burden from digestive diseases is in excess of $60 billion per year, or roughly 10% of the total costs of all illnesses.

Selected Readings

Lembo AJ. The clinical and economic burden of irritable bowel syndrome. *Pract. Gastroenterol.* 2007;Sept:3–9.

Longstreth GF, et al. Functional bowel disorders. *Gastroenterology.* 2006;130:1480–1491.

Martin BC, et al. The annual cost of constipation in the U.S. ambulatory and inpatients settings [abstract]. *Gastroenterology.* 2005;128(suppl 2):A-283. Abstract M974.

Singh G, et al. Use of healthcare resources and cost of care for adults with constipation. *Clin. Gastroentrol Hepatol.* 2007;5:1053–1059.

Spiller K. Clinical update: irritable bowel syndrome. *Lancet.* 2007;369:1586–1588.

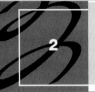

2   THE PATIENT'S COMPLAINTS

*S*urvival is the most important drive for human existence. Thus, eating, digesting, and eliminating are very important to human beings. Any disruption of any of these functions causes much concern to the individual.

Patient complaints may be directly related to gastrointestinal (GI) dysfunction, such as difficulty or painful swallowing, keeping foods down or difficulty in eliminating (i.e., having diarrhea or constipation). The complaints may be indirectly related to the GI system, such as pain in the chest from gastroesophageal reflux (GER), or pain in the abdomen or pelvis or from an intestinal disorder. Change in color, consistency, or shape of one's stool, unexplained weight loss, jaundice, or abdominal swelling may bring the patient to the health care professional.

A patient and a physician may differ in their perspectives on the patient's complaints. The physician's orientation generally is in terms of disease categories. The physician wants to make as accurate a diagnosis as possible and treat accordingly. On the other hand, the patient comes to the physician with one or several complaints that usually describe signs or symptoms perceived as "abnormal." A patient may complain of food sticking on swallowing; the physician thinks of an esophageal disease. A patient complains of yellow eyes or jaundice; the physician wonders if the patient has hemolysis or liver disease or biliary obstruction.

This divergence of orientation is sometimes a help and sometimes a hindrance. It is a help when the health care professional understands that diagnostic categories are merely aids to understanding and dealing with disease. It is a hindrance when the health care provider relies unquestioningly on an established or an apparent diagnosis and ignores other possibilities. For example, a 55-year-old woman with years of irritable bowel symptoms who develops pencil-thin stools should not simply be reassured and sent home; she needs an evaluation for carcinoma of the rectum or colon. On the other hand, the 45-year-old man with chest pain does not necessarily have coronary heart disease. His symptoms may be related to GER.

In the past 50 years, because of the diagnostic and therapeutic advances in medicine, and the wide availability of the Internet, the expectations of both patients and physicians have changed. Diagnostic tests have become much more sophisticated and accurate and available in most medical facilities. Special expertise in noninvasive or minimally invasive interventions has replaced invasive surgery as well as exploratory operations. Drugs specially designed to act on a specific target have replaced drugs with poorly understood and general effects. Many patients, before they consult their health care provider, go to the World Wide Web first and gather information on their complaints. This sophistication generates a milieu for preventive and early diagnostic and therapeutic measures.

Astute physicians and health care professionals are aware of their orientation and their shortcomings and listen carefully to patients' complaints. Sometimes the patient has a hidden agenda. A 42-year-old woman complains of recent abdominal pain and constipation. On additional inquiry, it is learned that her mother died recently of colon cancer. This patient is afraid that she also has cancer but may be reluctant to disclose that fear unless the physician asks her directly. In another patient, a 32-year-old man with a positive family history of early onset heart disease, the recent onset of epigastric or chest pain may be merely the overt manifestation of nearly overwhelming anxiety, which seems to be related to difficulties he is having at home and at work or exacerbation of gastroesophageal reflux disease (GERD) or recent onset of angina. The physician should not only listen carefully but also should be purposely redundant. It is helpful to review the same information several times, sometimes at different visits: "I know you told me about your abdominal pain last time, but I would like to go over the information again. When did you first notice the pain and what was it like?"

Selected Readings

Aziz Q, et al. Brain-gut axis in health and disease. *Gastroenterology.* 1998;114:599.

Bloomer JR, et al. Intermittent unexplained abdominal pain—is it porphyria? *Clin. Gastroentrol. Hepatol.* 2007;5(11):1255–1259.

Drossman DA, et al. Psychosocial factors in the case of patients with GI disorders. In: Yamada T, ed. *Textbook of Gastroenterology.* Philadelphia: Lippincott–Raven Publishers; 2003:636–654.

Knoll BM, et al. 56-year-old man with rash, abdominal pain and orthralgias. *Mayo Clin. Prac.* 2007;82(6):745–748.

Zinn W. The emphatic physician. *Arch Intern Med.* 1994;153:306–312.

3   EXAMINATION OF THE PATIENT

*B*ecause you are familiar with examining patients, this chapter is not intended to be comprehensive, but rather to orient you to the essential components of examining a patient with digestive complaints.

The physician should be sensitive to the patient's physical and emotional comfort. Is the patient in as comfortable a position as possible? Is the patient warm enough? Have you ensured the patient's privacy by closing doors and adjusting drapes? How does the patient feel about others in the room—colleagues, residents, students? Saying "This may be a little awkward or embarrassing for you" may reassure and relax the patient. As you conduct the examination, you should inform the patient of what you intend to do, particularly with regard to aspects of the examination that may be sensitive and embarrassing.

I. THE GENERAL PHYSICAL EXAMINATION. The physical examination of a patient with digestive complaints is not limited to the abdomen, although the abdominal examination is important. A general physical examination, including determination of vital signs, is indicated during the initial evaluation. In particular, is there pallor of the nail beds or conjunctivae? Is the tongue of normal color and texture? Is there any lymphadenopathy? What about changes in the color or texture of the skin? Is edema evident? Although abnormalities of the heart, lungs, or other organ systems may not be related directly to the patient's digestive complaints, they may be important considerations in the subsequent management of the patient.

II. THE ABDOMINAL EXAMINATION. The abdomen conventionally is divided into four quadrants: right upper, left upper, right lower, and left lower. It is also common, however, to refer to areas of the abdomen by more specific terms, such as epigastric, periumbilical, suprapubic, and right or left flank (Fig. 3-1).

  A. Patient position. The patient should lie in a supine position, although the head may be elevated slightly for comfort. Some patients lift their arms over their heads, which tightens the abdominal wall and makes palpation and interpretation of signs of peritoneal irritation difficult. The arms should remain at the patient's side. Flexion of the knees also may relieve abdominal tightness.

  B. Inspection

    1. Skin of the abdomen. Are there any scars, dilated veins, rashes, or other marks?

    2. Is the **umbilicus** normal? Is there an umbilical or abdominal wall hernia?

    3. Contour of the abdomen. Is the abdomen protuberant or concave? Are there any bulges?

    4. Can you see peristaltic movements or pulsations?

  C. Auscultation. In examining the abdomen, it is probably wise to listen before performing percussion and palpation because these maneuvers may alter the quality of bowel sounds.

    1. Bowel sounds. What is the character of the bowel sounds? In healthy people, the character and frequency of bowel sounds vary widely. In people who are hungry, bowel sounds may be active, whereas after a meal the abdomen typically becomes rather quiet. Bowel sounds may be increased in frequency and intensity in diarrheal conditions. Intestinal obstruction is characterized initially by increased bowel sounds that progress to high-pitched tinkling sounds and

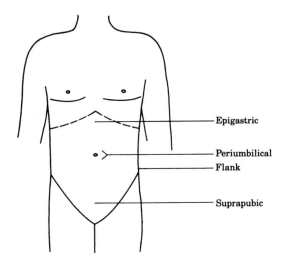

Figure 3-1. Areas of the abdomen.

rushes. On the other hand, bowel sounds become decreased or absent in conditions that cause paralytic ileus, such as peritonitis or electrolyte imbalance.

2. Other abdominal sounds. The physician should listen carefully also for sounds in the abdomen other than bowel sounds.

a. Arterial bruits may indicate narrowing or turbulence in the aorta or renal, iliac, or femoral arteries, depending on location. In some patients with renal artery stenosis, the bruit is heard best over the back in the lumbar area.

b. A venous hum is a soft sound in both systole and diastole that indicates increased collateral circulation between the portal and systemic venous systems. This rare finding usually is associated with cirrhosis of the liver.

c. A friction rub may be heard with respiration over the ribs that overlie the liver or spleen. The grating sound of a friction rub is caused by inflammation of the peritoneal surface, which may be caused by tumor, infection, or infarction.

D. Percussion and palpation. Most experienced physicians combine percussion and palpation in the examination of the abdomen. Because patients typically are somewhat tense during the abdominal examination, the examiner should avoid sudden movements. Much more information can be elicited by proceeding slowly and gently and sometimes firmly.

First, place one hand gently on the abdomen. This will tell you whether the abdomen is tense, firm, or soft and whether the patient is made uncomfortable by light pressure. Percuss the abdomen lightly in all four quadrants to determine tympany and dullness.

1. Liver. The size, shape, and consistency of the liver are best estimated by first percussing the upper and lower limits of liver dullness and then palpating the lower edge in both phases of respiration. Remember to feel for the liver not only in the right upper quadrant but also in the epigastrium. Some patients with hepatomegaly have predominantly left lobe enlargement, which may be evident only in the epigastrium. Occasionally, a markedly enlarged left lobe is mistaken for the spleen.

2. The **spleen** can be identified as an area of dullness just above the left costal margin posterior to the midaxillary line. In adults, the normal spleen usually cannot be palpated, although about 10% of teenagers and young adults have normal, palpable spleens. When the spleen enlarges, it expands anteriorly and toward the midline. In splenomegaly, the area of dullness moves anteriorly, therefore, the spleen may be palpated beneath the left ribs. A method of detecting a small degree of splenomegaly is to percuss at the junction of the left anterior axillary line and the costal margin. Normally the percussion note is tympanitic in both phases of respiration. Dullness to percussion at this point during inspiration may indicate early splenomegaly. Another method of palpating the spleen is to have the patient lie on the right side and lean slightly forward. This position allows the spleen to drop anteriorly and toward the midline. The examiner stands behind the patient, with fingers hooked beneath the ribs, and asks the patient to breathe in, thereby allowing the spleen to move down against the examining fingers.

3. **Other organs and masses** should be assessed for size, location, shape, and consistency. The aorta often is felt as a pulsatile mass in the upper abdomen, particularly in thin patients. Some estimation of the diameter of the aorta can be made by pressing firmly but gently on either side of the aorta with one or two hands. An enlarged, expansile aorta, sometimes accompanied by a bruit, indicates an aneurysm.

4. **Abdominal tenderness** may be superficial or deep, localized or focal.

   a. Guarding, particularly involuntary guarding, is usually a sign of peritoneal inflammation.

   b. **Rebound tenderness,** which also results from peritoneal inflammation, is elicited by slowly pressing the abdomen and quickly releasing the pressure. The examination for rebound tenderness usually is painful and should not be repeated by subsequent examiners merely for the purpose of documenting an interesting clinical sign.

E. **Detection of ascites.** A protuberant abdomen with bulging flanks may connote fluid within the peritoneal cavity. At this stage, however, the detection of ascites usually is not difficult, except perhaps in obese patients.

   1. **Shifting dullness** is identified by percussing the abdomen and noting the location of the border between the dullness of the ascitic fluid and the tympany of floating loops of bowel when the patient lies in a supine position, when the patient turns to one side or the other, the border of dullness shifts.

   2. **A fluid wave** is elicited when one flank is tapped briskly and the impulse is felt on the opposite flank. To prevent transmission of the wave through the fat of the abdominal wall, the patient or an assistant can press the edge of one hand firmly down along the midline of the abdomen. Some examiners with large hands are able to press along the midline with their own thumb and tap the flank with the small finger of the same hand.

   3. **The puddle sign,** although awkward to elicit, may detect small amounts of ascites. The patient assumes the knee–chest position on the bed or examining table. This position allows ascitic fluid to accumulate in the most dependent position of the abdomen, centering around the umbilicus. Tapping the abdomen while listening with the stethoscope under the umbilicus may produce a splashing sound. If the skin of the abdomen is scratched lightly, beginning from the periphery and moving toward the umbilicus, a change in the quality of the auscultated sound occurs at the border of the ascitic fluid.

III. **THE ANORECTAL EXAMINATION** is an important part of the general physical examination. It may be uncomfortable for the patient and cause embarrassment, but the discomfort and embarrassment can be ameliorated greatly by an understanding, unhurried, gentle attitude on the part of the physician.

A. **Patient position.** Most physicians ask the patient to lie on the left side with knees and hips flexed. Others prefer the patient to stand, leaning over an examining table. The former position is preferred and recommended.

B. **Perianal area.** The buttocks should be spread apart to allow inspection of the anus and perianal skin. Protuberant hemorrhoids, anal tags, fissures, or abscesses may be seen. The perianal area is palpated with a gloved finger. Tenderness and masses are noted.

C. Insertion. Before inserting a gloved index finger into the rectum, the physician lubricates both the finger and the anus well. Sometimes it is helpful to ask the patient to strain down gently, as if having a bowel movement. This maneuver relaxes the anal sphincter and allows easier penetration of the finger. The longitudinal axis of the anal canal is aimed roughly to the umbilicus; thus, the examiner gently presses the finger into the anal canal in the direction of the umbilicus. The rectum is found to turn posteriorly and open out into the hollow area formed by the sacrum and coccyx.

D. Examination of the rectum should be gentle. A tender anal canal may result from proctitis, inflamed or thrombosed hemorrhoids, a stricture, or a fissure. Note the tone of the anal sphincter. Palpate the lateral, posterior, and anterior walls of the rectum, noting any tenderness or nodularity. Anteriorly, in male patients, the prostate is felt as a bilobed structure with a median sulcus. What are the size, shape, and consistency? Is the prostate tender? Are there any nodules? In female patients, the cervix (and sometimes a vaginal tampon) can be felt as a firm mass through the anterior rectal wall.

Although most of the rectal wall that is accessible to the examining finger is below the peritoneal reflection, most examiners can reach above the peritoneal reflection anteriorly. Thus, tenderness of peritoneal inflammation or metastatic nodules may be identified.

E. Stool. On withdrawal of the finger, note the color and consistency of the stool. Is there any mucus or gross blood? If not, test the stool for occult blood.

Selected Reading

Bates B. The abdomen. In: Bates B, Hoeckelman RA, eds. *Guide to Physical Examination and History Taking.* 9th ed. Philadelphia: Lippincott Williams & Wilkins; 2007:339–368.

4 PSYCHOLOGICAL AND EMOTIONAL ASPECTS OF GASTROENTEROLOGIC DISORDERS

*T*he mind and body are not independent but parallel. "For there are not two processes, and there are not two entities; there is but one process . . . one entity, seen now inwardly as mind, now outwardly as matter, but in reality an inextricable mixture and unity of both. Mind and body do not act upon each other, because they are not other, they are one." Baruch Spinoza, as paraphrased by Will Durant, *The Story of Philosophy*, 1954.

An extensive review of the psychological and emotional aspects of digestive disorders is beyond the scope of this book. Because psychological factors do play an important role in gastroenterologic disorders, however, and patients certainly react emotionally to illness, we need to consider at least briefly the psychosomatic component of gastrointestinal disease.

Physicians tend to think of disorders as affecting organ systems and resulting in observable pathophysiologic changes. Most astute physicians and health care providers, however, either consciously or intuitively understand that a disorder is a complex interaction among pathophysiologic processes, the patient's emotional makeup, and the patient's perception of the disorder. A large number of factors may affect this interaction, including the patient's age, sex, socioeconomic and marital status, other "medical" disorders, emotional stress, family history, and society's view of the disorder. Additional complicating influences are the physician's view of the patient, the patient's disorders, and the options of managing the patient's problems.

There is more than a mere relation between the "psyche" and the "soma." Although there is a tendency to separate the psychological and somatic aspects of a disease, attach labels, and categorize, disorders exist as **inseparable entities** of psyche and soma. In some patients the psychological and emotional aspects seem to predominate and exert profound somatic effects, such as in bulimia, anorexia nervosa, and irritable bowel syndrome. Also, it is believed that exacerbations of some chronic diseases, such as Crohn's disease and ulcerative colitis, may be triggered by emotional factors, yet have their pathogenesis firmly rooted in the soma. In addition, in these chronic, sometimes devastating illnesses, it is easy to understand that patients also experience psychological trauma due to their illness.

Finally, no matter what the illness is and no matter how trivial it appears, illness of any degree represents a threat to the patient's integrity. An illness is never purely somatic—there is always a person who must experience the illness.

Selected Readings

DiBaise JK. Psychotherapy and functional dyspepsias: Brain-gut interactions. *Am J Gastroenterol.* 2001;96:278.

Drossman DA, et al. Psychosocial factors in the care of patients with GI disorders. In: Yamada T, ed. *Textbook of Gastroenterology.* Philadelphia: Lippincott–Raven Publishers; 2003:636–654.

Drossman DA. The physician-patient relationship. In: Corazziari E, ed. *Approach to the Patient with Chronic Gastrointestinal Disorders.* Milan: Messaggi; 1999:133–139.

Longstreth GF, et al. Severe irritable bowel and functional abdominal pain syndromes: Managing the patient and health care costs. *Clin Gastroenterol Hepatol.* 2005;3:397–400.

Talley NJ, et al. Practice Parameters Committee of the American College of Gastroenterology. Guidelines for the management of dyspepsia. *Am J Gastroenterol.* 2005;100:2324–2337.

Diagnostic and Therapeutic Procedures

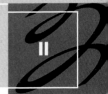

II

Since Hirschowitz and colleagues described the first flexible fiberoptic endoscopes, the technical explosion in fiberoptic endoscopy has produced instruments that are durable, safe, relatively comfortable, and capable of visualizing the gastrointestinal tract with great diagnostic accuracy.

The **typical modern fiberoptic endoscope** is a highly sophisticated instrument (Fig. 5-1). The shaft is 8 to 12 mm in diameter. The fiberoptic bundles pass through the shaft to transmit light to the tip and the image to the endoscopist. In the handle of the endoscope are controls for maneuvering the tip and buttons to regulate irrigation water, air insufflation, and suction for removing air, secretions, and blood. An instrument channel allows the passage of biopsy forceps, small brushes for obtaining cytology samples, snares for removing polyps and foreign bodies, and devices to control bleeding.

The adaptation of endoscopes to video monitoring systems has been developed using computer chip technology and now is in routine use in all endoscopy suites. The endoscopist conducts the examination by viewing the video screen, not by looking directly through the fiberoptic system of the endoscope. The video screen also allows a variable number of people, including the patient if desired, to observe what the primary endoscopist is seeing, and the procedure can be videotaped for clinical and educational purposes.

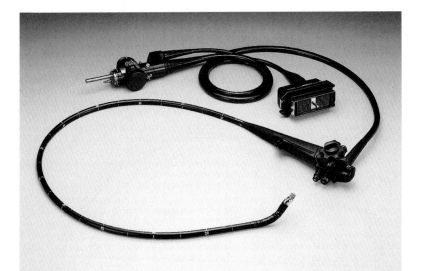

Figure 5-1. Flexible fiberoptic endoscope for examination of the upper gastrointestinal tract. An open biopsy forceps is shown at the tip of the endoscope, having been passed through the biopsy channel in the handle. This instrument also has been adapted to perform endoscopic ultrasonography by the addition of an ultrasound transducer at the tip. (GF-UE160-AL5, reprinted with Courtesy of Olympus®.)

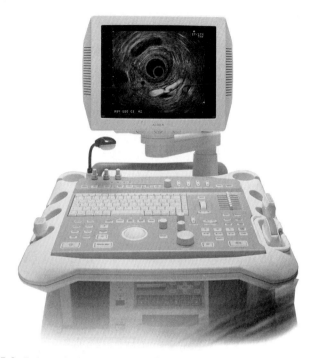

Figure 5-2. Endoscopic ultrasound system. The flexible endoscope on the right of the table has ultrasound transducers at the tip of imaging and fiberoptics that allow direct visualization of lesions. (SSD-ALPHA5, reprinted with Courtesy of Olympus®.)

During routine upper gastrointestinal endoscopy, the entire esophagus, stomach, and proximal duodenum are examined. Several therapeutic endoscopic techniques have been developed that allow endoscopists to treat bleeding lesions (see Chapter 14) and relieve esophageal obstruction caused by benign or malignant processes. Endoscopic placement of gastric feeding tubes—percutaneous endoscopic gastrostomy (PEG)—has largely replaced surgical gastrostomy.

A variation of upper gastrointestinal endoscopy, endoscopic retrograde cholangiopancreatography (ERCP), combines endoscopic and radiologic techniques to visualize the biliary and pancreatic ductal systems. ERCP methods also have been used therapeutically to perform sphincterotomy of the sphincter of Oddi, to remove common bile duct stones, and to place stents that bypass obstructing lesions.

During examination of the lower gastrointestinal tract by colonoscopy, a skilled endoscopist can reach the cecum in more than 95% of patients, and in many instances the terminal ileum can also be visualized. The major therapeutic capability of colonoscopy, popularized in the United States in the mid-1980s by President Ronald Reagan's experience with a cancerous polyp, is polypectomy, usually by electrocautery.

An important development in endoscopy is endoscopic ultrasonography (EUS) (Figs. 5-1–5-3). High-frequency, high-resolution ultrasound transducers that are built into the tip of the endoscope can be passed to sites that are relatively close to the target organ. Applications include evaluation of lesions involving the esophagus, mediastinum, stomach, duodenum, pancreas, colon, and rectum. EUS compares favorably with computerized tomography in tumor staging and determination of lymph node involvement. Indications for EUS are summarized in Table 5-1. Also, lymph nodes in the thorax and abdomen may be biopsied and pancreatic pseudocysts may be drained using EUS.

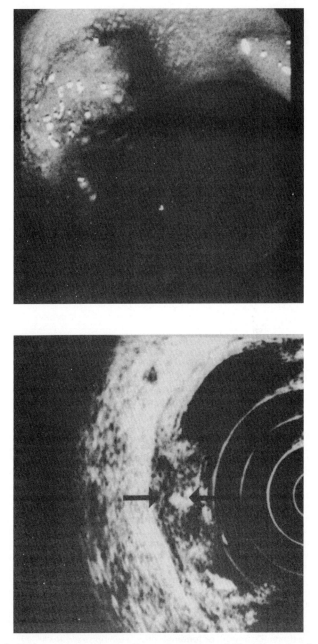

Figure 5-3. Endosonographic view of a villous adenoma (*arrows*). The tumor is invading the second hyperechoic layer (T_2 lesion).

TABLE 5-1	Indications for Endoscopic Ultrasonography
Esophagus	Esophageal cancer diagnosis and staging
	Anastomotic recurrence of cancer
	Submucosal tumors
	Mediastinal lymphadenopathy
	Esophageal varices
Stomach	Adenocarcinoma and lymphoma diagnosis and staging
	Submucosal tumors
	Gastric polyps
	Anastomotic recurrence of cancer
	Gastric ulcer healing
	Gastric varices
Duodenum	Submucosal tumors
	Ampullary carcinoma diagnosis and staging
Pancreas and biliary system	Pancreatic and biliary cancer diagnosis and staging
	Chronic pancreatitis and pseudocysts
	Biliary stone disease
	Endocrine tumors
Colon and rectum	Rectal and colon cancer diagnosis and staging
	Villous adenoma
	Recurrent colorectal cancer
	Benign perianal and perirectal disease

I. UPPER GASTROINTESTINAL ENDOSCOPY

A. Indications. Several conditions in which upper gastrointestinal endoscopy, also known as **esophagogastroduodenoscopy (EGD),** may be useful in making a diagnosis are listed Table 5-2. Opinions differ among physicians as to whether and when EGD should be performed for a given condition. For example, some physicians order an upper gastrointestinal x-ray series initially in the evaluation of a patient who has dyspeptic complaints. Other physicians treat a patient with dyspepsia empirically with antacids or some other acid-reducing medication without obtaining a diagnostic study, unless the patient is elderly or has evidence of gastrointestinal bleeding, weight loss, or vomiting, suggesting gastric outlet obstruction. An EGD might subsequently be arranged if the patient does not respond to treatment in a reasonable time or develops bleeding, weight loss, or vomiting.

B. Contraindications. EGD should not be performed if a perforated viscus is suspected or if the patient is in shock, is combative, or is unwilling to cooperate (Table 5-3).

C. Preparation of the patient. Elective EGD should be performed after the patient has fasted for 6 or more hours to ensure an empty stomach. However, this rule does not apply to emergent situations such as in acute upper gastrointestinal bleeding or with foreign body impaction of the esophagus or when food and clots may fill the esophagus and/or stomach and these may need to be immediately removed endoscopically.

In conscious patients, a topical anesthetic may be applied to the pharynx to numb the gag reflex. **Conscious sedation** (i.e., intravenous **midazolam [Versed], meperidine [Demerol], or fentanyl**) often is administered as a sedative. Tolerances for midazolam vary widely. Older and severely ill patients may become sedated or develop respiratory depression even at low doses. Thus, a test dose of 1 to 2 mg initially is advisable. Most patients require 2 to 5 mg to achieve adequate relaxation. The doses of meperidine and fentanyl also vary depending on the patient. Most patients require 12.5 to 100 mg. Because patients are likely to feel sleepy for

TABLE 5-2 Partial List of Conditions in Which Endoscopy May Be Useful in Making a Diagnosis

Condition	EGD	ERCP	Sigmoidoscopy or colonoscopy
Dysphagia	X		
Caustic or foreign body ingestion	X		
Dyspepsia	X		
Persistent nausea and vomiting	X		
Need to obtain small-intestinal biopsy	X		
Acute or chronic gastrointestinal bleeding	X		X
Inflammatory bowel disease	X		X
Chronic abdominal pain	X	X	X
Suspected polyp or cancer	X	X	X
Obstructive jaundice		X	
Change in bowel habits			X
Diarrhea longer than 1 wk			X

EGD, esophagogastroduodenoscopy (upper gastrointestinal endoscopy); ERCP, endoscopic retrograde cholangiopancreatography.

TABLE 5-3 Contraindications for Endoscopy

Perforated viscus suspected
Patient in shock
Combative or uncooperative patient
Severe inflammatory bowel disease or toxic megacolon (colonoscopy)

an hour or more after the procedure, it is required that the outpatients arrange for transportation home with an accompanying person after EGD.

Deep sedation, using **Propofol IV,** may be used in selective patients with medical or psychiatric comorbid conditions.

D. Therapeutic EGD. A number of methods have been used to treat actively bleeding lesions of the upper gastrointestinal tract. **Endoscopic band ligation and/or injection sclerotherapy** of esophageal varices is the most widely practiced therapeutic endoscopic method for the treatment of bleeding esophageal varices. Sclerotherapy or banding reduces both mortality and the frequency of rebleeding from esophageal varices. Other methods of controlling actively bleeding ulcers and erosions include **local injection of the bleeding site with epinephrine** or **hypertonic saline, electrocoagulation,** and/or **placement of clips on the bleeding lesion** and **laser photocoagulation.** These methods are described in more detail in Chapter 14. Endoscopic treatment of gastroesophageal reflux disease (GERD) will be discussed in Chapter 20.

E. Complications of upper gastrointestinal endoscopy. Endoscopy of the gastrointestinal tract is generally regarded as safe, but adverse events do occur (Table 5-4). Major complications of EGD—perforation of the esophagus or stomach, generation of new hemorrhage, pulmonary aspiration, serious cardiac arrhythmia—occur with a frequency of from 1 in 1,000 to 1 in 3,000 instances. Mortality ranges from 1 in 3,000 to 1 in 16,000 endoscopies. Sedation and inhibition of the gag reflex contribute to the risk of aspiration of blood, secretions, and regurgitated gastric contents.

TABLE 5-4	Complications of Endoscopy	

Complication	EGD	Colonoscopy
Perforation of viscus	X	X
Bleeding	X	X
Cardiac arrhythmias	X	X
Medication reactions	X	X
Vasovagal reactions	X	X
Pulmonary aspiration	X	
Cardiac failure (due to overhydration during bowel preparation)		X
Hypotension (due to underhydration during bowel preparation)		X

EGD, esophagogastroduodenoscopy.

Complications related to the topical anesthetic to the pharynx or to the intravenous midazolam are unusual. Fatalities reported from these agents usually are associated with large doses that have caused cardiac or central nervous system effects. Allergic reactions are rare. The major complication of intravenous midazolam and narcotics is respiratory depression. These drugs also may cause transient hypotension and obtundation. Patients at the highest risk are the elderly and those with advanced cardiac, pulmonary, hepatic, or central nervous system disease.

The frequency of complications associated with EGD can be reduced by anticipating problems and taking measures to prevent them. A complete history and physical examination are important, with special attention to history of allergic drug reactions, presence of bleeding disorders, and cardiac, pulmonary, renal, hepatic, or central nervous system disease. If a sedative is used, a small test dose should be administered initially, particularly in elderly or severely ill patients. The endoscopy assistant must suction secretions and regurgitated material when necessary from the pharynx. Nasal oxygen should be used to treat hypoxia, and resuscitation equipment should be available in the event of adverse cardiopulmonary reactions. After the procedure is completed, the patient should be observed for an adequate amount of time and for subsequent development of complications.

II. ENDOSCOPIC RETROGRADE CHOLANGIOPANCREATOGRAPHY (ERCP)

A. Evaluation of pancreatic and biliary ductal systems. ERCP usually is performed as an elective procedure to evaluate the pancreatic and biliary ductal systems. The endoscopic principles for ERCP are similar to those for routine EGD except that ERCP usually takes longer, patients are likely to be sedated more heavily, and a side-viewing instrument is used. The endoscope is passed into the second part of the duodenum, and the **ampulla of Vater** is visualized. The endoscopist then passes a catheter through the endoscope and maneuvers it into the orifice of the ampulla. Additional adjustment of the cannula allows it to enter the pancreatic duct or the common bile duct. After injection of radiocontrast material through the cannula, x-ray films are taken to identify the configuration of the biliary and pancreatic ductal systems (Fig. 5-4).

B. Sphincterotomy and calculus retrieval. In patients who have calculi in the common duct, endoscopic section (sphincterotomy) of the sphincter of Oddi allows access to the common duct bile and retrieval of the stones. The sphincterotomy device consists of a wire electrode within a plastic cannula. After the cannula has been inserted into the sphincter, the wire is elevated and the sphincter is cut by electrocautery. The stone passes spontaneously or may be crushed and/or extracted using a basketlike device that is passed through the endoscope.

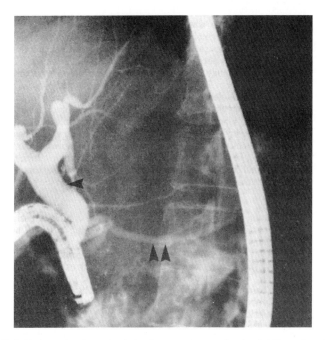

Figure 5-4. Endoscopic retrograde cholangiopancreatogram showing the fiberoptic endoscope in the second portion of the duodenum, a normal common bile duct (*single arrow*), and a normal pancreatic duct (*double arrow*). (Courtesy of John F. Erkkinen, M.D.; from Eastwood GL. Gastrointestinal endoscopy. In: Rippe JM, et al [eds.]. *Intensive Care Medicine.* Boston: Little, Brown; 1985:67–73. Reprinted with permission.)

    C. Stent insertion. Other techniques may also be used with ERCP to insert short tubes, or stents, through obstructing lesions, such as pancreatic or biliary cancer or strictures of the distal bile or pancreatic duct. The stents allow relief of the obstruction and may be used as definitive therapy in patients with inoperable disease or temporarily until the obstructive lesion is treated by irradiation or surgery.

III. CAPSULE ENDOSCOPY OR PILLCAM ENDOSCOPY. An orally ingested 2.3-by-0.8-cm capsule containing a computer chip has become a popular tool to visualize the gastrointestinal tract, especially the small intestine, by taking numerous pictures as it travels down the intestinal tract with peristalsis. The electronically recorded pictures are later reviewed by an experienced gastroenterologist or technician. This technique is most helpful in diagnosis of lesions in the small intestine that may be the cause of occult GI bleeding.

IV. LOWER GASTROINTESTINAL ENDOSCOPY
    A. Indications and contraindications. Indications for endoscopic examination of the lower gastrointestinal tract include active or occult bleeding, inflammatory bowel disease, suspicion of a polyp or cancer, unexplained abdominal pain, and change in bowel habits (Table 5-2). The contraindications are the same as those for EGD with the additional contraindications of active diverticulitis, severe inflammatory bowel disease and suspected toxic megacolon (Table 5-3).
    B. Proctosigmoidoscopy
        1. Instruments. The flexible **fiberoptic sigmoidoscope,** which measures up to 65 cm in length, is a short colonoscope and has replaced the 25-cm **rigid sigmoidoscope** for routine examinations. The flexible instruments are capable of

reaching the descending colon and may even reach the splenic flexure. Furthermore, patients tolerate flexible sigmoidoscopy better than rigid sigmoidoscopy.

2. **Preparation of the patient.** Tap water or commercial enemas (i.e., Fleet enemas) usually are sufficient preparation for either rigid or flexible sigmoidoscopy. However, the sigmoidoscopic examination should be performed without enema preparation when patients have watery diarrhea or suspected colitis. Most patients do not require conscious sedation. For flexible or rigid sigmoidoscopy, the patients are usually placed in the left lateral decubitus position.

3. **Biopsy and polypectomy.** As in EGD, the mucosa and lesions within the rectum or colon can be biopsied through the rigid or flexible instrument. Most endoscopists avoid biopsy immediately before barium enema because of the small chance of introducing air and barium into the mucosal defect caused by biopsy. Also, although polyps can be removed through either the rigid or flexible sigmoidoscope by standard electrocautery methods, this should not be done unless the entire colon has been properly prepared to avoid the possibility of gas ignition or explosion.

C. **Colonoscopy**

1. **Instruments.** Modern fiberoptic colonoscopes are similar in design to upper gastrointestinal endoscopes but are longer, ranging in length from 120 to 180 cm.

2. **Preparation of the patient.** Standard bowel preparation for colonoscopy is similar to the preparation for barium enema x-ray examination: 1 to 2 days of clear-liquid diet followed by a strong cathartic.

   Liquid preparations include a balanced electrolyte polyethylene glycol (PEG) lavage, exemplified by **GoLYTELY** or **Colyte.** Typically about 3.8 L of the solution must be consumed either orally or through a nasogastric tube over about 2 to 4 hours. The lavage solution is consumed 6 to 12 hours before the procedure. The advantages of this preparation are that it is quick, gentle and very effective in cleansing the bowel. The PEG solution also appears to be safe to use in anyone in whom it is safe to perform colonoscopy. One drawback is the difficulty some patients have in consuming a gallon of fluid over a few hours. Alternatively, 2 L of **HalfLytely** may be given after 4 Dulcolax tablets. **MoviPrep,** a newer, better tasting 2-L PEG solution, may be used instead without additional need for Dulcolax tablets.

   An easier colon preparation is **Fleet phospho-soda,** 1.5 oz. in 4 oz. of water taken twice, 6–8 hours apart, along with a clear-liquid diet. However, the safety of this preparation has been questioned due to the possibility of causing dehydration and renal insufficiency in some patients.

   Colon preparation has recently been further simplified by giving patients 28 to 32 tablets containing Fleet phospho-soda **(Visicol or Osmo-prep)** 6 to 12 hours prior to the procedure, along with a clear-liquid diet.

   Because colonoscopy generally takes longer and is more uncomfortable than flexible sigmoidoscopy, it is customary to administer intravenous medications such as **midazolam (Versed), meperidine hydrochloride (Demerol),** or **fentanyl** to promote relaxation and diminish discomfort. In some cases, intravenous **Propofol** may be administered by an anesthesiologist for deeper sedation.

3. **Biopsy and therapeutic procedures.** Colonoscopic biopsies of the mucosa and colonic lesions are obtained routinely for diagnostic purposes. The most common colonoscopic therapeutic procedure is polypectomy. Pedunculated polyps may be removed with a wire snare, which is maneuvered to encircle the stalk. After the snare is tightened, the stalk is severed directly or by passing electric current through the snare. Sessile polyps may be removed by polypectomy in several pieces or biopsied through the colonoscope. Raising a bleb with normal saline injection under a sessile polyp allows more complete removal as routine polypectomy. Some sessile lesions may require surgical removal. Bleeding lesions of the colon may be treated during colonoscopy in the same manner as upper gastrointestinal lesions.

D. **Complications of colonoscopy.** The two major complications of colonoscopy, perforation and hemorrhage, occur in less than 1% of instances. These are more likely to occur during colonoscopy with polypectomy. Other complications of colonoscopy include drug reactions, hypotension, vasovagal reactions, cardiac arrhythmias, and congestive heart failure complicated by over- or underhydration of a susceptive patient after bowel preparation (Table 5-4).

Colonoscopic complications are minimized by following most of the rules indicated for EGD. In addition, the colonoscope or sigmoidoscope should be advanced with care and overdistention of the colon should be avoided. Finally, the fluid and electrolyte status of elderly patients and those with renal and cardiac disease should be tended to during preparation of the bowel.

V. SMALL-INTESTINAL BIOPSY. Small-intestinal mucosal biopsy is a valuable aid in the evaluation of patients with malabsorption or diarrhea caused by small-intestinal mucosal disorders. In patients with Whipple's disease, for example, the biopsy is of critical importance in establishing the diagnosis. In celiac sprue, the diagnosis can be confirmed by a histologic appearance that is consistent with sprue. Also, the response to treatment with a gluten-free diet may be confirmed by subsequent biopsies. Although the diagnosis of giardiasis often can be made by examination of diarrheal stool samples, the small-bowel biopsy coupled with examination of luminal secretions remains the most accurate method of identifying *Giardia* organisms.

A. Indications and contraindications. Small-bowel mucosal biopsy is indicated in the evaluation of patients who may have a small-bowel mucosal disorder. These patients typically have diarrhea and malabsorption and some may present only with gas and bloating and abdominal pain. In the evaluation of a patient with suspected mucosal disease, the timing of a small-bowel biopsy is a matter of clinical judgment. Generally, the initial evaluation of such patients includes routine blood studies and several examinations of the stool for ova and parasites, bacterial pathogens, leukocytes, occult blood, and qualitative stool fat. Barium contrast studies of the upper and lower gastrointestinal tract, a xylose absorption test, and a quantitative stool-fat examination also may have been performed. The evaluation of specific disorders of the small intestine and the role of mucosal biopsy are discussed in subsequent chapters.

The contraindications to small-intestinal biopsy are few. History and clotting studies should indicate that there is no bleeding tendency, and the patient should be able to cooperate during the study.

B. Methods of obtaining small-intestinal mucosal biopsies

1. Endoscopic biopsies. Endoscopic biopsy of the small-intestinal mucosa has become preferred over the use of suction biopsy tubes. Endoscopic biopsies obtained with large (8-mm) forceps have been shown to be as diagnostically accurate as suction biopsies, provided they are taken from the distal duodenum, which avoids the variations in mucosal architecture that occur normally in the proximal duodenum, and they are oriented carefully. Also, endoscopic biopsies generally are technically easier to perform than biopsies using a suction tube.

2. Suction biopsies. The **Rubin tube,** also known as the **Quinton tube,** is one of several biopsy tubes available for obtaining suction mucosal biopsies of the small intestine. The tube is radiopaque and can be maneuvered under fluoroscopic control to the distal duodenum or proximal jejunum. The design of the biopsy capsule provides full-thickness mucosal samples without transecting larger blood vessels of the submucosa. These biopsies are easily oriented, which facilitates accurate histologic interpretation. This technique is no longer used except for research purposes.

C. Interpretation of the biopsy

1. Orientation. Proper orientation of the mucosal biopsy is crucial to obtain the maximal information from the biopsy. Proper orientation means that the plane of sectioning is along the axis of the villi and crypts (Fig. 5-5). Thus, villous height, crypt depth, and configuration of surface epithelial cells can be evaluated accurately.

2. Evaluating the biopsy. In evaluating small-bowel mucosal biopsies, one should look at two aspects: the mucosal architecture and the cellular elements.

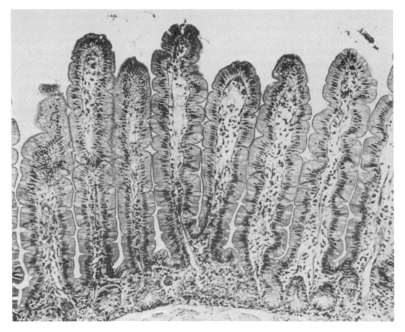

Figure 5-5. Photomicrograph of a normal human small-intestinal biopsy taken from the distal duodenum. (From Eastwood GL. *Core Textbook of Gastroenterology.* Philadelphia: Lippincott Williams & Wilkins; 1984:105. Reprinted with permission.)

a. **Architecture.** The normal villus-crypt ratio in well-oriented biopsies from the proximal jejunum of North Americans and Europeans is 4:1 or 5:1 (Fig. 5-4). Villi should be tall and narrow. A variable amount of submucosa may be present.

b. **Cellular elements.** Look carefully at the three elements of the mucosa: the epithelium, the lamina propria, and the muscularis mucosae.

   i. The **epithelium** is a single layer of columnar cells that lines the crypts and covers the villi. The four major epithelial cell types are columnar absorptive cells, mucous (goblet) cells, Paneth's cells, and enteroendocrine cells. Columnar absorptive cells are the most numerous. They are covered by a glycoprotein filamentous matrix, the so-called fuzzy coat seen by light microscopy, which is the site of many digestive enzymes such as the disaccharidases. Mucous cells, interspersed between the absorptive cells, contain abundant mucous granules, which in the aggregate have the appearance of a goblet and thus commonly are called goblet cells. Paneth's cells are found predominantly at the base of the crypts. Their function is unknown, but they appear to be secretory cells because of the eosinophilic granules they contain. Finally, the epithelium contains a wide variety of enteroendocrine cells that secrete numerous hormones, including gastrin, secretin, cholecystokinin, vasoactive intestinal peptide, somatostatin, and neurotensin.

   ii. Within the **lamina propria,** which forms the cores of the villi and lies between the crypts, are connective tissue elements, wisps of smooth muscle, lymphatics, blood vessels, macrophages, plasma cells, and lymphocytes. Normally neutrophils are not found in the lamina propria. Because increases in the number of cells within the lamina propria are characteristic of several mucosal diseases, some experience is necessary in viewing normal biopsies to determine whether the cellularity is increased or not.

    iii. The **muscularis mucosae** is a thin layer of muscle lying beneath the bases of the crypts and below which lays the submucosa.

3. Diagnostic value. The information that is obtained from the biopsy may make or refute a specific diagnosis or may be nonspecific but consistent with one or more diagnoses. The diagnostic value of small-intestinal biopsy can be categorized as follows (modified from Trier).

  a. Disorders in which the biopsy is invariably of diagnostic value include the following:

    i. Celiac sprue (the biopsy is nonspecific, but coupled with a clinical response to the elimination of dietary gluten, it is diagnostic)

    ii. Whipple's disease

    iii. Abetalipoproteinemia

    iv. Agammaglobulinemia

    v. *Mycobacterium avium-intracellulare*

  b. Disorders in which the biopsy may or may not be of specific value. (In these disorders, the lesion may be distributed in an irregular fashion; thus an abnormal biopsy may make a specific diagnosis, but a normal biopsy does not rule out the disorder.)

    i. Intestinal lymphoma

    ii. Intestinal lymphangiectasia

    iii. Eosinophilic enteritis

    iv. Systemic mastocytosis

    v. Parasitic infestation

    vi. Amyloidosis

    vii. Hypogammaglobulinemia

    viii. Dysgammaglobulinemia

  c. Disorders in which the biopsy may be abnormal but not diagnostic. (In these disorders, the biopsy findings are nonspecific.)

    i. Tropical sprue

    ii. Folate deficiency

    iii. Vitamin B_{12} deficiency

    iv. Irradiation enteritis

    v. Zollinger-Ellison syndrome

    vi. Small-bowel bacterial overgrowth

    vii. Drug-induced lesion

    viii. Malnutrition

    ix. Graft-versus-host reaction

    x. Viral enteritis

  d. Disorders in which the biopsy is normal.

    i. Pancreatic exocrine insufficiency

    ii. Cirrhosis

    iii. Postgastrectomy malabsorption (without intestinal disease)

    iv. Primary lactase deficiency

    v. Irritable bowel syndrome

VI. ENDOSCOPIC OR TRANSGASTRIC SURGERY is a new and very promising trend in abdominal and pelvic surgery. This technique allows surgical intervention without laparotomy or laparoscopy, thus much less invasive to the patient. The scope of this new technique is vast and rapidly expanding.

Selected Readings

Avunduk C, et al. Endoscopic sonography of the duodenum, pancreas, liver and the biliary tract: Findings in benign and malignant conditions. *Appl Radiol*. 1997;25–33.

Avunduk C, et al. Endoscopic Sonography of the stomach: Findings in benign and malignant lesions. *Amer J Roentgenol*. 1994;163:591–595.

Chak A, et al. Sedationless upper endoscopy. *Rev Gastroenterol Disord*. Winter 2006;6:13–21.

Cotton PB, et al. Comparison of virtual colonoscopy and colonoscopy in the detection of polyps/masses. *Gastrointest Endosc*. 2005;55:AB98.

Eliakim R, et al. A prospective study of the diagnostic accuracy of PillCam ESO esophageal capsule endoscopy versus conventional upper endoscopy in patients with chronic gastroesophageal reflux diseases. *J Clin Gastroenterol*. 2005;39:572–578.

Gress F. Endoscopic ultrasound-guided plexus neurolysis. *Gasterol. Hepatol*. 2007;3(4): 279–281.

Johnson JF, et al. A randomized, multicenter study comparing the safety and efficacy of sodium phosphate tablets with 26 polyethylene glycol solution plus bisacodyl tablets for colon cleansing. *Am J Gastroenterol*. 2007;102:2238–2246.

Kim OH, et al. CT colonography for the detection of advanced neoplasia. *N Eng J Med*. 2007;357:1403–1412.

Kovalak M, et al. Endoscopic screening for varices in cirrhotic patients: Data from a national endoscopic data base. *Gastrointest Endosc*. 2007;65:82–88.

Lamade W, et al. Transgastric surgery in the abdomen: The dawn of a new era? *Gastrointest Endosc*. 2005;62:293–296.

Leighton JA, et al. Capsule endoscopy: a meta-analysis for use with obscure gastrointestinal bleeding and Crohn's disease. *Gastrointest Endosc Clin N Am*. 2006;16:229–250.

Liu R. The future of surgical endoscopy. *Endoscopy*. 2005;37:38–41.

Paulsen SR, et al. CT enterography as a diagnstic tool in evaluating small bowel disorders: review of clinical experience with over 700 cases. *Radiographics*. 2006;26:641–57; discussion 657–62.

Ramirez FC, et al. Feasibility and safety of string, wireless capsule endoscopy in the diagnosis of Barrett's esophagus. *Gastrointest Endosc*. 2005;63:742–746.

Rex DK. Review article: moderate sedation for endoscopy; sedation regimens for non-anaesthesiologists. *Aliment Pharmacol Ther*. 2006;24:163–171.

Rockey DC, et al. Analysis of air contrast barium enema, computed tomographic colonography, and colonoscopy: Prospective comparison. *Lancet*. 2005;365:305–311.

Rossi A, et al. ASGE guidelines for the appropriate use of upper endoscopy: association with endoscopic findings. *Gastrointest Endosc*. 2002;56:714–719.

Sequeiros EV, et al. The role of endoscopic ultrasonography in the diagnosis, staging and management of pancreatic disease states. *Curr Gastroenterol Rep*. 2000;2:125.

Sotoudehmanesh R, et al. Role of endoscopic ultrasonography in prevention of unnecessary endoscopic retrograde cholangiopancreatography: a prospective study of 150 patients. *J Ultrasound Med*. 2007;26:455–60.

Sunada K, et al. Clinical outcomes of enteroscopy using the double-balloon method for strictures of the small intestine. *World J Gastroenterol*. 2005;11:1087–1089.

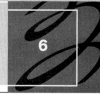

LAPAROSCOPY AND LAPAROSCOPIC SURGERY

6

$\mathcal{E}$xamination of the abdominal cavity and its organs by means of a laparoscope has been available for nearly a century. Until recently, laparoscopy was largely a diagnostic procedure; the instruments were used primarily to visualize and biopsy abdominal organs and other structures, although some treatment was possible in the form of aspiration of cysts and abscesses, lysis of adhesions, ligation of the fallopian tubes, and ablation of endometriosis or cancer by laser. In recent years, rapid and dramatic developments in operative laparoscopy have made laparoscopic cholecystectomy and appendectomy commonplace; other, more complicated operative procedures, such as partial gastrectomy and partial colectomy, have been described using laparoscopic methods.

I. LAPAROSCOPY

A. Indications. The reliance on diagnostic laparoscopy varies from one medical center to another. In some centers, laparoscopy is used routinely in evaluation of the abdominal conditions discussed in this chapter, whereas in other centers it is used rarely. This variability in the use of diagnostic laparoscopy can be attributed to the advances in computed tomography (CT) and other imaging techniques of the past decade, which have provided alternatives to laparoscopy that are either less invasive or more readily available. In hospitals and medical centers where diagnostic laparoscopy is available, it is usually performed for the following indications.

   1. Biopsy of the liver. This procedure may be done to evaluate a diffuse condition of the liver, such as cirrhosis or an infiltrating disease, or to biopsy a focal defect of the liver that has been identified by CT or ultrasound examination. During laparoscopy, the appearance of the liver also can be assessed; for example, the collateral vessels of portal hypertension or nodularity of cirrhosis or neoplasm may be evident.

   2. Determination of cause of ascites. When the cause of ascites is unknown, laparoscopic examination of the abdominal organs, the omentum, and the peritoneum may provide an answer. The most common causes are disseminated cancer, usually ovarian, and cirrhosis.

   3. Staging of Hodgkin's disease and non-Hodgkin's lymphoma.

   4. Evaluation of patients with fever of unknown origin.

   5. Evaluation of patients with chronic or intermittent abdominal pain. Diagnoses include abdominal adhesions, Crohn's disease, appendicitis, and endometriosis.

B. Contraindications include a perforated viscus, abdominal wall infections, diffuse peritonitis, and clinically significant coagulopathy. Chronic lung disease and congestive heart failure are relative contraindications. If laparoscopy is necessary in those instances, sedation should be minimized and the patient should have pulse oximetry and cardiovascular monitoring. Tense ascites interferes with adequate visualization and should be treated before attempting laparoscopy.

C. Technique. Most diagnostic laparoscopic procedures are performed electively in patients who have fasted and are under sedation and local anesthesia. A small skin incision is made, usually above and to the left of the umbilicus, avoiding surgical scars and abdominal masses. Nitrous oxide or carbon dioxide gas is introduced by a needle to distend the abdomen, and a trocar and cannula are passed through the incision into the peritoneal cavity. The laparoscope is inserted into the abdomen

25

and, by maneuvering the instrument or positioning the patient, most of the abdominal contents can be examined. Tissue samples can be obtained by brushes, needles, or forceps that are passed through the laparoscope. At the conclusion of the examination, the gas is withdrawn, the instrument is removed, and the small incision is closed with sutures or clips.

  D. Therapeutic laparoscopy. Some conditions can be treated by the laparoscopic techniques described. These treatments include aspiration of cysts and abscesses, lysis of adhesions, ligation of the fallopian tubes, and ablation of endometriosis or cancer by laser. However, the most dramatic advances in therapeutic laparoscopy have been in the area of operative laparoscopy, described in the following sections.

II. LAPAROSCOPIC SURGERY. The recent advances in laparoscopic surgery have been the result of two important contemporary factors: (a) the remarkable continuing developments in fiberoptic technology and (b) the strong economic incentives to minimize the duration of hospitalization and use of inpatient hospital facilities.

  A. Laparoscopic cholecystectomy

   1. Indications and **contraindications** for laparoscopic cholecystectomy are the same as for traditional operative cholecystectomy (Table 6-1).

   2. Technique. The equipment and instruments required to perform laparoscopic surgery are reviewed in the selected reading by Gadacz and associates. Briefly, the equipment includes a powerful (xenon) light source, a carbon dioxide insufflator, a high-resolution end-viewing camera with a high-resolution video monitor, an irrigation device that instills fluid at a high flow rate, and an electrocautery or laser device. A variety of instruments also are needed, including a Veress needle for insufflation, cannulas with trocars, endoscopes, retractors, graspers, dissectors, a clip applier, irrigation and aspiration catheters, coagulators, and catheters for performing cholangiography.

   Laparoscopic cholangiography and cholecystectomy can be performed under general or epidural anesthesia. Preoperative antibiotics generally are used at the discretion of the operator but are indicated in patients with recent cholecystitis, heart valve prostheses, and other medical risk factors. Before beginning

TABLE 6-1	Indications and Contraindications for Laparoscopic Cholecystectomy
Indications	Cholelithiasis and biliary colic
	Symptomatic gallbladder polyps
	Resolved gallstone pancreatitis
	Symptomatic chronic cholecystitis
Relative contraindications	Acute cholecystitis
	Previous upper abdominal operation
	Minor bleeding disorder
	Common duct stones
Absolute contraindications	Acute cholangitis
	Severe acute cholecystitis
	Acute pancreatitis
	Peritonitis
	Portal hypertension
	Pregnancy
	Serious bleeding disorder
	Morbid obesity

From Gadacz TR, et al. Laparoscopic cholecystectomy. *Surg Clin North Am.* 1990;70:1249. Reprinted with permission.

the procedure, the urinary bladder is drained with a Foley catheter, and the stomach is decompressed with a nasogastric tube. Two video monitors, one on each side of the operating table, allow all members of the operating team a view of the procedure. Several cannulas are inserted through the abdominal wall for insufflation and surgical manipulation; the surgical laparoscope is inserted just above the umbilicus. A detailed description of the laparoscopic cholecystectomy procedure is provided by Gadacz, et al.

3. **Results.** As experience with laparoscopic cholecystectomy increases, the procedure is recognized to be safe and effective. Operative time is less than 2 hours. Most patients are able to leave the hospital in fewer than 2 days and are able to return to work more quickly than after standard operative cholecystectomy. Thus, there are economic savings both in decreased hospital costs and in reduced time away from work. Fewer than 5% of patients require standard laparotomy because of a complication of the laparoscopic procedure, such as bleeding, bile duct leak, bile duct injury, or technical difficulties.

B. **Other laparoscopic operations.** Laparoscopic appendectomy and inguinal herniorrhaphy are performed routinely, and other more extensive abdominal operations, such as gastrectomy, colectomy, esophageal fundoplication, gastric stapling, and intestinal bypass are also performed, but require more advanced expertise. Laparoscopic techniques are also used to treat pulmonary and pericardial lesions in the chest. Intraluminal laparoscopic surgery via the lumena of the GI tract, e.g., stomach, is the promising new era of surgical management of intraabdominal diseases.

Selected Readings

Anvari M, et al. Five-year comprehensive outcomes evaluation in 181 patients after laparoscopic Nissen fundoplication. *J Am Coll Surg.* 2003;196:51–57.

Doherty GM, et al. *Current Surgical Diagnosis and Treatment.* 12th ed. New York, NY: McGraw-Hill; 2006:662–667.

Giger U, et al. Laparoscopic cholecystectomy in acute cholecystitis: indication, technique, risk and outcome. *Langenbecks Arch Surg.* 2005;390:373–80.

Gurusamy KS, et al. Early versus delayed laparoscopic cholecystectomy for acute cholecystitis. *Cochrane Database Syst Rev.* 2006;4:CD005440.

Iannelli A, et al. Therapeutic laparoscopy for blunt abdominal trauma with bowel injuries. *J Laparoendosc Adv Surg Tech A.* 2003;13:189–191.

Kalloo An, et al. Flexible transgastric peritoneoscopy: A novel approach to diagnostic and therapeutic interventions in the peritoneal cavity. *Gastrointest Endosc.* 2004;60: 114–117.

Kamoz T, Granderath F, Pontner R. Laparoscopic antireflux surgery. *Surg Endosc.* 2003;17:880–885.

Madan A. Laparoscopic bariatric surgery. *US Gastroenterol Rev.* 2000;1:29–33.

McQuay N, et al. Laparoscopy in the evaluation of penetrating thoracoabdominal trauma. *Am Surg.* 2003;69:788–791.

Polanivelu C, et al. Laparoscopic lateral pancreaticojejunostomy: A new remedy for an old ailment. *Surg Endosc.* 2006;20:458–461.

Roggin KK, et al. What is the long term safety and efficacy of laparoscopic resection for gastric and gastrointestinal stroma tumors? *Nat Clin Pract Gastroenterol Hepatol.* 2007;4:76–78.

Soper NJ, et al. Laparoscopic general surgery. *N Engl J Med.* 1994;330:409.

Tom J, et al. Laparoscopic surgery for Chron's disease: a meta analysis. *Dis Colon Rectum.* 2007;50(5):576–585.

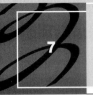
PERCUTANEOUS LIVER BIOPSY

*M*icroscopic or biochemical examination of liver tissue often provides the definitive diagnosis and leads to effective management of liver and systemic disorders. The liver tissue typically is obtained by percutaneous needle biopsy, either in hospitalized patients or in selected outpatients. The outpatient procedure is reserved for patients who do not have severe liver disease, a clotting disorder, or some other serious illness. Facilities must be available to observe the patients for 3 to 5 hours after the biopsy.

In recent years, percutaneous needle aspiration or biopsy of liver lesions under ultrasound or computed tomography (CT) scan guidance has obviated the need for obtaining a traditional "blind" liver biopsy in most patients. Automatic liver biopsy needles are used to obtain thin core biopsies of liver lesions or for sampling of the liver. Liver biopsy may also be obtained during laparoscopy.

I. **INDICATIONS AND CONTRAINDICATIONS.** The **major indication** for performing a liver biopsy is to clarify the nature of suspected liver disease. In some instances, liver biopsy is performed to determine the effect of treatment of known liver disease or to document the appearance of the liver before initiating therapy (usually for a nonhepatic disorder) with a potentially hepatotoxic drug.

Contraindications to percutaneous liver biopsy are listed in Table 7-1; some may not be absolute. For example, patients with severe liver disease commonly have clotting disorders. If a liver biopsy is believed to be necessary under those circumstances, patients can be prepared with infusions of fresh-frozen plasma and platelets. In patients with severe liver disease and coagulopathy, a transjugular venous liver biopsy may be the safer and the only alternative technique for obtaining a liver biopsy.

II. **TRADITIONAL METHOD OF PERFORMING THE BIOPSY**

A. **Prebiopsy care.** Patients should fast for at least 6 hours before the biopsy and, because they will have to remain in bed for several hours after the biopsy, they should be encouraged to void. Hemoglobin count, hematocrit, white blood cell count, platelet count, prothrombin time, and partial thromboplastin time should be determined several days before the biopsy.

B. **Choice of biopsy site.** The patient lies in a supine position near the right edge of the bed with the right hand under the head and the head turned toward the left. If the liver is not enlarged, an intercostal site is chosen that is within the area of

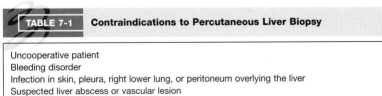

TABLE 7-1   Contraindications to Percutaneous Liver Biopsy

Uncooperative patient
Bleeding disorder
Infection in skin, pleura, right lower lung, or peritoneum overlying the liver
Suspected liver abscess or vascular lesion
Difficulty in determining liver location, as with ascites
Severe extrahepatic obstruction

maximal liver dullness between the anterior and midaxillary lines. If the biopsy is being done under ultrasound, the site is chosen by the radiologist.

C. Preparation of the biopsy site. Using sterile gloves, cleanse the biopsy site and surrounding skin with acetone-alcohol and iodine solutions, and arrange sterile drapes around the biopsy site. Infiltrate the skin with local anesthetic. The anesthetic also may be infiltrated beneath the skin to the liver capsule, with care taken to keep the needle at the upper edge of the rib to avoid the artery that runs below the rib.

D. Taking the biopsy. Make a 4-mm skin incision at the biopsy site with a no. 11 knife blade. Fill a 20-mL syringe with about 10 mL of sterile saline (avoid bacteriostatic preparations if you plan to culture the biopsy tissue), and attach the biopsy needle. (Generally, this is a Menghini or modified Menghini needle.) Insert the biopsy needle through the skin incision parallel to the surface of the bed, aiming toward the xiphoid. Advance the needle into the intercostal muscles, and flush the needle with 0.2 to 0.5 mL of saline.

Have the patient hold the breath at full expiration for the intercostal approach; at full inspiration for the subcostal approach. It is wise to have the patient practice this maneuver several times before the biopsy is obtained. Apply constant suction on the syringe and, in a rapid, smooth motion, advance and

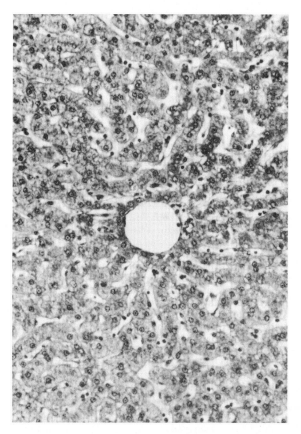

Figure 7-1. Photomicrograph of the liver, showing the central area of a classic lobule with a central vein. (From Snell RS. *Clinical and Functional Histology for Medical Students.* Boston: Little, Brown; 1984:479. Reprinted with permission.)

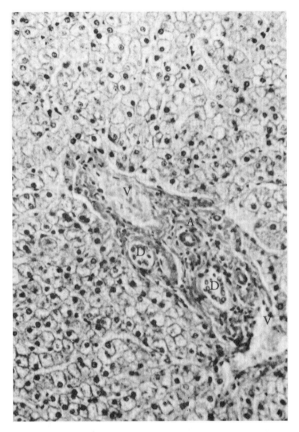

Figure 7-2. Photomicrograph of the liver, showing the peripheral area of a classic lobule with a branch of the hepatic artery (*A*), a branch of the portal vein (*V*), and a small bile duct (*D*). (From Snell RS. *Clinical and Functional Histology for Medical Students*. Boston: Little, Brown; 1984:479. Reprinted with permission.)

withdraw the needle 4 to 5 cm. The total duration of this movement should not exceed 1 second. Ask the patient to resume breathing. A second biopsy through the same incision at a slightly different angle will increase the diagnostic yield in patients with suspected cancer of the liver. The biopsy may be expelled from the needle temporarily into saline or directly into 10% formalin. Apply an adhesive bandage over the biopsy wound.

Percutaneous liver biopsies may also be obtained using **automatic biopsy needles.** These automatic needle "guns" are usually preferred by radiologists and

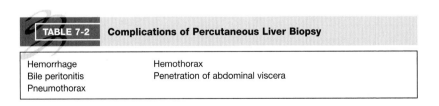

TABLE 7-2	Complications of Percutaneous Liver Biopsy
Hemorrhage	Hemothorax
Bile peritonitis	Penetration of abdominal viscera
Pneumothorax	

gastroenterologists obtaining liver biopsies under ultrasound or CT-scan guidance. The steps of the procedure are similar to the traditional biopsy technique.

E. Postbiopsy care. The patient should remain in bed for 4 to 6 hours. Some physicians advise patients to lie on their right side for the first 2 hours. After that time they may sit up in bed. Blood pressure and pulse should be checked frequently. One method is to obtain vital signs every 30 minutes for 2 hours, and every hour for 3 hours. Outpatients should be asked to communicate with a nurse or physician the next day. Patients may be allowed to drink clear liquids shortly after biopsy but should avoid solid food for several hours until it is clear that no serious complication has developed.

III. COMPLICATIONS FROM LIVER BIOPSY are infrequent but may be dramatic (Table 7-2 on page 30). Deaths have been reported in about 1 in 1,000 biopsies and major complications in about 3 in 1,000. Complications can be minimized by using a needle 1.2 mm in diameter or less, avoiding biopsy in high-risk patients, and adhering strictly to protocol for obtaining the biopsy.

IV. INTERPRETATION OF THE BIOPSY. The spectrum of pathologic changes is broad and cannot be discussed here at length. However, the approach to interpretation of a liver biopsy is similar to that for interpretation of a small-bowel mucosal biopsy: The observer looks for changes in cellularity and architecture.

The liver lobule contains a central (hepatic) vein surrounded by sinusoids (Fig. 7-1 on page 29). At the periphery of the lobule are several portal triads (Fig. 7-2 on page 30). Within the triads are bile ducts, portal vein, hepatic artery, connective tissue, and round cells. Pathologic changes may include expansion of the portal triads with inflammatory cells, accumulation of inflammatory cells and fibrosis between the triads (bridging), destruction of hepatic parenchymal cells, dropout of parenchymal cells, and distortion of the lobular architecture by inflammation and fibrosis.

Selected Readings

Bravo AA, et al. Liver biopsy. *N Engl J Med.* 2001;344:495.

Brunt EM, et al. Liver biopsy interpretation for the gastroenterologist. *Curr Gastroenterol Rep.* 2000;2:27.

Cjaza AJ, et al. Optimizing diagnosis from the medical liver biopsy. *Clin Gastroenterol Hepatol.* 2007;5(8):898–907.

Edmison JM, et al. How good is transjugular liver biopsy for the histologic evaluation of liver disease. *Nat Clin Pract Gastroenterol Hepatol.* 2007;4:306–308.

LefKowitch JH. Hepatobiliary pathology. *Curr Opin. Gastroenterol.* 2006;22:198–208.

Schiaro TD, et al. Importance of specimen size in accurate needle biopsy evaluation of patients with chronic hepatitis. C. *Clin Gastroenterol Hepatol.* 2005;3:930–935.

Sherman KE, et al. Liver biopsy in cirrhotic patients. *AJ Gastroenterol.* 2007;102:789–793.

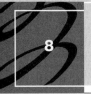

8   MANOMETRIC STUDIES

$\mathcal{T}$he gastrointestinal tract is a long, muscular tube in which the coordinated relaxation and contraction of smooth muscle, expressed as peristalsis, actions of various sphincters, and accommodation to the bulk of ingested food and secretions play an important role in normal digestive function. Increasingly, abnormalities in gastrointestinal neuromuscular activity are recognized as being responsible for clinical disorders.

I. ESOPHAGEAL MOTILITY STUDIES. The main purpose of the esophagus is to transport food and secretions to the stomach. It performs this task through a series of coordinated events that begins when a solid or liquid bolus is propelled to the back of the mouth and into the pharynx by the tongue. Thereafter, the process of swallowing becomes "automatic." First, the upper esophageal sphincter (UES), which constricts the esophagus just below the pharynx, relaxes as the pharynx contracts and the bolus passes into the upper esophagus. Next, a primary peristaltic contraction propels the bolus down the esophagus but usually is insufficient to carry the bolus the entire length of the esophagus.

Secondary peristaltic contractions are initiated when the esophagus is distended by the bolus, and these contractions finish moving the bolus to the stomach. Finally, as the bolus reaches the mid-to-lower esophagus, the lower esophageal sphincter (LES) relaxes to allow the bolus to pass into the stomach. The tonic contraction of the LES, which relaxes during swallowing, normally presents an effective barrier against reflux of gastric contents into the esophagus.

A. Indications and contraindications. Esophageal manometry is useful in diagnosing disorders of motility or a dysfunctional UES or LES (Table 8-1). Typically, patients with motility disorders complain of dysphagia, usually to both liquids and solids (see Chapter 20). Esophageal manometry also is useful in the evaluation of patients with noncardiac chest pain (see Chapter 21). Some of these patients can be shown to have esophageal spasm or a related motility disorder. Finally, esophageal manometry sometimes is used in the evaluation of patients with severe gastroesophageal reflux to document impairment of peristalsis or LES function (see Chapter 19). Patients with reflux symptoms usually do not require esophageal manometry, however.

Esophageal manometry should not be performed in a patient who is unwilling to cooperate in swallowing the tube or in a patient with severe mechanical esophageal obstruction.

B. Method of performing esophageal manometry. Patients are asked to fast for 6 to 8 hours before the study. Usually no sedatives or topical anesthetics are given because these medications may interfere with esophageal motor function. If the patient is unable to swallow the tube, however, a small amount of topical anesthetic may be applied to the pharynx or, if the tube is to be passed through the nose, to the internal nares. Patients may return to their usual activities and diet after completion of the study.

The **typical manometry tube** has three recording probes (either perfused catheter tips or solid-state transducers) arranged linearly toward the distal end of the tube (Fig. 8-1). The most proximal probe is 5 cm above the middle probe, which in turn is 5 cm above the distal probe. The tube is passed through either the nose or the mouth as the patient swallows and is positioned initially so that all three probes

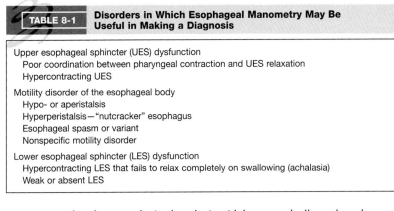

TABLE 8-1   **Disorders in Which Esophageal Manometry May Be Useful in Making a Diagnosis**

Upper esophageal sphincter (UES) dysfunction
  Poor coordination between pharyngeal contraction and UES relaxation
  Hypercontracting UES
Motility disorder of the esophageal body
  Hypo- or aperistalsis
  Hyperperistalsis—"nutcracker" esophagus
  Esophageal spasm or variant
  Nonspecific motility disorder
Lower esophageal sphincter (LES) dysfunction
  Hypercontracting LES that fails to relax completely on swallowing (achalasia)
  Weak or absent LES

are within the stomach. As the tube is withdrawn gradually, each probe passes through the LES. As the probes move up into the body of the esophagus, peristaltic contractions are recorded sequentially as they pass down the esophagus, first with the proximal probe, next the middle probe, and last the distal one. When the middle or distal probe lies within the LES, the relation between esophageal peristaltic contractions and sphincteric relaxation can be observed (Fig. 8-2). Similarly, when the upper probe lies in the pharynx and the middle probe is within the UES, the relation between pharyngeal contractions and UES relaxation can be recorded.

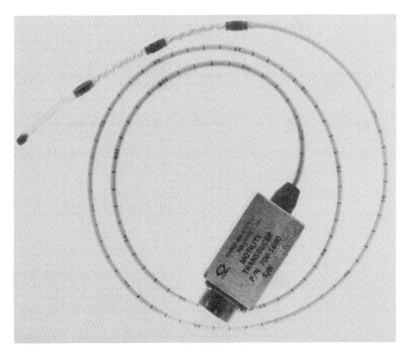

Figure 8-1. The esophageal manometry tube is coiled on a chart recorder. Note the three small transducers arranged serially, 5 cm apart, beginning 5 cm from the distal end of the tube.

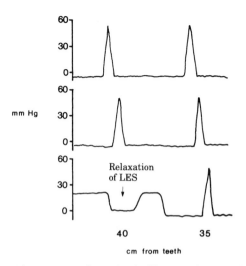

Figure 8-2. Manometric appearance of normal peristaltic contractions and relaxation of the lower esophageal sphincter (LES). The upper, middle, and lower probes are each separated by 5 cm. (From Eastwood GL. *Core Textbook of Gastroenterology.* Philadelphia: Lippincott Williams & Wilkins; 1984:27. Reprinted with permission.)

   C. Interpretation of manometric findings and the role manometry plays in the diagnosis of specific esophageal disorders are discussed in subsequent chapters. It is sufficient at this point to say that some conditions may have quite specific diagnostic findings by manometry, such as the hypercontracting LES of achalasia, which fails to relax completely on swallowing, whereas other conditions, such as esophageal motor disorders causing chest pain, may be accompanied by nonspecific or normal findings at the time of manometry; in these instances, manometry is of little diagnostic value.

II. pH TESTING. Measurement of esophageal pH by means of an intraesophageal pH electrode, which usually is positioned 5 cm above the LES, can be determined at the time of the esophageal motility study or over a 24-hour period.
   A. pH measurements after standard motility studies include testing for acid clearance in which 15 mL of 0.1 N HCl is infused into the lower esophagus. The patient is asked to dry-swallow every 30 seconds until the pH returns to the baseline value, which should occur within 15 swallows. Ineffective clearance of acid occurs in conditions that cause abnormal esophageal peristalsis, such as scleroderma, achalasia, and other esophageal motility disorders, and in conditions that decrease the volume of salivary secretion, such as scleroderma and the sicca complex.
      Measurements of lower esophageal pH also can be diagnostic of gastroesophageal reflux. Esophageal pH is documented with the patient supine, prone, and on the left and right sides; when relaxed and after performing the Valsalva maneuver; and after assuming the knee–chest position. After the patient is positioned, 300 mL of 0.1 N HCl is instilled into the stomach and pH measurements are repeated in all the positions. A drop in pH below 4.0 in any position in the basal state or in two positions after acid instillation is regarded as indicative of abnormal reflux of acid. Measurement of esophageal peristalsis during acid infusion (see Chapter 22, Section II.B.2.d, Bernstein test) may document a motility disorder that is responsible for the chest pain.
   B. Ambulatory pH measurements. Several ambulatory pH monitoring systems are available that allow continuous measurement of esophageal pH for up to 24 hours

under conditions that patients experience during their everyday lives. This procedure is particularly useful in documenting nocturnal reflux symptoms or symptoms that occur in relation to other experiences or activities. Patients are asked to keep a record of their symptoms. The best correlations with symptoms appear to be with total time that pH is less than 4.0 and with the number of times intraesophageal pH below 4.0 exceeds 5 minutes.

C. A **wireless pH monitoring (Bravo) device** has been developed to improve patient comfort and increase pH test sensitivity. It is placed endoscopically in the distal esophagus and allows for prolonged monitoring (48 hours vs. 24 hours). The extended monitoring period helps to better understand GER physiology by studying the day-to-day and moment-by-moment variability of GER. It may also be used to assess the effectiveness of acid suppressive therapy without the need for repeat testing.

D. **Multichannel intraluminal impedance (MII)** is a new technique for the evaluation of gastroesophageal reflux disease (GERD) and for esophageal motor function testing. It can assess esophageal bolus transit similar to barium swallow and the proximal extent of the reflux event. MII can be used in combination with esophageal manometry for concurrent assessment of esophageal motor function and motility.

E. **High-resolution manometry (HRM)** is solid-state manometry with 36 circumferential sensors spaced at 1-cm intervals (4.2-mm outer diameter). Each of these sensors contains 12 circumferentially isolated sensors that detect pressure over a 2.5-mm length of the esophagus.

The procedure involves placing the catheter in the esophagus and recording 10 swallows, then withdrawing. Pressures detected by each sensor are averaged to obtain a mean pressure measurement for each sensor, making each of the 36 sensors a circumferential pressure detector. The data obtained are then processed by a computerized program (ManoScan) to create high-resolution plots or conventual line traces.

HRM is simpler, faster, and more precise. It provides a complete observation of the esophageal motor function from the pharynx to the LES without the need for catheter reposition and gives accurate sphincter pressures and assessment of peristaltic performance.

III. **ANORECTAL MANOMETRY** may be useful in the evaluation of patients with constipation or stool incontinence. Measurements include documentation of baseline pressures of the internal and external anal sphincters and the relaxation response of the internal sphincter to distention of the rectal vault by stool or an inflated balloon. For example, in Hirschsprung's disease, the internal anal sphincter does not relax adequately in response to rectal distention.

Incontinence from internal anal sphincteric dysfunction can be caused by hemorrhoid surgery or neuromuscular disorders affecting smooth muscle. The internal anal sphincter is under autonomic control, whereas the external anal sphincter is under voluntary control. External sphincteric dysfunction may be related to sacral nerve disease and disorders of striated muscle.

IV. **MANOMETRY OF THE STOMACH, SMALL INTESTINE, AND COLON** is available in some institutions as a research tool to investigate clinical disorders of gut motility; however, the technique is not generally available. Conditions that may affect motility of the stomach and intestines include diabetes, autonomic neuropathy, vagotomy, connective tissue disorders, muscular disorders, and infiltrative disorders (e.g., amyloidosis).

Selected Readings

Adler DG, et al. Primary esophageal motility disorders. *Mayo Clin Proc.* 2001;76:195.

Fox M, et al. High-resolution manometry predicts the success of oesophageal bolus transport and identifies clinically important abnormalities not detected by conventional manometry. *Neurogastroenterol Motil.* 2004;16(5):533–542.

Kahrilas PJ. Esophageal motility disorders: current concepts of pathogenesis and treatment. *Can J Gastroenterol.* 2000;14:221–230.

Pandolfino J. Esophageal monitoring devices. *US Gastroenterol Rev.* 2007;(1)23–27.

Pandolfino J, et al. AGA medical position statement? Clinical use of esophageal manometry. *Gastroenterology.* 2005;128:107–108.

Park W, et al. Esophageal impedance recording: Clinical utility and limitations. *Curr Gastroenterol Rep.* 2005;7:182–189.

𝒥t is an unusual patient who, complaining of some digestive disorder, does not have a radiologic or ultrasound study sometime during the course of the evaluation. In the pre-endoscopic era, many gastroenterologists performed plain and barium-contrast radiographic studies in their own offices. Now the term *gastroenterologist* is virtually synonymous with *endoscopist*, and roentgenographic studies are performed (appropriately) by a radiologist. Nevertheless, all physicians who see patients with digestive complaints should be familiar with the radiologic, ultrasound, and radionuclide studies that are commonly available.

I. RADIOLOGIC AND ULTRASOUND STUDIES

A. Plain chest and abdominal films

1. **Chest films.** Sometimes physicians overlook the value of the plain chest and abdominal x-ray films. A widened mediastinum or an air-fluid level in the mediastinum may indicate an obstructed and dilated esophagus. Pleural effusions may accompany ascites or acute pancreatitis. Patients with pneumonia occasionally seek treatment for abdominal pain. In patients with suspected perforation of an abdominal viscus, the upright chest film is superior to abdominal films, which usually do not visualize the domes of the diaphragm, in identifying free air under the diaphragm.

2. **Abdominal films.** A complete set of plain abdominal films includes a supine view and an upright view. Sometimes the supine film is called the "**flat plate,**" a holdover from the early days of radiology when photographic plates instead of films were used. Another term in the medical jargon is **KUB,** an acronym for kidney, ureter, and bladder, although much more than these three organs are shown.

    a. **Both the soft tissue densities** and the **bony structures** should be examined carefully on the abdominal plain film. Accumulations of calcium may be seen in the pancreas or other organs, signifying chronic inflammatory disease. In atherosclerotic disease, calcium may outline the aorta and other vessels; an aortic aneurysm may first be suspected by careful examination of the abdominal plain film.

    b. The **distribution of air in the bowel** is of importance. Normally air is seen at various locations in the colon and rectum, and a small amount of air may appear in the small bowel. The air provides a natural contrast medium, which sometimes outlines mass lesions. Submucosal collections of blood, fluid, or inflammatory cells, which also protrude into the bowel lumen, may give a clue to the presence of a disorder such as ischemic bowel disease, lymphoma, or Crohn's disease. Dilatation of the small or large intestine occurs in bowel obstruction or ileus. A markedly dilated, ahaustral transverse colon is typical of toxic megacolon. Absence of bowel loops in a portion of the abdomen may indicate a large mass; the mass may distort the appearance of otherwise normal loops of bowel. The upright film (or a lateral decubitus film, if the patient cannot stand) may show air-fluid levels signifying obstruction or ileus. Rarely, an air-filled loop of bowel in the scrotum is seen, indicating a large inguinal hernia.

B. The **barium swallow** most often is ordered to evaluate disorders of swallowing, although it also may be useful in delineating size and configuration of the heart

chambers and other mediastinal structures. Occasionally an esophageal–tracheal fistula can be identified in this manner.

Views of the esophagus usually are included in a standard upper gastrointestinal (GI) series, but typically are limited to the middle and lower esophagus. During a barium swallow, the radiologist also obtains views of the pharynx and upper esophagus and looks carefully under fluoroscopy at the process of swallowing from initiation to completion. This step is facilitated by the use of a videotape of the swallowing action after the patient swallows both a liquid bolus and a solid bolus (e.g., barium-impregnated bread). This procedure allows the swallowing process to be scrutinized closely, using slow motion or stop-action when necessary.

C. **Upper gastrointestinal series.** The standard upper GI series includes views of the middle and lower esophagus, stomach, duodenum, and proximal jejunum. Although the upper GI series has less diagnostic accuracy than endoscopy, it plays a major role in the evaluation of digestive complaints. Gastrointestinal radiologists sometimes have the patient also swallow substances that release carbon dioxide, providing air contrast and improving diagnostic accuracy.

D. **Small-bowel series**

   1. The small-bowel series usually is a continuation of the upper GI series. In most radiology departments, however, the small-bowel series must be ordered specifically. After the patient has swallowed the requisite amount of barium to complete the upper GI series, delayed films are taken for up to 1 to 2 hours to visualize the loops of small bowel. Particular care is taken to identify the terminal ileum because of the predilection of Crohn's disease or lymphoma for that site. Sometimes, a reasonable view of the cecum and ascending colon can be obtained.

   2. An important variant of the small-bowel series is the **small-bowel enema, or enteroclysis.** In a small-bowel enema, the patient does not swallow barium; instead, a small tube is passed by mouth into the duodenum. Barium is injected through the tube to opacify the small intestine. This procedure has the advantage of allowing a smaller quantity of barium to be used, thereby not obscuring the loops of small intestine and thus focusing more specifically on that organ. Injection of air after the barium allows air-contrast films to be made and improves the diagnostic accuracy.

E. **Barium enema**

   1. The standard barium enema is performed after the colon has been evacuated with a conventional cathartic and enema preparation (usually preceded by a clear-liquid diet for 1 to 2 days) or a balanced electrolyte lavage solution. These bowel preparations are similar to those used before colonoscopy (see Chapter 5). Barium is subsequently allowed to flow by gravity into the colon through the rectum. Instillation of air improves the contrast. In most patients, barium refluxes into the terminal ileum.

   2. In general, a **sigmoidoscopy** should precede a barium enema. The two studies are complementary.

   3. In some clinical situations, a **limited barium enema** is performed **without a bowel preparation.** This would be the case when a bowel obstruction is suspected and a limited view of the colon is necessary. If the patient has an intussusception of the colon or a sigmoid volvulus, a carefully performed barium enema without preparation may correct these disorders. Finally, in the evaluation of suspected Hirschsprung's disease (aganglionosis of the rectum or distal colon), a limited barium enema in an unprepared colon has a greater likelihood of providing diagnostic information than examination of a colon empty of stool.

F. **Gallbladder and biliary studies.** A number of studies have been used to evaluate the gallbladder and biliary ductal system. These include oral cholecystography, intravenous cholangiography, percutaneous cholangiography, endoscopic retrograde cholangiopancreatography (ERCP) (see Chapter 5), computed tomography (CT) scan (see Section I.H), ultrasonography (see Section I.J), and the HIDA scan (see Section II.B).

   1. The **oral cholecystogram** has been available for decades to evaluate gallbladder function and diagnose gallstones. However, abdominal ultrasonography

(see Section I.J) has largely replaced oral cholecystography for identifying gallstones, although the two studies may be complementary in some patients. During oral cholecystography, radiopaque iodine-containing dye is ingested in the form of tablets, absorbed from the intestine, extracted by the liver, and excreted into bile, where it is concentrated in the gallbladder, which is then visualized radiographically. Usually the biliary ductal system is not opacified. Failure to see the gallbladder after a double-dose oral cholecystogram is a strong indicator of gallbladder disease. However, failure to opacify the gallbladder may also result from poor absorption of the dye, intrinsic liver disease, or a serum bilirubin level in excess of 3 mg/dL. Today, this technique is rarely observed.

2. During **intravenous cholangiography,** a radiopaque dye is injected by vein and, like the oral dye, is extracted by the liver and excreted in the bile. However, unlike oral cholecystography, both the major bile ducts and the gallbladder opacify during intravenous cholangiography. The study is severely limited when the serum bilirubin level is greater than 3 mg/dL. Furthermore, the extent and clarity of opacification of the bile duct system is considerably less than that achieved with ERCP or percutaneous cholangiography. Thus, currently there is little clinical use for intravenous cholangiography.

3. **Percutaneous transhepatic cholangiography (PTC)** is performed by passing a long, thin needle (about 23-gauge) through the skin into the liver. As the needle is withdrawn slowly, small amounts of radiopaque dye are injected until the bile duct is visualized. Sufficient dye is subsequently injected to opacify the biliary system. This test is more than 90% successful in patients with extrahepatic obstruction and dilated bile ducts. It is only 50% to 60% successful in patients with normal-size ducts. The ready availability of ERCP has decreased the frequency with which PTC is used. Often, when one of the two studies is unsuccessful, the other is successful in visualizing an obstructed biliary system.

G. **Intravenous pyelogram.** Although an intravenous pyelogram (IVP) is most commonly used in the evaluation of the genitourinary tract, it can be of help as an adjunct to the evaluation of some GI and other abdominal disorders. Retroperitoneal tumors and the inflammatory masses that occur in Crohn's disease may cause deviation or obstruction of the ureters. Similarly, masses may impinge on the bladder. Rarely, an enterovesical fistula can be visualized by IVP or by retrograde cystography.

H. **Computed tomography scan.** The nearly universal availability of computed tomography (CT) scanning has altered the diagnostic approach to many patients with abdominal complaints. The CT scan often aids in making a diagnosis quickly, abbreviating the diagnostic evaluation, shortening hospital stay, and avoiding unnecessary studies. For example, lesions in locations and in organs within the abdomen that formerly was obscure, such as the retroperitoneum and pancreas, now often can be readily visualized by CT scanning.

The CT scan has largely replaced the **radionuclide liver–spleen scan** for detecting masses of the liver because of its ability to resolve smaller lesions. In addition, the CT scan shows the size and shape of the liver more accurately and provides information about other abdominal organs that is not available by liver–spleen scan. Furthermore, the relative densities of mass lesions can be estimated by CT scanning to determine whether such lesions are solid or cystic.

The diagnostic accuracy of the CT scan is enhanced by the injection of contrast material intravenously to visualize the vascular system and by oral administration of contrast to delineate the GI tract.

The ability to obtain tissue samples by fine-needle aspiration has enhanced the diagnostic capability of CT scanning even more. In this manner, malignant lesions, abscesses, and benign cysts can be histologically and cytologically confirmed. Abscesses and infected cysts also can be drained and treated by CT-guided placement of drainage catheters.

CT colography has been developed for examination of the colon, especially for the detection of colonic polyps and neoplasms. The patients are prepared similarly as for colonoscopy. At the time of the scanning, air is introduced into the colon, and the colon is kept distended during the CT scanning. Patients do not receive any sedation and thus the procedure may be painful. Polyps larger than 7 to 10 mm are seen with acceptable accuracy; however, smaller polyps may be missed by this technique. If a polyp is found, patients are then referred for colonoscopy.

CT enterography is a newer technique gaining popularity used in the examination of the small intestine, especially for the detection of Crohn's disease and its complications. It is able to detect early lesions (i.e., aphthous ulcers, bowel wall inflammation and thickening, and early stricture and fistula formation).

I. **Angiography.** Selective arteriography of the celiac axis, superior mesenteric artery, inferior mesenteric artery, or their branches may reveal vascular tumors, document the effects of other tumors on abdominal organs, and identify sites of bleeding. For extravasation of dye to be seen at a bleeding site, it is estimated that the rate of bleeding must be at least 0.5 to 1.0 mL per minute.

Selective arteriography can also be therapeutic. Autologous clots or vasopressin can be injected into appropriate vessels. In patients with cancer, chemotherapeutic drugs can be delivered directly to the tumor. This procedure has been used particularly in the treatment of malignant lesions in the liver.

J. **Ultrasonography,** which depends on the reflection of sound waves to create an image rather than ionizing radiation, can visualize the organs of the abdomen with high accuracy by means of modern high-resolution equipment. Ultrasonography usually is less expensive than CT and is better in detecting some conditions, such as gallstones. Stomach or bowel gas may obscure visualization of the organs beneath.

The inclusion of an ultrasound device in the tip of an endoscope **(endoscopic ultrasound)** has produced a sophisticated technique for the examination of the GI tract and adjacent structures (see Chapter 5).

II. RADIONUCLIDE STUDIES

A. **Liver–spleen scan.** When a radiolabeled colloid, such as technetium Tc 99m sulfur colloid, is injected intravenously, it is taken up by the reticuloendothelial system of the liver, spleen, and bone marrow. Normally little, if any, radioactivity is detected over the bone marrow of healthy people because most of the colloid has been "filtered out" through the liver and spleen during the initial passages of the circulation. In moderate-to-advanced liver disease, however, when blood flow through the liver is impaired, relatively more colloid is removed in the spleen and bone marrow. This factor accounts for the increase in density of the spleen and bone marrow that is typical of chronic parenchymal liver disease. The liver–spleen scan can give some estimate of the size and shape of the liver and spleen and can indicate whether mass lesions are present. However, the lower limits of resolution for a mass lesion by radionuclide scan is about 1 to 2 cm, which is poorer than the resolving power of a CT scan—about 0.5 cm.

Indications for liver–spleen scanning have decreased since abdominal CT scanning has come into common usage. The liver–spleen scan is still a reasonable method of estimating the sizes of the liver and the spleen and of determining whether enough chronic liver disease is present to cause a shift of the colloid to the spleen and bone marrow.

B. **HIDA scan.** Technetium Tc 99m—dimethylphenylcarbamylmethyl-iminodiacetic acid (HIDA) is extracted from blood by liver parenchymal cells and excreted into bile. In this respect, it resembles oral cholecystography dye; because of nuclear imaging methods, however, the bile ducts and gallbladder can be visualized when the serum bilirubin is as high as 7 mg/dL. Other, related radiolabeled agents (i.e., PIPP DD) may be used when the serum bilirubin is as high as 10 to 15 mg/dL.

The major use of the HIDA scan is in making the diagnosis of acute cholecystitis. In acute cholecystitis, the gallbladder fails to visualize. HIDA scanning also has been used to implicate common bile duct obstruction when the radiolabel visualizes the bile ducts, but fails to enter the duodenum. However, other methods (e.g., ultrasonography, CT scanning, ERCP) are much more accurate in identifying obstruction of the common duct. Finally, HIDA scanning in conjunction with the injection of cholecystokinin (CCK) has been used as a test of gallbladder function. Some patients with an abdominal pain syndrome, but without gallstones, are believed to suffer from a dysfunctional gallbladder. Injection of CCK normally causes prompt but painless contraction of the gallbladder and relaxation of the sphincter of Oddi. If CCK injection during HIDA scanning causes reproduction of the patient's clinical pain and a delay in gallbladder emptying, it may indicate that gallbladder dysfunction is responsible for the patient's symptoms.

C. **Scans using radiolabeled blood cells and blood components**

   1. Scanning the abdomen after labeling the **red blood cells** or other blood components may indicate the site of bleeding. The rate of blood loss required to be evident by the scan is estimated to be about 0.1 mL per minute, much less than that required for selective arteriography. The value of the radionuclide scan for bleeding is not in making a specific diagnosis, but in suggesting the site of bleeding so that other diagnostic studies can be performed.

   2. Labeling the patient's **white blood cells** has been used in some institutions to help locate abscesses or tissue necrosis. A variant, the intravenous injection of gallium 67, can identify abscesses because of the binding of gallium to white cells. These techniques have been less useful since high-resolution CT scans have been available.

III. MAGNETIC RESONANCE IMAGING (MRI) depends on the magnetic properties of atomic nuclei with unpaired nucleons (i.e., an odd number of protons or neutrons). For clinical purposes, MRI uses the hydrogen atom, or proton. Protons are components of water and, to some extent, fats, which are found in all tissues. The MRI image is generated by placing the protons (tissue) in a strong magnetic field, which aligns them parallel to the magnetic field, and energizing the protons by the application of an appropriate radiowave. As the energized protons return to the former equilibrium state, they emit radiowaves, which are recorded as the MRI signal. The strength of the signal depends on the density of the protons, the blood flow, and the relaxation time constants, which are known as T1 and T2. The advantages of MRI over CT are that MRI uses no ionizing radiation, there is no bone artifact, and contrast agents usually are not required. The sensitivity and specificity of MRI is enhanced by intravenous contrast injection.

MRI has been used most extensively in neurodiagnostics, and its application to gastroenterology has been limited to imaging of the liver to characterize hepatic tumors, iron overload, and hepatic venous and portal venous occlusion. For the evaluation of the other abdominal organs and the retroperitoneum, CT is superior to MRI.

IV. POSITRON EMISSION TOMOGRAPHY (PET) uses positively charged electrons (positrons) that are emitted from natural elements, such as carbon 11, nitrogen 13, oxygen 15, and fluorine 18, to create images. These natural radioisotopes behave normally in the body and can be used to synthesize radiopharmaceuticals for specific purposes. An advantage of PET over CT and MRI is that it is more useful in evaluating organ function. Its clinical application has been largely in the evaluation of primary or metastatic cancer, recurrence, and for detection of cancer after surgery and/or chemoradiation therapy.

Selected Readings

Beebe TJ, et al. Assessing attitudes reward laxative preparation in colorectal cancer screening and effects on future testing: potential receptivity to computed tomographic colonography. *Mayo Clin Proc.* 2007;82:666–671.

Beets-tan R, et al. Preoperative MR imaging of anal fistulas: Does it really help the surgeon? *Radiology.* 2001;218:75.

Gourtsoyiannis NC, et al. Magnetic resonance imaging evaluation of small intestinal Crohn's disease. *Best Pract Res Clin Gastroenterol.* 2006;20:137–156.

Kim DH, et al. CT colonography versus colonoscopy for the detection of advanced neoplasia. *N Surg J Med.* 2007;357:1403–1412.

Klapman, JB, et al. Endoscopic ultrasound-guided fine-needle injection. *Gastrointest Endosc Clin North Am.* 2005;15(1):169–177.

Kochman, ML. EUS in pancreatic cancer. *Gastrointest Endosc.* 2002;56(20064):S6–12.

Lin C, et al. EUS for detection of occult cholelithiasis in patients with idiopathic pancreatitis. *Gastrointest Endosc.* 2000;51:28.

Paulsen SR, et al. CT enterography as a diagnostic tool in evaluation small bowel disorders: Review of clinical experience with over 700 cases. *Radio Graphics.* 2006;26:641–662.

Pickhardt PJ. Colonic preparation for computed tomographic colonography: Understanding the relative advantages of a noncathartic approach. *Mayo Clin Proc.* 2007; 82(6):659–661.

Pickhardt PJ. Screening for colorectal neoplasia with CT colonography: initial experience from the 1st year of coverage by third-party payers. *Radiology.* 2006 Nov;241: 417–425. Epub 2006 Sep 18.

Rockey DC, et al. Analysis of air contrast barium enema, computed tomographic colonography, and colonoscopy: prospective comparison. *Lancet.* 2005;365:305–311.

Shah JN, et al. Clinical impact of endoscopic ultrasonography on the management of malignancies. *Clin Gastroenterol Hepatol.* 2004;2(12):1069–1073.

Valls C, et al. Hepatic metastases from colorectal cancer: Preoperative detection and assessment of resectability with helical CT. *Radiology.* 2001;218:55.

Van Dam J, et al. Endosonography of the upper gastrointestinal tract. *New Engl J Med.* 2000;341:1745.

Nutritional Assessment and Management

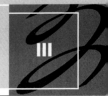

III

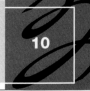
I. METABOLISM

A. Normal energy metabolism. Every day normal adults need roughly 25 to 30 kcal of fuel/kg of body weight. For a 70-kg person, this is about 2,100 kcal per day. A typical American derives 40% to 60% of daily calories from carbohydrates, 20% to 45% from lipids, and 10% to 20% from protein. Glucose is the body's preferred source of immediate energy. The healthy body manufactures glucose from carbohydrates, protein, and the glycerol backbone of triglycerides (TGs). Since very little carbohydrate can be stored in the body, most of the body's reserve energy stores are made up of lipids. There is no storage form of protein. Even though protein can be metabolized for energy, this results in wasting of lean body mass and negative nitrogen balance.

B. Metabolism of carbohydrates

1. **Glucose.** Most of the ingested carbohydrate is broken down to glucose, which enters the circulation. Glucose is taken up by all cells of the body and burned for immediate energy. Under normal, well-fed circumstances, the cells of the central nervous system depend on glucose for energy. However, neurons of the brain cortex and blood cells can use only glucose as fuel under all circumstances.

2. **Glycogen.** Glucose, fructose, and galactose can be converted to glycogen, a polymer of glucose, which is stored mainly in the liver (200 mg) and muscle (300 mg) as a readily available energy reserve. Liver glycogen can be converted directly to glucose for systemic distribution. However, muscle glycogen is burned by muscle itself. Total glycogen stores of the body can meet the body's energy needs for 36 to 48 hours.

   The body protects its glycogen stores for emergencies. At times of temporary glucose insufficiency, the body manufactures glucose by gluconeogenesis, from protein and glycerol of lipids. Also free fatty acids (FFAs) and amino acids are burned for direct energy. Excess dietary carbohydrate is converted to TGs for storage in the adipose tissue.

C. Metabolism of lipids. Lipids constitute the body's main energy reserve. A nonobese, 70-kg man has 12 to 18 kg of fat stores. This figure is somewhat higher for women. Fat supplies 9 kcal/g compared to 4 kcal/g from glucose or protein.

   Ingested lipids are hydrolyzed in the intestinal lumen, and then absorbed into enterocytes of the small intestine, where they are resynthesized into TGs. In the enterocytes, TGs made up of long-chain FFAs form chylomicrons by the addition of apoproteins. Chylomicrons are secreted into the intercellular space and are absorbed into the lymphatics. Short- and medium-chain FFAs are directly absorbed into the portal vein. Lipoprotein lipase of endothelial cells release FFAs from TGs, and FFAs enter cells of various tissues (e.g., heart and muscle), where they are oxidized for energy, and cells of adipose tissue to form TGs for storage. Adipose tissue can also convert carbohydrates and proteins into TGs by lipogenesis.

   Mobilization of TGs for energy by lipolysis begins with the hydrolysis of TGs into FFAs and glycerol. Glycerol may be either converted into glucose by gluconeogenesis or directly oxidized further. FFAs enter some tissue cells, are broken down to acetyl coenzyme A, and oxidized through the Krebs cycle. At times of starvation and lack of glucose as fuel, large quantities of FFAs enter tissue cells. The Krebs cycle may become overloaded, and FFAs may be incompletely oxidized.

Intermediate products in the form of acids and ketone bodies accumulate in the blood, leading to ketosis and acidosis.

D. Metabolism of protein. The body of a 70-kg man contains 10 to 14 kg of protein. Because there is no storage form of protein in the body, the protein compartment must be maintained by daily intake. A typical adult requires about 0.8 to 1.0 g of protein/kg of body weight per day. For a 70-kg man, this is about 65 to 70 g.

Ingested protein may be used for protein synthesis or fuel, especially if the body requires more energy than is supplied by carbohydrate and lipid intake. In this event, body protein may also be catabolized for energy. One third of the body's total protein is potentially available as an energy source in case of dire need. Further protein catabolism, however, severely jeopardizes health.

If protein is ingested in amounts greater than needed for protein synthesis and energy production, it is stripped of its nitrogen and converted to glucose, glycogen, and TGs for storage. Protein, besides being needed for structural purposes, is also needed for replacement, repair, and growth of tissue (cell components) and maintenance of circulating proteins (e.g., albumin, transferrin, coagulation proteins, enzymes, and antibodies).

E. Nitrogen balance. In a healthy adult, ingested protein must supply enough amino acids to maintain a constant level of body protein. Thus, the intake of protein must equal or exceed the breakdown of body protein. The effect of diet on the body's protein compartment may be approximated by nitrogen balance. Nitrogen balance is the difference between nitrogen intake and output.

   1. When protein synthesis is equal to protein degradation, one has a **neutral nitrogen balance.** In adults, this is a sign of health.
   2. Positive nitrogen balance occurs when protein synthesis exceeds protein degradation. This suggests tissue growth. This state is normal and expected in children. In adults, it may mean rebuilding of wasted tissue.
   3. In **negative nitrogen balance,** the protein breakdown is in excess of protein synthesis. This catabolic state usually occurs in sepsis, trauma, and burns, and when the carbohydrate and lipid intake is less than the body's energy needs, necessitating use of the body's own protein for fuel.
   4. Calculation of nitrogen balance. Nitrogen balance can be calculated with reasonable accuracy. Nitrogen makes up 16% of ingested protein. The division of protein intake in grams by 6.25 (the reciprocal of 0.16) will give nitrogen intake. Most of the nitrogen output from the body is into the urine as urea, which can be measured. Other excreted nitrogen is in feces and urine as nonurea nitrogen, amounting to about 4 g per day. The addition of 4 g to the urine nitrogen measured will give the daily nitrogen output. Thus, nitrogen balance can be calculated by subtracting nitrogen output from nitrogen input.

Nitrogen balance = nitrogen in − nitrogen out
          = protein intake − [daily urinary nitrogen + 4 g 6.25
          (for nonurea nitrogen)]

For example, if protein intake is 75 g, urine urea nitrogen is 500% or 5 g/L with 2,000-mL urine output per 24 hours.

Nitrogen balance = 75 g protein
          − [(5 g/L × 2 L) + 4]6.25 g protein/g nitrogen
          = 12 g nitrogen intake − 14 g nitrogen output
          = −22 g per day

F. Energy metabolism in starvation. During periods of starvation, when ingested nutrients are unavailable, the body goes through different stages of metabolic adaptation. Energy requirements are met by metabolism of substrates from the energy reserves, which are drawn on simultaneously, but not equally, following a careful sequence.

   1. For immediate use, the glycogen in the liver is depolymerized to glucose for systemic use. Muscle glycogen is oxidized locally. The lactate produced may be converted to glucose in the liver for systemic use. If used up entirely, the glycogen reserves are depleted in 36 to 48 hours.

2. **In early starvation,** glucose is produced from gluconeogenesis from amino acids, lactate, and glycerol, but within a week the amount available for fuel becomes severely limited. Its use is reserved exclusively for the central nervous system and glycolytic tissues: erythrocytes, leukocytes, and macrophages. Maintenance of this basal glucose production is essential. However, because its main source is amino acids derived from catabolism of the body's own protein, it jeopardizes the body's survival.

3. **After the first few days of starvation,** an adaptive response takes effect. Metabolic rate decreases. FFAs become the main source of energy. The heart, kidneys, and muscle take up and oxidize FFAs directly. Twenty-five percent of the FFA released from the adipose tissue is partially metabolized in the liver to form ketone bodies, which are readily used in peripheral tissues. There is also a recycling of lactate and pyruvate back into glucose by the Cori cycle. These changes decrease the protein requirements to about one third that of the non-adapted state.

4. **In prolonged starvation,** the brain also adapts to the use of ketone bodies for fuel. This further spares glucose and decreases protein breakdown. As the adipose tissue becomes depleted, the body is forced to use its own essential protein for energy, leading to loss of protein from muscle, liver, spleen, kidneys, gastrointestinal tract, and plasma. The heart, adrenals, and central nervous system are initially protected. However, weight loss in excess of 20% to 30% seriously increases mortality due to organ dysfunction, anemia, impaired immunity, ineffective wound healing, and decreased resistance to infection.

In contrast, the catabolic state in sepsis and injury induces an increase in protein requirements. Protein catabolism, as represented by urine urea nitrogen, may increase by 50% in patients with sepsis and may nearly double in those with severe trauma or burns. This increase in protein catabolism occurs without an adequate compensatory increase in protein synthesis. Mediators of this catabolic response include glucocorticoid, catecholamines, glucagon, and perhaps interleukin-1. These substances induce an increase in lipid mobilization and oxidation, skeletal muscle catabolism, and hepatic gluconeogenesis; they also induce a state of insulin resistance. The septic state is highly catabolic, with net catabolism even in the presence of abundant protein and calories.

II. **ASSESSMENT OF NUTRITIONAL STATUS.** Protein–calorie starvation is the progressive loss of lean body mass and adipose tissue because of inadequate intake of amino acids and calories. Anemia, malabsorption, and hypermetabolism are some of the causes of malnutrition in patients with a variety of subacute and chronic illnesses. Protein–calorie malnutrition, which increases morbidity and mortality, can be reversed by appropriate nutritional support by enteral and parenteral routes.

A. **Anthropometric measurements**

1. **Height, weight, triceps skinfold thickness** (for quantitative estimate of adipose tissue stores) and mid–upper arm circumference (for estimate of muscle mass [somatic protein]) are useful data in nutritional assessment. Each actual measurement can be compared to the standards (Tables 10-1–10-3) as follows:

$$\% \text{ standard} = \text{Actual measure/Standard} \times 100$$

2. **Body weight** below 90% of ideal is considered as protein–calorie undernutrition. However, due to pre-illness obesity and presence of edema, body weight may not be subnormal in the malnourished patient.

3. **Creatinine height index.** The most important laboratory test for detecting protein–energy undernutrition is the creatinine height index (CHI). The actual daily urinary creatinine excretion is compared with an ideal value to compute CHI.

Actual urinary creatinine/Ideal urinary creatinine $\times$ 100 = CHI

By expressing this index as a percentage of standards, the severity of the loss of muscle mass can be graded as mild, moderate, severe, or critical (Tables 10-4 and 10-5).

TABLE 10-1	Ideal Weight for Height*

Men					
Height (cm)	Weight (kg)	Height (cm)	Weight (kg)	Height (cm)	Weight (kg)
145	51.9	159	59.9	173	68.7
146	52.4	160	60.5	174	69.4
147	52.9	161	61.1	175	70.1
148	53.5	162	61.7	176	70.8
149	54.0	163	62.3	177	71.6
150	54.5	164	62.9	178	72.4
151	55.0	165	63.5	179	73.3
152	55.6	166	64.0	180	74.2
153	56.1	167	64.6	181	75.0
154	56.6	168	65.2	182	75.8
155	57.2	169	65.9	183	76.5
156	57.9	170	66.6	184	77.3
157	58.6	171	67.3	185	78.1
158	59.3	172	68.0	186	78.9
Women					
140	44.9	150	50.4	160	56.2
141	45.4	151	51.0	161	56.9
142	45.9	152	51.5	162	57.6
143	46.4	153	52.0	163	58.3
144	47.0	154	52.5	164	58.9
145	47.5	155	53.1	165	59.5
146	48.0	156	53.7	166	60.1
147	48.6	157	54.3	167	60.7
148	49.2	158	54.9	168	61.4
149	49.8	159	55.5	169	62.1

*This table corrects the 1959 Metropolitan Standards to nude weight and height without shoe heels.

From Blackburn GL, Bistrian BR, Maini BJ. Nutritional and metabolic assessment of the hospitalized patient. *J Parenter Enteral Nutr.* 1977;1:14. Reprinted with permission from the American Society for Parenteral and Enteral Nutrition.

TABLE 10-2	Arm Circumference—Adults

	Arm circumference (cm)				
Sex	Standard	90% of standard	80% of standard	70% of standard	60% of standard
Male	29.3	26.3	23.4	20.5	17.6
Female	28.5	25.7	22.8	20.0	17.1

From Keenan RA. Assessment of malnutrition using body composition analysis. *Clin Consult Nutr Support.* 1981;1:10. Reprinted with permission.

TABLE 10-3	Triceps Skinfold—Adult

		Triceps skinfold (mm)			
Sex	standard	90% of standard	80% of standard	70% of standard	60% of standard
Male	12.5	11.3	10.0	8.8	7.5
Female	16.5	14.9	13.2	11.6	9.0

From Keenan RA. Assessment of malnutrition using body composition analysis. *Clin Consult Nutr Support.* 1981;1:10. Reprinted with permission.

TABLE 10-4	Ideal Urinary Creatinine Values

Men[a]		Women[b]	
Ideal		Ideal	
Height (cm)	Creatinine (mg)	Height (cm)	Creatinine (mg)
157.5	1288	147.3	830
160.0	1325	149.9	851
162.6	1359	152.4	875
165.1	1386	154.9	900
167.6	1426	157.5	925
170.2	1467	160.0	949
172.7	1513	162.6	977
175.3	1555	165.1	1006
177.8	1596	167.6	1044
180.3	1642	170.2	1076
182.9	1691	172.7	1109
185.4	1739	175.3	1141
188.0	1785	177.8	1174
190.5	1831	180.3	1206
193.0	1891	182.9	1240

[a]Creatinine coefficient (men) = 23 mg/kg of ideal body weight.

[b]Creatinine coefficient (women) = 18 mg/kg of ideal body weight.

From Blackburn GL, Bistrian BR, Maini BJ. Nutritional and metabolic assessment of the hospitalized patient. *J Parenter Enteral Nutr.* 1977;1:15. Reprinted with permission of the American Society for Parenteral and Enteral Nutrition.

4. **Creatinine total arm-length ratio.** The measurement of total arm length is an alternative to height for use in nutritional assessment because of the variability of height in elderly patients. This measurement works equally well in younger patients.

B. **Biochemical data** such as serum albumin, transferrin, total lymphocyte count, delayed hypersensitivity skin response to common antigens, and nitrogen balance are useful indices for visceral protein status. Deficiency of visceral protein levels is found in patients with advanced protein depletion.

The serum albumin concentration may be a simple and reliable measurement for predicting outcome in critically ill patients in the intensive care unit (ICU) setting. In a study from the Mayo Clinic, serum albumin level correlated with the number of ICU days, with the number of days on a ventilator, and with the number of hospital days. It was the only measurement that correlated with the development of both a new infection and ventilator dependency.

C. Rate of nutritional depletion. Not only is the severity of the protein-intake depletion important, but also its rate of progression. Ingestion of less than 30 g per day of protein and less than 1,000 kcal per day means that protein–calorie undernutrition will progress rapidly. Associated fever, infection, trauma, or malabsorption will further accelerate the rate of nutritional depletion. It is important to note that the stress of sepsis induces an obligatory protein loss regardless of the provision of nutrients. Thus, nutritional status in these patients needs to be closely monitored.

III. NUTRITIONAL REQUIREMENTS. The body needs seven groups of nutrients: **carbohydrates, lipids, proteins, vitamins, electrolytes, trace elements,** and **water.** The calorie and energy requirements of healthy individuals vary depending on age, body size, and level of physical activity. Calorie intake should balance energy expenditure to maintain body weight. The energy requirements of seriously ill or injured patients are different than in health and depend on the nature and severity of the illness.

A satisfactory estimate of basal calorie requirement or basic energy expenditure (BEE) can be calculated from the Harris–Benedict equation, which takes into account sex, height, age, and weight (Table 10-5). For most patients, the Harris–Benedict equation provides an adequate estimate of caloric needs. However, in some clinical situations (e.g., impending respiratory failure, active weaning from mechanical ventilation), a more individualized and accurate estimate is needed. Indirect calorimetry is useful in such instances.

Indirect calorimetry is a method of determining caloric expenditure in different metabolic situations. The carbon dioxide and oxygen levels in inspired and expired air are measured and compared. The average of several measurements taken over a 10- to 20-minute period gives a close approximation of caloric expenditure.

Indirect calorimetry also provides the respiratory quotient (RQ), which reflects the number of carbon dioxide molecules produced per molecule of oxygen consumed. The RQ varies, depending on the metabolic substrate. For example, the RQ is 1.0 for pure carbohydrate metabolism, 0.8 for protein, and 0.7 for fat. Because respiratory effort may decrease as carbon dioxide production drops, patients with respiratory distress may benefit from a reduction in carbon dioxide production achieved by lowering the RQ.

Lowering the RQ involves two principles: avoidance of excess calories and substitution of fat for carbohydrate. A common error is to assume that providing additional fat calories will reduce the RQ. On the contrary, excess calories may cause the RQ to increase above 1.0, possibly to as high as 4.0, depending on the amount of excess calories.

TABLE 10-5	Harris–Benedict Equations for Calculation of Basal Energy Expenditure

Women: BEE = 655 + (9.6 × W) + (1.8 × H) − (4.7 × A)   **Men:** BEE = 66 + (13.7 × W) + (5 × H) − (6.8 × A)   Multiply resting energy expenditure value by stress or activity factor (ranging from 1.1 to 1.4) to obtain daily caloric requirements.
BEE, basal energy expenditure; W, actual or usual weight in kilograms; H, height in centimeters; A, age in years.
From Blackburn GL, Bistrian BR, Maini BJ. Nutritional and metabolic assessment of the hospitalized patient. *J Parenter Enteral Nutr.* 1977;1:14. Reprinted with permission of the American Society for Parenteral and Enteral Nutrition.

A. Proper use of indirect calorimetry and the RQ requires recognition of the following factors:

1. Excess calories tend to greatly increase the RQ and production of carbon dioxide.
2. When the RQ is greater than 1.0, total calories should be decreased initially to approximate the caloric requirement; indirect calorimetry may then be repeated.
3. When the RQ is less than 1.0 but greater than 0.85 and further reduction of the RQ is deemed beneficial, fat calories may be substituted for carbohydrate calories; however, simply adding fat calories is counterproductive.
4. Lowering the RQ is beneficial only when respiratory failure is impending or when weaning from mechanical ventilation is difficult. Patients undergoing long-term ventilatory support or who will not undergo weaning for several days do not benefit from high-fat feedings or a reduction in RQ.

B. If **lipid substitution** is desired, a dietitian can be helpful in making appropriate changes in enteral feeding or in adjusting glucose calories and substituting lipid in parenteral feedings. Although lipid substitution can be beneficial, studies have shown that intravenous administration of lipid has potentially adverse effects. Despite these reports, intravenous lipid feedings of 50 g per day or less have no definitive adverse effects. This amount is present in a standard 500-mL unit of 10% intravenous lipid and provides 450 kcal.

IV. GUIDELINES FOR NUTRITIONAL SUPPORT
A. Calorie and protein requirements

1. **Well-nourished patients without sepsis or injury.** Nutritional support is not needed for short-term problems. If normal eating is likely to resume within 5 days, no specialized feeding should be initiated. The risks of nutritional support outweigh any potential benefit. During observation or diagnostic testing, providing water and electrolytes is sufficient.
2. In **nondepleted, postoperative patients,** the goal of nutrition is to prevent loss of body protein. If the patient is unable to eat after surgery, the patient should be given 20% more calories than the BEE indicates ($1.2 - 1.5 \times$ BEE), which will provide about 35 to 40 kcal/kg of body weight. In addition, 0.8 to 1.0 g of protein per kg of body weight is required.
3. **Malnourished patients** without sepsis or injury. In this state of simple starvation, protein and caloric requirements are reduced. Increased nutrient intake is necessary for repletion, but caution is needed to avoid the refeeding syndrome.
4. **Refeeding syndrome.** Patients who are malnourished, commonly because of alcoholism or chronic insufficient protein and caloric intake, are at risk for the refeeding syndrome. When these patients receive carbohydrate or protein, the activation of anabolic enzymes and pathways may rapidly deplete the available cofactors. Profound hypophosphatemia and hypomagnesemia may occur, requiring prompt repletion. Daily assessment of serum phosphate, calcium, magnesium, and other electrolytes during the first few days of feeding and provision of adequate but not excessive calories should prevent the potentially dire consequences of the refeeding syndrome.
5. In **nutritionally depleted patients,** the protein intake should correspond to 1.5 to 1.8 g/kg of body weight, and the amount of calories should be 50% above the estimated BEE, or about 40 to 50 kcal/kg of actual body weight.
6. In **hypermetabolic patients,** the goal is to provide 2 g of protein per kilogram of body weight and a total energy intake of twice the BEE, about 50 kcal/kg of body weight.
7. **Well-nourished or malnourished patients** with sepsis or injury. An altered metabolic state exists initially and is characterized by hypermetabolism, increased endogenous protein breakdown, and a tendency for lipid oxidation and insulin resistance. Unless adequate calories and protein are provided, profound muscle catabolism and weight loss may result. Well-nourished patients may do well without feeding for a few days, but malnourished patients should receive prompt, consistent nutritional support.

8. **Calorie and nitrogen sources.** Calorie sources used in nutritional support regimens are carbohydrate solutions and lipid emulsions. Intact proteins, peptides, or crystalline amino acid solutions are used as nitrogen sources.

9. **Essential amino acids.** In addition to the general requirement for protein, the body needs the daily intake of essential amino acids, which the body cannot synthesize. These are leucine, isoleucine, lysine, methionine, phenylalanine, threonine, tryptophan, and valine. Histidine, arginine, and glutamine are considered essential in infants and possibly for healing in adults.

Glutamine is an amino acid synthesized in most body tissue. However, in catabolic states in critical illness, it may become an essential amino acid. It functions as a nitrogen transporter, a glycogenic precursor, and a high-energy source. Oxidation of glutamine yields 30 molecules of adenosine triphosphate (ATP). It is an important fuel for replicating cells (such as cells involved in immunity and gastrointestinal mucosal cells) and contributes considerably to gut growth. During catabolic states, glutamine and alanine are released in large quantities

| TABLE 10-6 | Recommended Daily Allowances of Essential Nutrients for Healthy Adults |

Nutrient	Recommended daily allowance
Water	1 mL/cal
Energy	1,800–2,500 kcal
Protein	45–56 g
Linoleic acid	4–6 g
Vitamin A	2,640–3,000 IU
Vitamin D	200 IU
Vitamin E	8–10 IU
Vitamin K	0.5–1.0 mg/kg
Ascorbic acid	60 mg
Folic acid	400 µg
Niacin	6.6 mg/1,000 kcal
Riboflavin	1.2–1.6 mg
Thiamine	0.5 mg/1,000 kcal
Vitamin B_6 (pyridoxine)	2.2 mg
Vitamin B_{12}	3.0 mg
Pantothenic acid	5–10 mg
Biotin	100–200 mg
Calcium	800 mg
Phosphorus	800 mg
Iodine	100–130 µg
Iron	10–18 mg
Magnesium	300–350 mg
Zinc	15 mg
Copper	2 mg
Potassium	2,500 mg[a]
Sodium	2,500 mg[a]
Chloride	2,000 mg[a]
Chromium	50–120 µg[a]
Manganese	6–8 mg[a]
Molybdenum	400 µg[a]
Selenium	50–100 µg[a]

[a]Recommended daily allowance not established. Values are those provided in a normal diet.

Adapted from Food and Nutrition Board, Recommended Daily Allowances. Washington, D.C., 1974; National Academy of Sciences, National Research Council.

from muscle, taken up by the splanchnic bed, and delivered to the gut and liver. In the gut, glutamine is converted to glutamate and enters the Krebs cycle. The liver metabolizes it to glucose, ketones, and ammonia. Glutamine supplementation of external and parenteral solutions seems to improve gut mass function and limit bacterial translocation from the gut to the circulation in critically ill patients.

B. Fluid and electrolytes. The fluid and electrolyte requirements of individuals vary depending on the disease process. Therapy should be tailored to the patient's individual needs and requirements based on appropriate clinical and laboratory evaluations. In general, the patient should receive maintenance requirements of water and electrolytes. Previous and ongoing losses should be replaced with attention to the patient's cardiopulmonary and renal status. A convenient method for **calculating maintenance fluid requirements** is as follows:

1. First 10 kg of body weight = 1,000 mL.
2. Next 10 kg of body weight = 500 mL.
3. Each kilogram of body weight thereafter = 20 mL.

C. Vitamins and trace elements serve as parts of enzymes or coenzymes and are needed by the body in small quantities each day. These should be included in the patient's daily diet (Table 10-6).

Selected Readings

Banh L. Serum Proteins as Markers of Nutrition: What are we treating? *Practical Gastroenterol.* 2006;xxx(10):46.

Heller AR, et al. Omega-3 fatty acids improve the diagnosis–related clinical outcome. *Crit Care Med.* 2006;34:972–979.

Heyland DK, et al. Antioxidant nutrients: a systematic review of trace elements and vitamins in the critically ill patient. *Intensive Care Med.* 2005;31:327–337.

Holick MF, et al. Vitamin D deficiency. *N Eng. J Med.* 2007;357:266–281.

Krystofiak C. Gastrointestinal Disease. In *The A.S.P.E.N. Nutrition Support Core Curriculum: A Case-Based Approach—The Adult Patient.* Edited by Gottschlich MM. Silver Spring, MD: American Society for Parenteral and Enteral Nutrition; 2007:163–186.

Ockenga J, et al. Glutamine-enriched total parenteral nutrition in patients with inflammatory bowel disease. *Eur J Clin Nutr.* 2005;59:1302–1309.

Wooley JA, et al. In *Nutrition Support Core Curriculum*, edn 2. Edited by Gottschlich MM. Silver Spring, MD: ASPEN; 2007:19–32.

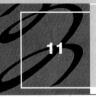

11 ENTERAL NUTRITION

I. PATIENT SELECTION. Patients with established protein–calorie malnutrition or those whose condition will result in protein–calorie undernutrition are candidates for nutritional support. The enteral route should be preferred in any patient with a functional gastrointestinal (GI) tract over the parenteral routes because of its relative simplicity, safety, and economy. Some indications for the use of enteral hyperalimentation are listed in Table 11-1. Enteral feeding is contraindicated in patients with severely compromised GI function, where access to the GI tract is not feasible, and in patients with severe vomiting, intestinal obstruction, ileus, or GI bleeding.

Nutritional support by the enteral route is not a single entity. It encompasses a wide range of techniques and products for use in the clinical spectrum of undernutrition. At one extreme, it may be the addition of a nutritional supplement to the patient's orally consumed diet; at the other extreme, it may provide the patient with the complete nutritional requirements. In some cases, a satisfactory level of nutritional support may not be achievable by the enteral route alone, and combination of this method with parenteral intravenous alimentation may be necessary.

II. ENTERAL FORMULAS. Three types of enteral mixtures differing in osmolality, digestibility, caloric density, lactose content, fat content, and cost (Table 11-2) are available: formulas with intact nutrients, formulas with predigested nutrients (elemental diets), and feeding modules.

A. Formulas with intact nutrients

1. Blenderized feedings are equivalent to a meat-based meal that has been prepared in a blender. They are nutritionally complete if sufficient calories are given and generally provide 1 kcal/mL. However, they tend to be viscous and do not flow well in the newer, narrower, soft feeding tubes, and most contain lactose.

TABLE 11-1	**Some Indications for the Use of Enteral Nutritional Support**

Anorexia	Major burns
Malabsorption syndromes	Severe trauma
Chronic malnutrition	Multiple fractures
Gastrointestinal tract fistulas (low)	Head and neck surgery
Partial obstruction of the gastrointestinal tract	Anorexia nervosa
Ulcerative colitis	Hepatic failure
Crohn's disease	Renal failure
Bowel irradiation	Prolonged ventilatory support
Pancreatic disease	Cerebrovascular accident
Short-bowel syndrome	Prolonged coma
Presurgical nutritional replenishment	Neurologic trauma
Postoperative nutritional support	Organic brain syndrome
Inflammatory bowel disease	Sepsis
Carcinoma	Multiple organ system failure

TABLE 11-2 Selected Enteral Nutritional Supplements

Product description	Calories	mOsm/kg	Protein g/L (%)	Nitrogen content g/L (%)	CHO g/L (%)	Fat g/L (%)	% MCT	Volume to meet 100% for USRDA vitamins & minerals	Source
Lactose-free formulas with intact nutrients									
Isocal	1/mL	300	34 (13)	5	133 (50)	44.3 (37)	20	1,877	Mead Johnson
Precision Isotonic	1/mL	300	7.5	5	37.5 (60)	7.8 (28)	28	1,800	Doyle
Osmolite	1/mL	300	37	6	145 (55)	38.4 (31.5)	50	2,000	Ross
Enrich (with fiber)	1.1/mL	300	40	—	162 (52)	37.1 (30)	—	—	Ross
Jevity (with fiber)	1/mL	310	44.3	—	151.4	36.7	—	—	Ross
Precision (low residue)	1.1/mL	530	26 (9.5)	4	248 (89)	1.6 (1.3)	—	1,710	Sandoz
Meritine	1/mL	600	(24)	10	(46)	(30)	—	—	Ross
Ensure	1/mL	450	37 (14)	6	145 (55)	37 (31.5)	—	1,391	Ross
Ensure Plus HN	1.5/mL	600	(17)	9	(53)	(30)	—	—	Ross
Sustacal	1/mL	625	(24)	10	(55)	(21)	—	—	Mead Johnson
Magnacal	2/mL	590	(27)	11	(50)	(23)	—	—	Organon

(continued)

TABLE 11-2 Continued

Product description	Calories	mOsm/kg	Protein g/L (%)	Nitrogen content g/L (%)	CHO g/L (%)	Fat g/L (%)	% MCT	Volume to meet 100% for USRDA vitamins & minerals	Source
Elemental									
Vivonex TEN	1/mL	630	38 (15) (30% branched-chain AA)	7	206 (82)	2.8 (2.5)	—	2,000	Norwich Eaton
Travasorb HN	1/mL	560	45 (18)	7	175 (70)	13.5 (12)	60	2,000	Travenol
Criticare HN	1/mL	650	38 (14)	6	222 (83)	3.4 (3)	—	1,900	Mead Johnson
Vital HN	1/mL	500	42 (18)	7	185 (78)	10.8 (5)	—	—	Ross
Modular									
Casec	3.7/g		(95)	(5)	—	—	—	—	Mead Johnson
Propack	4/g		(76)	(18)	(6)	—	—	—	Sherwood Medical
Polycose	3.8/g		—	—	(100)	—	—	—	Ross
SLD	3.65/g		20.4	(0.3)	(74.2)	—	—	1,022	Ross
MCT	9.0/g		—	100	—	—	100	—	Ross

CHO, carbohydrates; MCT, medium–chain triglycerides; USRDA, United States Recommended Daily Allowance; AA, amino acids; HN, high nitrogen; TEN, total enteral nutrition.

2. **Lactose-free feedings (1 kcal/mL).** These products have become the standard tube-feeding preparations. They are prepared from isolated nutrients rather than whole foods. They consist of polymeric mixtures of proteins, fats, and carbohydrates in high-molecular form. Thus, they are lower in osmolality (300–350 osm/L isotonic to plasma) than are formulas supplying equivalent amounts of calories in lower molecular weight substrates. Since these mixtures are prepared from undigested nutrients, patients who are receiving them must have intact digestive and absorptive capabilities. They are nutritionally complete if sufficient calories are given. Their sodium, potassium, lactose, and residue contents are low. Essential fatty acid insufficiency is not a problem. With these products, 30% to 40% of the calories are provided as fat, 50% to 70% as carbohydrate, and 3% to 10% as protein. Because these formulas are unflavored and generally taste like chalk, they are recommended for tube feeding only, not for oral intake. Two new enteral formulas are available that contain soy polysaccharide as a fiber source (Jevity and Enrich). These formulations may help decrease the incidence of diarrhea in tube-fed patients.

3. **Nutrient-dense feedings.** These formulas are virtually identical in composition to 1 kcal/mL products except that they are more concentrated and have high osmolality. They are nutritionally complete and provide 1.5 to 2.0 kcal/mL. They are also more flavorful and may be used as oral feedings and supplements.

B. **Formulas with predigested nutrients (elemental diets)**

1. **Nutritionally complete feedings.** These formulas are prepared from amino acids or small peptides, simple glucose polymers (oligosaccharides) rather than complex carbohydrates (polysaccharides), medium-chain triglycerides, and minimal amounts of fat. They are hypertonic and uniformly unpalatable. Elemental diets, because of their simple nutrients that do not require digestion, have been recommended for use in patients with digestive or absorptive abnormalities, such as patients with short-bowel syndrome, low intestinal fistulas, inflammatory bowel disease, acute and chronic pancreatitis, and malabsorptive states. Recent research has shown that di- and tripeptides are more readily absorbed than single amino acids by the normal or inflamed intestine. Digestion of fats containing long-chain triglycerides requires pancreatic lipase for hydrolysis, bile salts for water solubility, and an intact lymphatic system for intestinal absorption. Medium-chain triglycerides do not require pancreatic lipase, bile salts, or lymphatics because they are hydrolyzed by intestinal cell lipase and absorbed directly into the portal venous system.

   The use of oligosaccharides rather than polysaccharides as well as crystalline amino acids and small peptides increases the osmotic load of these formulas. Hypertonic solutions tend to induce osmotic diarrhea, leading to dehydration and serum electrolyte abnormalities. The high simple-sugar content increases the risk of hyperglycemia and hyperosmolar state, especially in patients with glucose intolerance (overt or latent). Essential fatty acid deficiency may result with prolonged use of some formulas with low long free fatty acid content. In such cases, essential fatty acids and linoleic and linolenic acids should be supplied by another source and means.

   These "elemental" formulas should be restricted to use in patients showing definite evidence of maldigestion and malabsorption.

2. **Disease-specific feedings.** Some formulas are designed for use in patients with renal failure, respiratory insufficiency, or hepatic encephalopathy. They are formulated with amino acid mixtures that are intended to modify the metabolic abnormalities associated with these disease states. Some of these formulas are nutritionally incomplete and should not be used alone for nutritional support. Thus, whenever possible, standard formulations are preferable.

   a. **Renal formulations (e.g., amino-acid)** are a mixture of carbohydrates, fats, and essential amino acids with a minimal amount of electrolytes. Theoretically, the body can convert the carbohydrate precursors of nonessential amino acids to the actual amino acids by recycling urea nitrogen, thus slowing down the rate of rise of blood urea nitrogen.

> **b. Hepatic formulas (e.g., Hepatic-Acid)** are enriched with branched-chain amino acids and are low in aromatic amino acids and methionine. It has been postulated that alterations in amino acid balance may contribute to the abnormal central nervous system function in patients with hepatic encephalopathy.
>
> **c. In patients with diabetes mellitus,** selection of a product low in simple sugars and with up to 50% of total calories in complex carbohydrates will keep insulin needs in moderation.
>
> **d. In patients with respiratory disease** with carbon dioxide retention, a formula with high-fat content (respiratory quotient [carbon dioxide produced/oxygen consumed] = 0.7 for fats vs. 1.0 for carbohydrate) is preferred. The complete oxidation of fat produces less carbon dioxide on a per-calorie basis than does the complete oxidation of either glucose or protein. Replacing carbohydrate calories with fat calories has been shown to reduce carbon dioxide production, oxygen consumption, and minute ventilation. These effects may aid in weaning patients from ventilatory support; however, high-fat enteral diets tend to produce diarrhea in some patients. Thus, initially, a 30% fat polymeric diet may be used; if tolerated, then the fat content may be raised to 50% of the total calories. In intolerant patients, enteral formulas may be supplemented with parenteral fat emulsion infusions.

C. Feeding modules are concentrated sources of one nutrient (e.g., fat: Lipomul, MCT Oil; carbohydrate: Polycose; and protein: Pro-Mix). These modules can be added to formula diets to increase specific components that are deficient or to yield a small-volume, high-calorie mixture (1.5–2.0 kcal/mL) for patients in whom fluids should be restricted.

III. CALORIC REQUIREMENTS

A. Using the Harris-Benedict equation (see Chapter 10, Table 10-6):
   1. The *enteral maintenance requirement* = 1.2 × basic energy requirements (BEE)
   2. The *enteral anabolic requirement* = 1.5 × BEE
   3. The energy in kilocalories, the nitrogen content, and the protein content of each enteral feeding formula per milliliter is given in the contents table of the product provided by the manufacturer. Once the number of kilocalories and the required amount of protein per day are determined, the number of milliliters per day that will yield these amounts can be calculated.

IV. METHODS OF ADMINISTRATION

A. Feeding tubes. Feeding tubes (e.g., Keofeed or Dobbhoff tubes) made of silicone or polyurethane plastics have several advantages over the polyvinyl plastic nasogastric tubes. They are thinner and more flexible and do not stiffen or become brittle in the GI tract. Many of these are weighted at the tip, serving as an anchor or as a leading end for easier passage of the tube.
   1. **Nasogastric feeding** uses the stomach as a reservoir and the pylorus to control the entry of the feedings into the intestine, diminishing the risk for diarrhea from osmotic causes and malabsorption.
   2. **Nasoduodenal tubes** offer more protection for the patient against aspiration than do nasogastric tubes because of the presence of the pylorus acting as another sphincter between the area of the tube feeding and the lungs.
   3. **Surgical placement of feeding tubes** may be indicated in some patients who require long-term enteral nutritional support. Most commonly, gastrostomy, jejunostomy, or needle–catheter jejunostomy is used.
   4. **Percutaneous endoscopic gastrostomy (PEG)** provides a less invasive alternative to laparotomy for placement of a gastrostomy tube. These tubes may be converted to jejunostomy tubes in selected patients.

   Prolonged use (>1 month) of nasogastric or nasoduodenal tube feedings is inconvenient, necessitating frequent changes of tubes, and may result in gastric and esophageal injury due to mechanical trauma from the tube.

The same nutrient formulas may be used with PEG tubes as with nasogastric or nasoduodenal tubes.

B. Types of infusion

1. **Continuous drip infusion** is the method of choice in initiating tube feedings; a defined amount is given continuously every hour with the use of an infusion pump. Although large volumes may be administered over 24 hours, the amount entering the GI tract at any given time is quite small. This method minimizes the potential for aspiration, abdominal distention, and diarrhea.

   a. **For most patients,** tube feedings are started at 50 mL/hour using a lactose-free, 1 kcal/mL formula with intact nutrients. Thereafter, the rate is increased by increments of 25 mL/hour daily until the desired rate is achieved.

   b. If a **nutrient-dense or elemental formula** is used, the initial starting dilution should be at least isotonic to plasma. Hypotonic and isotonic solutions behave almost identically in terms of small intestinal flux of fluid, and thus there is no advantage to overdiluting a feeding product.

   c. When **feeding into the small bowel,** isotonic solutions (3,000 mOsm) are started at a continuous rate of 25 to 50 mL/hour every 8 hours until the needed volume is reached. Osmolarity is then increased until the patient's nutrient requirements are reached.

   d. **Patient position.** The patient's head and shoulders must be kept at a 30- to 45-degree elevation to minimize the risk of aspiration.

2. The **"cyclic" method of drip infusion** may be used once a patient has been stabilized on maintenance therapy to provide the patient "flat-in-bed" time by increasing the rate of infusion per hour during the day and stopping the infusion at night, thus still delivering the same volume of nutrients to the patient over the 24 hours. The patient's head and shoulders must be elevated during feeding and 1 hour after the feeding has been stopped to ensure that gastric emptying has occurred. Gastric residuals must be measured 2 to 3 hours after the feeding is stopped.

V. COMPLICATIONS

A. Mechanical complications

1. **Tube clogging.** Viscous preparations may obstruct the lumen of the feeding tube. This can be prevented by flushing the tube every 4 to 8 hours with 20 mL of water or cranberry juice.

2. **Pharyngeal irritation** and esophageal erosion are rare with the softer tubes.

3. **Tracheoesophageal fistula** may occur in patients with endotracheal or tracheostomy tubes receiving mechanical ventilation.

4. **Aspiration** is the most serious problem with tube feedings. It may be minimized by placement of the tube well beyond the pylorus into the duodenum, by keeping the gastric volumes less than 100 mL, and by elevation of the patient's head and shoulders at 30 to 45 degrees while the patient is being fed.

B. Gastrointestinal complications. Patients may have nausea, vomiting, crampy abdominal pain, distention, flatulence, bloating, and diarrhea.

It is not unusual for tube-fed patients to have no bowel movements for 3 to 5 days because most commercial formulas are low in residue. Likewise, it is not unusual for patients to have loose stools. As long as the volume of the stools is not large, this may be tolerated. Diarrhea can result from gut atrophy, osmotic overload, malabsorption, lactose intolerance, concurrent medications (e.g., antibiotics, nonsteroidal antiinflammatory drugs, and magnesium-containing antacids), additives, or vehicles added to medications and fecal impaction with the liquid feces escaping around the impaction.

Starting patients on slow, continuous infusion of tube feeding without lactose, with gradual increase in concentration and rate of delivery, or the use of formulas with fiber, minimizes this problem. If diarrhea continues, DTO (deodorized tincture of opium) may be added to the tube feedings with care that ileus does not develop.

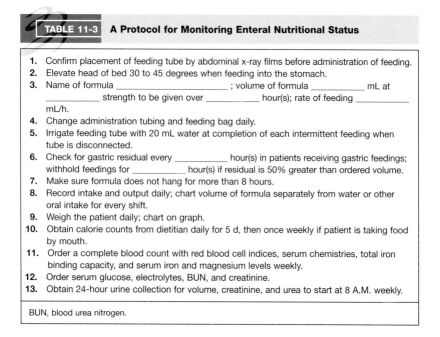

TABLE 11-3 **A Protocol for Monitoring Enteral Nutritional Status**

1. Confirm placement of feeding tube by abdominal x-ray films before administration of feeding.
2. Elevate head of bed 30 to 45 degrees when feeding into the stomach.
3. Name of formula _____ ; volume of formula _____ mL at _____ strength to be given over _____ hour(s); rate of feeding _____ mL/h.
4. Change administration tubing and feeding bag daily.
5. Irrigate feeding tube with 20 mL water at completion of each intermittent feeding when tube is disconnected.
6. Check for gastric residual every _____ hour(s) in patients receiving gastric feedings; withhold feedings for _____ hour(s) if residual is 50% greater than ordered volume.
7. Make sure formula does not hang for more than 8 hours.
8. Record intake and output daily; chart volume of formula separately from water or other oral intake for every shift.
9. Weigh the patient daily; chart on graph.
10. Obtain calorie counts from dietitian daily for 5 d, then once weekly if patient is taking food by mouth.
11. Order a complete blood count with red blood cell indices, serum chemistries, total iron binding capacity, and serum iron and magnesium levels weekly.
12. Order serum glucose, electrolytes, BUN, and creatinine.
13. Obtain 24-hour urine collection for volume, creatinine, and urea to start at 8 A.M. weekly.

BUN, blood urea nitrogen.

C. Metabolic complications. Fluid and electrolyte imbalances may occur, especially in compromised patients. Patients may also develop edema, hyperglycemia, hyperammonemia, azotemia, and essential fatty acid deficiency. Thus, strict monitoring of patients is mandatory.

VI. MONITORING OF PATIENTS ON TUBE FEEDINGS. Patients on tube feedings should be continuously monitored for mechanical aspects of the feeding: patient position, tube position and patency, and gastric residual. In addition, the patient's daily weight, serum electrolytes, chemistries, nitrogen balance, nutritional status, and progress need close attention by both the physicians and the paramedical staff caring for the patient. A monitoring protocol (Table 11-3) helps ensure that the specified nutritional goals are met.

Selected Readings
Bruder EA, et al. Colonmetric carbon dioxide detection of enteral feeding tube placement. *US Gastroenterol Rev.* 2007;1:17–19.

DeLegge MH, et al. Randomized prospective comparison of direct percutaneous endoscopic jejunostomy (DPEJ) vs. percutaneous endoscopic gastrostomy with jejunal extension (PEG-J) feeding tube placement for enteral feeding. *Gastrointest Endosc.* 2004;59:I58(A).

DeLegge MH. Endoscopic options for enteral feeding. *Gastroenterol Hepatol.* 2007;3(9):690–692.

Guidelines for the use of parenteral and enteral nutrition in adult and pediatric patients. *J Parenter Enteral Nutr.* 2002;26:1–138.

Ho KM, et al. A comparison of early gastric and post pyloric feeding in critically ill patients: a meta-analysis. *Intensive Care Med.* 2006;32:639–649.

Javid PJ, et al. The role of enteral nutrition in the reversal of parenteral nutrition-associated liver dysfunction in infants. *J Pediatr Surg.* 2005;40:1015–1018.

Marin M, et al. Enteral formulations. In: Merritt R, ed. *The ASPEN Nutrition Support Practice Manual.* 2nd ed. Silver Spring, Md.: American Society for Parenteral & Enteral Nutrition; 2005:63–75.

Mizock BA. Risk of aspiration in patients on enteral nutrition: frequency, relevance, relation of pneumonia, risk factors, and strategies for risk reduction. *Curr Gastroenterol Rep.* 2007;9(4):338–344.

Uklej A. Gastric versus post-pyloric feeding: relationship to tolerance, pneumonia risk, and successful delivery of enteral nutrition. *Curr Gastroenterol Rep.* 2007;9(4):309–316.

Zhou M, et al. Immune-modulating enteral formulations: optimum components, appropriate patients, and controversial use of arginine in sepsis. *Curr Gastroenterol Rev.* 2007;9(4):329–337.

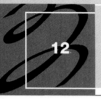

12 PARENTERAL NUTRITION

I. DEFINITION. Parenteral nutrition (PN) is defined as the administration of nutrients directly into the venous system. PN can be given peripherally into the veins of the arm or centrally into the subclavian or internal jugular vein or vena cava.

The decision to use peripheral parenteral nutrition (PPN) rather than central or total parenteral nutrition (CPN or TPN, respectively) is based on the number of calories to be given as well as the duration of the nutritional support. Concentrated solutions of carbohydrates (CHOs) and amino acids (AAs) providing a large number of calories are hypertonic and cannot be given into the peripheral veins. Due to their small size and relatively low blood flow, peripheral veins are irritated by hypertonic solutions and tend to develop thrombophlebitis. In the larger central veins, the hypertonic solutions are quickly diluted by the rapid blood flow, decreasing the risk of inflammation and venous thrombosis. Both forms of PN can be used in conjunction with enteral feedings.

II. INDICATIONS. PN should be considered in any patient who cannot ingest or absorb sufficient calories through the gastrointestinal tract. Table 12-1 lists some of the disease categories with indications for PN.

III. CENTRAL OR TOTAL PARENTERAL NUTRITION
   A. Administration. PN is rather complex. To be practiced successfully and safely, it should be administered by a trained TPN team using a strict protocol. An effective TPN team consists of a physician, nutritionist, pharmacist, and nurse.
   B. Placement of the central venous catheter
      1. Percutaneous subclavian or internal jugular catheter is used for short-term therapy. The placement of the central line should be done by an experienced physician using standard protocol.
      2. Hickman and/or Groshong-Broviac soft catheters for long-term therapy (>1 month) are silicone (Silastic) catheters with single- or double-lumen tubing and externally needled Luer-Lok caps, which are inserted by an experienced physician under fluoroscopy. They are tunneled and anchored subcutaneously with a polyester (Dacron) cuff.
   C. Mechanical complications of central catheterization. Each of the following complications should be expected and handled expediently by the TPN team:
      1. Pneumothorax
      2. Hemothorax, hydrothorax, or chylothorax
      3. Pericardial effusion with tamponade
      4. Arterial puncture
      5. Brachial plexus injury
      6. Catheter embolism
      7. Air embolism
      8. Venous thrombosis and thrombophlebitis
   D. Catheter care. Patients receiving TPN often have an increased risk of infection. The predisposing factors include malnutrition, immune incompetence, steroid treatment or chemotherapy, concomitant infections, broad-spectrum antibiotic therapy, and presence of a foreign body (the catheter) in the vascular system. TPN-related infection may result from contamination of the catheter by skin flora, contamination of the TPN solution or tubing, or bacteremia originating from another source in the body.

TABLE 12-1	Indications for Parenteral Nutrition

Gastrointestinal disease
  Inflammatory bowel disease
  Radiation enteritis
  Short-bowel syndrome
  Severe malabsorption state
  Intestinal fistula
  Pancreatitis
  Diverticulitis
  Intestinal obstruction
Preoperative preparation of malnourished patients
  Carcinoma of the head and neck
  Esophageal stricture or carcinoma
  Tracheoseophageal fistula
  Gastric outlet obstruction
  Severe peptic ulcer disease
  Inflammatory bowel disease
Postoperative surgical complications
  Paralytic ileus
  Gastrointestinal tract fistula
  Enterocutaneous fistula
  Pancreatic or biliary fistula
Miscellaneous
  Extensive burns or trauma
  Cancer patients receiving radiation or chemotherapy
  Anorexia nervosa
  Some forms of liver disease
  Renal failure

Most pathogens responsible for infected catheters originate from superficial sites such as tracheostomies or abdominal wounds. The most common organisms associated with catheter infections are: *Staphylococcus epidermidis, Staphylococcus aureus, Klebsiella pneumoniae,* and *Candida albicans.*

A specific procedure using aseptic technique must be followed in the care of the catheter and dressing. The catheter should be used exclusively for TPN and not for any other purpose (e.g., blood drawing; central venous pressure measurement; administration of drugs, antibiotics, or blood products).

E. Caloric requirements. Nutritional support regimens are usually based on estimates of energy expenditure. These estimates were thought to be increased substantially in patients with severe trauma or sepsis because of a presumed hypermetabolic state. However, using actual energy expenditure measurements, a large increase in the metabolic rate has not been seen in stressed patients. Excessive caloric intake can produce complications such as hepatomegaly and liver dysfunction due to fatty infiltration of the liver, respiratory insufficiency due to excessive carbon dioxide production during increased lipogenesis, and hyperglycemia with osmotic diuresis due to glucose intolerance.

   1. A patient's energy requirements depend on a number of factors, including age, sex, height, and degree of hypermetabolism. Resting energy expenditure (REE) may be measured using the principles of indirect calorimetry from measurements of carbon dioxide production and oxygen consumption. If metabolic nutritional analysis is not available, it is possible to estimate the basal energy expenditure (BEE) using the Harris–Benedict equation.

2. The **Harris–Benedict equation** offers a reasonable estimate of energy expenditure but generally overestimates at smaller body sizes and smaller body energy expenditures (W = weight in kilograms, H = height in centimeters, A = age in years).

    a. Men. BEE = 66 + (13.7 × W) + (5 × H) − (6.8 × A)

    b. Women. BEE = 655 + (9.6 × W) + (1.7 × H) − (4.7 × A)

3. Most studies now suggest that a 12% to 40% increase over estimated BEE is an appropriate adjustment for **septic or injured or critically ill patients** requiring mechanical ventilation. One must increase the BEE by an additional 15% to account for the calories required for utilization of TPN.

4. **In summary,** if a patient is not stressed by sepsis or trauma, a 15% increase in BEE is needed to provide the energy necessary to utilize the nutrients provided by TPN. If the patient requires mechanical ventilation, a 20% to 25% increase in BEE is needed, and if the patient has evidence of hypermetabolism from sepsis or injury, an increase of 30% to 40% in BEE may be required.

F. **Protein and nitrogen requirements.** The healthy individual needs 0.8 g of protein per kilogram of ideal body weight. Needs may increase up to 2.5 g/kg because of stress. To replace protein lost because of stress or to promote anabolism, 1.2 to 1.5 g/kg is frequently used.

    Another common way of estimating protein needs is to use the nonprotein calorie-to-nitrogen ratio. The ratios of 100 to 150 kcal:1 g of nitrogen in stressful conditions to promote anabolism and 250 to 300 kcal:1 g of nitrogen for normal body maintenance are often used. The nonprotein calorie-to-nitrogen ratio is based on the premise that sufficient calories must be ingested before protein will be used for tissue maintenance and repair, that is, 100 to 150 kcal is needed to lay down 1 g of nitrogen.

$$\text{Ideal calorie–nitrogen ratio} = 150{:}1$$
$$\text{Protein (gm)}/150 = 6.25 \times \text{energy requirement in kilocalories}$$
$$1 \text{ g of nitrogen} = 6.25 \text{ g of protein}$$

    AAs are administered as a substrate for anabolism rather than as an energy substrate except in patients with burns or severe sepsis who cannot utilize lipid or glucose effectively and require AA as a substrate for both energy and anabolism.

    AA solutions containing a higher concentration of the branched-chain AAs (BCAA), leucine, isoleucine, and valine, may be metabolized more effectively in patients with hypercatabolic states, such as sepsis and trauma. In some studies, it was noted that septic or injured patients treated with BCAA rather than a conventional AA solution had more rapid improvements in nitrogen balance, total lymphocyte count, and delayed hypersensitivity. Because BCAA solutions require a hypermetabolic state to exert their beneficial effects, they should not be used routinely.

G. **Nutrient sources.** Balanced intake of seven groups of nutrients is needed daily. These are CHOs, lipids, proteins, electrolytes, trace elements, and water. These are ordered by the physician daily.

    Glucose solutions and lipid emulsions are calorie sources (energy substrate) used in PN except in patients with burns or severe sepsis who are unable to utilize lipid or glucose effectively. In these patients AAs, preferably BCAAs, are used as both an energy source and a substrate for anabolism. If glucose is used as the exclusive energy substrate in TPN solutions, carbon dioxide production increases markedly with increased glucose loading (>40 kcal/kg per day) because there is increased lipogenesis (net fat synthesis) relative to glucose oxidation. In addition to increased carbon dioxide production, resulting in an increase of the respiratory quotient above 1, there is also an increase in oxygen consumption because fat synthesis requires energy. Therefore, large amounts of glucose may constitute a metabolic stress and cause carbon dioxide retention where respiratory function is impaired. Using lipids plus glucose, instead of isocaloric amounts of glucose alone, decreases the respiratory workload in patients with compromised pulmonary function. Fat is the favored energy source in sepsis, in which glucose utilization is depressed with increased insulin resistance. It is recommended that in the septic hypermetabolic patient, glucose intake be restricted to one half or less of the REE.

IV. TPN SOLUTIONS

    A. Dextrose solutions (CHO source). Commonly used dextrose solutions are 5% (170 kcal/L), 10% (340 kcal/L), 50% (1,700 kcal/L), and 70% (2,380 kcal/L).

    B. Protein solutions. Commonly used AA solutions are 3.5%, 8.5%, 10%, and 11.4%.

    C. Lipid emulsions. Lipid 10% (500 mL [1.1 kcal/mL]) or 20% (500 mL [2.0 kcal/mL]).

V. CALCULATIONS OF NUTRIENT VALUES FOR TPN

    A. CHO

        1. CHO (g) = dextrose 50%(mL) $\times$ 0.5 or dextrose 70%(mL) $\times$ 0.7

        2. CHO (kcal) = 3.4 $\times$ CHO(g) or 3.4 kcal/g of CHO
            Dextrose 50% = 1.7 kcal/mL or 1,700 kcal/L
            Dextrose 70% = 2.38 kcal/mL or 2,380 kcal/L

        3. Maximum glucose utilization rate = 5 mg/kg per minute or 40 kcal/kg per 24 hours

    B. Protein

        1. Protein (g) = 10% AAs = 0.1 g protein/mL
                     = 3.5% AAs = 0.03 g protein/mL
                     = 8.5% AAs = 0.085 g protein/mL
                     = 11.4% Novamine = 0.114 g protein/mL
                     = 6.9% FreAmine HBC = 0.069 g protein/mL
                     = 8.0% Hepatamine = 0.08 g protein/mL

        2. 1 g of protein = 4.3 kcal

    C. Fat

        1. Lipids are available as emulsions of cottonseed, soy, and safflower oils and of glycerol. These emulsions are isotonic and may be administered peripherally or centrally.

        2. The maximum fat allowance = 2.5 g/kg per day.

        3. Not more than 60% to 70% of total calories per day should be from fat.

        4. Lipid is given daily to most patients on TPN to supply 30% to 50% of the total energy requirements and essential fatty acids. In most medical centers, 20% lipid solutions are preferred, and the lipid is directly added to the CHO and protein solutions. The combined mixture is administered to the patient.

        5. In a minority of patients, acute respiratory distress, hypoxemia, and cyanosis may develop at the initial exposure to lipid emulsions. The rate of administration of the initial dose of lipid should be 1 mL per minute for 30 minutes. If no problems occur, the infusion rate may be increased up to 100 mL per hour. Serum triglyceride and cholesterol levels should be determined before and 4 hours after the onset of the infusion to document the utilization of the lipid.

    D. TPN nutrient composition is determined by the extent of the patient's ability to utilize lipid as an energy source. The TPN solution in a septic or injured patient should provide an energy–nitrogen ratio of 80 to 200 kcal/g of energy to 13 to 32 kcal/g of protein. An energy–protein ratio of 24 kcal/g of energy to 150 kcal/g of nitrogen may be ideal in hospitalized patients.

    E. Maintenance fluid requirements

        1. First 10 kg of body weight = 1,000 mL.

        2. Next 10 kg of body weight = 500 mL.

        3. Each kilogram of body weight thereafter = 20 mL.

        4. In critically ill patients who are receiving TPN, close attention must be given to the patient's volume status. Strict monitoring of the intake, output, daily weight, and hemodynamic status is essential. In most patients, total fluid intake may be calculated as equal to output plus 500 to 800 mL per day to cover the insensible losses. This additional amount may not be necessary in patients on ventilation.

VI. EXAMPLES OF CALCULATIONS FOR TPN IN DISEASE STATES

A. Sepsis
1. Calories = BEE
2. Provide 50% of calories as fat and 50% of calories as CHO. Maximum glucose utilization rate = 4 mg/kg per minute or 25 kcal/kg per 24 hours
3. Protein. 100 to 150:1 = calorie–nitrogen ratio
4. 2 g protein/kg of ideal body weight

B. Respiratory failure
1. Calories = 1.5 × BEE
2. Provide 50% of calories as fat and 50% as CHO
3. Maximum glucose utilization rate = 4 mg/kg per minute or 25 kcal/kg per 24 hours
4. Protein. 100 to 150:1 = calorie–nitrogen ratio
5. 1.5 to 2.0 g protein/kg of ideal body weight

C. Renal failure
1. Calories: maintenance to anabolic as needed
2. Protein
   a. Without dialysis, 20 to 60 g per day depending on blood urea nitrogen, creatinine, and body weight
   b. With dialysis, 701 g per day depending on blood urea nitrogen, creatinine, and body weight
   c. 1.0 to 1.2 g protein/kg of ideal body weight can be provided as
      i. AA solution
      ii. Solution containing essential AAs (e.g., Nephramine)

D. Hepatic failure
1. Calories = 1.5 × BEE (maintenance requirements)
2. Provide 50% or more of calories as fat and 50% or less as CHO.
3. Protein can be provided as
   a. Standard AA solution
   b. AA solution containing branched-chain AAs (e.g., Hepatamine) at 701 g of protein per day

VII. EXAMPLE. Patient is a 30-year-old woman with Crohn's disease who has an ileocolic fistula and requires TPN prior to surgery: weight (W) = 50 kg (110 lbs), height (H) = 166.4 cm (5 ft 1/2 in.)

A. Energy requirements per day
1. BEE = 655 + (9.6 × W) + (1.7 × H) − (4.7 × age)
   For this patient:
   BEE = 655 + (9.6 × 50) + (1.7 × 166.4) − (4.7 × 30) = 1,300 kcal per day
2. Parenteral anabolic requirements = 1.8 × BEE
   = 1.8 × 1,300 kcal per day
   = 2,300 kcal per day

B. Protein requirements per day
1. Ideal kcal per nitrogen ratio = 150:1
2. 1 g nitrogen = 6.25 g of protein
3. Protein (g) = $\dfrac{6.25 \times \text{energy requirement per day}}{150}$
4. This patient needs

$$\text{Protein (g)} = \frac{6.25 \times 2,300 \text{ kcal per day}}{150}$$
$$= 100 \text{ g}$$

5. To provide 100 g of protein per day, 1,000 mL of 10% aminosyn solution is needed.

C. Fluid requirements per day
1,000 + 500 + 20 (30) = 2,100 mL per day

D. Maximum fat allowance per day

$2.5 \times 50 \times 9 = 1,125$ kcal per day

For this patient, this is approximately 50% of the total daily calories.

E. Final TPN solution per day

**1. **

Solution	Volume (mL)	Kcal
10% AA	1,000	0[1]
50% dextrose	1,000	1,700[2]
20% lipid	300	600
Total	2,300	2,300

2. If more of the calories are to be given as fat, then use

Solution	Volume (mL)	Kcal
10% AA	1,000	0[1]
50% dextrose	700	1,200[2]
20% lipid	550	1,100
Distilled water	50	0
Total	2,300	2,300

3. As can be seen in **1** and **2,** the volume of CHO and lipid solutions can be manipulated, and other permutations can be worked out to achieve the total number of calories and total volume of fluid.

4. When the fluid volume needs to be restricted, as in patients with heart failure or renal insufficiency, more concentrated solutions, for example, 70% dextrose, 11.4% AA, and 20% lipid, may be used.

5. Distilled water can be added to the final solution to bring the volume to the desired amount.

VIII. ADDITIVES. The basic TPN solution does not contain electrolytes, trace elements, or vitamins. The electrolyte additives to TPN must be individualized to prevent fluid and electrolyte abnormalities.

A. Electrolytes (Table 12-2)

1. Sodium (Na), the principal extracellular cation, must be administered in sufficient quantities to provide for maintenance needs and to replace any existing deficits or ongoing losses. The quantity of Na added to TPN is determined by the patient's extracellular fluid volume status and serum Na concentration. Patients

TABLE 12-2 **Electrolytes**

Additives	Usual daily requirements
Sodium chloride ⎫ Sodium acetate ⎰	60–200 mEq Na
Potassium chloride ⎫ Potassium acetate ⎰	50–150 mEq K
Sodium phosphate ⎫ Potassium phosphate ⎰	50–150 mM PO_4
Magnesium sulfate	8–24 mEq Mg
Calcium gluconate	8–32 mEq Ca

Na, sodium; K, potassium; Mg, magnesium; Ca, calcium.

---

[1] Calories from AAs are not used in calculation for energy.
[2] See section V.A for calculation of CHO calories from dextrose solutions.

with hyponatremia should receive larger quantities of Na to limit free water administration (e.g., 75 to 120 mEq/L of TPN), whereas patients with hypernatremia or extracellular fluid excess require less Na (e.g., 30 mEq/L of TPN). Na may be administered as the chloride, phosphate, acetate, or bicarbonate salt.

2. **Chloride (Cl),** the predominant extracellular cation, is given as sodium and potassium salts. Chloride excess in TPN may cause hyperchloremic metabolic acidosis.

3. **Acetate** is metabolized to bicarbonate in the body and should be included in the TPN solution to counteract acidosis at doses of 50 to 120 mEq per day.

4. **Potassium (K)** is the major intracellular cation. It is needed in large amounts during anabolism. Hypokalemia readily develops in patients receiving TPN. K is lost with diuresis resulting from hyperglycemia induced by TPN. Increased plasma insulin concentration during TPN is associated with activation of the Na-K–ATPase pump, resulting in the shift of K from the extracellular space to the intracellular space. Beta-adrenergic stimulation and administration of vasopressors and inotropic agents also activate the Na-K–ATPase pump and may lead to clinically significant hypokalemia mediated by transcellular shifts of K.

   Patients with a normal plasma potassium level when TPN is initiated may receive 20 to 30 mEq of K per liter of TPN initially. Subsequent changes should be made according to the serum K level. K may be administered as the Cl or the phosphate salt depending on the serum phosphate concentration.

5. **Magnesium (Mg)** deficiency may occur in patients with history of alcoholism, malabsorption, malnutrition, or parathyroid disease and due to magnesia urea accompanying aminoglycoside therapy. During TPN, Mg is incorporated into newly synthesized muscle tissue and bone stores. It should be provided in the TPN solutions with special attention to the patient's renal status since Mg is excreted by the kidneys. Patients with mild hypomagnesemia with serum Mg levels of 1.2 to 1.8 mEq/L should receive 2.5 to 5.0 mEq (1–2 mL) of a 50% solution of Mg sulfate in each liter of TPN. More severe Mg deficiency needs additional intravenous (IV) supplementation.

6. **Phosphate** is a component of nucleic acids, phosphoproteins, and lipids and is needed to form high energy bonds and 2,3-diphosphoglycerate in red blood cells and for bone metabolism. Hypophosphatemia and total body phosphate depletion often complicate stress-starvation and refeeding states. The hypermetabolism seen in sepsis and injury results in skeletal muscle catabolism and depletion of intracellular phosphate stores. Hypophosphatemia may be exacerbated during TPN, with glucose infusions resulting in shifts of phosphate from extra- to intracellular space, similar to that seen with K.

   Phosphate should be included in the daily TPN orders. A reasonable initial dose of phosphate for septic or injured patients receiving TPN is 15 to 30 mmol per day. Phosphate may be administered as either an Na or a K salt depending on the serum K concentration.

7. **Calcium (Ca),** like magnesium, should be provided daily. Hypercatabolic states (e.g., sepsis or injury) may be associated with increased excretion of Ca. Mobilization of Ca from bone results in reductions in total body Ca. Vitamin D deficiency also leads to Ca deficiency. Because Mg is required for the secretion and end-organ effect of parathyroid hormone, hypocalcemia may result from hypomagnesemia. Approximately 50% to 60% of serum Ca is bound to albumin. In hypoalbuminemic patients, serum Ca concentrations may be falsely low. To adjust the measured serum Ca for hypoalbuminemia, the following formula may be used:

   Serum Ca + 4.0 − serum albumin (0.8 g/dL) = corrected serum Ca

   Patients with corrected low serum Ca levels should receive 5 mEq of Ca as the gluconate or the gluceptate salt in each liter of TPN solution.

8. **Buffers.** Metabolic acidosis may develop during TPN therapy. The oxidation of cationic and sulfur-containing AAs results in the production of hydrogen ions. When serum bicarbonate or total carbon dioxide binding capacity falls below 20 mEq/L, a portion of the Na in the TPN solution (e.g., 25–30 mEq/L)

may be administered as acetate. Acetate is metabolized by the liver to yield bicarbonate. In patients with hepatic dysfunction, sodium bicarbonate (e.g., 25–50 mEq/L) may be used to correct the metabolic acidosis.

B. **Vitamins.** Water-soluble forms of vitamins A, D, and E along with vitamin C, B vitamins, biotin, folate, and B_{12} (packaged as multivitamins-12) 5 mL should be added daily in amounts exceeding the recommended daily allowances to the TPN solutions. Vitamin K 10 to 25 mg weekly is given intramuscularly separately and should not be given to patients receiving anticoagulants. Patients requiring hemodialysis should receive 1 mg/dL of folic acid, because folic acid is removed by dialysis.

C. **Trace elements.** Chromium, manganese, copper, selenium, and zinc are needed daily and should be added to the TPN solution as trace elements (3–5 mL). Some authors advocate the administration of a unit of plasma every 3 to 4 weeks to provide undefined cofactors.

D. **Heparin.** Use of heparin, 1,000 U/L of TPN solution, has been shown to enhance vein and line patency and is recommended.

E. **Albumin.** In states of severe protein depletion (serum albumin <2.0 g/dL), the administration of salt-poor albumin may be helpful.

F. **Regular insulin** in crystalline form may be added to the TPN solution to cover patients with persistent hyperglycemia or glycosuria. It is generally not needed as an additive in the average patient.

Hyperglycemia may develop during TPN therapy even in previously nondiabetic patients. The serum glucose concentrations should be maintained at 100 to 200 mg/dL. When a patient has hyperglycemia greater than 200 mg/dL, regular human insulin should be added to the TPN solution in an initial dose of 5 to 10 U/L. The rate of TPN administration should not be altered to treat the hyperglycemia; rather, the hyperglycemia should be controlled with either IV or subcutaneous regular insulin, using a sliding scale based on the serum glucose concentration. Regular insulin may be administered IV every 2 to 3 hours. An example of a sliding scale is as follows:

Serum Glucose Level	Regular Insulin
200 to 300 mg/dL	2 to 3 units
300 to 400 mg/dL	3 to 5 units
400 + mg/dL	5 to 10 units

If hyperglycemia cannot be controlled by intermittent IV insulin, insulin may be infused continuously to control the patient's serum glucose level. One adds 250 units of insulin to 250 mL of normal saline; infusion may be started at a rate of 3 units per hour and adjusted according to the patient's serum glucose concentration. The regular insulin dose may be increased once each day until the serum glucose stabilizes at 100 to 200 mg/dL. The increase in insulin dose may be calculated as one half the IV dose of the previous 24 hours.

IX. INITIATING, TAPERING, AND DISCONTINUING TPN SOLUTION

A. **The initiation of TPN therapy** should be done gradually according to the patient's glucose tolerance and individual requirements. On the first day, 1,000 mL may be given, then 2,000 mL the second day, and 3,000 mL or more the third day.

B. **When stopping TPN solutions,** it is recommended the solution be tapered over 48 hours. However, TPN solutions can be reduced to a drip rate of 50 mL per hour. After 30 to 60 minutes at this rate, the solution can be discontinued. Rarely, a patient may experience hypoglycemia.

C. TPN solutions are commonly infused at a continuous rate evenly over 24 hours. **If infusion falls behind,** it should not be caught up rapidly. This may cause glycosuria and diuresis. It is usually possible to increase the drip rate by 10% to 20% in catch-up situations.

Example: A 52-year-old man is admitted to the intensive care unit with ileus and multilobar pneumonia requiring ventilatory support. He has severe protein–calorie malnutrition with a total lymphocyte count of 800 and a serum albumin level of 1.8 g/dL. His serum chemistries are:

Na: 133 mEq/L   Cl: 96 mEq/L   Creatinine: 1.1 mg/dL
K: 3.4 mEq/L HCO_3^-: 19 mEq/L   BUN: 13
W: 80 kg   H: 180 cm   Age (A): 52 years

$$BEE = 66 + (13.7 \times W) + (5 \times H) - (6.8 \times A)$$
$$= 66 + (13.7 \times 80) + (5 \times 180) - (6.8 \times 52) \text{ years}$$
$$= 1,708 \text{ kcal}$$

This patient has sepsis and requires mechanical ventilation. REE should exceed BEE by 30%.

$$REE = BEE \times 1.3$$
$$= 1,708 \times 1.3 - 2,221 \text{ kcal}$$

Minimal protein requirement = 1.0 to 1.5 kg per day

TPN Solution

1 L AA 10%	100 g protein (16 g nitrogen)
1 L 50% D/W	500 g dextrose 175 kcal
500 mL 10% Intralipid	550 kcal
Total kcal per day	2,300 kcal

This formula provides 44.2 kcal/kg (76% glucose, 24% lipid)

Energy–nitrogen ratio = 144 kcal/g nitrogen
    = 23 kcal/g, protein

Electrolytes to be added to each liter of TPN:

Sodium chloride (NaCl): 50 mEq
Potassium chloride (KCl): 20 mEq
Magnesium sulfate ($MgSO_4$): 5 mEq
Na acetate: 25 mEq KPO_4: 10 mEq

Administration Orders

Day 1 (infuse over 24 hours)

AA 10%	500 mL
50% D/W	500 mL
Electrolytes (as above)	
Multivitamins	5 mL
Trace elements	5 mL
Lipid emulsion 10%	500 mL

Day 2 (infuse over 24 hours)

AA 10%	1,000 mL
50% D/W	1,000 mL
Electrolytes (as above)	
Multivitamins	5 mL
Trace elements	5 mL
Lipid emulsion 10%	500 mL

X. MONITORING OF THE PATIENT ON TPN

   A. Monitor patient's intake and output.
   B. Obtain baseline weight and height. Check weight daily at the same time of day.
   C. Check vital signs every 4 hours. If the temperature exceeds 38°C, the physician should be notified.
   D. Laboratory evaluation. Obtain baseline laboratory values for 24-hour urine for creatinine and urea nitrogen, serum chemistries (SMA-12), electrolytes, magnesium, transferrin, triglycerides, complete blood count with differential, and platelet count.

After the TPN is initiated, the concentrations of serum electrolytes and phosphorus should be determined twice a day until daily requirements are ascertained. Serum glucose concentration should be measured every 4 to 6 hours. Serum Ca, Mg, creatinine, and blood urea nitrogen (BUN) should be determined daily. When the patient is stabilized on TPN, serum electrolytes, creatinine, and BUN should be measured every other day. Ca and Mg levels may be measured twice weekly. Serum transaminase, alkaline phosphate, and bilirubin levels should be measured weekly to facilitate early diagnosis of hepatic steatosis.

To determine the efficacy of TPN therapy, the total lymphocyte count and serum albumin and transferrin levels should be measured on a weekly basis. The optimal method for assessing the adequacy of TPN is through nitrogen balance studies. A 24-hour urine sample is collected for the urea and creatinine determinations. To calculate a patient's nitrogen balance see section III.F.

If lipids are given in addition to the TPN on a daily basis, serum triglyceride levels should be measured daily for several days to document that the lipid load is not exceeding the patient's metabolic capabilities. Serum triglyceride concentrations may be measured weekly when patients are on a stable TPN regimen.

XI. COMPLICATIONS OF TPN

A. Hyperglycemia. Patients with overt or latent diabetes, liver disease, or acute or chronic pancreatitis are at risk of development of hyperglycemia and glycosuria. This may result in hyperosmolar nonketotic coma and dehydration. Slow infusions of TPN initially with frequent glucose determinations should minimize this complication.

B. Hypoglycemia. Abrupt cessation of TPN may precipitate this condition. Peripheral 10% glucose should be given for treatment.

C. Hypo- and hyperkalemia, calcemia, magnesemia, and phosphatemia should be avoided by administration of adequate amounts of these minerals with regular measurement of serum values.

D. Azotemia. The delivery of a high nitrogen load may lead to a modest elevation of the blood urea nitrogen. Dehydration and prerenal states should be avoided.

E. Acute thiamine deficiency may complicate TPN in patients with chronic alcohol abuse, sepsis, or injury who are not receiving multivitamins in the TPN solution. Acute thiamine deficiency is characterized by severe lactic acidosis refractory to bicarbonate therapy, high output, cardiac failure, confusion, and hypotension. The lactic acidosis responds only to thiamine infusions.

F. Adverse reactions to lipid infusions. Long-term adverse reactions to a lipid infusion, especially if it exceeds 2.5 g/kg per day, include lipid accumulation in the lungs, decreasing oxygen diffusing capacity, and in the liver, impairment of biliary function. Fat infusions greater than 4 g/kg per day may lead to a bleeding diathesis (fat-overload syndrome). Thrombocytopenia, platelet dysfunction, and bleeding tendency are reversible with reduction of the infusion rate.

G. Acute fatty infiltration of the liver or hepatic steatosis may complicate TPN with glucose-predominant regimens. The glucose in such formulations is converted by the hepatocytes to fat and deposited in the liver parenchyma. Patients with hepatic steatosis exhibit cholestatic jaundice with elevations of serum alkaline phosphatase and bilirubin levels. Lipid-predominant or mixed lipid-glucose formulations rarely lead to hepatic steatosis.

Calculous and acalculous cholecystitis occurs in approximately 45% of patients undergoing long-term TPN. Impaired biliary motor function, stasis, sludge formation, and stones contribute to the pathogenesis. This complication is more prevalent in patients with hematologic malignancies.

H. Taurine deficiency. Parenteral solutions do not contain this nonessential AA. Reduced taurine levels may be found in children and adults on long-term home TPN. Taurine deficiency causes retinal dysfunction, and its addition to TPN solutions reverses this condition.

I. Carnitine deficiency. Carnitine may be required during metabolic response to injury. It is required for fatty acid oxidation in skeletal and cardiac muscles. In deficiency states, hyperbilirubinemia, generalized muscle weakness, and reactive hypoglycemia have been reported. Red cell carnitine and plasma carnitine should be measured.

J. Biotin deficiency. Hair loss, eczematous dermatitis, waxy pallor of skin, lethargy, depression, and anemia has been reported with biotin deficiency in patients on long-term TPN.

K. Selenium deficiency. A dilated cardiomyopathy associated with diffuse focal myocardial necrosis and conduction defects has been reported due to deficiency of selenium. Gastrointestinal fluid losses enhance selenium losses.

L. Respiratory complications. Protein–calorie malnutrition may be associated with respiratory muscle failure. Ventilator-dependent patients are more likely to be weaned successfully from ventilators after nutritional deficits are corrected.

AA infusions may increase ventilatory responsiveness to carbon dioxide. High-glucose TPN regimens are associated with an increased respiratory quotient and carbon dioxide production. These patients should receive TPN regimens that contain a larger fraction of lipid as energy substrate because lipid has a lower respiratory quotient than glucose and results in less carbon dioxide production.

M. Protein-calorie mismatch. Most TPN regimens provide an energy–nitrogen ratio of 80 to 200 kcal/g of nitrogen or 13 to 32 kcal/g of protein. If inadequate energy source in the form of glucose or lipid is administered, the patient utilizes AAs as an energy source. The metabolism of the AAs results in progressive increases in BUN levels out of proportion to creatinine levels. Protein–calorie mismatch may occur in patients with burns, severe hypermetabolism, or renal failure. This complication is managed by increasing the energy–nitrogen ratio either by reducing the administered amount of AA or increasing the level of nonprotein energy substrate.

N. Catheter infection. Sepsis occurs in fewer than 5% of all patients undergoing TPN. The incidence is clearly related to the catheter, dressings, and solutions. Catheter sepsis should be suspected whenever there is unexplained fever and leukocytosis in the absence of other sources. Blood, urine, sputum, and wound cultures should be obtained. The TPN bottle and tubing should be changed and cultured with each fever spike. A blood culture should be drawn through the TPN catheter. The catheter should be removed and the tip cultured if the blood culture is positive. The catheter should not be reinserted for 24 to 48 hours to allow the bloodstream to clear. Dextrose 10% should be administered peripherally during this time. Treatment involves coverage of the patient for the causative organism with intravenous antimicrobials.

XII. PERIPHERAL PARENTERAL NUTRITION

A. Indications. PPN can be used for
  1. Patients in whom a central line is precluded.
  2. Patients in whom short-term nutritional support is important (e.g., selected pre- and postoperative patients).
  3. Patients who are eating but not getting sufficient calories.

B. Advantages of PPN
  1. Placement of a peripheral intravenous line is safer than the placement of a central line.
  2. Infection control at infusion site is easier.
  3. Nursing care is less complicated.
  4. The complications of hyperosmolar glucose are avoided.

C. Disadvantages of PPN
  1. Hyperosmolar solutions cannot be used in PPN because they irritate the peripheral veins and cause thrombophlebitis.
  2. The volume of solution required to deliver an adequate number of calories may be too high, thus limiting the number of calories given.
  3. The number of calories that can be given may be inadequate for long-term anabolism.

D. PPN solutions. A mixture of dextrose and AA solutions is used. A major portion of nonprotein calories can be provided by the use of lipid emulsions. Peripheral vein tolerance for osmolality is about 800 mOsm/L. The osmolality of a solution can be calculated as follows:

$$\text{Osm (mOsm/L)} = 10 \times \text{protein (g)} + 6 \times \text{CHO (g)}$$
$$+ (0.3 \times \text{mL 20\% Intralipid}) \text{ total fluid (liter)}$$

E. Example. For the patient receiving the TPN solution described in section VII.E
   1. The osmolality of the TPN solution can be calculated as follows:

$$\text{Protein} = 100 \text{ g, CHO} = 1{,}700 \text{ kcal} = 500 \text{ g}^3$$

$$\frac{\text{Osm (mOsm/L)}}{2.3} - 10(100) + 6(353) + 0.3(550) = 1{,}427$$

This solution is too hyperosmolar to be used in PPN.
   2. The osmolality can be decreased by increasing the total volume of the solution. Because 800 mOsm/L is the desired osmolality, we can solve for total volume needed to give osmolality of 800 mOsm/L.

$$800 = 10(100) + 6(353) + 0.3(550)$$

total fluid volume in liter

Total volume = 4 L

   3. Most patients cannot tolerate such high volumes of IV fluids; thus PPN can only deliver maintenance amounts of calories.
   4. For this patient the **maintenance energy requirement** is

$$\text{BEE} \times 1.5 = 1.5 \times 1{,}300 = 1{,}900 \text{ kcal per day}$$

   5. The **maintenance protein requirement** is

$$\text{Protein} = \frac{6.25 \times 1{,}900 = 80 \text{ g per day}}{150}$$

   6. Maximum fat allowance 1,125 kcal per day
   7. Final PPN solution per day:

Solution	Volume (mL)	Kcal
10% AA	800	—
50% dextrose	470^3	800
20% Intralipid	550	1,100
Total	1,820	1,900

   8. Total volume to allow 800 mOsm/L

$$\frac{10(80) + 6(235) + 0.3(550)}{800} = 3 \text{ L}$$

   9. To bring the total volume of PPN solution to 3 L, we need to add 1,180 mL of distilled water.
   10. Adequate electrolytes, vitamins, and trace elements as in TPN are added to the final solution if the patient is not receiving these nutrients enterally.
        In many instances, if the PPN is to be administered for a short time a more simplified PPN solution may be made from:

Solution	Volume (mL)	Kcal	Amount (g)	Osmolality (mOsm/L)
8.5 % AA	1,000	340	85	850
10% Dextrose	1,000	340	100	505
10% Lipid	500	550	50	260
Total	2,500	1,230	235	595

F. Method of administration. The protein and CHO solution may be given simultaneously with the lipid emulsion. The infusion sets are connected by a Y-connector

---

$^3 \dfrac{\text{CHO (g)}}{3.4}$ = kcal (see section V.A).

that delivers the lipid emulsion to the vein in a piggybacked fashion. This method seems to "soothe" the vein and decrease the incidence of phlebitis. In most medical centers, the PPN solutions contain the lipid, CHO, and protein solutions mixed together into an emulsion. This eliminates the need for piggybacking of the lipid emulsion. The management and monitoring of patients receiving PPN are the same as for those receiving TPN, and the same meticulous care and team approach are necessary to give the best results.

Selected Readings

Bistrian BR, et al. Nutritional and metabolic support in the adult intensive care unit: Key controversies. *Crit Care Med.* 2006;34:1525–1531.

Cheung NW, et al. Hyperglycemia is associated with adverse outcomes in patients receiving total parenteral nutrition. *Diabetes Care.* 2005;28:2367–2371.

Heller AR, Rossler S, Litz RJ, et al. Omega-3 fatty acids improve the diagnosis-related clinical outcome. *Crit Care Med.* 2006;34:972–979.

Huschak G, et al. Olive oil based nutrition in multiple trauma patients: a pilot study. *Intensive Care Med.* 2005;31:1202–1208.

Krein SL, et al. Use of central venous catheter-related bloodstream infection prevention practices by US hospitals. *Mayo Clin Proc.* 2007;82:672–678.

Kudsk KA. Immunonutrition in surgery and critical care. *Annu Rev Nutr.* 2006;26:463–479.

Marik PE. Maximizing efficacy from parenteral nutrition in critical care: appropriate patient population, supplemental parentral nutrition, glucose control, parenteral glutamine, and alternative fat sources. *Curr Gastroenterol Rep.* 2007;9(4):345–353.

Sacks GS, et al. Parenteral nutrition implementation and management. In: Merritt R, ed. *The ASPEN Nutrition Support Practice Manual.* 2nd ed. Silver Spring, Md.: American Society for Parenteral & Enteral Nutrition; 2005:108–117.

van der Voort PH, et al. Intravenous glucose intake independently related to intensive care unit and hospital mortality: an argument for glucose toxicity in critically ill patients. *Clin Endocrinol.* 2006;64:141–145.

Waitzberg DL, et al. Postsurgical infections are reduced with specialized nutrition support. *World J Surg.* 2006;30:1592–1604.

Gastroenterologic Emergencies 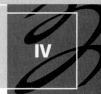 IV

THE ACUTE ABDOMEN

13

$\mathcal{T}$he term **acute abdomen** evokes an image of a patient suffering from sudden, severe abdominal pain, perhaps accompanied by vomiting, attentively surrounded by physicians and surgeons who are earnestly deciding whether to take the patient to the operating room. Indeed, many instances of acute abdomen are surgical emergencies. However, the differential diagnosis is extensive, and the management of an acute abdomen varies according to the diagnosis.

I. **DIFFERENTIAL DIAGNOSIS.** The differential diagnosis in a patient with an acute abdomen may be broad or narrow, depending on the clinical signs and symptoms. For example, a 12-year-old boy whose generalized abdominal pain has intensified and become localized to the right lower quadrant very likely has acute appendicitis, but acute Crohn's disease and mesenteric lymphadenitis must also be considered. On the other hand, severe midabdominal pain in a 65-year-old man with ascites may indicate spontaneous bacterial peritonitis, intestinal ischemia, a perforated ulcer, or a leaking aortic aneurysm, among other possibilities.

   A partial list of the diagnostic considerations for an acute abdomen is found in Table 13-1.

II. **CLINICAL PRESENTATION**
   A. **History**
      1. **Pain**
         a. **Types.** Abdominal pain is an invariable feature of an acute abdomen and presents as one or a combination of three types.
            i. **Visceral pain** develops from stretching or distending of an abdominal viscus or from inflammation. The pain is diffuse and poorly localized. It generally has a gnawing, burning, or cramping quality.
            ii. **Somatic pain** arises from the abdominal wall, the parietal peritoneum, the root of the mesentery, or the diaphragm. It is more intense and better localized than visceral pain.
            iii. **Referred pain** is felt at a site distant from the source of the pain but shares the same dermatome or neurosegment. Referred pain is usually sharp and well localized; thus, it resembles somatic pain.
         b. **The onset of pain** may be instantaneous, or the pain may develop over minutes or even hours. Sudden severe pain characterizes such events as a perforated ulcer, a ruptured viscus, a ruptured ectopic pregnancy, a spontaneous pneumothorax, or a dissecting aortic aneurysm. On the other hand, more gradual development of pain is typical of acute pancreatitis, acute cholecystitis, intestinal obstruction, bowel perforation, diverticulitis, and intraabdominal abscess.
      2. **Vomiting** usually accompanies an acute abdomen to a variable degree. A clinical rule is that pain precedes vomiting in disorders requiring surgical treatment, whereas vomiting precedes pain in medically treated disorders. Vomiting can be persistent, as with intestinal obstruction. Long-standing obstruction may result in feculent vomiting due to the proximal growth of colonic bacterial flora. Vomiting of bloody material suggests that the bleeding lesion is above the ligament of Treitz.
      3. **Other historical aspects.** A history of a known disorder, such as pancreatitis or peptic ulcer, makes that diagnosis more likely as the cause of the current

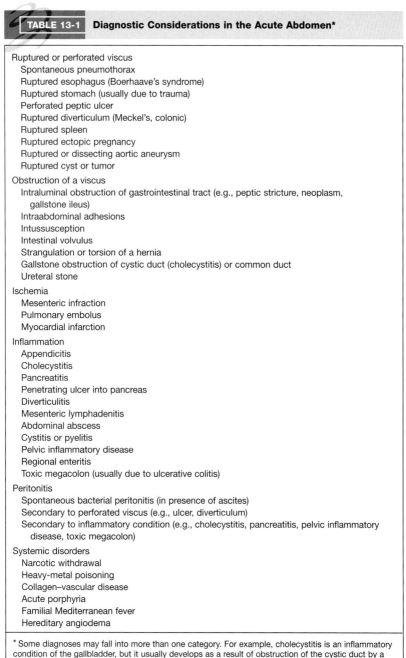

TABLE 13-1 Diagnostic Considerations in the Acute Abdomen*

Ruptured or perforated viscus
  Spontaneous pneumothorax
  Ruptured esophagus (Boerhaave's syndrome)
  Ruptured stomach (usually due to trauma)
  Perforated peptic ulcer
  Ruptured diverticulum (Meckel's, colonic)
  Ruptured spleen
  Ruptured ectopic pregnancy
  Ruptured or dissecting aortic aneurysm
  Ruptured cyst or tumor
Obstruction of a viscus
  Intraluminal obstruction of gastrointestinal tract (e.g., peptic stricture, neoplasm,
    gallstone ileus)
  Intraabdominal adhesions
  Intussusception
  Intestinal volvulus
  Strangulation or torsion of a hernia
  Gallstone obstruction of cystic duct (cholecystitis) or common duct
  Ureteral stone
Ischemia
  Mesenteric infraction
  Pulmonary embolus
  Myocardial infarction
Inflammation
  Appendicitis
  Cholecystitis
  Pancreatitis
  Penetrating ulcer into pancreas
  Diverticulitis
  Mesenteric lymphadenitis
  Abdominal abscess
  Cystitis or pyelitis
  Pelvic inflammatory disease
  Regional enteritis
  Toxic megacolon (usually due to ulcerative colitis)
Peritonitis
  Spontaneous bacterial peritonitis (in presence of ascites)
  Secondary to perforated viscus (e.g., ulcer, diverticulum)
  Secondary to inflammatory condition (e.g., cholecystitis, pancreatitis, pelvic inflammatory
    disease, toxic megacolon)
Systemic disorders
  Narcotic withdrawal
  Heavy-metal poisoning
  Collagen–vascular disease
  Acute porphyria
  Familial Mediterranean fever
  Hereditary angioedema

* Some diagnoses may fall into more than one category. For example, cholecystitis is an inflammatory condition of the gallbladder, but it usually develops as a result of obstruction of the cystic duct by a gallstone.

event. If the patient has had abdominal surgery, intraabdominal adhesions become a consideration. Alcohol abuse may suggest pancreatitis or gallstone disease.

B. Physical examination

1. **Vital signs.** Temperature elevation suggests sepsis from intraabdominal inflammation and infection. Tachycardia typically accompanies an acute abdomen. Blood pressure may also be elevated, although hypotension and shock may develop in patients with a perforated viscus or severe sepsis.

2. **Inspection**

   a. **Patient position.** A patient with peritonitis is likely to lie quietly with knees flexed. A patient with acute pancreatitis finds it uncomfortable to lie on the back and may assume the fetal position. A patient with colicky pain typically cannot lie still.

   b. **The abdomen** may be distended due to ascites or intestinal obstruction. In thin patients with complete obstruction, hyperperistalsis may be visible on the abdominal wall. Ecchymosis in the flanks (Grey Turner's sign) or around the umbilicus (Cullen's sign) may indicate hemorrhagic pancreatitis or a ruptured ectopic pregnancy.

3. **Auscultation.** Peristalsis is increased in partial or complete bowel obstruction; typically there are rushes and high-pitched sounds. Hypo- or aperistalsis develops in intestinal ileus from a variety of causes, including peritonitis, electrolyte imbalance, severe inflammation (e.g., toxic megacolon, pancreatitis), and long-standing intestinal obstruction.

   The examiner should listen for vascular bruits and friction rubs. The former may suggest an aneurysm, whereas the latter can develop after rupture of the spleen or rupture of a lesion of the liver.

4. **Percussion.** Tympany typically is present in the distended abdomen of intestinal obstruction or toxic megacolon. Percussion can help in outlining the liver and may indicate enlargement of other organs.

5. **Palpation**

   a. Patients with an acute abdomen typically have **abdominal tenderness.** If peritonitis is present, either localized or generalized, there may be guarding and rigidity. Localized tenderness may provide a clue to the diagnosis. Rebound tenderness should be elicited by gently depressing the abdominal wall with one or two fingers, then quickly releasing the pressure. Sharp pain on release of the pressure indicates peritoneal inflammation. Because this maneuver often is so uncomfortable to the patient, it should not be repeated indiscriminately by subsequent examiners.

   One should remember that the signs of peritonitis may be blunted in elderly or severely ill patients. Thus, presence of little or no tenderness does not exclude peritonitis in these patients.

   b. Gentle palpation also may identify **organ enlargement or mass lesions.** An expansile, midabdominal mass may indicate an aortic aneurysm. Patients with acute Crohn's disease often have a tender mass in the right lower quadrant.

6. **Rectal and pelvic examinations.** Examination of the rectum and pelvis may provide valuable information about the pelvic organs and perirectal tissues. Tumors, inflammatory masses, abscesses, and pelvic inflammatory disease may be evident.

III. EVALUATION AND MANAGEMENT OF THE PATIENT

A. Laboratory studies. Laboratory examination of blood and urine may help in establishing a diagnosis and managing the patient with an acute abdomen (Table 13-2).

1. **Complete blood count.** White blood cell count (WBC) is usually elevated in patients with an acute abdomen, particularly in inflammatory and infectious conditions. WBC may be depressed in severe sepsis, in viremia, and in association with immunosuppressive therapy. A low hematocrit and hemoglobin count may reflect chronic anemia or may result from recent bleeding or rupture of a blood-filled viscus. Thrombocytopenia may contribute to abdominal bleeding or

TABLE 13-2	Laboratory and Radiologic Studies in the Evaluation of the Acute Abdomen

Blood studies
  Complete blood count
  Electrolytes
  Calcium and magnesium
  Amylase
  Bilirubin, SGOT, SGPT, alkaline phosphatase
  Arterial blood gases
Urinalysis
Electrocardiogram
Chest x-ray films
Abdominal x-ray films (flat and upright or decubitus)
Additional studies that may be indicated
  Ultrasound scan
  CT scan
  HIDA scan
  Intravenous pyelogram
  Diagnostic paracentesis

SGOT, serum glutamic-oxaloacetic transaminase; SGPT, serum glutamic-pyruvic transaminase; CT, computed tomography; HIDA, hepatoiminodiacetic acid.

result from sepsis. Either thrombocytosis or thrombocytopenia can be associated with a malignancy.

2. **Serum electrolytes** (sodium, potassium, chloride, bicarbonate) and calcium and magnesium levels should be determined periodically because of the fluid and electrolyte shifts that may occur in patients with an acute abdomen.

3. **Arterial blood gases** also are important to monitor in acutely ill patients.

4. **Serum amylase level** may be elevated in acute pancreatitis and in bowel obstruction and ischemic bowel disease. Other conditions causing hyperamylasemia that are not associated with an acute abdomen include salivary gland disease, renal insufficiency, and the benign condition macroamylasemia.

5. **Elevations in serum bilirubin, aspartate aminotransferase (AST; or serum glutamic-oxaloacetic transaminase, SGOT), alanine aminotransferase (ALT; or serum glutamic-pyruvic transaminase, SGPT), and alkaline phosphatase levels** may indicate liver or biliary disease. Elevations in alkaline phosphatase in particular may be an early indicator of obstruction of the biliary tract, either within the liver or in the extrahepatic bile ducts.

6. **Urinalysis** may indicate pyuria caused by acute pyelonephritis or hematuria due to a renal stone.

7. **An electrocardiogram** should be performed in all patients to establish a baseline tracing and to look for acute changes of myocardial injury.

B. **Radiologic studies** (Table 13-2; see also Chapter 9)

1. **The chest x-ray should** not be omitted. Pneumonia, pulmonary embolus, subdiaphragmatic free air, or a widened mediastinum of a dissecting aneurysm may be evident. Plain films of the abdomen, supine and erect or decubitus may indicate air-fluid levels, free intraabdominal air, or calcification. Loops of bowel may be displaced by an abscess or other mass. Marked dilatation of the bowel may indicate obstruction or toxic megacolon.

2. **Ultrasound scan, computed tomography scan, HIDA scan, and intravenous pyelography** may give additional valuable information. (See Chapter 9 for full descriptions of these studies.)

C. **Diagnostic paracentesis.** In some patients with an acute abdomen, withdrawal of fluid already within the abdomen or withdrawal of instilled fluid is helpful in making a diagnosis. Patients with infected ascites have an elevated ascitic WBC and often have positive bacterial cultures. Fluid that contains blood suggests hemorrhage from a viscus, infarction, or hemorrhagic pancreatitis. An elevated amylase level may be found in pancreatitis or bowel infarction.

The **safest site** for a closed (needle) paracentesis is in the midline about 2 cm below the umbilicus, where the abdominal wall is relatively avascular. However, care should be taken not to puncture a distended urinary bladder. Also, a midline abdominal wound from previous surgery precludes the use of this site. An open paracentesis using a small paramedian incision and a dialysis catheter may be safer and more accurate than a needle paracentesis.

D. **Treatment** includes measures that are applied to all patients plus specific therapies that depend on the underlying cause.

1. **The general approach** to patients with an acute abdomen includes intravenous fluids, nothing by mouth, and in most instances nasogastric suction to decompress the stomach and prevent additional air from entering the bowel. In some patients, it may be necessary to pass an additional long tube to decompress the bowel. Careful attention to volume of fluid intake and urine output is important. As previously indicated, serum electrolytes and arterial blood gases should be monitored.

2. **Specific treatment** depends on the cause of the acute abdomen and is discussed in the appropriate subsequent chapters. (See particularly Chapter 37 for management of toxic megacolon, Chapter 44 for management of intestinal ischemia, Chapter 46 for management of severe pancreatitis, and Chapter 49 for management of acute cholecystitis.) A major decision in the management of a patient with an acute abdomen is whether the patient needs surgery. Patients who have a ruptured viscus need prompt surgical intervention. Unresolved ischemia, which has progressed or will progress to tissue necrosis as a result either of vascular infarction or strangulation of a viscus, demands surgical treatment. Some inflammatory conditions, such as acute appendicitis, necrotizing pancreatitis, necrotizing cholecystitis, and toxic megacolon, which have not responded to medical therapy within 24 to 48 hours, also require surgical attention. Finally, some acute conditions, such as acute cholecystitis or acute diverticulitis, resolve with medical management but may be treated subsequently under elective conditions by surgery.

Selected Readings

Al-Salamah SM, et al. Role of ultrasonography, computed tomography and diagnostic peritoneal lavage in abdominal blunt trauma. *Saudi Med J.* 2002;23:1350–1355.

Brown TA, et al. Acute appendicitis in the setting of clostridium difficile colitis. *Clin Gastroenterol Hepatol.* 2007;5(8):969–971.

Fry LC, et al. The yield of capsule endoscopy in patients with abdominal pain or diarrhea. *Endoscopy.* 2006;38:498–502.

Iancelli A, et al. Therapeutic laparoscopy for blunt abdominal trauma with bowel injuries. *J Laparoendosc Adv Surg Tech A.* 2003;13:189–191.

Khawaja FJ, et al. 86-year-old woman with abdominal pain and diarrhea. *Mayo Clin Proc.* 2007;82(4):487–489.

Knoll BM, et al. 56-year-old man with rash, abdominal pain and orthralgias. *Mayo Clin Proc.* 2007;82(6):745–748.

Maglinte DD, et al. Current concepts in imaging on small bowel obstruction. *Radiol Clin North Am.* 2003;41:263–283.

Ng B, et al. 49 year old woman with acute abdominal pain and nausea. *Mayo Clin Proc.* 2001;76:649.

Poulin EC, et al. Early laparoscopy to help diagnose acute non-specific abdominal pain. *Lancet.* 2000;355:861.

Wolfe JM, et al. Analgesic administration to patients with acute abdomen: A survey of emergency medicine physicians. *Am J Emerg Med.* 2000;18:250.

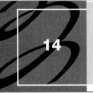

14 ACUTE GASTROINTESTINAL BLEEDING

*A*cute gastrointestinal bleeding ranges in severity from a single, nearly inconsequential bleeding episode, perhaps resulting in vomiting of "coffee-ground" material or the brief passage of red-colored stool, to massive hemorrhage and shock. Chronic or occult gastrointestinal bleeding is discussed in Chapter 44.

Gastrointestinal bleeding is generally classified as either upper or lower in origin (Table 14-1) simply because the source of bleeding is only rarely in the jejunum or ileum and also because the presenting signs and symptoms frequently are characteristic of either an upper or a lower gastrointestinal source. Regardless of the source, however, the principles of the initial management of all patients with acute gastrointestinal bleeding are generally the same (Table 14-2). Because patients vary in the severity of bleeding, the orderly sequence of history taking, physical examination, diagnostic evaluation, and treatment may have to be altered to meet the immediate demands.

I. INITIAL MANAGEMENT
A. History
1. **Vomiting or passage of blood per rectum.** The action of gastric acid on blood quickly forms dark particles that resemble coffee grounds. Vomiting of red blood (hematemesis) or of coffee-ground-appearing material usually signifies a source of bleeding in the esophagus, stomach, or duodenum, but it can result from swallowed blood from the respiratory tract. On the other hand, passage of red- or maroon-colored stool per rectum (hematochezia) usually indicates that the source is in the rectum, colon, or terminal ileum.

TABLE 14-1 Diagnostic Considerations in Acute Gastrointestinal Bleeding

Upper gastrointestinal bleeding	Lower gastrointestinal bleeding
Bleeding from nose or pharynx	Hemorrhoids
Hemoptysis	Anal fissure
Esophagogastric (Mallory-Weiss) mucosal tear	Inflammatory bowel disease (proctitis or colitis)
Esophageal rupture (Boerhaave's syndrome)	
Inflammation and erosions (esophagitis, gastritis, duodenitis)	Neoplasm (carcinoma or polyps)
	Diverticulosis
Peptic ulcer of esophagus, stomach, duodenum, or surgical anastomosis	Ischemic enteritis or colitis
	Angiodysplasia
Dieulafoy's lesion (ruptured mucosal artery)	Antibiotic-associated colitis
Varices of esophagus, stomach, or duodenum	Radiation colitis
Neoplasm (carcinoma, lymphoma, leiomyoma, leiomyosarcoma, polyps)	Amyloidosis
	Meckel's diverticulum
Hemobilia	Vascular-enteric fistula
Vascular-enteric fistula (usually from aortic aneurysm or graft)	Brisk bleeding from an upper gastrointestinal source

TABLE 14-2	**Principles of the Initial Management of Acute Gastrointestinal Bleeding**

I. Perform in order determined by activity of bleeding
  A. History
  B. Vital signs, including postural signs
  C. Physical examination, including rectal examination
  D. Insertion of large-bore peripheral venous catheter and, if necessary, a central venous line
  E. Withdrawal of blood for initial laboratory studies
  F. Administration of intravenous electrolyte solutions and blood
II. Pass a nasogastric tube
  A. If clear initially or clears promptly with lavage, remove
  B. If bloody, leave in to monitor gastrointestinal bleeding and to provide access to the gastrointestinal tract
III. Survey for concomitant heart, lung, renal, liver, or central nervous system disease
IV. Consult a gastroenterologist, a surgeon, and, if indicated, a radiologist
  V. Make a diagnosis (see section II and Figs. 14-1 and 14-2)

However, an important exception is the upper gastrointestinal lesion that bleeds profusely, such as a ruptured esophageal varix or an eroded vessel within a peptic ulcer, in which a large volume of blood passes rapidly through the intestines and appears as hematochezia. The passage of black stool (melena) usually indicates a more moderate rate of bleeding from an upper gastrointestinal source, sometimes as little as 50 mL per day, although bleeding from the terminal ileum or ascending colon can result in melena.

2. Age of patient. Advanced age worsens the prognosis of acutely bleeding patients. The age of the patient also makes some diagnoses more or less likely, particularly with regard to lower gastrointestinal bleeding. The differential diagnosis of acute lower gastrointestinal bleeding in people over age 60 includes ischemic colitis, carcinoma of the colon, arteriovenous malformation, and diverticulosis, whereas none of these is a serious consideration in a 25-year-old. On the other hand, bleeding from inflammatory bowel disease or a Meckel's diverticulum is more likely in a child or young adult.

3. Ingestion of gastric mucosal irritants. The recent ingestion of aspirin, other nonsteroidal antiinflammatory drugs, or alcohol raises the possibility that erosive gastritis or other mucosal injury has developed. Aspirin not only causes direct mucosal injury, but also interferes with platelet adhesion; thus, bleeding lesions in patients who take aspirin are less likely to clot.

4. Associated medical conditions. The number of associated medical conditions directly increases the risk of mortality in acute gastrointestinal bleeding. Mortality in patients with no accompanying medical conditions is about 1%, whereas the risk of dying in patients with four or more associated illnesses is more than 70%.

Patients with liver disease are at risk to develop esophageal varices, which could bleed. Although acute upper gastrointestinal bleeding in patients known to have esophageal varices is most likely caused by the varices, other sources must be considered.

Previous abdominal or pelvic irradiation raises the possibility that lower gastrointestinal bleeding is caused by radiation enteritis or colitis. Gastrointestinal bleeding may develop from the acute effects of irradiation on the gut, or bleeding may occur months to years later. The latter situation represents a form of ischemic colitis that is accelerated by the perivascular inflammation that results from the effects of irradiation.

Knowledge of serious cardiovascular, pulmonary, liver, renal, or neurologic disease may be valuable in guiding medical and, if necessary, surgical decisions during subsequent treatment of the patient.

B. Physical examination
1. The physical examination is unlikely to indicate a precise cause of bleeding. However, coolness of the extremities, palmar creases, and pallor of the conjunctivae, mucous membranes, and nail beds may be evident as a result of blood loss and peripheral vasoconstriction. The signs of chronic liver disease or abdominal tenderness may provide relevant information.
2. **The rectal examination** is important and should not be omitted, even in seemingly obvious upper gastrointestinal bleeding. The anus, perianal area, and lower rectum can be assessed, as can the character and color of the stool.

   Occult blood in the stool can be detected with as little as 15 mL of blood loss per day. Stools may remain positive for occult blood for nearly 2 weeks after an acute blood loss of 1,000 mL or more from an upper gastrointestinal source.
3. **Postural signs.** As the patient loses intravascular volume due to blood loss, cardiac output and blood pressure fall, and pulse rate increases. Under conditions of severe volume loss, postural compensation of blood pressure and pulse are inadequate. Thus, so-called postural signs are present if, when the patient sits from a supine position, the pulse rate increases more than 20 beats per minute and the systolic blood pressure drops more than 10 mmHg. Under these circumstances, it is likely that blood loss has exceeded 1 L. However, age, cardiovascular status, and rate of blood loss all influence the development of postural signs.

C. Fluid, electrolyte, and blood replacement
1. A large-bore intravenous catheter should be inserted promptly into a peripheral vein. Blood can be drawn at this time for laboratory studies (see section I.D). In a profusely bleeding patient, a single peripheral intravenous catheter may not be sufficient to provide adequate blood replacement; two or more intravenous catheters may be required. In an acute emergency in which a peripheral vein is not available, venous access should be established via a jugular, subclavian, or femoral vein.
2. **Infusion of fluids and blood.** Normal saline is infused rapidly until blood for transfusion is available. In patients who have excess body sodium, such as those with ascites and peripheral edema, the physician may be reluctant to infuse large amounts of saline. In those instances, the restoration of hemodynamic stability should take precedence over other considerations. In other words, if the patient is bleeding profusely and blood for transfusion is not yet available, saline should be infused without regard for the patient's sodium balance. If bleeding is less severe, hypotonic sodium solutions may be infused until blood for transfusion arrives. Appropriate treatment of acute gastrointestinal bleeding includes not only replacement of blood, usually in the form of packed red cells, but also infusion of supplemental electrolyte solutions and, when necessary, clotting factors.
3. **A central venous pressure catheter or Swan-Ganz catheter** may be necessary to evaluate the effects of volume replacement and the need for continued infusion of blood, particularly in elderly patients or patients with cardiovascular disease.
4. **Monitoring of urine output** provides a reasonable indication of vital organ perfusion. In severely ill patients, a urinary catheter may be necessary.

D. Laboratory studies
1. **Initial blood studies** should include a complete blood count (CBC) and levels of electrolytes, blood urea nitrogen (BUN), creatinine, glucose, calcium, phosphate, and magnesium; blood should be drawn for typing. Hemoglobin and hematocrit levels usually are low, and the level of these measures may have some relation to the amount of blood loss. However, some patients bleed so rapidly that there is insufficient time for the blood volume to equilibrate, and the hemoglobin and hematocrit levels are normal or only slightly reduced. In acutely bleeding patients, changes in blood pressure and pulse and the direct

evidence of continued bleeding via the nasogastric tube or per rectum are better indicators than the hemoglobin and hematocrit levels for determining the administration of electrolyte solutions and the replacement of blood. Clotting status should be assessed with platelet count, prothrombin time, and partial thromboplastin time. Depending on the clinical presentation, other blood studies may be important, such as serum amylase, liver tests, and cardiac enzymes. In severely ill patients, arterial blood gases should be monitored.

2. **Leukocytosis,** usually not in excess of 15,000/μL, can accompany acute gastrointestinal bleeding. However, an elevated white blood cell count should not be attributed to acute blood loss without a search for sources of infection.

3. **Elevated BUN** in a patient whose BUN has recently been normal or whose serum creatinine level is normal suggests an upper gastrointestinal bleeding source. The rise in BUN results from the hypovolemia of acute blood loss, but digestion of blood proteins in the small intestine and the absorption of nitrogenous products can also contribute. In patients with impaired liver function, the increased protein load may be sufficient to induce or aggravate hepatic encephalopathy. The magnitude of the protein load can be calculated roughly by multiplying the grams of hemoglobin and serum protein per deciliter of blood by the estimated volume of blood lost. For example, if a patient has an initial hemoglobin level of 13 g/dL and serum protein of 7 g/dL and loses 1,000 mL (or 10 dL) of blood, approximately 200 g of protein is presented to the small intestine ([13 g + 7 g] $\times$ 10 = 200 g). Thus, gastric lavage and control of bleeding are additionally important in patients with liver disease.

4. **Later studies.** Because of rapid fluid shifts during gastrointestinal bleeding and the infusion of blood, blood products, and other fluids, frequent assessment of serum electrolytes, calcium, phosphate, and magnesium levels is necessary. Extensive transfusion dilutes platelets and clotting factors, particularly factors V and VII. This condition can be treated by infusion of fresh-frozen plasma and platelets as necessary. Also, a high proportion of patients who bleed while taking therapeutic anticoagulants do so from a clinically significant lesion. Thus, it is important to evaluate these patients for gastrointestinal pathology in addition to correcting their clotting status. Most patients who receive blood transfusions do not need calcium supplements, although hypocalcemia as a result of binding of calcium by anticoagulants in banked blood may occur after massive transfusions. Patients who receive more than 100 mL of blood per minute may be given 0.2 g calcium chloride ($CaCl_2$) via another intravenous line during the time the blood is infusing. Measurement of the ionized calcium and monitoring of the electrocardiographic QT interval are recommended during the rapid infusion of anticoagulated blood.

E. **Nasogastric intubation and gastric lavage.** A nasogastric (NG) tube should be passed in all patients with acute gastrointestinal bleeding unless the source is obviously the lower gastrointestinal tract. Blood from an esophageal or gastric source pools in the stomach, and in more than 90% of bleeding duodenal ulcers the blood refluxes back across the pyloric channel into the stomach. If the aspirate is clear or clears readily with lavage, the NG tube may be removed. If there is fresh blood or a large amount of old blood or retained material, the stomach should be lavaged by means of a large-bore sump tube (20–24 French) or an Ewald tube. Removal of as much of the gastric contents as possible facilitates subsequent endoscopy and may contribute to hemostasis by allowing the walls of the stomach to collapse. Because of its adverse effects, the NG tube should be removed promptly when it no longer fulfills a useful purpose.

1. **Benefits of NG intubation**
   a. To document the presence of blood
   b. To monitor the rate of bleeding
   c. To identify recurrence of bleeding after initial control
   d. To lavage and decompress the stomach
   e. To remove gastric acid

    2. Adverse effects of NG intubation
      a. Patient discomfort
      b. Predisposition to gastroesophageal reflux and pulmonary aspiration
      c. Irritation of the esophageal and gastric mucosae, creating mucosal artifacts and aggravating existing lesions
  F. Consultations. The appropriate management of acute gastrointestinal bleeding typically involves a team of physicians. Specific diagnostic studies usually require the expertise of a gastroenterologist or a radiologist. The surgeon, when consulted early, may offer valuable assistance in managing the patient and is in a much better position to make a decision regarding operative intervention.

II. DIAGNOSTIC AND THERAPEUTIC STUDIES. Schemes for the diagnostic evaluation of acute upper and lower gastrointestinal bleeding are shown in Figs. 14-1 and 14-2, respectively.
  A. Endoscopy. Gastrointestinal endoscopy, of both the upper gastrointestinal tract and the colon and rectum, is discussed in Chapter 5 with regard to diagnostic capability and methods of performing the procedures.
    1. Upper gastrointestinal bleeding
      a. Diagnostic endoscopy. Endoscopy usually is recommended as the initial diagnostic procedure in acute upper gastrointestinal bleeding because

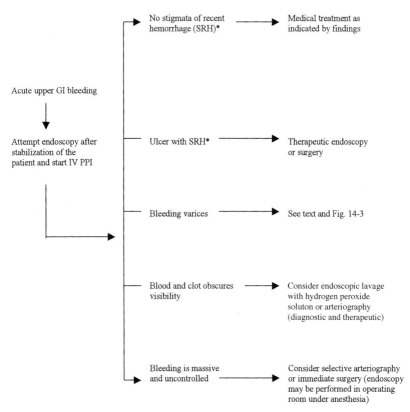

Figure 14-1. Scheme for the diagnostic evaluation of acute upper gastrointestinal bleeding. (*Stigmata of recent hemorrhage are a visible vessel, fresh blood clot, black eschar, or active bleeding.)

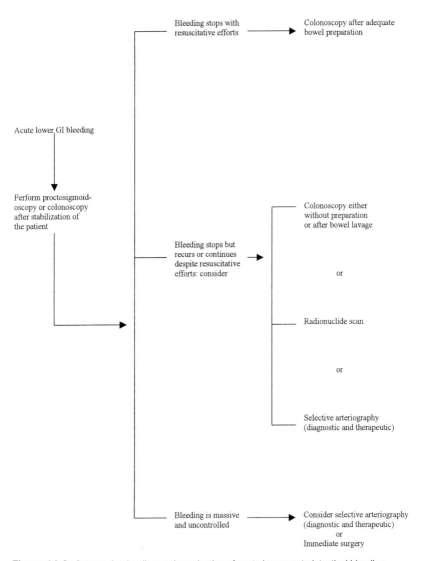

Figure 14-2. Scheme for the diagnostic evaluation of acute lower gastrointestinal bleeding.

knowledge of the specific diagnosis may dictate a specific treatment regimen. For example, the treatment of bleeding esophageal varices (see section IV.A) is likely to be quite different from the treatment of a bleeding peptic ulcer, hemorrhagic gastritis, or a Mallory-Weiss tear of the esophagogastric junction. The appropriate treatment of a peptic ulcer that stops bleeding includes acid-inhibiting drug therapy for several weeks, whereas hemorrhagic gastritis, if caused by aspirin ingestion or alcohol abuse, typically heals rapidly after withdrawal of the offending agent, and administration of acid-inhibiting drug therapy. A Mallory-Weiss tear may be expected to heal in several days without specific therapy. Furthermore, the endoscopic identification of the so-called **stigmata of recent hemorrhage (SRH)** within an ulcer crater may have some prognostic and therapeutic significance. SRH include a protruding visible vessel, an adherent clot, a black eschar, and actual oozing or spurting of blood. Patients with SRH are more likely to have uncontrolled bleeding or recurrent bleeding and to require intervention by therapeutic endoscopic methods or surgery.

   b. Therapeutic endoscopy. Methods of treating peptic ulcer bleeding through the endoscope have included thermal electrocoagulation, laser photocoagulation, injection of epinephrine, ethanol or hypertonic solutions, and placement of clips on the bleeding vessels or ulcer. Experience to date has shown the following:

     i. Bipolar electrocoagulation, laser photocoagulation, injection of various agents, and placement of clips all appear to be capable of controlling acute bleeding. The combination of two of these techniques seems to yield better and more lasting results (less rebleeding).

     ii. Laser photocoagulation and electrocoagulation has been shown to reduce the need for emergency surgery and improve survival.

     iii. Laser therapy is less available and the most difficult to learn, whereas injection therapy is the least difficult and readily available in most hospitals.

     iv. Injection therapy (epinephrine 1/10,000 or normal saline) appears to be the safest and the least expensive.

     v. Combining injection therapy with electrocoagulation may have added benefits and is currently being widely used (Table 14-3). In the endoscopic treatment of bleeding esophageal varices, endoscopic banding is preferred over injection sclerosis (see section IV.A).

  2. Lower gastrointestinal bleeding. The initial diagnostic procedure for acute lower gastrointestinal bleeding is proctosigmoidoscopy, preferably with a flexible fiberoptic instrument. If the bleeding seems to be occurring above the reach of the sigmoidoscope, emergency colonoscopy may be performed after the colon is cleaned with osmotically balanced electrolyte solutions (e.g., GoLYTELY or Colyte) administered orally or by nasogastric tube. If colonoscopy is not feasible, selective arteriography may be performed both for diagnostic and possible therapeutic measures.

B. Radionuclide scanning of the abdomen after labeling of the patient's red blood cells or other blood components may indicate the site of bleeding (see Chapter 9, section II.C). A positive scan may point the way to more definitive diagnostic or therapeutic procedures. The radionuclide scan appears to be more sensitive than

---

TABLE 14-3   **Endoscopic Treatment of Bleeding Ulcers**

Characteristic	Electrocoagulation	Laser photocoagulation	Injection therapy
Controls bleeding	Yes	Yes	Yes
Reduces need for surgery	Yes	Yes	?
Reduces mortality	Yes	Yes	?
Difficulty to learn	Intermediate	Most	Least
Safety	Intermediate	Least	Most
Expense	Intermediate	Most	Least

From Eastwood GL. Endoscopy in gastrointestinal bleeding: Are we beginning to realize the dream? *J Clin Gastroenterol.* 1992;14:187. Reprinted with permission.

selective arteriography in detecting active bleeding; a "positive" scan requires a lower rate of bleeding (0.1 mL per minute vs. 0.5–1.0 mL per minute) but is less specific than arteriography in locating the site of bleeding.

C. Selective arteriography of the celiac axis, superior mesenteric artery, inferior mesenteric artery, or their branches can be both diagnostic and therapeutic.

   1. Diagnosis. A focal extravasation of dye usually indicates an arterial bleeding source. A diffuse blush in the region of the stomach may be found in hemorrhagic gastritis. During the venous phase, esophageal, gastric, or intestinal varices may be seen, although actual variceal bleeding cannot be documented by arteriography.

   2. Treatment. Injection of autologous clot or small pieces of gelatin sponge (Gelfoam) has been used to embolize arteries supplying localized bleeding sites. Infusion of vasopressin, 0.1 to 0.5 units per minute, into the arterial supply of the bleeding site also has been effective in controlling bleeding. Variceal bleeding may be controlled by vasopressin infusion into the superior mesenteric artery, thereby diminishing splanchnic blood flow and reducing portal venous pressure. Administration of vasopressin by peripheral vein at a rate of 0.3 to 1.0 units per minute is as effective as intraarterial vasopressin in the control of variceal bleeding. Moreover, the frequency of cardiovascular side effects after peripheral venous versus arterial vasopressin infusion is similar. In most patients who receive vasopressin for the control of variceal bleeding, therefore, a peripheral venous route is preferred. Intravenous infusion of nitroglycerin may reduce the hazard of vasopressin in patients at risk for ischemic cardiovascular disease. Intravenous infusion of octreotide is as effective and safer than vasopressin and is preferred.

D. Barium-contrast radiographic studies. Upper gastrointestinal series and barium enema usually provide a lower diagnostic yield than endoscopic studies. In addition, the presence of barium in the stomach or intestine can make endoscopic visualization of the mucosa difficult and can render an arteriogram uninterpretable. For these reasons, barium-contrast studies are not recommended in the initial diagnostic evaluation of patients with acute gastrointestinal bleeding.

III. GASTRIC AND ANTISECRETORY AGENTS. Because gastric acid plays a pathogenic role in many causes of upper gastrointestinal bleeding, it is reasonable to inhibit acid secretion with antisecretory agents such as histamine-2 (H_2) antagonists, or proton-pump inhibitors (PPIs). The intent is to maintain the intraluminal gastric pH above 4.0. This is difficult to achieve with the use of H_2 antagonists. PPIs inhibit gastric acid secretion much more effectively and at adequate doses increase the gastric pH to above 4. In the United States, pantoprazole sodium (Protonix), esomeprazole (Nexium), and lansoprazole (Prevacid) are available in intravenous form as well as in an oral formulation.

   The reduction of intraluminal acid may be effective in two ways. First, the direct, harmful effects of acid and pepsin on the bleeding lesion are diminished. Second, a less acid environment allows platelets to aggregate and thus promotes clotting. After the NG tube is removed, the patient is treated with an antisecretory agent, preferably with a PPI. A bolus of 80 mg of intravenous PPI is administered, followed by a continuous infusion at 80 mg an hour up to 72 hours.

IV. SPECIAL CONSIDERATIONS

A. Esophageal varices. The treatment of bleeding esophageal varices differs substantially from the treatment of other bleeding lesions of the upper gastrointestinal tract. Moreover, patients with esophageal varices typically have severe liver disease and thus are likely to suffer from poor nutrition, blood clotting disorders, and encephalopathy, all of which can adversely affect morbidity and mortality.

   1. Initial treatment. Figure 14-3 outlines a scheme for the management of bleeding esophageal varices. There is no single correct approach to the control of variceal hemorrhage; although in most institutions endoscopic band ligation or injection sclerosis are the initial choices of treatment. These procedures are

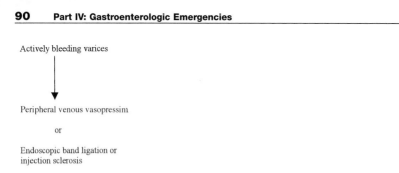

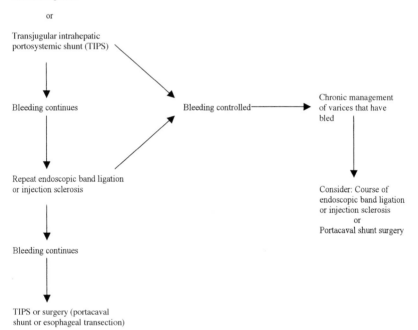

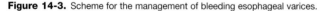

Figure 14-3. Scheme for the management of bleeding esophageal varices.

equally effective or better tolerated than surgical procedures such as portosystemic shunts and esophageal transection in controlling acute variceal bleeding.

Endoscopic band ligation of esophageal varices has been shown to be as effective as **injection sclerosis** in controlling bleeding: It eradicates the varices more rapidly than sclerosis and reduces the adverse side effects, such as fever, chest pain, esophageal ulceration, and pleural effusion that have been associated with sclerotherapy. **Infusion of octreotide (a synthetic analog of somatostatin)** has been shown to be effective in controlling esophageal varied bleeding. Octreotide given as 50 μg bolus, then 50 μg per hour administered intravenously for 2 to 5 days has replaced vasopressin as the medical therapy of choice for acute variceal bleeding. In some studies, **the combination of octreotide and**

endoscopic therapy has been shown to improve outcome as compared to endoscopic therapy alone.

2. **Balloon tamponade by Sengstaken-Blakemore tube.** The triple-lumen Sengstaken-Blakemore (SB) tube is representative of several tubes that can compress gastroesophageal varices by balloon tamponade. One lumen is used to evacuate the stomach. The second and third lumens lead to the gastric and esophageal balloons, respectively. Because use of the SB tube has been associated with serious complications, including occlusion of the airway by the esophageal balloon, pulmonary aspiration of secretions and blood from the esophagus, and ischemic necrosis of the esophageal mucosa due to prolonged compression by the balloon, the following steps are recommended:

   a. Use a new SB tube in each patient.

   b. Before passing the SB tube, fill the balloons with sufficient air to test for leaks.

   c. Deflate the balloons, lubricate well, and pass the tube through either the nose or the mouth into the stomach.

   d. After inflating the gastric balloon with 100 mL of air, pull it up firmly against the gastroesophageal junction and inject another 150 to 200 mL of air into the balloon, bringing the total amount of air to 250 to 300 mL.

   e. Secure the SB tube externally by taping the tube to the nose or mouth or to the bar of a football helmet or baseball catcher's face mask worn by the patient. This type of traction may be termed passive traction. It serves to maintain traction on the gastric balloon but, in the event of deflation, does not pull the tube up to occlude the airway. Never apply active traction such as might be accomplished by tying the external end of the SB tube to a weight hanging over a pulley.

   f. Pass an accessory sump tube into the esophagus to suction blood and secretions. (Some SB-type tubes already have a fourth lumen that permits esophageal suction.) If no fresh blood is aspirated from the esophagus, either the bleeding originates below the esophagus or bleeding from esophageal varices has stopped. If no fresh blood is aspirated from the intragastric lumen of the SB tube under these circumstances, one can presume that the bleeding originated from varices in the gastric cardia that are being compressed by the gastric balloon.

   g. If fresh blood is aspirated from the esophagus, inflate the esophageal balloon to a pressure of 35 to 40 mmHg. This is accomplished by connecting the external lumen of the esophageal balloon via a Y-connector to a blood pressure manometer. Continue to suction secretions from the esophagus above the balloon by means of the accessory sump tube or, if present, the fourth lumen.

   h. Deflate the esophageal balloon for about 30 minutes every 12 hours.

   i. Tape a scissors to the wall beside the patient's head. If the tube needs to be removed emergently or after it is no longer needed, it can be cut as it exits the nose or mouth, thereby instantly deflating the balloons and facilitating prompt removal. The scissors also serve as a visible reminder of the dangers of the SB tube.

   j. In most patients, use of the SB tube does not exceed 48 hours. By that time, bleeding has been controlled or more definitive therapy by means of endoscopic sclerosis or portosystemic shunt surgery has been instituted.

3. **Transjugular intrahepatic portosystemic shunt (TIPS).** Patients who continue to bleed despite endoscopic therapy or have bleeding gastric varices may require a portosystemic shunt. Since surgical morbidity and mortality are very high in open portosystemic shunt procedures, TIPS has been developed as a less invasive procedure often performed by interventional radiologists. TIPS has been shown to decrease rebleeding more effectively than endoscopic therapy, band ligation, or injection sclerotherapy. However, most patients with TIPS experience shunt stenosis within 1 to 2 years and require reinstrumentation, and many patients develop hepatic encephalopathy. Thus, TIPS is preferred for

patients with severe liver disease and for those who may require liver transplantation. Patients with compensated cirrhosis may be better treated with distal splenorenal shunt-type portosystemic shunt surgery.

4. **Long-term management.** After acute variceal bleeding has been controlled by endoscopic variceal banding or injection sclerosis, octreotide infusion, or balloon tamponade, a decision regarding long-term management of the varices must be made. Some physicians elect no specific therapy, hoping that bleeding will not recur. Because the risk of rebleeding is high, however, some form of treatment usually is indicated. The daily oral administration of beta-blockers (e.g., nadolol) and nitrates (e.g., isosorbide dinitrate) has been shown to reduce portal hypertension in patients and decrease the risk of rebleeding. Because long-term survival appears to be increased after repeated endoscopic band ligation or injection sclerosis to eradicate the varices or portosystemic shunt surgery, most patients should be considered for one of these treatments. Total health care costs are probably less and the risk of encephalopathy is lower in patients who undergo band ligation or injection sclerosis. Thus, repeated endoscopic band ligation or injection sclerosis, consisting of repeated injections separated by 1 to 4 weeks for several months, is a reasonable first choice.

   Complications of endoscopic band ligation and injection sclerosis include acute perforation of the esophagus, mucosal ulceration and necrosis, and stricture formation. Patients who have recurrent variceal bleeding despite band ligation and injection sclerotherapy and whose risk of surgery is acceptable may benefit from portosystemic shunt surgery.

B. **Mallory-Weiss gastroesophageal tear.** Bleeding from a Mallory-Weiss mucosal tear at the esophagogastric junction traditionally has been associated with repeated vomiting or retching before the appearance of hematemesis. However, in a large review of patients with documented Mallory-Weiss lesions, such a history was obtained in less than one third of the patients. The diagnosis of Mallory-Weiss mucosal tear must be made by endoscopic visualization of the lesion. Most patients stop bleeding spontaneously. In those with active bleeding, endoscopic placement of clips, bipolar electrocautery or injection of epinephrine may be used successfully.

C. **Aortoenteric fistula.** Patients with an aortoenteric fistula typically have massive hematemesis or hematochezia. The bleeding may stop abruptly; if it recurs, it often is fatal. This is a surgical emergency and immediate surgical intervention is necessary.

Selected Readings

Angtuaes TL, et al. The utility of urgent colonoscopy in the evaluation of acute lower gastrointestinal tract bleeding: A 2-year experience from a single center. *Am J Gastroenterol.* 2001;96:1782.

Bardou M, et al. Meta-analysis proton pump inhibition in high-risk patients with acute peptic ulcer bleeding. *Aliment Pharmacol Ther.* 2005;21:677–686.

Bianco MA, et al. Combined epinephrine and bipolar coagulation vs. bipolar coagulation alone for bleeding peptic ulcer: A randomized, controlled trial. *Gastrointest Endosc.* 2004;60:910–915.

Chan FK, et al. Preventing recurrent upper gastrointestinal bleeding in patients with *Helicobacter pylori* infection who are taking low-dose aspirin or naproxen. *N Engl J Med.* 2001;344:967.

Chan FKL, et al. Combination of a cyclo-oxygenase 2 inhibitor and a proton-pump inhibitor for prevention of recurrent ulcer bleeding in patients at very high risk: a double-blind, randomised trial. *Lancet.* 2007 May 12;369:1621–6.

Cipolletta L, et al. Endoclips versus heater probe in preventing early recurrent bleeding from peptic ulcer: A prospective and randomized trial. *Gastrointest Endosc.* 2001; 53:147–151.

Corely DA, et al. Octreotide for acute esophageal variceal bleeding: A meta analysis. *Gastroenterology.* 2001;120:946.

A 40-year-old woman with epistaxis, hematemesis, and altered mental status. Case records of the Massachusetts General Hospital. *N Engl J Med.* 2007;356:174–182.

Geier A, et al. Profuse rectal bleeding of no visible cause. *Lancet.* 2007;369:1664.

Gerson LB, et al. Endoscopic band ligation for actively bleeding Dieulafoy's lesions. *Gastrointest Endosc.* 1999;50:454.

Howarth DM. The role of nuclear medicine in the detection of acute gastrointestinal bleeding. *Semin Nucl Med.* 2006;36:133–46.

Lau JY, et al. Oweprazole before endoscopy in patients with gastrointestinal bleeding. *N Eng J Med.* 2007;356:1631–1640.

Lau JUW, et al. Effect of intravenous omeprazole on recurrent bleeding after endoscopic treatment of bleeding ulcers. *N Engl J Med.* 2000;343:310.

Leontiadis GI. Proton pump inhibitor treatment for acute peptic ulcer bleeding. *Cochrane Database Syst Rev.* 2006;1:CD002094.

Park JJ. Meckel diverticulum: the Mayo Clinic experience with 1476 patients (1950–2002). *Ann Surg.* 2005;241:529–33.

Sanyal AJ. Octreotide and its effects on portal circulation. *Gastroenterology.* 2001;120:303.

Schmulewitz N, et al. Dieulafoy lesions: A review of 6 years of experience at a tertiary care center. *Am J Gastroenterol.* 2001;96:1688.

Sharara AI, et al. Gastroesophageal variceal hemorrhage. *N Engl J Med.* 2001;345:669, 2001.

Sung JJY, et al. The effect of endoscopic therapy in patients receiving omeprazole for bleeding ulcers with nonbleeding visible vessels or adherent clots. A randomized comparison. *Ann Intern Med.* 2003;139:237–243.

Villanueva C, et al. Endoscopic ligation compared with combined treatment with nadolol and isosorbide mononitrate to prevent recurrent variceal bleeding. *N Engl J Med.* 2001; 345:647.

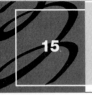

15 FOREIGN BODIES IN THE GASTROINTESTINAL TRACT

*F*oreign bodies may be deliberately or accidentally swallowed or introduced into the lower gastrointestinal tract from the rectum. The most frequent victims are young children, persons with dentures, and individuals who are inebriated or mentally impaired.

There are no controlled studies for the management of foreign bodies in the gastrointestinal tract. Each situation needs to be evaluated depending on the nature of the foreign body, the symptoms, the condition of the patient, and the organs involved. Most ingested foreign bodies pass safely through the intestinal tract between 48 hours and 1 month after ingestion. Some objects may result in obstruction or perforation and may require endoscopic or surgical intervention. Sharp objects such as pins, toothpicks, and bones may cause perforation, especially in the esophagus and the ileocecal area. Patients may have pain, sepsis, mediastinitis, peritonitis, hemorrhage, abscess, or abdominal mass.

I. **ESOPHAGUS.** Foreign bodies may cause obstruction above the upper esophageal sphincter and may compromise the airway. These patients should be urgently handled by ear, nose, and throat specialists.

Most obstructions from foreign body ingestions involve the esophagus; many occur above a benign or malignant stricture, web, or ring. The four areas of physiologic narrowing in the esophagus—the cricopharyngeal muscle, the aortic arch, the left main-stem bronchus, and the gastroesophageal junction—are also common sites for obstruction. Sharp objects such as fish or poultry bones, pins, or toothpicks may perforate the esophagus, resulting in sepsis or hemorrhage. Button (miniature, 7.9–11.6 mm) battery ingestions are not uncommon in children. Most of these spontaneously pass; however, those with larger diameters (15.6–23.0 mm) may impact in the esophagus, causing tissue necrosis, perforation, or hemorrhage.

A. **Clinical findings**
   1. **Signs and symptoms.** Acute esophageal obstruction may result in substernal pain at the level of obstruction or be referred to the sternal notch. The pain may be mild or severe or may mimic a myocardial infarction. There may be profuse salivation and regurgitation. In patients who have ingested a sharp object like a fish bone, odynophagia and a sensation of the object lodged in the esophagus may be present.
   2. **Physical examination** is usually unrewarding. When perforation is suspected, subcutaneous air in the soft tissues should be sought by looking for crepitus by palpation of the upper thorax and neck.

B. **Diagnostic tests**
   1. **Radiographic techniques**
      a. **Photographic densities.** Plain x-rays are frequently used in the detection of foreign bodies. However, not all foreign bodies are radiopaque due to differences in their densities.
         i. **Foreign bodies of high density** are highly radiopaque and have low photographic density on a radiograph. If the object is of adequate size, it is easily differentiated from the surrounding tissues. Common examples include objects made of iron, steel, and some alloys, as in nails, screws, chips, bullets, and many coins.
         ii. **Foreign bodies with physical densities somewhat higher than body tissues** (e.g., glass, aluminum, chicken bones, plastics) have photographic densities slightly less than body tissues and form more subtle images.

    iii. Body-density foreign bodies possess the same photographic density as the surrounding body tissues and are virtually impossible to detect in radiographs. Thorns, cactus needles, sea- and freshwater animal spines, some plastics, and wood that has been in the body for more than 48 hours are common examples.

    iv. When the density of the object is less than the density of surrounding body tissues, it appears darker. Some examples of this type of foreign body are wood immediately after introduction into the body, materials containing air, and some plastics.

    v. Glass, contrary to the general assumption that it is radiolucent, is in fact radiopaque compared to body tissues. Leaded crystal and optical glass are highly radiopaque.

    vi. Aluminum is of low physical density and may be difficult to detect radiographically. Aluminum alloy, pennies, and pull-top rings of aluminum soda cans are commonly ingested and may not be detected in plain films.

    vii. Wood, when dry, immediately after ingestion appears radiolucent due to its lower physical density than body tissues. However, within 24 to 48 hours it absorbs water, becomes isodense to body tissues, and may not be visible on the plain films.

  b. X-ray views. When the location of a foreign body is to be determined radiographically, two views at 90 degrees to each other (e.g., anteroposterior and lateral films) are recommended with techniques used for evaluation of bones. Additional tangential views may be obtained to gain more information about the depth of the foreign body.

  c. Contrast studies. When the information from the plain radiographs is inadequate, the use of contrast media may be required. Water-soluble contrast agents or barium may be used. Because barium may interfere with proper visualization of the object at endoscopy, however, a water-soluble contrast agent such as Gastrografin is preferred. If perforation is suspected, the leak may also be evaluated using a water-soluble contrast study.

2. Endoscopy. Esophageal foreign bodies may be directly visualized by flexible endoscopy after adequate sedation of the patient. Intravenous glucagon may be necessary to relax the esophagus.

C. Management

  1. Esophageal relaxation. After a detailed history regarding the nature and timing of the ingestion is obtained, if no complications are suspected, mild sedation and esophageal relaxation with intravenous glucagon may allow spontaneous passage of the foreign body. The patient should be kept in an upright posture, or the head of the bed should be elevated. In cases of obstruction, a nasogastric tube may be placed in the esophagus above the object, and secretions may be suctioned to decrease the risk of aspiration. Intravenous fluids should be used to prevent dehydration of the patient.

  2. When a meat bolus is lodged in the distal esophagus, enzymatic dissolution with papain has been used (e.g., Adolph's Meat Tenderizer). Papain, however, may lead to esophageal wall digestion and perforation or pulmonary aspiration; thus, we do not recommend its use.

  3. Endoscopy. Food boluses or other foreign bodies may be removed endoscopically using forceps, snares, or baskets. An overtube, placed around the intraesophageal portion of the endoscope and the object, will protect the esophageal mucosa and the airway as the object is pulled out in the endoscope. General anesthesia may be necessary in children and uncooperative patients. Sharp objects and those that are embedded in the esophageal wall may require surgical removal.

II. STOMACH

  A. Clinical findings. Foreign bodies in the stomach usually do not cause any symptoms. The presence of nausea and vomiting may indicate pyloric obstruction; pain, bleeding, and fever may suggest mucosal injury or perforation.

B. Diagnosis

1. **Chest and abdominal radiographs** help in determining the location and nature of the swallowed object. Contrast studies may be needed if the object cannot be visualized by plain films or if there is a question of perforation. The presence of air under the diaphragm also should be ascertained.

2. **Endoscopy** visualizes the foreign object, but this may be difficult when the stomach is full of food.

C. Management. Most ingested objects that have made their way into the stomach pass through the pylorus and the rest of the gastrointestinal tract. Most coins, such as dimes and nickels, do not cause obstruction, but quarters may not pass in children. With rounded objects, it is thought to be safe to wait several days for the spontaneous passage of the foreign body. The progress is followed by daily x-rays. Because objects may become embedded in the wall of the stomach after several days, endoscopic removal is advised. However, bones, denture fragments, pencils, toothpicks, needles, razor blades, and other sharp objects should be removed immediately, endoscopically or surgically. Induced vomiting, especially in intoxicated persons and in children, carries the risk of aspiration of the gastric contents and the foreign body and is not recommended.

III. SMALL BOWEL

A. Most objects that have passed through the pylorus will also pass through the small bowel and the ileocecal valve. Long, thin objects may hang up in the angulations of the duodenum, the angle of Treitz, and the ileocecal area.

B. Management. Objects beyond the second portion of the duodenum cannot be retrieved endoscopically. Their progress may be followed radiologically. If pain, fever, distention, vomiting, or bleeding develops, the patient should be surgically explored. Stimulation of bowel motility by laxatives and cathartics may be harmful, especially when the object is sharp. Mineral oil, stool softeners, or bulking agents may be useful, but their efficacy has not been studied.

IV. COLON AND RECTUM

A. Occasionally, **swallowed** objects may hang up in the cecum or the sigmoid colon. These objects may be retrieved with the colonoscope.

B. Many objects have been **inserted** into the rectum and sigmoid colon for sexual stimulation, or by individuals who are mentally impaired. Most of these objects may be retrieved using flexible or rigid sigmoidoscopic techniques. Patients may need general anesthesia for cooperation and for relaxation of the anal sphincter. If perforation or mucosal injury is suspected, surgical intervention may be necessary.

Selected Readings

Athanassiadi K, et al. Management of esophageal foreign bodies: A retrospective review of 400 cases. *Eur J Cardio Thorac Surg.* 2002;21:653–656.

Focht D, Kaul A. Food impaction and eosinophilic esophagitis. *J Ped.* 2005;147:540.

Janik JE, et al. Forceps extraction of upper esophageal coins. *J Pediatr Surg.* 2003;38: 227–229.

Jeen YT, et al. Endoscopic removal of sharp foreign bodies impacted in the esophagus. *Endoscopy.* 2001;33:518–522.

Lam HC, et al. Esophageal perforation and neck abscess from ingested foreign bodies: Treatment outcomes. *Ear Nose Throat J.* 2003;82:786–794.

Mosca S, et al. Endoscopic management of foreign bodies in the upper gastrointestinal tract: Report on a series of 414 adult patients. *Endoscopy.* 2001;33:692–696.

Panda NK, et al. Management of sharp esophageal foreign bodies in young children: A cause for worry. *Int J Pediatr Otorhinolaryngol.* 2002;64:243–246.

Soprano JV, et al. Four strategies for the management of esophageal coins in children. *Pediatrics.* 2000;105:e5.

Vanelli PM, et al. Exploring the link between eosivephilic esophagitis and esophageal foreign bodies in the pediatric population. *Pract Gastroenterol.* 2007;xxx1(10):81–85.

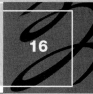

CAUSTIC INGESTION   16

$\mathcal{T}$he ingestion of caustic chemicals may cause tissue injury on contact with the oropharynx, esophagus, stomach, and duodenum. Accidental ingestion of these caustic or corrosive substances is most frequent in small children and inebriated individuals. Intentional ingestion occurs more commonly in persons who are suicidal.

Caustic substances can be divided into acids and alkalis. Many household and industrial products contain acids or alkalis in liquid or solid form (Tables 16-1 and 16-2).

I. ALKALI INGESTION. Alkalis (e.g., lye–sodium or potassium hydroxide) are ingested more frequently than acids. Alkalis produce injury by liquefaction necrosis, which allows deep penetration into the tissues, resulting in full-thickness tissue burns.

TABLE 16-1   Common Alkalis

Sodium or potassium hydroxide (lye)
   Detergents and washing powders
   Paint removers
   Drain cleaners (Drano [granular and liquid], Liquid Plumr, Plunge, Open-Up)
   Oven cleaners (Easy-Off, Mr. Muscle)
   Clinitest tablets
   Denalan denture cleanser (NaOH is formed *in vivo*)
Sodium hypochlorite
   Bleaches (Clorox)
   Cleansers
Sodium borates, carbonates, phosphates, and silicates
   Detergents
   Electric dishwashing preparations
   Water softeners
   Purex bleach
Ammonia
   Toilet bowl cleaners (Lysol)
   Metal cleaners and polishers
   Hair dyes and tints
   Antirust products
   Jewelry cleaners
Sodium permanganate
   Illegitimate abortifacient medical applications (topical)
Phosphorus
   Matches
   Rodenticides
   Insecticides
   Fireworks

NaOH, sodium hydroxide.

TABLE 16-2	Common Acids

Hydrochloric acid (muriatic acid)
  Metal cleaners (Quaker House Steam Iron Cleaner)
  Toilet bowl cleaners (Lysol liquid toilet bowl cleaner, Sno Bol)
  Swimming pool cleaners
Sulfuric acid
  Battery acid
  Drain cleaners (Mister Plumber, Rooto)
Sodium bisulfite
  Toilet bowl cleaners (Sani Flush [granular], Varnish [granular])
Oxalic acid
  Disinfectants
  Furniture polish
  Zud Rust and Stain Remover (granular)
Hydrofluoric acid
  Antirust products
Formaldehyde (formic acid)
  Deodorizing tablets
  Plastic menders
  Fumigants
  Embalming agents
Carbolic acid (phenol-creosol, creosote)
  Antiseptics
  Preservatives

A. **The severity of the tissue injury** after caustic ingestion depends on the nature, concentration, and quantity of the caustic substance and the duration of tissue contact. The higher the pH, the more destructive is the alkaline agent. The critical pH that causes esophageal ulceration is 12.5. Most cases of deep ulceration that progress to stricture formation involve lye solutions of pH 14.0.

B. **Areas of injury.** The oropharynx and esophagus are most commonly injured in alkali ingestions. Twenty to thirty percent of the patients who have esophageal injury also have gastric injury. The severity of the injury varies from inflammation and ulceration to necrosis and perforation of the viscera.

  1. **Solid alkali ingestion.** Alkali swallowed in solid form adheres on contact to mucous membranes of the oropharynx or esophagus, usually sparing the stomach. If solid alkali is swallowed with water, it is carried further down the digestive tract.

  2. **Liquid alkali ingestion,** especially of lye, exposes most of the mucosal surface of the oropharynx and upper gastrointestinal tract to the caustic substance. The esophagus is the most commonly injured organ. The stomach is also usually injured. In addition to ulceration and necrosis of the affected tissues, bleeding may occur after liquid-lye ingestion. Respiratory distress secondary to soft-tissue swelling of the epiglottis, larynx, vocal cords, or trachea may occur due to aspiration of lye. Tracheoesophageal fistulas may develop after severe injury. The most common delayed complication of lye ingestion is esophageal stricture formation. Strictures may involve a variable length of the esophagus, ranging from a focal narrowing to complete stenosis of the entire esophagus. Antral scarring and pyloric stenosis also have been reported.

II. ACID INGESTION

A. Types of acids. A number of commercially available household substances contain caustic acids (e.g., toilet bowl cleaners, disinfectants, automobile battery acids, soldering fluxes). These substances may contain hydrochloric, sulfuric, nitric, phosphoric, and trichloroacetic acids as well as phenol, zinc chloride, mercurial salts, and formaldehyde (formic acid). Sulfuric acid is the most corrosive of these acids. However, hydrochloric and nitric acids are volatile and may predispose the patient to chemical pneumonitis in addition to gastrointestinal tract injury.

B. Tissue injury. Caustic acids produce coagulation necrosis, forming a firm protective eschar that may limit deep-tissue injury. They tend to pass rapidly through the esophagus and usually produce shallow burns, except in cases where there are anatomic or motility disorders. In the stomach, the acids usually flow along the lesser curve to the pylorus. Pylorospasm results in pooling of the acid in the antrum, where the worst of the damage occurs. The range of tissue injury is diffuse gastritis, hemorrhagic ulceration, and necrosis leading to perforation of the stomach. Gastric perforation may lead to mediastinitis, peritonitis, and shock.

III. CLINICAL EVALUATION

A. History. A detailed history should be obtained from the patient or family to determine the type of caustic agent ingested, the time and quantity of ingestion, whether the patient took anything by mouth before or after the ingestion, and whether vomiting has occurred. If possible, the container and contents should be examined and the pH of the substance determined.

B. The physical examination should include vital signs, attention to respiratory status, and signs pertaining to possible perforation of the esophagus or stomach. The presence of fever, respiratory distress, subcutaneous air, or signs of peritoneal irritation should be noted.

IV. INITIAL MANAGEMENT

A. If **cardiovascular or respiratory distress** is present, a central venous line should be placed immediately, the airway should be protected, and the patient resuscitated. Arterial blood gases and a complete blood count should be obtained, and a surgeon should be notified.

B. In the event of respiratory distress with **swelling of soft tissues of the upper airway,** tracheostomy may be necessary because blind nasotracheal intubation may cause perforation.

C. Upright x-ray films of the chest and abdomen should be obtained and examined for signs of aspiration and perforation of the esophagus or stomach.

D. Initially, patients should receive **nothing by mouth.** Gastric lavage or emesis is contraindicated due to the risks of aspiration, reexposing the damaged tissues to the caustic agent, and perforation.

E. The use of **diluents** is controversial. Neutralization of alkali with acid or acids with alkali commonly results in an exothermic reaction. The resulting heat may produce thermal injury and further tissue damage. Water and milk have been shown to cause minimal temperature elevation, but they may contribute to increased esophageal and gastric volume and motility and may increase the already existing tissue damage. Thus, their use and the use of activated charcoal and cathartics are not recommended.

F. Morphine sulfate or **meperidine hydrochloride** may be used for pain control after the patient's condition is stabilized.

V. DIAGNOSIS OF TISSUE INJURY

A. Barium or soluble contrast studies of the esophagus and stomach do not accurately demonstrate the degree and extent of initial tissue injury. Adherent barium also may obscure the mucosa from endoscopic observation. Thus, contrast radiologic studies are not recommended for initial diagnostic evaluation. If a perforation is suspected, however, a radiologic study using a soluble contrast material may be performed to localize the site of perforation. After 1 to 2 months, the extent of fibrosis and stricture formation may be assessed periodically by radiocontrast studies.

B. Endoscopy of the upper gastrointestinal tract within the first 24 hours of ingestion is recommended to establish the extent and severity of the tissue damage and to remove by suction any remaining caustic material from the stomach. Rigid scopes should not be used. Endoscopes with diameters less than 1 cm are safe in experienced hands. If esophageal or gastric perforation is suspected clinically or from plain films, endoscopy should not be performed.

C. The severity of tissue injury is classified by endoscopic appearance.

Grade 0: Normal endoscopic examination

Grade I: Edema and hyperemia of the mucosa

Grade IIa: Friability, hemorrhages, erosions, blisters, whitish membranes or exudates, superficial ulcerations

Grade IIb: Grade IIa plus deep discrete or circumferential ulcerations

Grade IIIa: Grade II plus multiple ulcerations and small scattered areas of necrosis (areas of brown-black or grayish discolorations)

Grade IIIb: Grade II plus extensive necrosis

VI. THERAPY

A. Patients with grade 0 and grade I injuries are expected to heal with no specific therapy. They should receive nothing by mouth until they can eat without discomfort. A barium swallow and upper gastrointestinal series may be done after 1 to 2 months to look for scarring and strictures.

B. Patients with grade IIa and some patients with grade IIb injuries recover rapidly and may be discharged from the hospital within 5 to 12 days. Healing usually occurs by the third or fourth week without sequelae. Some grade II and all grade III injuries heal with scarring. Complications such as hemorrhage and perforation should be carefully looked for in patients with grades IIb and III injuries. Most patients with grade IIIb injury require immediate surgical attention.

C. Patients with **more extensive tissue injury** should be treated in the intensive care unit with special attention to the possibility of viscous perforation. To protect the injured tissues, the upper gastrointestinal tract should not be used. Total parenteral nutrition should be started immediately. Intravenous histamine-2 (H_2)-blocker therapy may be used to reduce gastroduodenal acidity to prevent further acid–peptic injury.

D. Steroids. In pharmacologic doses, corticosteroids impair wound healing, depress immune defense mechanisms, and mask the signs of infection and viscous perforation. They cannot salvage an already injured organ. Because the risks outweigh the possible benefits, their use is not recommended.

E. Antibiotics. Serious infections are infrequent with caustic injury. In first- or second-degree burns, antibiotics should be withheld until evidence of infection is present. In patients in whom the possibility of perforation exists, antibiotics are recommended to reduce the risk of infectious mediastinitis or peritonitis.

F. Surgery. The coordinated intensive efforts of both medical and surgical teams are necessary for the best outcome in patients severely injured with caustic ingestion. In the event of extensive tissue necrosis, perforation, peritonitis, or severe hemorrhage, emergency surgery may be necessary.

In severe gastric burns, antral and pyloric stenosis may require partial or total gastrectomy. Total gastrectomy and esophageal replacement may be necessary in cases of simultaneous severe esophageal and gastric injury.

G. Stricture formation is usually noted 2 to 8 weeks after a second- or third-degree caustic injury with circumferential lesions.

  1. Dilatation. Single and minor strictures usually respond to repeated dilatation. However, because early dilatation increases the risk of perforation, it should be delayed until after the acute injury has healed.

  2. Surgery. Extensive esophageal strictures may require surgical resection with transposition of a segment of jejunum or colon. Placement of an intraluminal silicone stent under endoscopic guidance for 4 to 6 weeks has been used to prevent severe stricture formation.

H. Long-term follow-up. Esophageal and gastric cancer may develop in the scarred mucosa 10 to 15 years after the initial injury. These patients require ongoing clinical and endoscopic surveillance and follow-up.

Selected Readings

Bernhardt J, et al. Caustic acid burn of the upper gastrointestinal tract: First use of endosonography to evaluate the severity of injury. *Surg Endosc.* 2002;16:1004.

Boukhir S, et al. High doses of steroids in the management of caustic esophageal strictures in children. *Arch Pediatr.* 2004;11:13–17.

Erdogan E, et al. Esophageal replacement using the colon: A 15-year review. *Pediatr Surg.* 2000;16:546–549.

Hamza AF, et al. Caustic esophageal strictures in children: 30-year experience. *J Pediatr Surg.* 2003;38:828–833.

Katzka DA, et al. Caustic injury to the esophagus: Current treatment options. *Gastroenterology.* 2001;4:59–66.

Kukkody A, et al. Long-term dilation of caustic strictures of the esophagus. *Pediatr Surg Int.* 2002;18:486–490.

Nunes AC, et al. Risk factors for stricture development after caustic ingestion. *Hepatogastroenterology.* 2002;49:1563–1566.

Zwischenberger JB, et al. Surgical aspects of esophageal disease. Perforation and caustic injury. *Am J Repir Crit Care Med.* 2001;164:1037–1040.

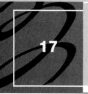

17 FULMINANT HEPATIC FAILURE AND ENCEPHALOPATHY

*F*ulminant hepatic failure (FHF), acute hepatic failure, and **fulminant hepatitis** all refer to acute severe impairment of liver function accompanied by coagulopathy, advanced stages encephalopathy, and coma in patients who have had liver disease for less than 8 weeks. FHF, in most instances, is complicated by multiorgan failure and cerebral edema, lasts 1 to 4 weeks, and ends fatally in 60% to 95% of patients. FHF is a rare condition with an incidence of 2,000 cases per year in the United States.

In a subgroup of patients, the duration of illness before the onset of encephalopathy is more prolonged **(subacute FHF)** but as in FHF, there is no evidence of previous liver disease. In patients with late-onset hepatic failure, hepatic encephalopathy and other evidence of hepatic decompensation appear between 8 and 24 weeks after the first symptoms. Patients with late-onset disease are significantly older than those who have FHF; median ages of onset are 44.5 years and 25.5 years, respectively.

Liver transplantation may be the ultimate solution in FHF.

New terminology has been introduced and is based on the interval from the onset of jaundice to the development of encephalopathy.

> **Hyperacute liver failure,** with an interval of <7 days
> **Acute liver failure,** with an interval of 8–28 days
> **Subacute liver failure,** with an interval of 4–12 weeks.

I. ETIOLOGY. Table 17-1 outlines the numerous causes of FHF.

   A. Hepatitis. FHF is most commonly seen with viral and toxic hepatitis. In fact, viruses are implicated in 75% of instances.

      1. FHF is most commonly seen with **hepatitis B virus (HBV)** infection; 1% of patients acutely infected with HBV may develop the syndrome. Thirty to forty percent of these patients may be infected concomitantly with the hepatitis delta virus (HDV). Infection with hepatitis A virus (HAV), and rarely hepatitis C virus (HCV), herpes simplex virus (HSV), cytomegalovirus (CMV), and parvovirus B19 also may lead to FHF. Enterically transmitted hepatitis E virus may cause FHF in pregnant women, especially in the third trimester.

      2. Acute toxic hepatitis may result from an idiosyncratic hypersensitivity reaction to a drug (e.g., halothane, isoniazid, rifampin, alpha-methyldopa) or from substances that are intrinsically toxic to the liver (e.g., acetaminophen, hydrocarbons, white phosphorus, some poisonous mushrooms).

      3. These toxic agents and viral infections cause **panlobular hepatic necrosis resulting** in FHF.

   B. Hepatic ischemia resulting from severe hypoxemia, hypotension, cardiac failure, or acute Budd-Chiari syndrome may cause extensive centrilobular hepatic necrosis and FHF.

   C. Wilson's disease may present as FHF accompanied by acute intravascular hemolysis.

   D. FHF may result from a group of disorders characterized by **acute extensive infiltration of hepatocytes with microdroplets of fat and minimal hepatocellular necrosis.** These disorders include Reye's syndrome, tetracycline induced fatty liver, fatty liver of pregnancy, fatty liver after jejunoileal bypass surgery, and acute alcoholic hepatitis. Dideoxyinosine (DDI) used in the treatment of acquired immunodeficiency syndrome (AIDS) also may cause this condition.

TABLE 17-1	Causes of Fulminant Hepatic Failure

Viral agents	
Hepatitis A virus	Herpes viruses
Hepatitis B virus	Adenovirus
Hepatitis C virus	Cytomegalovirus
Hepatitis D virus	Paramyxovirus
Hepatitis E virus	Epstein-Barr virus
Toxic substances	
Acetaminophen	Valproic acid
Halothane	Disulfiram
Isoniazid	Nortriptyline
Rifampicin	White or yellow phosphorus
Amine oxidase inhibitors	Emetic toxin of *Bacillus cereus*
Hydrocarbons	Mushroom poisoning (*Amanita phalloides*)
Carbon tetrachloride	Some herbal medicines
Nonsteroidal antiinflammatory drugs	Dideoxyinosine
Ischemic liver necrosis	
Wilson's disease with intravascular hemolysis	Shock (hypotension hypoxemia)
Acute Budd-Chiari syndrome	Autoimmune hepatitis
Congestive heart failure	Heat stroke
Acute steatosis syndromes	
Reye's syndrome	
Acute fatty liver of pregnancy	
Tetracycline	
Massive blastic infiltration of the liver	Hodgkin's lymphoma
Lymphoreticular malignancies	Burkitt-type lymphoma
Malignant histiocytosis	
Non-Hodgkin's lymphoma	
Acute leukemia	
Acute phase of chronic myelogenous leukemia	
Acute monoblastic leukemia	
Metastatic liver disease from primary lung or breast cancer and melanoma	

E. Rarely, FHF may develop in patients who have one of the **hematolymphoid malignancies,** such as malignant histiocytosis, Burkitt's lymphoma, the acute phase of chronic myelogenous leukemia, acute monoblastic leukemia, and Hodgkin's and non-Hodgkin's lymphomas. Massive infiltration of hepatic parenchyma with malignant cells results in infarction and necrosis, leading to FHF.

II. DIAGNOSIS. Serum aminotransferase (aspartate aminotransferase [AST], alanine aminotransferase [ALT]) and bilirubin levels may provide useful clues regarding the cause of FHF. In toxic or viral FHF, the serum aminotransferases are significantly elevated due to injury to the hepatocytes. In instances of acute fatty infiltration and mitochondrial damage, aminotransferases are only moderately elevated.

The presence in serum of IgM antibody to HAV supports the diagnosis of acute hepatitis A. The presence of hepatitis B surface antigen (HBsAg) or IgM antibody to hepatitis B core particle (HBcAb) or both and HBV-DNA in a patient with FHF favors hepatitis B as the etiologic agent. IgM antibody to the delta virus can be detected by serologic study only in patients carrying HBsAg. Antibody to hepatitis C may help in establishing the diagnosis of hepatitis C but may not be detectable in the acute phase of the disease. A mutant form of hepatitis B and rarely hepatitis C is implicated in most instances of late-onset hepatic failure. Determination of viral DNA or RNA titers of hepatitis B and C viruses by polymerase chain reaction respectively may give information that is more accurate in the cases of viral hepatitis B or C.

Liver biopsy may be helpful in establishing a diagnosis but may be difficult to perform because of the severe coagulopathy, which is not correctable with replacement of clotting factors.

III. PROGNOSIS. Survival from FHF depends on the ability of the liver to regenerate with restitution of the normal hepatic function. Prothrombin time greater than 100 seconds, regardless of the stage of encephalopathy or the presence of any three of the following findings, indicates a poor prognosis in FHF caused by viral hepatitis or drug toxicity excluding acetaminophen toxicity:

> Arterial pH <7.3
> Age <10 or >40 years
> Jaundice >7 days before the onset of encephalopathy
> Prothrombin time >50 seconds
> Serum bilirubin >18 mg/dL

Prognosis in FHF depends on the age of the patient, cause of the acute liver failure, clinical course, occurrence of secondary complications, and duration and severity of the coma.

A. Causes of death in FHF are neurologic complications (67%), gastrointestinal hemorrhage (13%), bacterial and/or fungal infection and sepsis (13%), hemodynamic complications (8%), and progressive respiratory and renal failure.

IV. CLINICAL SYNDROME

A. The encephalopathy of FHF may begin with mild confusion, irrational behavior, euphoria, or psychosis. It is usually associated with a widely fluctuating but progressive deterioration of the mental state. Coma may develop rapidly within several days of onset of symptoms.

1. The pathogenesis of hepatic encephalopathy (HE) is unknown, but there are several theories. HE is a potentially reversible metabolic disorder of the brain in the milieu of hepatic failure.

a. "Neurotoxic" substances. The ability of the liver to remove toxic substances from the circulation is important in the maintenance of normal brain function. In liver failure, it is assumed that neurotoxic substances normally extracted from portal venous blood and metabolized in the liver gain access to the systemic circulation and reach the brain parenchyma through a more permeable blood–brain barrier. These substances may be directly toxic to the neurons or may modulate neuronal function by causing changes in the metabolism of neurotransmitters or the functional status of the neurotransmitter receptors. The toxic substances most commonly implicated in hepatic failure are ammonia (NH_3), γ-aminobutyric acid (GABA), endogenous "benzodiazepines and opioids," mercaptans, **and fatty acids.**

b. "False neurotransmitters." Another theory implicates the accumulation of false neurotransmitters in the brain. In liver failure, the plasma ratio of aromatic amino acids (phenylalanine, tyrosine, and tryptophan) to branched-chain amino acids increases because of the impaired capacity of the liver to remove aromatic amino acids. It is thought that this circumstance permits greater entry of aromatic amino acids into the brain and promotes the synthesis of serotonin and false neurotransmitters (e.g., octopamine) at the expense of the true neurotransmitters (e.g., dopamine, norepinephrine) by competitive inhibition. The increase of inhibitory neurotransmitters and the deficiency of excitatory neurotransmitters may induce encephalopathic coma.

c. Multifactorial causes. Most likely the cause of HE in FHF is multifactorial with synergistic interactions among the various factors. Other causes of coma, such as hypoglycemia, hypoperfusion, anoxia, electrolyte disturbances, and brain edema, may contribute to its pathogenesis.

   d. Arterial NH₃. It has been customary to use arterial NH_3 levels to follow the course of hepatic encephalopathy. Even though the level of NH_3 does not correlate with the stage of encephalopathy in each patient, the levels help to establish trends. One must remember, however, that elevation of NH_3 may be an epiphenomenon that reflects the concentration of other neuroactive nitrogenous substances such as GABA that are involved in hepatic encephalopathy and coma.

  2. Neurologic assessment. Daily assessment of neurologic function is important in following the patient's course and therapy.

   a. A clinical coma scale (Tables 17-2 and 17-3) separately appraises the state of six brain and brainstem functions. There is a high correlation between best–worst initial coma scores and outcomes and the day-to-day changes in the score with improvement or deterioration. The presence or absence of oculovestibular reflexes has been the best predictor of outcome.

TABLE 17-2   **A Clinical Coma Profile for Bedside Use**

Verbal response	Oculocephalic–oculovestibular reflexes
None	No reaction
Incomprehensible	Partial or dysconjugate
Confused	Full
Normal	Normal
Eye opening	Best motor response
None	None
Noxious stimuli only	Abnormal extensor
Verbal stimuli	Abnormal flexor
Spontaneous	Withdraws or localizes
Pupils	Obeys commands
Nonreactive	Respiration
Sluggish	Nil or ventilator
Brisk	Irregular
	Regular >22 breaths/min
	Regular <22 breaths/min

TABLE 17-3   **Hepatic Encephalopathy Scale**

Grade	Neurologic status
0	No abnormality detected
1	Trivial lack of awareness, shortened attention span, impairment noted on arithmetic testing
2	Lethargy, disorientation in time, clear personality change, inappropriate behavior
3	Very drowsy, semicomatose but responsive to stimuli, confused, gross disorientation in time or space, bizarre behavior
4	Comatose, unresponsive to painful stimuli with or without abnormal movements (e.g., decorticate or decerebrate posturing)

  b. The electroencephalogram (EEG) pattern changes in a predictable way parallel with the neurologic state. Initially there is a slowing of the alpha rhythm. With increasing drowsiness, this phenomenon is replaced by lower frequency theta activity. As coma deepens, high-amplitude delta waves become prominent, and the characteristic triphasic waves appear. Preterminally the amplitude of these waves decreases, and finally the EEG becomes isoelectric.

  c. Visual-evoked potentials have been found to be superior to the EEG in terms of specificity and ease of quantitation of central neuronal activity associated with hepatic coma. However, auditory, somatosensory, and visual-evoked potentials are not widely available clinically.

  d. Assessment of cerebral edema. Cerebral edema, which may result in cerebellar or uncal herniation or both, is a frequent complication of FHF. The exact stage at which cerebral edema develops is difficult to determine clinically. Papilledema is seldom present. Findings from computed tomography or magnetic resonance imaging (MRI) scan of the head are usually normal. However, loss of definition between gray and white matter may be diagnostic of early cerebral edema. In advanced disease, the first clinical sign may be sudden respiratory arrest along with fixed and dilated pupils and absent brainstem reflexes, indicating tentorial herniation.

B. Renal, electrolyte, and acid-base abnormalities. Microvascular obstruction with cellular debris from the damaged liver affects most organs and especially the kidneys.

 1. Renal abnormalities. Renal failure is common in patients with FHF. Acute tubular necrosis with high urine sodium concentration (>20 mmol/L) and isosmolar urine occurs in some patients. Hepatorenal syndrome develops in about one half of the patients; it is characterized by low urine sodium concentration (<10 mmol/L), a hyperosmolar urine, and oliguria. This form of renal dysfunction does not improve unless there is simultaneous improvement in hepatic function. Renal dialysis in FHF has a high frequency of complications. Peritoneal dialysis is associated with peritonitis and intraperitoneal hemorrhage. Hemodialysis may lead to hypotension and gastrointestinal hemorrhage caused by the use of heparin. The most common indications for dialysis are volume overload, acidosis, and hyperkalemia.

 2. Electrolyte abnormalities are common in FHF. Hypokalemia is seen in the early stages. Hyponatremia is often associated with high renal retention of sodium and water and decreased free water clearance. Hypernatremia may follow multiple transfusions of fresh-frozen plasma or the use of osmotic diuretics.

 3. Alkalosis. Respiratory alkalosis is common in FHF and is thought to be central in origin. Metabolic alkalosis may be caused by hypokalemia. Gastric aspiration may potentiate this problem.

 4. Lactic acidosis is common, especially in patients with peripheral circulatory failure. If it is also associated with hypoglycemia, it may be caused by both failure of hepatic gluconeogenesis and increased anaerobic metabolism.

C. Respiratory disorders. Acute respiratory distress syndrome (ARDS) and unexpected respiratory arrest may occur at any time in FHF. Endotracheal intubation may facilitate delivery of oxygen when hypoxia supervenes and protect the airway from aspiration.

D. Cardiovascular disorders. An increased cardiac output is common. Central vasomotor depression with hypotension, cardiac arrhythmias including ventricular ectopy, heart block, and bradycardia may also occur.

E. Coagulation disorders. In FHF, hepatic protein synthesis is impaired. The synthesis of the proteins of the clotting cascade, the fibrinolytic proteins, and the inhibitors of the activated factors are all deranged. Because hepatic clearance is also impaired, coagulopathy is nearly impossible to correct with factor repletion. Disseminated intravascular coagulation (DIC) also occurs and may be accentuated by infection and endotoxemia.

F. **Gastrointestinal and other bleeding.** More than half of the patients with FHF have severe gastrointestinal bleeding from acute erosions in the stomach and esophagus. Coagulopathy, thrombocytopenia, abnormal platelet function, and DIC contribute to the bleeding propensity of these patients. Because gastric acid plays a major role in the formation of erosions and ulcers, prophylactic use of intravenous proton pump inhibitors or histamine-2 (H_2)-receptor antagonists has been shown to decrease the frequency of upper gastrointestinal bleeding.

Retroperitoneal hemorrhage, epistaxis, or bleeding into the lungs may also occur. Prophylactic use of fresh-frozen plasma is not of proven benefit. In bleeding patients, however, maintenance of the blood volume by the use of blood products and correction of clotting factor deficiencies should be tried.

G. **Hypoglycemia** is common in patients with FHF and may lead to abrupt deepening of coma. Blood sugar needs to be closely monitored.

H. **Sepsis** usually complicates FHF due to leukocyte and macrophage dysfunction, bacterial gut translocation, decreased opsonin function and complement, release of endotoxin and cytokines, as well as iatrogenic causes such as placement of nasogastric tubes, catheters, and central lines. Prophylactic antibiotics are not generally recommended, but if sepsis is suspected, cultures should be obtained and sepsis promptly treated.

V. MANAGEMENT

A. **General measures.** If hepatic regeneration occurs, complete recovery from FHF is theoretically possible. The major factors that affect progression of liver injury are intercurrent infections and respiratory and hemodynamic instability, resulting in alterations of cerebral and hepatic perfusion. Vigorous maintenance of vital functions and prompt identification and treatment of all anticipated complications, particularly of cerebral edema to prevent brain damage, are essential. The patient should be treated in an intensive care unit, where monitoring personnel are in constant attendance and prepared for emergencies.

The patient's vital signs and cardiac rhythm should be monitored continuously. A nasogastric tube, passed to decompress the stomach and monitor for gastrointestinal bleeding, may be used as an access to give oral medicines. Close attention should be given to the patient's fluid balance. A urinary catheter and a central venous catheter should be placed. It may be necessary to monitor the plasma glucose as frequently as hourly. Hemoglobin level, blood urea nitrogen (BUN), and electrolytes should be checked every 12 hours. Measurement of arterial blood gases is essential in determining the acid–base status and oxygenation. The usual indications for endotracheal intubation and assisted ventilation should be observed. Frequent surveillance for infection is necessary. The prophylactic use of antibiotics is not recommended.

Patients should not be given prophylactic infusions of fresh-frozen plasma or concentrates of clotting factors to treat the coagulopathy without any evidence of bleeding. Daily administration of parenteral vitamin K is appropriate. Suppression of gastric acid secretion, maintaining the intragastric pH above 5.0, has been shown to be effective in preventing upper gastrointestinal bleeding and reducing the requirements for blood transfusions in patients with FHF. Hypothermia should be avoided. In patients with delirium or convulsions, intravenous diazepam may be used cautiously.

Acetylcysteine may be given intravenously in a dose of 150 mg/kg of body weight in 250 mL of 5% dextrose over a period of 15 minutes and then in a dose of 50 mg/kg in 500 mL of 5% dextrose over a period of 4 hours. This regimen has been shown to increase survival of patients with established liver damage induced by acetaminophen even when administered more than 15 hours after the acetaminophen overdose. This beneficial effect seems to result from an increase in tissue oxygen transport (delivery and consumption) in response to acetylcysteine. The beneficial effect was also seen in eight persons with FHF from other causes.

Penicillin and silibinin infusions may be effective in mushroom poisoning with *Amanita phalloides*. Penicillin works as an antagonist of amatoxin and silibinin blocks hepatocyte uptake of amatoxin.

Various treatment modalities have proven ineffective in FHF. These include exchange transfusion, insulin and glucagon infusion, prostaglandin E_2 infusion, and charcoal hemoperfusion and hyperimmune globulin infusion for FHF resulting from HBV infection.

The use of **corticosteroids** to reduce hepatic inflammation in patients with FHF has not been substantiated. Corticosteroids in these patients are associated with a significant increase in the BUN concentration thought to be caused by steroid-augmented protein catabolism in the peripheral tissues. This situation results in increased NH_3 formation in the intestine, contributing to the encephalopathy. The immunosuppressive and ulcerogenic potential of corticosteroids may predispose these patients to increased risk of sepsis and gastrointestinal bleeding. Currently, corticosteroid therapy is contraindicated in the management of patients with FHF.

B. Nutritional support. Parenteral nutrition is essential in these very ill patients to provide adequate calories and to minimize the obligatory protein breakdown (see Chapter 11, section I.2.b, and Chapter 12, section VI.D). Intravenous lipid preparations may not be well tolerated. In addition to dextrose, the total parenteral nutrition (TPN) solutions rich in branched-chain amino acids and low in aromatic acids and methionine are efficacious and help maintain a positive nitrogen balance. The usual additives to the TPN solution and supplements of vitamin K (15 mg daily), thiamine hydrochloride (100 mg twice daily), folic acid (1 mg daily), and ascorbic acid (500 mg daily) should be given.

C. Treatment of hepatic encephalopathy. The main points in the treatment of hepatic encephalopathy are to identify, correct, and treat any of the precipitating factors and to minimize the interactions between nitrogenous substances and the enteric bacterial flora.

1. Gastrointestinal tract cleansing. No protein or amino acids are given by mouth. The gastrointestinal tract is evacuated by giving a balanced electrolyte solution (e.g., GoLYTELY, NuLytely, or Colyte) or cathartics such as oral or nasogastric instillation of magnesium citrate or lactulose and enemas with proper positioning of the patient to fill the entire colon. If the patient has ileus, a balanced electrolyte solution may be instilled into the duodenum via a nasogastric tube to clean out the small and large bowel.

2. Oral antibiotics. The enteric bacterial flora may be suppressed by oral administration of poorly absorbed antibiotics such as **neomycin,** which also may be given as an enema. Oral **metronidazole** also may be used in the treatment of acute and chronic encephalopathy and may be preferred because of its lack of nephro- and ototoxicity. The **combination of the two antibiotics** may be even more efficacious in some instances. A **combination of lactulose and neomycin** has been used when either agent alone was unsatisfactory.

Rifaximin, a nonabsorbable gut specific antibiotic, taken orally, is a safer and much better tolerated alternative. It compares favorably to other antibiotics and lactulose in the treatment of hepatic encepahlopathy.

D. Treatment of cerebral edema. Frequent assessment of the clinical neurologic status using the criteria outlined in Tables 17-2 and 17-3 is necessary. Early diagnosis and treatment of cerebral edema is essential. Papilledema is an inconstant sign. Signs of a deteriorating brainstem, including sluggish pupillary reaction, slow oculovestibular reflexes, or absent ciliospinal reflexes, should be serially assessed. However, these signs are not sensitive and may be misinterpreted. Direct monitoring of intracranial pressure through a burr hole using a stable, drift-free intracranial transducer attached to a flat-bed recording system is desirable but not possible in all patients. As an alternative to direct intracranial pressure monitoring, extradural, epidural, and subdural catheters may be used. Subdural catheter intracranial pressure monitors are thought to be more accurate than epidural catheters. Extradural catheters may be safer and may have fewer complications with infections and hemorrhage. Intravenous glycerol or corticosteroids are not effective in reducing the cerebral edema of FHF.

Intravenous **mannitol** (0.3–0.4 g/kg body weight) given as a 20% solution with rapid infusion has been effective in most patients in reducing cerebral edema. Because the response is variable and at times adverse, mannitol therapy should be used in conjunction with intracranial pressure monitoring. Renal failure precludes the use of mannitol in these patients. **Thiopental** (250 mg) infusion may be used, but its efficacy is still controversial. When cerebral edema progresses despite medical therapy, decompressive craniectomy may be considered, especially in instances of Reye's syndrome and acetaminophen overdose.

E. **Temporary hepatic support,** if possible, provides a desirable milieu and time for the massively damaged liver to regenerate and resume normal function. Many different methods have been tried. These include exchange blood transfusions, plasmapheresis, and total body washout, cross-circulation with another human or animal, dialysis using various membranes, hemoperfusion through isolated liver or liver cell cultures, and hemoperfusion through columns of adsorbents. None of these methods has been shown to be effective in FHF. The early use of charcoal hemoperfusion with concomitant infusion of prostacyclin to inhibit platelet aggregation and release has been beneficial in a few patients. In dogs with acetaminophen-induced FHF, the use of an extracorporeal liver-assist device has been associated with the reversal of FHF. This device consists of a highly differentiated human liver cell line cultured in a hollow fiber cartridge. Even in the presence of severe liver injury, the device used in this trial was capable of supporting total liver function for 48 hours.

F. **Liver transplantation.** Liver transplantation may be a lifesaving procedure for patients with FHF, and delays in implementing this therapy can be fatal. Because mortality and long-term morbidity of liver transplantation are substantial, early prognostic indicators and clear guidelines are necessary to select the patients most likely to benefit at a time in the course of their disease when liver transplantation is still feasible. A significant relation exists between the survival of patients maintained with intensive medical therapy and the cause of FHF. In a study involving 137 patients with FHF, the survival rate for patients with acetaminophen overdose was 52.9%; hepatitis A, 66.7%; hepatitis B, 38.9%; and halothane or drug reactions, 12.5%. In the last three instances, therefore, liver transplantation should be considered early in the course of FHF.

In most centers, worsening hepatic encephalopathy, clinical evidence of cerebral edema, and increasing prolongation of the prothrombin time after 24 to 48 hours of intensive medical treatment are used as the key factors for recommending liver transplantation. The 1-year survival rate for such patients after liver transplantation is 65%. The outcome of liver transplantation also depends on graft quality, because grafts from incompatible blood groups, steatotic grafts, or partial or reduced-size grafts do not produce as favorable results. Unfortunately, in patients infected with hepatitis B or C viruses, the allograft also becomes infected despite interferon therapy.

Axillary liver transplantation has been introduced as an alternative treatment option in patients with FHF caused by toxins, drugs, or vascular insufficiency. In these patients, the native liver, which is left in place, may recover if a transplanted axillary liver provides temporary support. In those patients who recover, immunosuppression is withdrawn and the donor liver is left to atrophy or may be removed surgically.

In conclusion, patients with FHF require accurate assessment of their critical condition and of the cause of the FHF, intensive medical management with strict and persistent attention to the vital functions and complications of the disease, and treatment of the complications as early as they are identified. Patients who are candidates for liver transplantation need to be identified early and transferred to the transplantation center for early and appropriate liver transplantation.

Selected Readings

Albataineh H, et al. Acute liver failure secondary to Clarithromyah: A case report and literature review. *Pract Gastroenterol.* 2007; xxx1(7):87–89.

Keefe EB. Acute liver failure. In: McQuaid KR, Friedman SL, Grendell JH, eds. *Current Diagnosis and Treatment in Gastroenterology.* 2nd ed. New York: Lange Medical Books/McGraw-Hill; 2003:536–545.

Khashab M, et al. Epidemiology of acute liver failure. *Curr Gastroenterol Rep*. 2007; 9:66–73.

Montalti R, et al. Liver transplantation in fulminant hepatic failure: experience with 40 adult patients over a 17-year period. *Transplant Proc*. 2005;37:1085–1087.

O'Grady JG. Acute liver failure. *Post Grad Wed J*. 2005;81:148–154.

Ostapowicz G, et al. Results of a prospective study of acute liver failure at 17 tertiary care centers in the United States. *Ann Intern Med*. 2002;137:947–954.

Polson JL. AASL position paper: the management of acute liver failure. *Hepatology*. 2005;41:1179–1197.

Riordan SM, et al. Fulminant hepatic failure. *Clin Liver Dis*. 2000;4:24–45.

Riordan SM, et al. Use and validation of selection criteria for liver transplantation in acute liver failure. *Liver Transplant*. 2000;6:170–173.

Schiodt FV, et al. Etiology and outcome for 295 patients with acute liver failure in the United States. *Liver Transplant Surg*. 1999;5:29–34.

Voquero J, et al. Mild Hypothermia for the treatment of acute liver failure. *Nat Clin Pract Gastroenterol Hepatol*. 2007;4(10):528–529.

GASTROINTESTINAL AND HEPATOBILIARY DISEASES IN PREGNANCY

$\mathcal{P}$regnant women may present with specific diseases that occur exclusively during pregnancy as well as those that are present at the time of pregnancy and those that occur coincidentally with pregnancy. In this chapter, only the diseases that occur exclusively in pregnancy will be discussed.

I. HYPEREMESIS GRAVIDARUM

  A. Definition and epidemiology. Hyperemesis gravidarum involves intractable vomiting during pregnancy that may lead to electrolyte abnormalities, dehydration, and malnutrition. It is more common in the first trimester, in women younger than 25 years of age, and with multiple gestations. Incidence in the United States may be as high as 6 in 1,000 deliveries.

  B. Clinical findings. Patients usually present with nausea, vomiting, dysphagia, odynophagia, epigastric pain, and dehydration. Fifty percent of patients may have elevations in the serum aminotransaminases (alanine aminotransferase and aspartate aminotransferase) as well as, occasionally, also of bilirubin and alkaline phosphatase levels. There may be concomitant gastroesophageal reflux disease (GERD) and in the severely malnourished patient, esophageal candidiasis, or herpes simplex virus (HSV) infection. Some patients may have hyperthyroidism.

  C. Treatment. Most patients do well with intravenous hydration and antiemetics. Some patients may require gastric acid suppressive drugs such as proton-pump inhibitors (PPIs) or histamine receptor blockers to control GERD, and esophagitis. While no formal studies of these drugs have been performed on pregnant women, there have been no reports of adverse effects to the mothers or fetuses during clinical use. Prokinetic drugs such as metoclopramide hydrochloride (Reglan) 10 to 20 mg intravenously or by mouth four times daily may be used concomitantly with PPIs. Antiemetics (i.e., ondansetron [Zofran] 4–5 mg) may be given by mouth three to four times a day or 8 mg intravenously every 4 to 8 hours.

  In refractory cases, upper gastrointestinal (UGI) endoscopy may be required to document UGI mucosal injury due to peptic and/or infectious (candida or HSV) concomitant disease. A minority of patients may require total or peripheral parenteral nutrition.

II. INTRAHEPATIC CHOLESTASIS OF PREGNANCY

  A. Definition and epidemiology. A cholestatic syndrome is more commonly seen during the second and third trimesters of pregnancy, with elevations in serum bile acid levels but normal γ-glutamyltransferase (GGT) and alkaline phosphatase levels in most cases. It is more common in women with a family history of intrahepatic cholestasis of pregnancy (IHCP), with a history of intrahepatic cholestases during use of estrogen or birth control pills, and with use of progesterone during pregnancy.

  B. Clinical findings. The predominant symptom is pruritus. Patients may present with skin excoriations due to inadvertent scratching. Jaundice may follow the onset of pruritus. Elevation of serum transaminase, cholesterol, and triglyceride

111

levels may be present. For early diagnosis, the specific biochemical marker of the change of 3β-hydroxysteroid-sulfate ratio of progesterone metabolites may be used.

C. Clinical outcome. Mothers do well in nearly in all cases; however, fetal outcome may be complicated by prematurity, prenatal death, fetal distress, and meconium staining of the amniotic fluid.

D. Treatment. Symptomatic treatment of pruritus addresses increased serum bile salt concentration.

  1. Cholestyramine resin (Questran) (4 mg, 1–4 times daily before meals) works by intraluminal binding of bile salts.

  2. Ursodeoxycholic acid (Actigall) (300 mg, 3–4 times daily) works by modification of the serum bile acid concentrations by inhibiting the absorption of more hydrophobic bile acids that are thought to be more pruritic.

  3. Dexamethasone (2 mg per day) may be used in refractory cases. Its mode of action is not well delineated.

III. ACUTE FATTY LIVER OF PREGNANCY

A. Definition and epidemiology. In acute fatty liver of pregnancy (AFLP), microvascular fatty infiltration of the hepatocytes leads to progressive liver failure. Incidence in the United States is 1 in 7,000 to 15,000 deliveries. AFLP is more common in cases of multiple gestations, male fetuses, and in first pregnancies. It generally occurs in the third trimester, as early as 26 weeks of gestation.

B. Clinical findings. Presenting symptoms include nausea, vomiting, headache, malaise, and abdominal pain (diffuse, right upper quadrant, or epigastric). Jaundice may follow initial symptoms. Serum alkaline phosphatase, bilirubin, and transaminase levels are mildly to moderately elevated. Hyperuricemia may occur in 80% of patients. Hypoglycemia may be present. Preeclampsia may occur in 20% to 40% of patients. Progressive liver failure may occur with coagulopathy, encephalopathy, and renal failure.

C. Diagnosis. Diagnosis should be prompt with high clinical awareness. Abdominal ultrasound shows diffusely increased echogenicity of the liver. Computed tomography scan of the abdomen may be more sensitive than abdominal ultrasound.

D. Treatment and outcome. Treatment is rapid delivery of the fetus. If fulminant hepatic failure develops, liver transplantation may be lifesaving. Maternal mortality is reported to be 8% to 18% and fetal morality 18% to 23%.

IV. HELLP SYNDROME

A. Definition and epidemiology. Hemolytic anemia elevated liver chemistry tests, and low platelets. Occurs in the third trimester (25–32 weeks' gestation) in 0.1% to 0.6% of pregnancies. It may accompany acute fatty liver of pregnancy, preeclampsia, or eclampsia. It is more common in multiparous women older than 25 years. It also may occur postpartum within 2 days of delivery or later.

B. Clinical findings. Patients may complain of nausea and vomiting, epigastric pain, headache, edema, and visual changes. Patients usually present with hypertension microangiopathic hemolytic anemia with decreased haptoglobin levels and increased indirect bilirubin and lactate dehydrogenase (LDH) levels and proteinuria. Platelets may be less then 10,000/mm³. In patients with preeclampsia, a positive d-dimer test may help diagnose the onset of HELLP.

C. Treatment. Initial trial of glucocorticoids maybe attempted; however, in patients with severe symptoms and/or fetal distress, immediate delivery is indicated. Plasma exchange may be beneficial in postpartum patients.

D. Outcome. The maternal mortality rate is 1% to 3.5%, and the infant mortality rate is 10% to 60%. There is increased risk of intrauterine growth retardation, infant prematurity, disseminated intravascular coagulation (DIC), and thrombocytopenia. There is also increased risk of maternal DIC, abruptio placentae, and cardiopulmonary, renal, and hepatic failure. HELLP may recur in 4% to 27% of cases and the risk of preeclampsia increases by 2% to 40% in subsequent pregnancies.

V. PREECLAMPSIA AND ECLAMPSIA

A. **Definition and epidemiology.** Preeclampsia is a disease with hepatic hematologic, renal, central nervous system, and placental–fetal involvement, characterized by hypertension, edema, and proteinuria.

B. **Eclampsia.** Eclampsia differs from preeclampsia by the added complications of seizures and/or coma that may occur after delivery. Eclampsia most commonly occurs in primigravidas, usually in the second or third trimester (after 20 weeks of gestation). Preeclampsia may occur in 5% to 10% of pregnancies and eclampsia in 1% to 2%. There is an increased incidence in patients younger than 20 and older than 45 years and in those with obesity, hypertension, or diabetes mellitus. Additional risk factors include family history of preeclampsia/eclampsia, hydatidiform mole, polyhydramnios, fetal hydrops, multiple gestations, inadequate prenatal care, and cigarette smoking. There may be a genetic inheritance pattern involving an autosomal recessive single gene.

C. **Clinical findings.** Blood pressure is elevated to more than 140/90 mmHg but may rise above 160/110 mmHg. Patients usually present with headache, visual changes, congestive heart failure, respiratory distress, abdominal pain, and oliguria. If the patient develops seizures or coma, eclampsia is diagnosed. Diagnosis is based on clinical findings including elevated transaminase levels (5–100 times) with a moderate increase in bilirubin level. Microangiopathic hemolytic anemia and thrombocytopenia may also be present.

D. **Treatment.** Management of patients who are remote from term is controversial, but in those who are near term, rapid delivery is recommended.

E. **Outcome.** Increased perinatal morbidity and mortality in the mother and fetus correlate with the severity of the preeclampsia and preexisting maternal medical conditions. The most common causes of maternal death are cerebral involvement and hepatic rupture. Risks to the fetus include fetal growth retardation, abruptio placentae, prematurity, and low birth weight.

VI. HEPATIC RUPTURE

A. **Definition and epidemiology.** The partial or complete fracture of the maternal liver is rare (1 in 50,000–250,000 deliveries) and is most commonly seen in the third trimester of pregnancy and near term. Hepatic rupture may occur in patients with AFLP, HELLP, preeclampsia, or eclampsia as well as in patients with hepatic, hemangioma, abscess, adenoma, or hepatocellular carcinoma.

B. **Clinical findings.** Patients present with a sudden onset of severe right upper quadrant or diffuse abdominal pain, abdominal distention, nausea, vomiting, hypotension, and shock. Serum transaminase levels are elevated (2–100 above normal range) with concomitant anemia, thrombocytopenia, and coagulopathy. The diagnosis is based on clinical findings, which may be supplemented by abdominal ultrasound and computed tomography.

C. **Treatment.** Early clinical recognition and diagnosis is essential, followed by delivery of the infant and additional surgical or radiologic intervention as necessary for the mother.

D. **Outcome.** The maternal mortality rate ranges from 50% to 75%, and fetal mortality rate ranges from 50% to 60%.

Selected Readings

Bor S, et al. Association of heartburn during pregnancy and the rise of gastroesophageal reflux disease. *Clin Gastroenterol Hepatol.* 2007;5:1035–1039.

Floreami A, et al. Intrahepatic cholestatis of pregnancy: three novel MDR3 gene mutations. *Ailment Pharmacul Ther.* 2006;23:1649–1653.

Lammernt F, et al. Intrahepatic cholestasis of pregnancy: Molecular pathogenesis, diagnosis and management. *J Hepatol.* 2000;33:1012–1021.

Mazzella G, et al. Ursodeoxycholic acid administration in patients with cholestasis of pregnancy: Effects on primary bile acids in babies and mothers. *Hepatology.* 2001;33: 504–508.

O'Brien J, et al. Impact of high dose corticosteroid therapy for patients with HELLP (hemolysis, elevated liver enzymes and low platelet count) syndrome. *Am J Obstet Gynecol.* 2000;183:921–924.

Pauli-Magnus C, et al. Sequence analysis of bile salt export pump (ABC B11) and multi drug resistance p-glycoprotein 3 (ABC B4, MDR3) in patients with intrahepatic cholestasis of pregnancy. *Pharmacogenetics.* 2004;14:91–102.

Statea T, et al. Orthotopic liver transplantation for complicated HELLP syndrome: Case report and review of the literature. *Arch Gynecol Obstet.* 2000;264:108–111.

Specific Complaints and Disorders

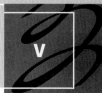

V

$\mathcal{T}$he esophagus is rarely infected in immunocompetent persons but is a common site of infection in patients with immune defects. Normal host defenses of the esophagus are the salivary flow, an intact mucosa, normal esophageal motility, and normal gastric acidity with the absence of excessive gastroesophageal reflux.

Humoral immunity including secretory IgA is important in protecting the mucosal integrity. However, based on the observation that patients with neutropenia and obvious defects in cell-mediated immunity have higher rates of esophageal infections, it seems likely that a major protective mechanism in the esophagus is cell-mediated immunity.

The esophagus can be involved with infections by bacteria, fungi, and viruses. Most esophageal infections are fungal (*Candida albicans*) or viral (herpes simplex virus [HSV] or cytomegalovirus) or a combination of the two. Diagnosis of the specific etiologic agent is essential because of the availability of effective antiviral, antifungal, and antibacterial therapy.

I. **FUNGAL ESOPHAGITIS.** *C. albicans* is the most common fungus recovered from patients with fungal esophagitis. However, other species have been isolated and implicated as etiologic agents of such infections. These are *Candida tropicalis, Candida parapsilosis, Candida glabrata, Histoplasma capsulatum, Blastomyces dermatitidis, Aspergillus,* and *Torulopsis glabrata.*

C. albicans is found in the oropharynx of approximately 50% of the healthy population. It is also found in the skin and the bowel of immunocompetent persons. Patients with defects in cellular immunity and those treated with antibiotics may have sufficient alteration in their normal bacterial flora to have luminal candidal overgrowth. It is thought that patients with physical or chemical damage to the esophageal mucosa (e.g., acid reflux) may be at increased risk for developing candidal overgrowth and subsequent invasive disease. Indeed, the worst lesions visible in many instances of *Candida* esophagitis are in the distal esophagus, the area most likely to suffer from reflux damage. The mechanisms responsible for permitting mucosal adherence and subsequent invasion are unknown.

Candidiasis is by far the most common esophageal infection. In fact, it is a rather common disease with a varying spectrum of severity. It can be an asymptomatic incidental finding during endoscopy as well as an overwhelming infection causing death. In one study, 90% of the HIV-infected patients with oral thrush who underwent endoscopy had mucosal lesions caused by *Candida*. Larger series have not confirmed this high figure; however, many of the treatments effective for oral thrush are also effective in most instances of *Candida* esophagitis, suggesting that diagnostic evaluation such as endoscopy might best be reserved for patients who do not respond to initial topical antifungal therapy.

In addition to acute manifestations of the disease, late sequelae can develop. Mucosal sloughing caused by an intense inflammatory response, esophageal perforation, and stricture formation have been reported.

While *Candida* esophagitis can occur in any patient, certain conditions seem to predispose to it.

A. **Predisposing factors.** These factors include HIV infection, neutropenia, hematologic and other malignancies, organ transplantation, and immunosuppressive agents including corticosteroids, antineoplastic chemotherapy, radiation therapy, broad-spectrum antibiotics, diabetes mellitus, renal failure, alcoholism, malnutrition, old age, and chronic mucocutaneous candidiasis (CMC). In CMC, esophageal candidiasis may occur in addition to the chronic involvement of the nails, skin, and oral cavity. These patients have defective cellular immunity. However, since the wide use of highly active antiretroviral therapy (HAART), the incidence of opportunistic infections has been drastically reduced.

B. Diagnosis
   1. Clinical presentation
      a. Dysphagia and odynophagia. The most common symptoms of esophageal candidiasis are dysphagia and odynophagia; fever may be present. Pain may be substernal and radiate to the back. In some patients, odynophagia may be experienced only when they drink hot or cold beverages, and in others, it may be so severe that they may not be able to eat at all. The symptoms may be absent in 20% to 50% of the patients, especially those with mild infection, patients who are severely debilitated, and those with CMC.
      b. Oral thrush may be present in children and in HIV-infected individuals with esophageal candidiasis, but it is usually absent in immunocompetent adults. The plaques adhere to the underlying mucosa but can be dislodged at endoscopy revealing an inflamed, friable mucosa underneath. *Candida* can coexist with other pathogens in up to 30% of patients, and reliance on the endoscopic appearance alone may result in failure to identify a concomitant viral or bacterial infection. Multiple biopsies are essential to exclude coexisting disorders. During endoscopy, mucosal lesions should be brushed and submitted for cytologic evaluation and biopsied for histologic examination. Cytologic examination of brushings is more sensitive than histologic examination of the biopsy specimens since organisms may be washed off the mucosa in superficial *Candida* infections during the processing of the biopsy specimens.

      In addition to cytologic evaluation, material obtained from esophageal brushings may be placed on a microscopic slide, and a drop of potassium hydroxide may be added to lyse the epithelial cells. Both yeast and hyphae of *C. albicans* can be demonstrated in this manner. Because mycelia are not found in the normal esophagus, their presence in the brushings strongly suggests the diagnosis. A Gram's stain of esophageal brush specimens can also demonstrate the presence of yeast, hyphae, and bacteria.

      Biopsy specimens should be stained with hematoxylin-eosin to assess the severity of the inflammation. Silver and periodic acid–Schiff stains of biopsy specimens may confirm the presence of fungal elements.

      In patients with AIDS, concomitant infection with viruses (e.g., cytomegalovirus, HSV) may be present. Cytoplasmic and nuclear inclusion bodies and other findings suggestive of viral infection also should be looked for in both biopsy and brush specimens. Figure 19-1 is an algorithm that may be used as a diagnostic approach.
   2. Diagnostic studies
      a. Endoscopy. Fiberoptic endoscopy is the most useful method in the diagnosis of *Candida* esophagitis. Direct observation of the esophageal mucosa may allow the differentiation of *Candida* esophagitis from other infections (e.g., herpes) and from varices, carcinoma, or peptic disease, which may have a similar radiologic picture. The endoscopic appearance of esophageal candidiasis is graded on a scale from I to IV. The lesions range from small raised white plaques to ulceration and confluent plaque formation appearing as friable pseudomembranes.
      b. Radiologic studies. If a barium swallow is performed, the esophagram is normal in most patients. When radiologic abnormalities are found, the infection is usually severe. A double-contrast esophagram may increase the yield of positive findings. The esophagus usually has a "shaggy" appearance due to superficial ulcerations, but deep ulcerations may also be present. Abnormal motility with diminished peristalsis and occasional spasm may be seen. Esophageal stricture is commonly present in CMC.

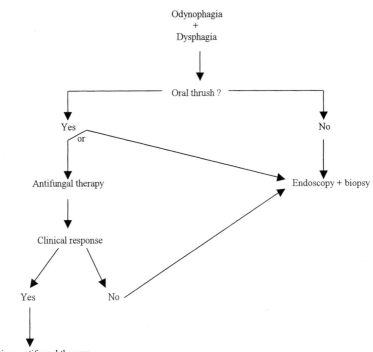

Figure 19-1. Algorithm depicting diagnostic approach in patients with suspected fungal esophagitis.

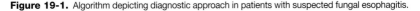

This may be a focal narrowing in the upper esophagus or may involve the entire length.

C. Treatment

1. Before the initiation of any specific therapy for esophageal candidiasis, the underlying predisposing factor should be identified.

2. Patients with AIDS and mild-to-moderate symptoms who have oral thrush may be treated initially with one of the topical agents such as **nystatin** (Mycostatin) **suspension, clotrimazole troches,** or one of the **"azoles"** may be an alternative form of therapy before undergoing a diagnostic procedure (Table 19-1).

3. Patients with leukopenia or with severe symptoms or systemic signs should undergo endoscopy to obtain biopsy and brushing specimens for fungi, viruses, and bacteria.

4. Orally administered systemic antifungal agents include the azoles and polyene antibiotics. The most commonly used azoles include ketoconazole (Nizoral), fluconazole (Diflucan), and itraconazole (Sporanox). All are effective in treating esophageal candidiasis.

    Ketoconazole may be used at high doses. However, its gastrointestinal side effects; decreased absorption in achlorhydric patients or patients on acid antisecretory drugs such as histamine-2 (H_2) blockers, proton-pump inhibitors, and prostaglandin analogs; and hepatotoxicity may limit its usefulness.

    Fluconazole is extremely efficacious in treating oral candidiasis and *Candida* and other fungal esophagitis with or without tissue invasion. Fluconazole may be administered via oral or parenteral routes. Its oral absorption is efficient and does not require the presence of gastric acid. It is minimally metabolized and excreted by the urine. Drug interactions have been demonstrated between fluconazole

TABLE 19-1	Available Agents for the Treatment of Fungal Esophagitis

Agent	Treatment schedule
Topical	
Nystatin	1–3 million units (10–30 mL) 4–5 times daily; swish and swallow for 5–10 days
Clotrimazole	1 troche (10 mg) 5 times daily for 5–10 days
Systemic	
Amphotericin B	0.3–0.6 mg/kg/d intravenously
Ketoconazole	200–400 mg once daily, orally for 5–10 days
Fluconazole	50–200 mg once daily, orally for 5–10 days
	100–200 mg twice daily intravenously for 5–10 days
Itraconazole	200 mg once daily for 5–10 days

(and the other azoles) and other medications, including phenytoin, oral antico-agulants, sulfonylureas, cyclosporin A, rifampin, and barbiturates. Fluconazole augments the effects of warfarin, necessitating careful observation of patients receiving both of these agents. Fluconazole may increase serum levels of cyclosporin A. Serum cyclosporin A and creatinine levels must be monitored carefully in patients receiving both of these drugs. Fluconazole and the other azoles also appear to increase the serum levels of phenytoin and oral hypo-glycemic agents. Fluconazole appears to have minimal antisteroidogenic effects in humans at currently recommended doses. This results from fluconazole highly specific affinity for fungal cytochrome P-450 enzymes, with virtually no affinity for the mammalian system. This is an important advantage of fluconazole over ketoconazole in patients with AIDS, who often have adrenal insufficiency sec-ondary to adrenal cytomegalovirus (CMV) infection.

    Itraconazole has a longer half-life than ketoconazole, but its absorption is also reduced by hypochlorhydria. These two azoles are metabolized by the liver and excreted in the bile. Dose adjustments are not required in the patient with renal failure. Total treatment dosage is about 100 to 200 mg.

5. Intravenous (IR) **amphotericin B** should be considered in symptomatic patients who fail to respond to the above regimen and in those in whom sys-temic involvement is suspected. In the absence of systemic *Candida* infection, a low-dose regimen of 10 to 20 mg per day for 10 days may be given. The dosage may be increased if the patient does not respond favorably. If systemic infection is present, the dosage should be increased gradually to 0.5 mg/kg per day. Most patients are treated for 6 weeks. The major serious side effect of amphotericin is renal toxicity, which is usually reversible.

6. A major problem in the treatment of esophageal candidiasis is relapse after therapy is discontinued, especially in patients with AIDS, in whom immuno-suppression is unrelenting. If the underlying predisposing factors persist, the chances for permanent cure are low, and maintenance therapy may be neces-sary (e.g., fluconazole 100 mg/day). However, in patients with reversible predisposing conditions (e.g., radiotherapy, steroid use), a single course of therapy for 10 to 21 days should be successful.

7. **Nutritional support** of the patient is very important. If the patient can swal-low, the diet should be supplemented with liquid enteral formulas to ensure that adequate calories are received. If the patient is unable to swallow, par-enteral nutrition should be given until the patient can receive enteral feedings.

II. **VIRAL ESOPHAGITIS** is also a common esophageal disorder, especially in immuno-compromised patients, which may clinically mimic *Candida* esophagitis. The herpes viruses are the most common etiologic agents of viral esophagitis, with **HSV** and **CMV** predominating. In patients with AIDS, **Epstein-Barr virus (EBV), varicella zoster virus,** and **HIV-1** also have been implicated in esophageal ulcerations.

A. HSV esophagitis. Herpetic esophagitis may be seen in healthy, normal individuals, especially after strenuous physical exertion and stress. The infection in such individuals is self-limited and resolves in approximately 7 to 10 days. Recovery generally indicates intact humoral and cellular immunity. Persistence or recurrence of the disease may be a sign of acquired immunodeficiency, requiring further workup of the patient.

1. Predisposing factors

   a. Immunocompromise

      i. Malignancy, mainly of the hematopoietic and lymphoreticular systems

      ii. Transplantation

      iii. Immunosuppressive drugs, steroids

      iv. Antineoplastic chemotherapy

      v. AIDS

   b. Severe debilitation

      i. Elderly

      ii. Burns

   c. Antecedent trauma

      i. Nasogastric tubes

      ii. Tracheal intubation

      iii. Gastroesophageal reflux disease and peptic esophagitis

2. Diagnosis

   a. Clinical presentation. Herpetic infection of the esophagus usually presents as a triad of fever, odynophagia, and substernal pain that increases with feeding. The pain may radiate to the back. Patients may complain of pain on palpation of the xiphoid process. Gingival stomatitis may be present. Disseminated HSV infection is seen in 30% of the patients. Multiple organ involvement with the virus (e.g., gastric and respiratory infection) is usually life-threatening. Simultaneous infection with other organisms (bacteria, fungi, and other viruses) is common. Severely debilitated patients may not complain of pain; therefore, a high index of suspicion should be present if these patients have dysphagia and decreased oral intake.

   b. Diagnostic studies

      i. Endoscopy. Endoscopic examination of the esophagus is the preferred diagnostic approach in these patients. Biopsies and brushings of the affected mucosa should be obtained. Biopsies should be obtained from the edge of the ulcers.

         a) The endoscopic appearance varies according to the stage of the viral infection.

            1) Early—vesicles of various sizes.

            2) Mid—small, punched-out superficial ulcers covered with yellow, fibrinous exudates.

            3) Late—coalescing ulcers forming a diffuse, erosive esophagitis with large areas of shallow ulceration.

         b) The lesions often become overgrown with *Candida* and bacteria. The virus may be cultured from ulcer margins and vesicles. A smear of the ulcer base should be processed for *Candida*. Histologically, the epithelial cells at the border of the ulcers contain inclusion bodies. The chromatin of the infected nuclei is displaced toward the periphery of the nucleus, giving a "rim" appearance. Multinucleated giant cells are often present.

      ii. Barium swallow. Double-contrast radiography may show ulcers or plaques. The picture may be indistinguishable from that of *Candida* esophagitis.

   c. Diagnosis of herpes esophagitis is often difficult because the characteristic nuclear inclusions or multinucleate giant cells of HSV infection may be absent in endoscopic biopsy specimens. Immunoperoxidase and in situ hybridization techniques may be used to detect the HSV when nuclear inclusions are not readily apparent in infected epithelium. In situ hybridization and immunoperoxidase techniques should be used also to detect other viruses such as CMV, Epstein-Barr, and HIV-1. The diagnosis of HSV esophagitis may still be missed when no infected epithelium is present in the biopsy specimen. The presence of aggregates of large mononuclear cells (macrophages) with convoluted nuclei adjacent to infected epithelium in the exudates of herpetic esophagitis seems to be a characteristic inflammatory response in ulcerative herpetic esophagitis. The presence of these mononuclear cells in a biopsy specimen that initially does not show herpetic inclusions warrants additional studies to rule out herpes virus infection.

   d. Both brushings and biopsy specimens may be cultured for HSV to increase the diagnostic yield.

 3. Treatment

   a. Supportive measures. Patients may benefit from viscous lidocaine swallows for local anesthesia, especially before eating. Patients who have severe, unremitting odynophagia may require intravenous hyperalimentation.

   b. Acyclovir (Zovirax) has been shown to be effective in the prompt resolution of symptoms. The dosage used is usually 6.2 mg/kg intravenously every 8 hours, for a 10- to 14-day course. Acyclovir 200 mg, five times a day by mouth, may be used in mild-to-moderate disease.

   Valacyclovir (1,000 mg three times a day for 7 days) and **famciclovir** (500 mg orally twice a day for 7 days) seem to have similar efficacy as acyclovir, but may be administered three times a day.

B. Cytomegalovirus esophagitis. CMV is one of the most common opportunistic infectious agents causing disease in patients with AIDS. In the gastrointestinal tract, it most often infects the colon and esophagus.

 1. Clinical presentation. CMV esophagitis may mimic HSV, *Candida*, and peptic esophagitis. Patients may seek treatment for odynophagia, dysphagia, fever, nausea, vomiting, or decreased oral intake. Hemoptysis, hematemesis, melena, or esophageal perforation and sepsis may occur.

 2. Diagnostic studies

   a. Endoscopy. The endoscopic appearance of CMV esophagitis may resemble that of HSV or *Candida* esophagitis. Discrete, deep ulcers may be present. Biopsies should be taken from the center of the lesions.

   b. Pathology. Histologic diagnosis of CMV infection is made with hematoxylin-eosin stain by identifying typically enlarged cells with characteristic intranuclear and intracytoplasmic inclusion bodies. More sensitive techniques such as in situ DNA hybridization and immune histochemical staining using CMV-specific antibodies have increased the diagnostic yield. Infected cells are often identified in the granulation tissue and in stromal papillae of the mucosa and the endothelium, but never in the squamous epithelium. Thus, deep biopsies are necessary for diagnosis.

   Viral cultures of the brushings and biopsies should be done to increase the diagnostic accuracy and yield. Because multiple infections may coexist in these patients, other agents such as bacteria, fungi, and other viruses should be excluded.

 3. Treatment. Ganciclovir sodium (5 mg/kg IV body weight twice daily for 14–21 days) has been used successfully in severely ill patients with improvement in the symptoms of esophagitis. However, patients may require long-term maintenance therapy and are subject to the myelosuppressive toxicity of the drug. **Foscarnet (foscavir)** (60 mg/kg IV or 90 mg IV twice a day) is used in refractory diseases or when side effects of gancyclovir sodium are limiting. It is effective in clinically resistant cases of CMV. Its major side effect is reversible renal insufficiency. **Cidofovir,** due to its long half-life, may be administered once weekly. It also causes reversible renal insufficiency. Relapse rate is 50% in patients with AIDS, especially those who are not on HAART.

III. IDIOPATHIC ESOPHAGEAL ULCER (IEU) related to primary HIV infection. Large, deep ulcers resembling CMV or HSV ulcers may occur in patients with AIDS and, when other etiologies are excluded are attributed to HIV. Endoscopic cure may be obtained with treatments with oral prednisone or thalidomide.

IV. BACTERIAL ESOPHAGITIS may be a distinct clinical and pathologic entity in immunocompromised patients. In a neutropenic patient with either fever or a bacteremia of unknown source, esophagitis must be considered as a possible cause. In some patients with bacteremia, the same organism may be seen on endoscopic biopsy specimens from the esophagus. Most of the organisms isolated from tissue specimens and blood in these patients are gram-positive cocci or rods and enteric gram-negative bacilli. Antibiotics should be directed at the specific pathogen isolated.

V. ESOPHAGEAL TUBERCULOSIS. Involvement of the esophagus with **tuberculosis** is rare. The condition may result from reactivated lung disease or direct extension of the infection from adjacent mediastinal or hilar lymph nodes, vertebral bodies, aortic aneurysms, pharynx, or larynx. Disease can also occur when a patient with active pulmonary tuberculosis swallows large numbers of organisms that colonize preexisting mucosal disease. However, most patients with tuberculous esophagitis have no evidence of active pulmonary involvement on chest x-ray.
  A. Clinical presentation. Epigastric pain and dysphagia are the most common presenting symptoms. The symptoms in some patients are vague and nonspecific.
  B. Diagnosis
    1. Radiologic findings are usually diverse and may include extrinsic compression by lymph nodes, ulceration, and stricture resembling esophageal malignancy.
    2. Endoscopy. The endoscopic lesion is ulcerative, with shallow, smooth edges; granular with small mucosal miliary granulomas; or hyperplastic, with fibrosis, luminal narrowing, and stricture formation. Biopsies may show caseating granulomas with or without acid-fast bacilli.
    3. Sputum cultures may grow *Mycobacterium tuberculosis* even in patients with normal chest x-rays.
    4. An **intermediate-strength tuberculin skin test** is usually positive and should be compared with other, control antigens.
  C. Treatment. A 9-month course of multidrug regimen including isoniazid, rifampin, and ethambutol hydrochloride has been used to cure esophageal tuberculosis.

Selected Readings

Bini EJ, et al. Natural history of HIV-associated esophageal disease in the era of protease inhibitor therapy. *Dig Dis Sci.* 2000;45:1301–1306.

Denning DW. Echinocardin anti fungal drugs. *Lancet.* 2003;362:1142–1452.

Kearney DJ, et al. Esophageal disorders caused by infection, systemic illness, medications, radiation and trauma. In: Feldman M, Freedman LS, Schlessinger MH, eds. Philadelphia: WB Saunders; 2002:623–646.

Keate RF, et al. Lichen planus: Report of three patients with oral tacrolimus or intraesophageal corticosteroid injection or both. *Dis Esophagus.* 2003;16:47–53.

Pappas PG. et al. Guidelines for treatment of candidias. *Clin Infect Dis.* 2004;38:161–189.

Ramanthan J, et al. Herpes simplex esophagitis in the immunocompetent host: An overview. *Am J Gastroenterol.* 2000; 95:2171–2176.

Rebolic AC, et al. Anidula fungia versus flucarazole for invasive candidiasis. *N Eng J Med.* 2007;356:2472–2482.

Walsh TJ. Echinocardins—an advance in the primary treatment of invasive candidiasis. *N Eng J Med.* 2006;354:1215–1256.

20 GASTROESOPHAGEAL REFLUX DISEASE

I. DEFINITIONS

A. Gastroesophageal reflux (GER) occurs when gastric contents escape into the esophagus. This process may or may not produce symptoms. The most common symptoms are heartburn, regurgitation, chest pain, and dysphagia.

B. Reflux esophagitis can be defined as esophageal inflammation caused by refluxed material.

C. Gastroesophageal reflux disease (GERD) includes the constellation of symptoms and consequences to the esophagus from reflux damage.

II. PATHOGENESIS.

The extent and severity of esophageal injury due to GER depend on the frequency and the duration of esophageal exposure to the refluxed material, the volume and potency of gastric juice available for reflux, and the ability of the esophageal mucosa to withstand injury and to repair itself.

The pathogenesis of reflux esophagitis or GERD is a multifactorial process. The following factors all contribute to the development of GERD:

A. Antireflux mechanisms. A positive pressure gradient exists between the abdomen and the thorax. If there were no physiologic barrier at the area of the gastroesophageal junction, GER would occur continuously, especially with increases in intraabdominal pressure or changes in gravitational position and during events associated with abdominal muscle contraction, such as coughing, sneezing, straining, bending, turning in bed, and exercise. The antireflux barrier can be divided into two categories.

1. **Anatomic factors extrinsic to the lower esophageal sphincter (LES) that augment the LES to prevent GER** include a distal esophageal mucosal flap, the acute esophagogastric angle, compression of the esophagogastric junction by gastric sling fibers, the diaphragmatic crus acting as pinchcock, a hiatal tunnel, the sling action of the right diaphragmatic crus, and the intraabdominal junction of the esophagus. The longer the intraabdominal segment, the less likely reflux is to occur.

   The presence of hiatal hernia with loss of the abdominal esophageal segment supported by the diaphragm and the normal acute esophagogastric angle may lead to GER. However, a direct causal relationship has not been found between hiatal hernia and GER. Nevertheless, a hiatal hernia generally (90%) accompanies reflux esophagitis. It is possible that hiatal hernia enhances the likelihood of LES dysfunction due to the loss of angulation at the esophagogastric junction and the direct transmission of intragastric pressure to the infrathoracic LES. Also, the hiatal hernia may act as a reservoir of refluxate and impair esophageal clearance in the recumbent position, thus promoting esophageal injury.

2. **The closure strength and efficacy of LES**

   a. LES corresponds to the 2- to 4-cm zone of asymmetrically thickened smooth muscle at the esophagogastric junction.

   b. LES maintains a high-pressure tone during resting conditions and relaxes with swallowing, esophageal distention, and vagal stimulation. These properties are independent of the diaphragm and persist even when the LES is in the thorax, as in patients with hiatal hernia.

c. LES is innervated by both excitatory and inhibitory autonomic nerves carried in the vagi to the esophageal plexuses. The major function of the LES inhibitory nerves is to mediate sphincter relaxation in response to swallowing.

d. LES pressure (LESP) is controlled by neural (most likely cholinergic), hormonal, and myogenic factors.

e. Resting LES pressure is not constant and varies from minute to minute in the awake state. During sleep, this variability is diminished.

f. The intrinsic tone (the resting LESP) is one of the major factors that prevent spontaneous GER.

g. In general, patients with GER have lower LESPs than controls. A minimum resting LESP in the range of 6 to 10 mmHg prevents GER even during transient increases in intraabdominal pressure.

h. Changes in resting LES pressure occur throughout the day, especially during the postprandial period. In addition, transient episodes of LES relaxation occur not only in response to swallowing but also spontaneously, a process referred to as "inappropriate LES relaxation" or "transient LES relaxation" (TLESR). In "physiologic refluxers," most reflux events occur during the relaxation events. In "pathologic refluxers" (i.e., patients with reflux disease), other mechanisms of reflux also occur, including gradual decreases in resting pressure and episodes of increased intragastric pressure. However, most reflux events continue to occur during TLESR.

TLESR appears to represent a physiologic response to increased gastric distention to relieve intragastric pressure.

i. Some GER occurs in all individuals with normal or lower-than-normal LESP throughout the day. The frequency of GER increases for 2 hours postprandially. However, patients with esophagitis have significantly more and longer episodes of GER than controls.

j. Low resting LESP seen in patients with esophagitis may be primary or secondary to injury from reflux and inflammation.

k. LESP is affected by various drugs and hormones (Table 20-1). Avoidance of agents that decrease the LESP and use of agents that increase LESP can be helpful in diminishing GER symptoms and esophageal damage.

B. Gastric factors

1. Gastric volume

a. **The occurrence of GER** depends on an available reservoir of gastric fluid.

b. **The probability and rate** of GER are related to gastric volume.

c. **The rate of reflux and the volume of the refluxate** increase with incremental increases in gastric volume, intragastric pressure, and the pressure gradient between the stomach and the esophagus.

d. **Gastric volume** is determined by several factors.
   i. Volume and composition of ingested materials
   ii. Rate and volume of gastric secretion
   iii. Rate and efficiency of gastric emptying
   iv. Frequency and volume of duodenogastric reflux

e. One or more of the factors in **d** that favor an increase in gastric volume also favor the occurrence of GER.

f. **Pyloric channel or duodenal ulcers** may result in delayed gastric emptying and predispose to increased GER and GERD.

g. **Delayed gastric emptying** due to neuromuscular abnormalities such as in collagen vascular diseases, diabetes mellitus, and hypothyroidism or mechanical gastric outlet obstruction may also predispose to GERD.

2. Irritant potency of the refluxed material

a. **The composition of the material refluxed** into the esophagus is important in determining the nature and extent of esophageal injury.

b. **Gastric acid** causes esophageal injury by protein denaturation and back diffusion of hydrogen ion into deeper layers of the esophageal wall to cause deeper injury.

TABLE 20-1	Agents Affecting Lower Esophageal Sphincter Pressure

Increase LESP	Decrease LESP
Gastrin	Secretin
Pitressin	Cholecystokinin
Angiotensin II	Glucagon
Cholinergics (e.g., bethanechol)	Vasoactive intestinal polypeptide
Gastric alkalinization	Progesterone (birth control pills)
Metoclopramide	Theophylline
Anticholinesterases	Caffeine
Protein meal	Gastric acidification
Prostaglandin $F_{2\alpha}$	Fatty meals
	Chocolate (xanthines)
	Carminatives (spearmint, peppermint)
	Smoking
	Ethanol
	α-Adrenergic antagonists
	β-Adrenergic agonists
	Anticholinergics
	Calcium channel blockers
	Nitrates
	Prostaglandin E_2, prostaglandin A_2
	Morphine, meperidine
	Diazepam, other benzodiazepines

LESP, lower esophageal sphincter pressure.

      c. Pepsin, a protease, digests esophageal epithelial intercellular substance, causing shedding of epithelial cells.

      d. Duodenogastric reflux, especially postprandially, introduces bile salts and pancreatic enzymes into the stomach, which may then reflux into the esophagus. Bile salts may result in micellar dissolution of the lipids in the esophageal epithelial cell membranes and increase the permeability of the esophageal mucosa to hydrogen ion back diffusion. Pancreatic enzymes may cause proteolytic injury.

      e. Pancreatic digestive enzymes and bile salts may be the significant agents of esophageal injury in patients with gastric hypochlorhydria and near-neutral pH.

C. Esophageal clearance

   1. The severity of esophageal injury from GER depends on the irritant potency of the refluxed material and its contact time with the esophagus.

   2. The rate of esophageal clearance determines the duration of the exposure of the esophageal mucosa to the refluxed material.

   3. Esophageal clearance of the refluxed material involves three mechanisms:

      a. Volume clearance involves the emptying out of the esophagus of the volume of the refluxed material. It is facilitated by gravity, esophageal motor activity, and salivation.

         i. Normal esophageal motor activity (peristalsis) is required for esophageal clearance.

         ii. Primary peristalsis is initiated by swallowing, and the contraction wave progresses in a sequential fashion throughout the entire length of the esophagus, resulting in esophageal emptying into the stomach.

Normally, primary peristalsis occurs about once a minute while an individual is awake. It is the main esophageal motor event that clears the esophagus of refluxed material. The absence of swallowing and esophageal peristalsis during sleep impedes esophageal clearance of refluxed material and predisposes to esophageal injury. Similarly in patients with abnormal esophageal motility, increased nonperistaltic contractions lead to increased reflux injury to the esophagus.

    iii. Secondary peristalsis is elicited with distention of the esophagus by a bolus of food or refluxed fluid. It has a limited effect on volume clearance, because it does not result in a complete stripping peristaltic wave.

  b. Acid clearance involves the disappearance of the hydrogen ion from the esophageal mucosa after the reflux of acid fluid. It is accomplished by a neutralizing action of swallowed saliva.

  c. Saliva is the third factor that contributes to esophageal clearance.

    i. Normal awake individuals generate 0.5 mL of saliva per minute.

    ii. Salivation stops during sleep.

    iii. Salivation stimulates swallowing.

    iv. Stimuli that increase salivary secretion include sucking, eating, intubation, and cholinergic agents.

    v. Under basal conditions, saliva has a pH of 6 to 7 due to the presence of bicarbonate ion as the major buffer.

    vi. During stimulation, both the salivary volume and the bicarbonate ion concentration increase.

    vii. Normal salivary flow effectively neutralizes small volumes (<1 mL) of refluxed acid.

    viii. Salivation, by promoting swallowing and primary stripping peristalsis, clears the esophagus of the main volume of the refluxed material. Subsequently saliva itself clears the acid from the esophageal mucosa by its neutralizing action.

    ix. Diminished salivation, primary (e.g., in Sjögren's syndrome) or secondary (e.g., due to anticholinergic drugs) causes delayed acid clearance and promotes esophageal injury.

D. Tissue resistance of the esophageal mucosa. The esophageal mucosa itself has intrinsic protective mechanisms that resist and limit mucosal injury.

  1. Preepithelial defenses

    a. The luminal surface of esophageal epithelium is lined by a **layer of mucus** that serves as both a lubricant and a protective barrier against noxious and irritant luminal contents. This viscous gel layer prevents large protein molecules like pepsin from contacting the underlying epithelium directly and slows down hydrogen ion back diffusion.

    b. Underneath the mucous layer, there is an area of low turbulence called the **unstirred water layer,** which is rich in bicarbonate. This layer establishes a protective alkaline microenvironment on the epithelial surface, neutralizing the hydrogen ion that penetrates the mucous layer.

    c. Mucus and bicarbonate are secreted by salivary glands and submucosal glands located just below the upper esophageal sphincter and near the esophagogastric junction. The rate of secretion of these glands increases with vagal stimulation and with prostaglandins.

  2. Postepithelial defenses. As in all tissues, adequate blood flow and normal tissue acid–base status are essential for the maintenance of a healthy epithelium. Blood flow provides the epithelium with oxygen, nutrients, and bicarbonate (HCO_3^-) as buffer and removes injurious waste products.

E. Epithelial regeneration. Despite the intrinsic ability of the esophageal mucosa to resist injury, prolonged exposure to noxious substances results in epithelial cell necrosis. Cell death further increases epithelial permeability, setting up a vicious circle for further damage. The replicating cells of the stratum basale along the basement membrane need to be protected for epithelial regeneration. The destruction of this layer appears to be necessary for the development of esophageal ulcers, strictures, and Barrett's epithelium. There is evidence that epithelial cell turnover and replication is increased after hydrogen (H^+) injury. Basal cell hyperplasia seen in mucosal biopsies of patients with reflux esophagitis lends further support to this finding. Normal turnover rate for esophageal epithelium is 5 to 8 days. This rate seems to be increased to 2 to 4 days with injury. This will allow for epithelial renewal and repair in a short time if further injury is prevented.

F. **Summary.** Patients with reflux esophagitis have heterogeneous abnormalities that contribute to the development of esophagitis. Because patients have different underlying abnormalities responsible for their reflux esophagitis, correct diagnosis of the specific abnormalities involved allows for designing and selecting appropriate therapy. Thus, therapy may be individualized and directed toward increasing the LES pressure, enhancing esophageal clearance, promoting salivary output, improving gastric emptying, suppressing gastric acidity, binding bile salts and proteolytic enzymes, and promoting intrinsic epithelial defenses. **Nighttime GER** is most deleterious to the esophageal mucosa and it should be considered with each patient and addressed therapeutically.

III. DIAGNOSIS

A. **Clinical presentation.** The prevalence of heartburn, the most common clinical manifestation of GER, is difficult to determine. Most people consider this sensation normal and do not seek medical attention. It is estimated that at least one third to one half of the U.S. population experience heartburn at least once a month and up to 20% of the population experience heartburn daily. The most common symptoms of GERD are as follows:

1. **Heartburn (pyrosis).** A substernal burning pain, radiating upward. Ingestion of antacids usually relieves this symptom within 5 minutes.

2. **Regurgitation.** Reflux of sour or bitter material into the mouth usually at night, while lying down, or when bending over. It suggests severe reflux.

3. **Dysphagia.** Difficulty in swallowing. Dysphagia usually indicates a narrowing or stricture of the esophagus; however, it may occur due to inflammation and edema, which may resolve with aggressive medical therapy of the GERD.

4. **Odynophagia.** Pain on swallowing, which sometimes accompanies severe esophagitis.

5. **Water brash.** Filling of the mouth suddenly with a clear, slightly salty fluid, which comes in large quantities. The fluid is not refluxed from the stomach but is secreted by the salivary glands in response to GER.

6. **Chest pain.** Resembling angina of cardiac origin, chest pain is an atypical presentation of GERD. This pain may result from acid-induced irritation of the nerve endings in the elongated rete pegs protruding into the surface epithelium or from GER-induced esophageal spasm or GER-induced angina pectoris.

   In a study of the cardiovascular effect of reflux, esophageal acid perfusion produced an increase in cardiac workload in patients with angiographically proven coronary artery disease. Some patients had ischemic changes on electrocardiography during acid perfusion. This suggests that esophageal and cardiac disease not only may coexist, but also may interconnect. The standard clinical approach aimed at distinguishing between esophageal and cardiac pain may represent a serious oversimplification.

7. **Hemorrhage** may be the first clinical manifestation of esophagitis. It may be brisk, bright red, or slow and may result in iron-deficiency anemia.

8. **Pulmonary symptoms** may be the only manifestation of GER and include chronic cough, hoarseness of voice, wheezing, hemoptysis, asthma, and recurrent aspiration pneumonia. Although it is often assumed by clinicians that pulmonary symptoms associated with reflux result from aspiration, reflux may increase airway resistance without aspiration, apparently through vagus-mediated neural reflexes.

9. **Other symptoms** such as sleep apnea, poor sleep/insomnia, and daytime sleepiness may result from nighttime GER.

B. Diagnostic studies. When a patient describes recurrent retrosternal burning or regurgitation that is worse after eating, lying down, or bending but is relieved with antacids, clinical diagnosis of GERD can easily be made. However, when the presentation is atypical and GERD is suspected, further testing may be required to establish the diagnosis and determine the severity and extent of the disease.

  1. **Usefulness of tests in GERD.** The tests of GERD can be divided into three subgroups.

  a. **Tests indicating possible GER**
      i. Barium swallow, upper gastrointestinal (GI) series
      ii. Endoscopy
      iii. Manometry, measurement of LES pressure

  b. **Tests showing results of GER**
      i. Bernstein test
      ii. Endoscopy
      iii. Mucosal biopsy
      iv. Double-contrast barium esophagram

  c. **Tests measuring actual GER**
      i. Barium swallow and esophagram
      ii. Standard acid reflux test
      iii. Prolonged pH monitoring of the esophagus
      iv. GE scintiscan

  2. **Barium esophagram and upper GI series.** Radiologic examination of the esophagus, stomach, and proximal duodenum is one of the first and most common tests ordered in patients with upper GI complaints. The demonstration of barium reflux during this study is not specific, and many patients with GERD may not show reflux during the time of study.

  GER damage to the esophageal mucosa is usually not detected by single-contrast esophagrams. The double-contrast studies may not show mild degrees of inflammation but are more sensitive for severe grades of esophagitis. Positive signs include contour irregularity, erosions, ulcerations, longitudinal fold thickening, incomplete esophageal distensibility, and stricture formation. An upper GI series will also help to rule out other upper gastrointestinal lesions, such as peptic ulcer disease. It is a poor test in assessing esophageal motor dysfunction but should be obtained in all patients with dysphagia to look for anatomic causes.

  3. **GE scintiscan.** In this test, 300 mL of normal saline containing technetium 99m–sulfur colloid is placed into the stomach, and counts over the stomach and esophagus are measured at 30-second intervals while abdominal pressure is increased incrementally using an abdominal pressure cuff. A reflux index is calculated as the number of counts over the esophagus for given 30-second intervals as a percentage of the number of counts initially present over the stomach. The sensitivity and specificity are considered to be 90%. Because external pressure is applied to the abdomen, however, it is not certain that this technique approximates the physiologic situation.

  4. **Esophageal manometry** has limited usefulness in the routine evaluation of patients with GERD. It is helpful in evaluating the atypical patient with chest pain, patients in whom medical therapy has failed, and those being considered for antireflux surgery. It is a poor test in predicting GER unless the LES pressure is less than 6 mmHg.

  5. **High-resolution manometry (HRM)** offers a more precise and more complete observation of esophageal motor function from the pharynx to the LES and more accurate sphincter and peristaltic pressures.

  6. **Prolonged pH monitoring.** In recent years, prolonged esophageal pH monitoring has become the gold standard for measurement of acid GER. This test provides the most physiologic measurement of acid reflux over 12 to 24 hours in relation to meals, body position, activity, and sleep.

  A pH electrode is placed 5 cm above the LES, and the pH is charted electronically by a system similar to the Holter monitoring of cardiac rhythm.

Patients follow a normal diet with the exception of foods with pH below 5.0. Patients are asked to write down their symptoms and their body position (upright or supine) during the test period. Reflux is defined as the point at which the pH drops to less than 4.0. Each patient's reflux status is assessed by a composite score that incorporates six components:

a. Percentage of time of total acid exposure of the esophagus.

b. Percentage of acid exposure in upright and recumbent positions.

c. Presence of reflux episodes.

d. Total number of reflux episodes.

e. Number of reflux episodes longer than 5 minutes.

f. The longest reflux (time). This test is excellent in identifying acid GER but does not detect "alkaline" reflux. Prolonged pH monitoring has also been helpful in documenting the suspected association between GER and pulmonary disease.

7. **Wireless pH monitoring (Brano) device** which is placed endoscopically in the distal esophagus allows for prolonged monitoring (2–4 days) and better understanding of the day-to-day variability of GER as well as assessing the effectiveness of acid suppressive therapy without performing a second test.

8. **Multichannel intraluminal impedance (MII)** is used to assess GER, esophageal bolus transit (peristaltic function), and the proximal extent of the reflux event. MII may be used in combination with esophageal manometry and pH testing. It is helpful in documenting GER regardless of the pH of the refluxate.

9. **Esophagogastroduodenoscopy and mucosal biopsy.** Flexible fiberoptic endoscopy has become the most widely used method to examine the mucosal surface of the esophagus for evidence of esophagitis. Endoscopic forceps biopsies are adequate for evaluating histologic changes of GERD. Even when endoscopic appearance of the esophagus is normal, histologic examination of the biopsies may confirm the presence of GERD.

   Findings of esophagitis by endoscopy are as follows:

   a. Mild. Erythema; edema of the mucosa with obliteration of small, linear blood vessel; mild friability; and increased irregularity of the Z line.

   b. Moderate-severe. Round and longitudinal superficial ulcers or erosions, diffusely hemorrhagic mucosa with exudates, and deep, punched-out esophageal ulcers and strictures.

10. **Histology.** In patients with GERD, there is a hyperplasia of the basal cell layer of the squamous epithelium. This layer constitutes more than 15% of the epithelial thickness. The dermal papilla extends more than 65% of the distance to the epithelial surface. Polymorphonuclear leukocytes and eosinophils may be seen in the lamina propria and may invade the epithelium. Ingrowth of capillaries is also seen in the lamina propria.

    In about 10% to 20% of the patients with chronic GERD, a specialized columnar metaplastic epithelium (Barrett's epithelium) is present. Endoscopic examination of the stomach and the duodenum can rule out other possible lesions in these areas.

11. **Summary. For the diagnosis of GERD,** most patients with the classic symptoms of GERD of heartburn or regurgitation are given an empiric trial of medical therapy without further investigation. Endoscopy and mucosal biopsies are recommended in patients with refractory symptoms, odynophagia, dysphagia, and atypical symptoms and in patients when Barrett's esophagus is suspected (e.g., those patients with GER symptoms for more than 5 years). Prolonged pH monitoring and manometry are reserved for patients with atypical symptoms and pulmonary complaints.

IV. COMPLICATIONS OF GERD

A. Strictures. An esophageal peptic stricture is thought to result from fibrosis when inflammation and injury extend below the mucosa as consequences of chronic GER. Up to 11% of patients with GERD seem to develop strictures. Factors predisposing to stricture formation include prolonged GER, reflux while supine, nasogastric intubation, duodenal ulcer disease, gastric hypersecretory states, postgastrectomy states, scleroderma, and treated achalasia. Ringlike stricture in the distal esophagus at the E-G junction is called Schatzki's ring.

1. **Location.** Strictures are usually located in the distal third of the esophagus. In the barium esophagogram, they usually have a smooth, tapered appearance and are of variable lengths. In some instances of Barrett's esophagus, the stricture is located in the middle third or, less commonly, in the proximal third of the esophagus.

2. **Symptoms.** Peptic strictures usually produce no symptoms until the esophageal intraluminal diameter is decreased to less than 12 mm. Initially dysphagia is mostly for solids, but with progressive narrowing, swallowing of liquids also becomes a problem. It is not uncommon for the patient to notice improvement in the usual reflux symptoms as dysphagia develops with narrowing of the strictured area. Some patients do not recall even having GER symptoms.

3. **Treatment.** After appropriate diagnostic tests (barium esophagram, endoscopy, and biopsies) have been performed to ensure that the stricture is not due to a malignant process, intensive medical therapy is begun for reflux esophagitis. With resolution of edema and inflammation, some patients may have relief of their symptoms. However, most patients require additional therapy in the form of dilatations, surgery, or both.

   a. **Dilatation.** Progressive dilatations with graded mercury-filled rubber bougies (Maloney or Hurst dilators) have been used in the past for symptomatic relief. Savary dilators passed over a guidewire or inflatable balloon dilators with endoscopic guidance offer safer and more effective means of dilatation.

      Savory dilators come in graded sizes. The guide wire is passed through the biopsy channel of the endoscope and advanced into the stricture, then into the stomach. The endoscope is then removed. The savory dilator is then "threaded over" the guide wire and gently advanced into the lumen of the stricture to dilate it. Afterward, it is withdrawn, then a larger-sized savory dilator is advanced. Similarly, the process is repeated with larger dilators until the stricture is adequately dilated and/or "blood" is seen on the dilator. The dilators should never be forced into the stricture to avoid perforation. Many gastroenterologists use savory dilators with the aid of fluoroscopy.

      Endoscopic balloon dilators allow endoscopic visualization during the entire procedure of dilatation. Each balloon catheter can be inflated to three enlarging sizes that allow progressive dilatation with one insertion. During the EGD the balloon dilatator catheter is introduced via the biopsy channel into the esophageal lumen, then into the stricture. The balloon at the end of catheter is then dilated progressively until the stricture is dilated to the desired size.

      The **major complications of dilatations** are **perforation** and **bleeding**. **Perforations** are rare but should be suspected if the patient complains of persistent pain after dilatation. Perforations are identified by a radiologic contrast study. Patients are treated with intravenous nutrition and antibiotics to cover for organisms from the mouth flora. Surgical drainage and repair should be considered early, since mortality associated with large esophageal perforations is high.

      Dilatation of the stricture and medical therapy for reflux yield good results in 65% to 85% of patients. The patency of the esophageal lumen is maintained by additional dilatations at intervals of weeks to months.

   b. **Surgery.** For the 15% to 40% of patients in whom dilatation and medical therapy fail, surgery is indicated. The preferred surgical approach to strictures is pre- or intraoperative dilatation combined with an antireflux operation, such as the Nissen fundoplication. If the stricture cannot be dilated or is too extensive, resection and end-to-end anastomosis or interposition of a segment of colon or small bowel may be used. These may be combined with a Nissen fundoplication to avoid anastomotic leaks or recurrence of the strictures.

B. Esophageal ulcers and bleeding. A small percentage of patients with GERD, in addition to severe esophagitis, have deep peptic ulcers penetrating into the muscular layers. These ulcers occasionally perforate or cause massive bleeding.

Most of these ulcers respond to intensive medical therapy, but some require surgery. Often, deep ulcers are found in metaplastic Barrett's epithelium. These ulcers should be biopsied prior to therapy to rule out the possibility of malignancy.

C. Pulmonary manifestations. Respiratory problems attributable to GER include laryngitis, hoarseness, chronic cough, asthma, bronchitis, bronchiectasis, aspiration pneumonitis, atelectasis, and hemoptysis. Although most of these patients experience GER symptoms, these symptoms are not always present.

   1. Diagnosis. Documentation of pulmonary aspiration of gastric contents is difficult. Radionuclide scintiscanning of the lungs may be used to document pulmonary aspiration following the placement of technetium 99m–sulfur colloid in the stomach. If a positive result is found, it may be helpful; however, a negative result does not rule out aspiration or absence of a relationship between the pulmonary disease and GER. Prolonged pH monitoring may be helpful in some patients. Numerous studies have demonstrated an increased frequency of reflux in patients with acute and chronic obstructive pulmonary disease. It is accepted that GER with or without aspiration produces an increased airway resistance often requiring strict antireflux therapy with constant suppression of gastric acid secretion with the use of high-dose proton-pump inhibitors (PPIs). Fundoplication may be necessary in some patients (e.g., refractory asthma, GER-related apnea, recurrent aspiration pneumonitis).

   2. Treatment. Intensive therapy of GER may be beneficial in these patients. Many of the medications used to treat asthma lower LES pressure and increase the chance for GER. Thus, the medications used in these patients should be closely monitored. In addition, patients should be discouraged from smoking. Patients who do not improve with medical therapy with PPIs may require antireflux surgery.

D. Barrett's esophagus. In some patients, chronic reflux esophagitis results in replacement of the normal squamous epithelium of the distal esophagus with metaplastic specialized columnar epithelium called **Barrett's epithelium.** Depending on the length of the abnormal tissue, Barrett's esophagus may be subclassified as **short segment** (if it is less than 2 cm) or **long segment Barrett's esophagus.** The prevalence of Barrett's esophagus may be as high as 20%. Even though Barrett's esophagus may be seen at any age, most instances come to medical attention after the fourth decade of life. It is more common in patients with nighttime GER.

Barrett's epithelium consists of a complex mixture of varying cell types, glands, and surface architecture that is normally seen in the small bowel with varying degrees of atrophy.

   1. Complications. Peptic **ulceration, strictures,** and **adenocarcinoma** are complications associated with Barrett's esophagus. Strictures are characteristically found in the mid to lower esophagus with squamous epithelium above and columnar epithelium below the stricture.

     Dysplasia and **adenocarcinoma** of the esophagus have been recognized arising in Barrett's epithelium with a reported prevalence of 3% to 9%. The neoplastic changes may be multifocal and may represent a major pathway in the genesis of adenocarcinoma of the lower esophagus and gastric cardia. The presence of a malignant lesion should be suspected in any patient with mid-esophageal narrowing and stricture formation. However, dysplastic and malignant changes may be present in any patient with Barrett's esophagus. Periodic (e.g., every 1–5 years) multiple endoscopic biopsies and brush cytology should be performed in these patients, especially in patients with histologic dysplasia, to monitor for malignancy. The frequency of endoscopic surveillance of

Barrett's esophagus is controversial. However, if **low-grade dysplasia** is found, yearly EGD and biopsies are recommended. If high-grade dysplasia is found. EGD and biopsies should be repeated every 3 to 6 months. Some experts even suggest therapeutic modalities to eradicate the highly dysplastic tissue and/or consider surgery.

2. **Treatment.** Most patients with Barrett's esophagus are treated medically for reflux esophagitis with high-dose PPIs. Despite strict intensive medical therapy, regression of this metaplastic change has not been documented. **Esophagectomy** or **mucosal ablation therapy** is recommended if severe dysplasia is found. Mucosal ablation may be accomplished by endoscopic mucosal resections, photodynamic therapy followed by laser ablation, or by laser, or bipolar heater probe cautery. These procedures are still not widely accepted or available except in special tertiary medical centers.

V. TREATMENT OF GERD. GERD is a chronic disorder. It is important to educate the patients to modify their lifestyle and habits that may promote GER and encourage them to adopt new habits that will bring long-term beneficial results.

A. Medical therapy

1. Dietary and lifestyle changes recommended include the following:

a. Elevation of the head of the bed (15.2 cm [6 in.]), especially for patients with regurgitation, may be achieved by the placement of 15.2-cm (6-in.) blocks under the head of the bed or a 15.2-cm (6-in.) foam-rubber wedge in place of or under the pillow.

b. Avoid
   i. Smoking
   ii. Fatty and fried foods
   iii. Chocolate
   iv. Alcohol
   v. Tomato products
   vi. Citrus juices and fruits
   vii. Coffee, tea, and carbonated beverages
   viii. Carminatives (spearmint, peppermint)
   ix. Large meals that would distend the stomach

c. Encourage
   i. High-protein, low-fat diet.
   ii. Three small-to-moderate-sized nutritionally balanced meals a day. The evening meal should be light and easy to digest.

d. No eating 4 to 5 hours prior to reclining or going to sleep.

e. Weight loss, if overweight.

f. Avoid using tight belts or girdles that increase intraabdominal pressure.

g. Avoid drugs that promote GER (reduce LES pressure and esophageal clearing):
   i. Progesterone or progesterone-containing birth control pills
   ii. Anticholinergics
   iii. Sedatives/opiates
   iv. Tranquilizers
   v. Theophylline
   vi. Beta-adrenergic agonists
   vii. Nitrates
   viii. Calcium channel blockers

2. **Pharmacologic therapy**

a. **Antacids.** Frequent use of antacids and lozenges (e.g., every 2 hours) is recommended. The most effective and commonly used antacids are those that contain a combination of magnesium and aluminum hydroxides. For patients with renal failure, only aluminum hydroxide-containing antacids are recommended since magnesium may accumulate in the blood. Low-sodium preparations (e.g., Riopan) are available for patients on severe sodium restriction.

b. **Drugs that decrease gastric acid output.** Those most commonly used drugs are **histamine-2 (H$_2$) blockers.** For patients with intermittent, infrequent or mild symptoms of GER, H$_2$ blockers may be prescribed. These drugs are usually effective in controlling symptoms of mild to moderate GER, but have not been shown to effectively heal erosive esophagitis. H$_2$-blockers do not suppress gastric secretions completely. They decrease gastric acid secretion by binding to the histamine receptor on the parietal cell in a competitive fashion. When their concentration decreases around the parietal cell, histamine binds to the parietal cell receptor and acid secretion is resumed. Thus, regular and frequent dosing is essential. H$_2$ blockers also have very limited acid suppressive ability at times of eating and the gastric pH rarely rises above 2 to 3. Because GER occurs most commonly during and after eating, acid and pepsin activity is not eliminated with H$_2$ blockers and their effectiveness is thus limited.

   i. Cimetidine (Tagamet), 300 mg q.i.d. or 400 to 800 mg q12h a.c. and h.s.

   ii. Ranitidine (Zantac), 150 to 300 mg q12h

   iii. Famotidine (Pepcid), 20 to 40 mg at h.s.

   iv. Nizatidine, 150 to 300 mg q12h

   Note: Tagamet, Zantac, and Pepcid are also available at lower doses as over-the-counter medications.

c. **Proton-pump inhibitors.** The final step of gastric acid secretion by the parietal cell involves the extrusion of a proton or a hydrogen ion (H$^+$) into the gastric lumen in exchange of a potassium ion (K$^+$), which enters the parietal cell via the H$^+$ K$^+$-ATPase or the "proton pump." PPIs are a group of drugs designed to inhibit acid secretion by forming a covalent bond within the proton pump and, thus, inhibiting the exchange of (H$^+$) and (K$^+$) ions permanently by that proton pump. These drugs are extremely effective in inhibition of gastric acid secretion for 19 to 24 hours and allow the gastric pH to rise above 4 or 5, thus, also eliminating the pepsin activity. PPIs have been shown to effectively heal erosive esophagitis, diminish the formation of esophageal strictures, and control most symptoms and signs of GERD. PPIs, when used continuously, prevent recurrence of erosive esophagitis. As a group of drugs, they are safe and have minimal side effects. In most instances, they are used as first line therapy for GERD.

   Currently, there are six commercially available PPIs approved by the U.S. Food and Drug Administration (FDA) for healing erosive GERD. These are **omeprazole (Prilosec),** 20 to 40 mg p.o. (q.d. or b.i.d.); **lansoprazole (Prevacid),** 15 to 30 mg p.o. (q.d. or b.i.d.); **rabeprazole sodium (AcipHex),** 20 mg orally (once daily); **pantoprazole (Protonix),** 40 mg p.o. (q.d.); **esomeprazole magnesium (Nexium),** 20 to 40 mg p.o. (q.d.); and **omeprazole sodium bicarbonate (Zegerid),** 40 mg p.o. (q.d.). All PPIs are most effective if taken 15 to 30 minutes before breakfast or dinner. Omeprazole, lansoprazole, pantoprazole, and esomeprazole magnesium are excreted in the urine. Rabeprazole sodium is mostly excreted in bile. No dose adjustments are necessary in renal or hepatic insufficiency. Omeprazole, esomeprazole magnesium, lansoprazole, and rabeprazole sodium are metabolized by the p450 system in the liver and may have minor drug–drug interactions with some drugs; however, these have not been shown to be clinically significant. Pantoprazole has no known drug–drug interactions. Pantoprazole, esomeprazole, and lansoprazole are also available in intravenous (IV) formulation and have been FDA-approved for in patients with GERD who are unable to receive medications by the oral route.

   Side effects of PPIs are rare and include minor headaches, diarrhea, and nausea. PPIs have revolutionized the treatment of GERD and most of its complications. These drugs have been noted to be safe and free of long-term complications. Initial concerns about gastric bacterial overgrowth, Vitamin B$_{12}$ and iron malabsorption, and causation of gastric carcinoid tumors have not been clinically observed. A retrospective observational study suggests that patients taking PPIs for many years may have decreased calcium absorption. Thus it may be prudent to encourage patients on prolonged PPI therapy to take calcium supplements.

   d. Drugs that increase LES pressure and esophageal clearance

   i. Metoclopramide hydrochloride, a dopamine antagonist, has been shown to increase LES pressure and to improve esophageal and gastric emptying. It counteracts the receptive relaxation of the gastric fundus and increases duodenal and small-bowel motility. It is also a centrally active antiemetic. This drug is especially helpful in patients with GERD and abnormalities of gastric emptying. Since metoclopramide crosses the blood–brain barrier, 10% of patients seem to experience psychotropic side effects (e.g., somnolence, lassitude, restlessness, anxiety, insomnia, and, rarely, extrapyramidal reactions). These side effects are reversible with cessation of the drug. Elevated prolactin levels may occur and cause galactorrhea. The usual dosage is 10 to 20 mg q.i.d., 15 to 30 minutes a.c. and h.s.

   ii. Other prokinetic drugs such as **domperidone** and **cisapride** do not cross the **blood–brain barrier** and have only the peripheral effects of metoclopramide. These drugs have excellent promotility qualities and have been used successfully in the treatment of GERD.

   However, cisapride, due to its drug–drug interactions with those drugs that prolong the Q-T interval (on electrocardiogram) and the possibility of precipitating cardiac arrhythmias, has been removed from the market in the United States by the manufacturer. Cisapride and domperidone are available in Canada and other countries.

   e. Drugs that enhance mucosal resistance. As the importance of mucosal resistance is appreciated, drugs that potentiate cytoprotection and mucosal resistance are being added to the medical armamentarium of acid-peptic disease.

   i. Sucralfate (Carafate), an aluminum sucrose polysulfate shown to be effective in healing duodenal ulcers due to its cytoprotective action, has not been shown to be highly effective in patients with esophagitis. However, sucralfate suspension seems to give symptomatic and possibly therapeutic benefit to patients with erosive esophagitis. Dose is 1 g 1–4 times daily.

   ii. Prostaglandin analogs (e.g., misoprostol) have also been shown to be cytoprotective and effective in the treatment of peptic ulcer disease, but have not been found highly effective in the treatment of GERD.

   f. The results of maintenance therapy with H_2-receptor antagonists are disappointing. Neither twice-daily nor single-dose-bedtime regimens of cimetidine or ranitidine are significantly more effective than placebo in preventing symptomatic or endoscopic evidence of relapse. However, maintenance therapy with 20 mg of omeprazole daily sustains endoscopic healing in most patients with severe, recalcitrant esophagitis. In some patients, the dosage needs to be increased to 40 mg. Significant and persistent elevations in fasting serum gastrin concentrations may occur in a minority of patients. It is important to note that up to 90% of patients who healed with omeprazole treatment had recurrence of their esophagitis within 6 months of stopping treatment, indicating that some form of chronic treatment is needed. Similar excellent results have also been achieved with the other PPIs (lansoprazole, rabeprazole sodium, pantoprazole, and esomeprazole magnesium) at the same doses used to heal erosive esophagitis.

B. Phase III, endoscopic interventional and/or surgical therapy, is reserved for patients in whom intensive medical therapy has failed and those with complications such as a nonhealing or bleeding esophageal ulcer or a refractory stricture. Surgery for Barrett's esophagus is still controversial.

   Endoscopic treatment of GERD has been attractive as an alternative to surgery by providing a less invasive solution to GER refractory to medical therapy.

The initial procedures involved **injection of collagen circumferentially at the LES (Enteryx)** which created a "tighter" LES and the **Stretta procedure** which places minute areas of thermal injury in the muscle of the lower esophageal sphincter and cardia using radio frequency waves. These procedures have shown improvement in GERD symptoms, but have not shown a consistent reduction in esophageal acid exposure or improved LES tone. Serious complications have been reported and both of these procedures have been abandoned.

Endoscopic suturing devices, which place submucosal sutures in the gastric cardia, and **endoscopic plicators,** which place transmural staples around the LES, are still in evolution and offer promise. Both of these procedures decrease the luminal size of the distal esophagus and gastric cardia to decrease GER and regurgitation.

The **preferred antireflux operation** is the **Nissen fundoplication**, in which the LES is reinforced with a 360-degree gastric wrap for a distance of about 5 cm around the lower esophagus, which is secured below the diaphragm. If a hiatal hernia is present, it is reduced. An adequate esophageal lumen is secured with a 60-French, mercury-filled bougie placed in the esophageal lumen during the surgical procedure. Nissen fundoplication performed by a competent surgeon has been shown to be successful with lasting effects. It should be considered in young patients for long-term relief of GERD. This procedure is currently widely available as a **laparoscopic procedure (laparoscopic Nissen fundoplication)** with much lower morbidity and, in good hands with equivalent effectiveness to the open Nissen fundoplication.

Selected Readings

Abid S, et al. Pill-induced esophageal injury: Endoscopic features and clinical outcomes. *Endoscopy.* 2005;37:470–474.

Abou-Rebych H, et al. Long-term failure of endoscopic suturing in treatment of gastro-esophageal reflux: A prospective follow-up study. *Endoscopy.* 2005;37(3):213–216.

Boolchard V, et al. Risk for Carcenin Barrett's esophaus: medical versus surgical therapy. *Cur Gastroenterol Hepatol.* 2007;9:189–194.

Byrne P, et al. Comparison of transoesophageal endoscopic plication (TEP) with laparoscopic Nissen fundoplication (LNF) in the treatment of uncomplicated reflux disease. *Am J Gastroenterol.* 2006;101:431–436.

Charbel S, et al. The role of esophageal pH monitoring in symptomatic patients on PPI therapy. *Am J Gastroenterol.* 2005;100:283–289.

Chejtec G, et al. Gastroesophageal reflux disease—A review. *US Gastroenterol Rev.* 2007; 1:84–87.

DeVault KR, et al. Updated guidelines for the diagnosis and treatment of gastroesophageal reflux disease. *Am J Gastroenterol.* 2005;100:190–200.

Domagh D, et al. Endoluminal gastroplasty (EndoCinch) versus endoscopic polymer implantation (Enteryx) for treatments of gastroesophageal reflux disease: 6 month results of a prospective, randomized trial. *Am J Gastroenterol.* 2006;101:422–430.

Fass R, et al. Treatment of patients with persistent heartburn symptoms: A double-blind randomized trial. *Clin Gastroenterol.* 2006;4:50–56.

Fernando HC, et al. Outcomes of laparoscopic Toupet compared to laparoscopic Nissen fundoplication. *Surg Endosc.* 2002;16:905–908.

Hirano I. Review article: Modern technology in the diagnosis of gastroesophageal reflux disease—Bilitec, intraluminal impedance and Bravo capsule pH monitoring. *Aliment Pharmacol Ther.* 2006;23(suppl 1):12–24.

Kikendall JW. Pill induced esophagitis. *Gastroenterol Hepatol.* 2007;3(4):275–276.

Lagergren J, et al. Symptomatic gastroesophageal reflux as a risk factor for esophageal adenocarcinoma. *N Engl J Med.* 1999;340:825.

Martinez SD, et al. Non-erosive reflux disease (NERD), acid reflux and symptom patterns. *Aliment Pharmacol Ther.* 2003;17:537–545.

Oleynikov D, et al. Total fundoplication is the operation of choice for patients with gastroesophageal reflux and defective peristalsis. *Surg Endosc.* 2002;16:909–913.

Overholt BF, et al. Photodynamic therapy for Barrett's esophagus follow-up in 100 patients. *Gastrointest Endosc.* 1999;49:1.

Pandolfino JE, et al. Ambulatory esophageal pH monitoring using a wireless technique. *Am J Gastroenterol.* 2003;98:545–550.

Remedios M, et al. Eosinophilic esophagitis in adults: clinical, endoscopic histologic findings, and response to treatment with fluticasone propionate. *Gastrointest Endose.* 2006;63(1):3–12.

Richter JE. Gastroesophageal reflux disease and asthma: The two are directly related. *Am J Med.* 2000;108(suppl 4a):1535.

Richter JE. Gastroesophageal reflux disease and esophageal cancer: New respect for an old disease. *Curr Gastroenterol Rep.* 2000;2:1.

Sgouros SN, et al. Eosinophilic esophagitis in aduts: what is the clinical significance? *Endoscopy.* 2006;38:515–20.

Shah A, et al. Treatment of eosinophitic esophagitis: Drugs, diet or dilation? *Cur Gastroenterol Rep.* 2007;9:181–188.

Sifrim D, et al. Acid, non-acid, and gas reflux in patients with gastroesophageal reflux disease during ambulatory 24-hour pH-impedance recordings. *Gastroenterology.* 2001; 120:1588–1598.

Spight DH, et al. Defining risk for early detection of esophageal adenocarcinoma—finding the needle in the haystack. *US Gastroenterol Rev.* 2007;1:94–96.

21 DYSPHAGIA

I. ESOPHAGUS
A. Anatomy
1. **The esophagus** is a muscular tube measuring about 25 cm (40 cm from the incisor teeth) extending from the pharynx at the cricoid cartilage to the cardia of the stomach. It pierces the left crus of the diaphragm and has an intraabdominal portion of about 1.5 to 2.5 cm in length.
2. **The esophageal mucosa** consists of a nonkeratinizing squamous epithelium, lamina propria extending into the basal layer as rete pegs, and muscularis mucosa, which is sparse and thin in the upper portion but thicker near the gastroesophageal junction.
3. **The submucosa** contains mucous glands and an extensive lymphatic plexus in a connective tissue network.
4. Between the submucosa and muscularis propria are the cell bodies of secondary neurons forming the **Auerbach's plexus.**
5. The muscularis propria, the main muscle layers of the esophagus, is composed of inner circular and outer longitudinal coats. In the upper part, these are striated. There is a gradual change to smooth muscle in the middle. In the lower third of the esophagus, both of these coats are entirely composed of smooth muscle.
6. Between the muscle layers, the **myenteric plexus** contains the cell bodies of other secondary neurons.
7. The esophagus does not have a serosal layer.
8. **Lower esophageal sphincter.** The distal 3 to 4 cm of the esophagus constitutes a zone of increased resting pressure in an asymmetric fashion. This area, called the lower esophageal sphincter (LES), behaves both physiologically and pharmacologically as a distinct entity from the esophageal smooth muscle immediately adjacent to it. Basal LES pressure is normally 10 to 25 mmHg higher than intragastric pressure and drops promptly (within 1–2 seconds) with swallowing. The LES control remains poorly understood but is thought to involve the complex interaction of neural, hormonal, and myogenic activities.

B. Physiology of esophageal function.
The function of the esophagus is to transport food and secretions from the mouth to the stomach. This coordinated process operates regardless of the force of gravity.
1. **A swallow** begins when a liquid or solid bolus is propelled to the back of the mouth into the pharynx by the tongue. The upper esophageal sphincter (UES), the cricopharyngeus, which is just below the pharynx, relaxes, allowing the bolus to pass into the upper esophagus. In response to swallowing, an orderly, progressive contraction of the esophageal body occurs (primary peristalsis), propelling the bolus down the esophagus. When the esophagus is distended by a bolus (i.e., with regurgitation), secondary peristaltic contractions are initiated. The LES relaxes as the bolus reaches the lower esophagus, allowing passage of the food into the stomach.
2. **The relaxation of the UES and peristalsis in the upper esophagus** are initiated by the voluntary act of swallowing, controlled by the swallowing center in the brainstem and the fifth, seventh, ninth, tenth, eleventh, and twelfth cranial nerves. These nerves coordinate the movement of the bolus to the hypopharynx,

closure of the epiglottis, relaxation of the UES, and contraction of the striated muscle of the upper esophagus. The sequential nature of this function is due to progressive activation of nerve fibers carried in the vagus nerve controlled through a central mechanism.

3. **The peristalsis in the smooth-muscle portion of the esophagus** is regulated by activation of neurons located in the myenteric plexus with cholinergic neural transmission. The vagi innervate the upper esophagus in its striated muscle portion only. If the vagi are cut below the level of mid esophagus, peristalsis in the lower half of the esophagus and the function of the LES remain intact.

II. DYSPHAGIA

A. Definition

1. **Dysphagia** is difficulty in swallowing. Clinically, it includes the inability to initiate swallowing and/or the sensation that the swallowed solids or liquids stick in the esophagus.

2. **Odynophagia** refers to pain with swallowing. In some disorders, odynophagia may accompany dysphagia.

3. **Globus hystericus** describes the sensation of the presence of "a lump in the throat" that is relieved momentarily by swallowing.

B. Preesophageal or oroesophageal dysphagia.
Patients with this disorder have problems with the initial steps of swallowing. They may have difficulty in propelling food to the hypopharynx. If the food passes normally to the hypopharynx, the presence of pain, intra- or extraluminal mass lesion, or a neuromuscular disorder may interfere with the orderly sequence of pharyngeal contraction, closure of the epiglottis, UES relaxation, and initiation of peristalsis by contraction of the striated muscle in the upper esophagus.

1. **Signs and symptoms.** These patients usually cough and expel the ingested food through their mouth and nose or aspirate when they attempt to swallow. Their symptoms are worse with liquids than with solids. They may have a "wet" voice quality, reduced cough, upper airway congestion, and aspiration pneumonitis.

2. **Causes**

   a. **Central nervous system conditions.** Cerebral vascular accidents (bulbar or pseudobulbar palsy), multiple sclerosis, amyotrophic lateral sclerosis, Wilson's disease, Parkinson's disease, Friedreich's ataxia, tabes dorsalis, brainstem tumors, paraneoplastic disorders, reaction to drugs or toxins, other congenital and degenerative disorders of the central nervous system.

   b. **Peripheral nervous system conditions.** Poliomyelitis (bulbar), diphtheria, rabies, botulism, diabetes mellitus, demyelinating diseases, Guillain-Barré syndrome.

   c. **Disorders of the myoneural junction.** Myasthenia gravis, Eaton-Lambert syndrome.

   d. **Muscular disorders.** Dermatomyositis, muscular dystrophies, myotonic disorders, congenital myopathies, metabolic myopathies (thyrotoxicosis, hypothyroidism, hyperthyroidism, steroid myopathy), collagen vascular diseases, amyloidosis.

   e. **Toxins.** Tetanus, botulism, tic paralysis, arsenic, lead, mercury poisoning.

   f. **Local structural lesions.** Conditions involving the mouth, pharynx, and hypopharynx.

      i. **Infection or inflammation.** Abscess; tuberculosis; syphilis; viral, bacterial, and fungal infections; Lyme disease; diphtheria; rabies.

      ii. **Space-occupying lesions.** Neoplasms, congenital webs, Plummer-Vinson syndrome.

      iii. **Extrinsic compression.** Cervical spine spurs, lymphadenopathy, thyromegaly, Zenker's diverticulum.

      iv. **Trauma.** Surgical repair, foreign body ingestion, caustic injury.

   g. **Motility disorders of the upper esophageal sphincter.** Hypertensive UES, hypotensive UES with esophagopharyngeal regurgitation, abnormal

UES relaxation (incomplete relaxation: cricopharyngeal achalasia, premature closure, delayed relaxation).

C. Esophageal dysphagia describes difficulty with transport of food down the esophagus once the bolus has been successfully transferred into the proximal esophageal lumen. Any disorder, structural or neuromuscular, involving the body of the esophagus, the LES, or the gastroesophageal junction may result in dysphagia or the sensation of food being "stuck" behind the sternum. If the patient can localize the symptom to some point along the sternum, a good correlation with the anatomic site is possible. However, if the symptoms are felt at the sternal notch, the anatomic site of the lesion cannot be predicted.

1. Structural disorders are usually caused by a discrete lesion such as a neoplasm, stricture, or extrinsic compression that interferes with the transport of the swallowed bolus. Initially, dysphagia is noted with solid foods. However, as the lumen narrows with enlarging lesions, passage of liquids also becomes impaired.

a. Tumors (see also Chapter 23)

i. Squamous carcinoma accounts for approximately one third of all esophageal cancers. Excessive alcohol intake and cigarette smoking seem to increase the risk. Other predisposing factors include head and neck cancer, Plummer-Vinson syndrome (anemia and esophageal web), tylosis, achalasia, and lye stricture.

ii. Adenocarcinoma of the esophagus constitutes about two thirds of esophageal cancers. It is thought to arise from extension of gastric cardia carcinoma, from the esophageal glands or, more commonly, from the columnar metaplasia of the esophagus (Barrett's epithelium).

iii. Kaposi's sarcoma, lymphoma, melanoma, and metastatic tumors from the lungs, pancreas, breasts, and other structures may also involve the esophagus.

iv. Benign tumors of the esophagus are rare and account for less than 10% of esophageal tumors. These tumors most commonly arise from neuromesenchymal elements. Leiomyomas that arise from esophageal smooth muscle are the most common. These intramural lesions are covered by normal squamous epithelium of the esophagus. They protrude into the lumen, eventually causing narrowing of the passage. Other lesions such as fibroadenomas, though rare, may become very long and large and may cause obstruction.

b. Strictures

i. Peptic strictures. Most esophageal strictures are found in the distal or mid esophagus and are the result of chronic inflammation caused by gastroesophageal reflux. Peptic strictures are usually benign, but those associated with Barrett's epithelium may be malignant.

ii. Burns caused by ingestion of corrosive substances (e.g., strong alkali and acids) may result in esophageal strictures in single or multiple locations of the esophagus.

iii. Some **drugs in tablet form** may lodge in a segment of the esophagus and cause local inflammation, ulceration, and stricture.

iv. Foreign bodies (e.g., coins or button batteries) may be swallowed and cause obstruction or injury of the esophagus.

c. Rings and webs are usually thin, circumferential mucosal shelves that protrude into the esophageal lumen and cause intermittent dysphagia, especially to solids. Webs occur in the upper esophagus and may be associated with iron-deficiency anemia (Plummer-Vinson syndrome).

Rings (Schatzki) are most often found at the gastroesophageal junction. Schatzki's rings seem to be related to chronic gastroesophageal reflux. Most of these contain only mucosal elements; however, thicker ones may also contain a thickened muscle layer.

d. Eosinophilic esophagitis is an inflammatory condition of the esophagus anatomically characterized by the presence of multiple concentric firm rings throughout the entire length of the esophagus. It is also referred to as **corrugated esophagus, ringed esophagus, corrugated ringed esophagus,** and **congenital esophageal stenosis** occurring in children and young adults, especially males.

i. Dysphagia is the primary presenting symptom with occasional food impaction. Heartburn and GER is rare but may exist.

ii. Diagnosis: Barium swallow or UGI x-rays are usually too insensitive to show the rings; however, with the use of fluoroscopy, double contrast and a solid bolus, the corrugations may be demonstrated.

iii. Esophageal motility testing is normal or may show high amplitude contractions.

On **endoscopy,** the esophageal lumen appears generally narrow and the rings are clearly visible. There may be strictures. The esophageal mucosal biopsies show intense eosinophilic infiltration. The degree of eosinophilic infiltration may differ in patients however, the presences of more than 20 eosinophils per each high power filed is used as a guide in diagnosis. Eosinophilic infiltration, to a lesser degree, is also seen in other GI disorders including GFRD, parasitic infections, fungal infections, reaction to drugs, inflammatory bowel disease, scleroderma, Hodgkin's disease, and allergic vasculitis.

The **etiology** of eosinophilic esophagitis is thought to be due to a sensitization after an exposure to food or airborne allergen followed by an allergic reaction to subsequent exposures. However, the results of allergy testing are inconsistent. The anatomical structure may be congenital and/or inherited.

The treatment may involve esophageal dilation and elimination of offending foods identified by skin testing. Best results are obtained with the use of topical steroids used as an aerosol, four puffs twice daily applied without a spacer. Patients should not eat or drink for 3 hours after each treatment. The course of treatment is usually 6 weeks. The relief may last 4 to 6 months. Additional treatment may be needed intermittently.

e. Extrinsic compression. The esophageal lumen may be narrowed from compression by an external lesion. These lesions include the following:

i. Mediastinal tumors, primary or metastatic.

ii. Vascular lesions, such as aberrant right subclavian artery (dysphagia lusoria), a dilated aneurysmal aorta, or an enlarged cardiac chamber.

iii. Cervical osteoarthritis and bone spurs.

iv. Esophageal diverticula may cause dysphagia when they become large and distended with food and secretions. They tend to occur in three main parts of the esophagus: just above the UES (Zenker's), at the middle (traction), and near the diaphragm (epiphrenic). Zenker's and epiphrenic diverticula are thought to result from motor abnormalities of the esophagus. Even though midesophageal diverticula have been attributed to traction on the walls of the esophagus by external inflammatory and fibrotic processes (e.g., tuberculosis or sarcoidosis), they also may result from abnormal esophageal motility.

2. Gastroesophageal reflux (see Chapter 20). The reflux of the gastroduodenal contents into the esophagus may cause dysphagia in some patients, especially if severe inflammation, ulceration, or stricture develops. With resolution of the inflammation and edema, dysphagia may abate. In some patients, gastroesophageal reflux (GER) may result in esophageal motility disorders, which may contribute to dysphagia and chest pain.

3. Neuromuscular or motility disorders result in dysphagia to both liquids and solids due to aberrant peristalsis. These disorders are present in about half the patients who have dysphagia without an evident structural abnormality. In these disorders, peristalsis is either absent, weak, too strong and sustained, or uncoordinated. The LES function may also be abnormal. The resting LES pressure may be too high or low and the sphincter may not relax completely on swallowing.

a. Primary motor disorders

i. Achalasia is a disorder of esophageal smooth-muscle function with three diagnostic prerequisites. First, there is a complete absence of primary and secondary peristalsis in the smooth muscle of the esophagus. Skeletal muscle function is generally normal. Second, the LES does not relax completely with swallows. Third, the resting LES pressure is usually high. The lack of peristalsis and the sustained high-pressure zone at the gastroesophageal junction results in retention of ingested material and oral secretions in the esophagus with gradual loss of tone and progressive dilatation of the body of the esophagus.

    a) Cause. Achalasia is most likely the result of neuronal abnormalities rather than a primary myopathy. Lesions have been found in the dorsal vagal nucleus in the brainstem, in the vagal trunks, and in the myenteric ganglia in the esophagus. Secondary achalasia may resemble primary achalasia. It may result from tumor invasion of the LES region, constriction from malignant nodes, or paraneoplastic syndromes.

    b) Signs and symptoms. Patients with achalasia consistently have dysphagia to both solids and liquids. Occasionally, early in the disease and in patients with "vigorous achalasia," chest pain may occur. Regurgitation of esophageal contents often with tracheal aspiration is a common complication of the disease.

    c) Treatment of achalasia is designed to decrease the pressure in the LES. This allows the aperistaltic esophagus to empty in the upright position. LES myotomy may be accomplished surgically (open or laparoscope) or by forceful dilatation with an inflatable, pneumatic peroral balloon dilator or by intramucosal injection of Botulinum toxin endoscopically. Medical management of achalasia is usually unsuccessful. In some patients, calcium channel blockers may lower the LES pressure and produce transient symptomatic improvement.

ii. Diffuse esophageal spasm (DES). This entity accounts for about 10% to 15% of patients with esophageal motility disorders. Patients with this disorder have high-amplitude, simultaneous contractions in the smooth-muscle portion of the esophageal body. Skeletal muscle function is normal. The "spastic" waves are usually initiated by swallows but may occur randomly interspersed with normal-appearing peristalsis. The LES may have normal or high pressure and may not completely relax with swallowing.

    a) Signs and symptoms. In these patients, dysphagia is intermittent. It occurs with both liquids and solids. Sometimes it is exacerbated with hot or cold foods and may cause chest pain. In fact, the chest pain of DES is often confused with angina pectoris. Thus, it is important in these patients to exclude possible cardiac disease.

    b) Treatment of DES is generally directed toward decreasing the frequency and intensity of simultaneous contractions. Smooth muscle relaxants, including nitrates (e.g., nitroglycerin, 0.4 mg sublingually a.c. and p.r.n.); isosorbide dinitrate, 30 mg per os (p.o.) 30 minutes a.c.; hydralazine, 25 to 50 mg p.o. three times daily; calcium channel blockers (e.g., nifedipine, 10–20 mg, four times daily); psychotropic drugs (e.g., diazepam 1–5 mg p.o., four times daily; trazodone 50–100 mg p.o., twice daily; doxepin, 50 mg p.o., h.s.); and anticholinergics (e.g., dicyclomine 10–20 mg p.o., four times daily) have been tried with variable results.

        Because abnormal motility is not always documented in patients with dysphagia secondary to dysmotility, provocation of symptoms and manometric findings with drugs may be attempted. Edrophonium is the best tolerated and most effective of currently available drugs.

        Bougienage and pneumatic dilatation sometimes yield transient symptom relief. In difficult cases, surgical myotomy may be tried. The outcome is often variable, and successful relief of symptoms is rare.

c) **"Vigorous achalasia."** An overlap between DES and achalasia called vigorous achalasia has been observed in some patients. In this condition, in addition to simultaneous, high-amplitude contractions in the distal esophagus as in DES, the LES function is similar to that in achalasia. The symptoms are usually chest pain and dysphagia. This overlap, as well as a transition from DES to achalasia in some patients, suggests that these two disorders may be different manifestations of the spectrum of esophageal smooth muscle dysfunction.

iii. **Nutcracker esophagus** or "super squeezer" is a motility disorder found in approximately one half of the patients with chest pain of esophageal origin and one tenth of the patients with dysphagia. These patients have normal LES function and peristalsis; however, the contractile amplitude is usually two to three times the normal value. Most of these patients also have an abnormal prolongation of the peristaltic wave. A subgroup of patients with contraction waves of normal amplitude but prolonged duration also has been described.

The symptoms of patients with nutcracker esophagus are similar to those associated with DES. Patients may have prolonged chest pain, which may be nocturnal, and intermittent dysphagia. The nutcracker esophagus may evolve into DES, suggesting that these disorders are related. Treatment of nutcracker esophagus is similar to treatment of DES (see section II.C.3.b).

iv. **Nonspecific esophageal motor disorders (NEMD).** Most patients with symptoms of esophageal dysmotility cannot be classified neatly into specific groups. The incidence of these disorders of the peristaltic wave or LES function is at least five times that of achalasia and DES combined. The patients may have an isolated abnormality of the LES (increased pressure, incomplete relaxation, hypertensive LES) with or without abnormal esophageal contractions (increased amplitude or duration, simultaneous contractions, nonpropagated waves).

a) **Treatment.** There is no reliable therapy for patients with nonspecific esophageal motor disorders. Smooth-muscle relaxants have been tried as in DES, again with variable results. Bougienage may give transient relief in some patients.

b) Patients with **diabetes mellitus** may have abnormal esophageal motility such as poor propagation of the peristaltic wave and diffuse spasm, most likely due to visceral neuropathy.

b. **Secondary motor disorders.** Esophageal smooth-muscle dysfunction may be associated with a number of systemic disorders.

i. **Scleroderma.** Approximately 80% of the patients with scleroderma, particularly those who exhibit Raynaud's phenomenon, have decreased amplitude of peristalsis in the smooth-muscle portion of the esophagus with decreased resting LES pressure. Initially, the disorder seems to be neural; however, with progression of the disease, collagen deposition and fibrosis of the smooth muscle are observed. These patients are a setup for severe reflux esophagitis, which is frequently complicated by stricture formation and Barrett's esophagus.

ii. **Other diseases.** The abnormal esophageal motility associated with scleroderma has been reported in some patients with other collagen vascular diseases and those with Raynaud's phenomenon. Patients with polymyositis and lupus also may exhibit esophageal smooth muscle dysfunction.

iii. **Chagas' disease.** An achalasialike disease has been seen as a secondary disorder with Chagas' disease (infection with *Trypanosoma cruzi*).

iv. **Tumors** of the mediastinum, lower esophagus, gastroesophageal junction, and gastric cardia, as well as lymphoma, pancreatic, lung, and bronchogenic carcinoma may also present as achalasia. Tumors may invade the myenteric plexus or produce an obstruction at the gastroesophageal junction; thus, aperistalsis may be secondary to neural invasion or a response to LES obstruction.

v. Chronic idiopathic intestinal pseudoobstruction usually involves the esophagus as well as all other parts of the gastrointestinal tract. The esophageal abnormality includes aperistalsis and incomplete relaxation of LES, producing a functional obstruction. Patients with this disease usually have either congenital or acquired neuromuscular degeneration of the entire gut, affecting the neural plexuses and the myenteric ganglia.

c. Reflux esophagitis and esophageal dysmotility (see also Chapter 20). Patients with gastroesophageal reflux and reflux esophagitis have been shown to have a number of abnormalities of smooth-muscle function. These include a low resting LES pressure; abnormal, prolonged periods of relaxation of the LES; and decreased esophageal clearance due to disorder of primary and secondary peristaltic waves. It is difficult to determine whether these defects are a primary cause of reflux or a result of the associated esophagitis.

III. DIAGNOSTIC APPROACH

A. History. Differentiation of the major causes of dysphagia can be facilitated by eliciting the history on several critical points: consistency of the food causing symptoms, localization and duration of dysphagia, and presence of associated symptoms such as odynophagia, heartburn, cough, and weight loss.

1. Consistency of foods causing dysphagia. As mentioned before, a motility disorder usually causes dysphagia to both liquids and solids from the onset of the symptoms, whereas a structural disorder causes dysphagia to solids first and, if the lesion further compromises the esophageal lumen, progressively to semisolids and liquids.

2. The duration and constancy of the symptoms are also diagnostically pertinent. Intermittent dysphagia for solid foods only is typical of lower esophageal (Schatzki) ring. A patient with a long history of heartburn may notice its disappearance when a stricture develops, which may cause dysphagia, especially to solids. The patient with esophageal cancer typically has a more accelerated course of progressive dysphagia over several months, usually accompanied by weight loss and anorexia.

3. Other disorders. The possible presence of neurologic, muscular, connective tissue, or other systemic disorders and the use of drugs that may affect striated or smooth-muscle function of the esophagus should be determined.

B. The physical examination may be indirectly helpful in the diagnosis of dysphagia related to another disease such as a central nervous system, muscular, endocrine–metabolic, or connective tissue disorder. The presence of pharyngeal inflammation, a mass in the neck, an enlarged thyroid, a deviated trachea, cardiomegaly, or an epigastric mass may also be helpful in reaching the diagnosis.

C. Radiographic studies

1. The chest x-ray may be helpful indirectly in the diagnosis of the cause of dysphagia. In advanced achalasia with dilatation of the esophagus, patients may have a widened mediastinal shadow with an air-fluid level made up of food and secretions held up by the tight LES. Mediastinal masses or cardiomegaly with chamber enlargement may also be evident on a chest x-ray.

2. Barium swallow, cineesophagogram, and upper gastrointestinal series are usually the first specific diagnostic studies performed in the workup of dysphagia. The patient is asked to swallow liquid barium or a piece of bread dipped in barium. The movement of the bolus is then observed by the radiologist fluoroscopically and recorded on x-ray film or videotape (cineradiography). In this way, the course of the bolus is followed from the mouth to the stomach.

This test gives visual information about the preesophageal swallowing function, the nature of the peristaltic activity, and the presence of gastroesophageal reflux as well as information about the anatomy of the esophagus with respect to structural disorders, such as carcinoma, stricture, esophageal web or ring, or presence of extrinsic compression.

The barium study is less helpful in the diagnosis of motility disorders. However, in achalasia one may see a dilated esophagus with a "parrot beak" narrowing at the gastroesophageal junction. Tertiary or corkscrew contractions may suggest the diagnosis of diffuse esophageal spasm; however, this may be a normal finding, especially in elderly patients.

D. Upper gastrointestinal endoscopy. The direct visualization of the mucosa and lumen of the esophagus, stomach, and proximal duodenum is possible with flexible endoscopes. Structural and inflammatory lesions may be directly examined, and biopsies and cytologic specimens may be obtained. Intramural lesions such as leiomyomas may also be seen. Biopsies of these lesions are not recommended, since the scarred overlying mucosa may adhere to the movable tumor and prevent its easy surgical enucleation. Submucosal tumors may be examined using endoscopic ultrasonography (EUS).

E. Esophageal manometry is recommended when an esophageal motility disorder is suspected. In this test, intraesophageal pressures and peristaltic activity are recorded as a function of time with wet and dry swallows. This test yields information about the lower and upper esophageal sphincter function and the nature of the peristaltic wave.

The typical manometry tube consists of soft, flexible tubing that has three recording sensors arranged linearly 5 cm apart from one another in a spiral fashion at the distal end. The patient is asked to swallow the tube, which is then advanced into the stomach. As the tube is gradually withdrawn, each sensor passes through the LES, measuring its pressure. In the body of the esophagus, the peristaltic waves are recorded in a sequential manner as they progress down the esophagus, first with the proximal sensor, next with the middle, and last with the distal sensor. If peristalsis is progressive, this normal sequence is observed. If simultaneous, repetitive contractions are noted, their amplitude and duration will help in establishing the type of motility disorder. When the middle or distal sensor lies within the LES, the relationship between esophageal peristaltic contractions and sphincter relaxation can be observed. Similarly, when the upper sensor lies in the UES, the relationship between pharyngeal contractions and UES relaxation can be recorded.

In patients with achalasia, a careful examination of the distal esophagus and gastroesophageal junction is essential to rule out malignancy. Even benign appearing strictures should be biopsied and brushed to look for malignant cells. EUS may help in evaluation of strictures and give information on the extent of tissue involvement with malignant infiltration.

Evaluation of the stomach and duodenum may be helpful in eliminating diseases of these organs that may coexist or give symptoms that may be confused with those of esophageal disorders.

IV. TREATMENT

A. Oropharyngeal dysphagia. The treatment of oropharyngeal dysphagia depends on the specific cause.

1. Systemic disease (see section IV.B.1).

2. Neurologically impaired patients require special attention during feedings with respect to dietary texture; body, head, and neck position; size and frequency of food bolus administration; and aspiration precautions. Patients should sit fully upright in bed or in a chair while eating. The bolus size should be small in sips or bites. Foods with thicker textures (e.g., thick liquids and pudding textures) are often better tolerated than clear liquids. Spicy, acidic foods and coffee, tea, and alcohol should be avoided. After meals, patients should remain in the upright position for an additional 1 to 3 hours to minimize the risk of aspiration. The head of the bed should be elevated during resting and sleeping hours.

B. Esophageal dysphagia

1. Systemic disease. If the disorder is secondary to a systemic disease, the treatment needs to be directed to the primary disease. Infections and inflammatory lesions of the esophagus are discussed in Chapter 19.

2. **Rings, webs, and strictures.** Of the structural disorders, the treatment of rings and webs is the most gratifying to both the patient and the physician. Dilatation with a mercury-filled bougie usually relieves the symptoms. Esophageal strictures may also be dilated under endoscopic guidance with balloon dilators or savory dilators that allow progressively larger dilators to be passed over a guidewire. (For further discussion, see section II.C.1.)

3. **Motility disorders.** Treatment of motility disorders is difficult, and variable results are obtained (see section II.C.3).

Selected Readings

Adler DG, et al. Primary esophageal motility disorders. *Mayo Clin Proc.* 2001;76:195.

Fibbe C, et al. Esophageal motility in reflux disease before and after fundoplication: A prospective, randomized, clinical and manometric study. *Gastroenterology.* 2001;121:5.

Fox M, et al. High-resolution manometry predicts the success of oesophageal bolus transport and identifies clinically important abnormalities not detected by conventional manometry. *Neurogastroenterol Motil.* 2004;16:533–542.

Jayaderan R, et al. Dysphagia in the elderly. *Pract Gastroenterol.* 2001;25:75.

Lee JI, et al. The effect of silderafil on esophageal motor function in health, subjects and patients with nutcracker esophagus. *Neurogastroenterol Motil.* 2003;15:617–623.

Oelschlager BK. Surgical options for treatment of esophageal disorders. *Gastroenterol Hepatol.* 2007;3(9):687–689.

Oh TL, et al. Dysphagia in inflammatory myopathy: clinical characteristics, treatment strategies, and outcome in 62 patients. *Mayo Clin Proc.* 2007;82(4):441–447.

Rubenstein JH, et al. Dysphagia drives doctors to diagnose a disease: Pitfalls in interpreting observational studies. *Gastrointest Endosc.* 2005;61:809–811.

Shay S, et al. Twenty-four-hour ambulatory simultaneous impedance and pH monitoring: A multi-center report of normal values in 60 health volunteers. *Am J Gastroenterol.* 2004;99:1037–1043.

Straumann A, et al. Natural history of primary eosinophilic esophagitis: A follow-up of 30 adult patients for up to 11.5 years. *Gastroenterology.* 2003;125:1660–1669.

Tutuian R, et al. Clarification of the esophageal function defect in patients with manometric ineffective esophageal motility: Studies using combined impedance-manometry. *Clin Gastroenterol Hepatol.* 2004;2:230–236.

Varadarjullu S, et al. The yield and the predictors of esophageal pathology when upper endoscopy is used for the initial evaluation of dysphagia. *Gastrointest Endosc.* 2005; 61:804–808.

$\mathcal{T}$he term **noncardiac chest pain** generally means pain in the chest that mimics or may be confused with cardiac chest pain. Often the pain is caused by a disorder of the esophagus, stomach, or gallbladder. Diagnosis is particularly confusing in patients who have both cardiac and noncardiac chest pain. Much of the diagnostic confusion arises from the generous overlap in pain sensations entering the spinal cord from the heart, mediastinum, stomach, and other upper abdominal organs.

I. The **differential diagnosis** of noncardiac chest pain is outlined in Table 22-1. Although this chapter deals mostly with esophageal causes of chest pain, one cannot neglect the numerous other causes in evaluating patients with chest pain. Also, it seems an inherent contradiction to say that cardiac chest pain should be a consideration in the differential diagnosis of noncardiac chest pain; yet some patients who are referred because they are thought to have noncardiac chest pain, but have not had an adequate cardiac evaluation, eventually are found to have cardiac disease or a combination of cardiac and noncardiac chest pain.

II. **DIAGNOSIS.** Many patients with noncardiac chest pain already have had an evaluation for cardiac disease. This evaluation may have consisted of an electrocardiogram (ECG) only or may have been extensive, including stress testing and coronary arteriography. In any event, the patient's major concern usually is whether he or she has heart disease. If the pain can be attributed to a noncardiac cause, the patient often feels better, even though in some instances little can be done to relieve the pain.

Cardiac causes of chest pain must first be excluded. This cannot always be done with absolute certainty, and in some patients a diagnosis of both cardiac and noncardiac chest pain is made. Furthermore, it appears that, in some of these patients, noncardiac pain can stimulate cardiac chest pain.

A. **Clinical presentation**

1. **The character of the pain** may help differentiate cardiac from noncardiac pain. Cardiac pain typically is aggravated by stress and exercise and radiates to the neck, shoulder, and left arm. Chest wall and esophageal pain, however, also sometimes appear to be aggravated by stress and exercise. The pain of gastroesophageal reflux can radiate to the neck and jaw, but it rarely radiates down the arm.

2. **Accompanying symptoms and relation of the pain to other events** can help differentiate the cause. Dysphagia in association with the pain points to an esophageal origin (see Chapter 21). If the dysphagia is for both liquids and solids, an esophageal motility disorder is likely. Pain after eating can be cardiac, but it is more likely to be of esophageal or perhaps gallbladder origin. Pressure over the site of pain that aggravates the pain suggests a chest wall source such as costochondritis or trauma, although chest wall tenderness has been described in cardiac pain.

B. **Diagnostic studies**

1. **Exclusion of cardiac disease**

a. **X-ray and ECG.** All patients should be evaluated with a chest x-ray and ECG. Some patients require exercise stress testing using standard ECG monitoring or thallium scanning.

TABLE 22-1	Diagnostic Considerations in Noncardiac Chest Pain

I. Chest wall pain
  A. Costochondritis
  B. Trauma
II. Mediastinal pain
  A. Inflammation
  B. Tumor
III. Esophageal pain
  A. Motility disorders
      1. Achalasia (usually "vigorous" achalasia)
      2. Diffuse esophageal spasm
      3. "Nutcracker" esophagus
      4. Nonspecific motor disorder
  B. Mucosal disorders
      1. Gastroesophageal reflux with or without gross injury
      2. Viral or fungal infections
      3. Acid or alkali ingestion
      4. Cancer
IV. Gallbladder disease
V. Pancreatitis or pancreatic pseudocyst
VI. Peptic ulcer
VII. Cardiac chest pain (initial failure to diagnose)
  A. Coronary artery disease
  B. Pericarditis

    b. Coronary arteriography, CT, or MRI. Not every patient with chest pain requires coronary arteriography to exclude cardiac disease for practical clinical purposes. Some patients clearly have a noncardiac problem, such as gastroesophageal reflux or an esophageal motility disorder. In many patients, however, coronary disease must be excluded by coronary arteriography, CT, or MRI.

2. Esophageal studies

    a. Barium swallow radiography (see Chapter 9). X-ray films of the esophagus usually are not of much help in evaluating chest pain that mimics cardiac pain. However, obstructing lesions or severe esophagitis (reflux, monilial, or herpetic) may be evident from the static films. Furthermore, fluoroscopy or videotape of the swallowing function may suggest that a motility disorder is present.

    b. Endoscopy and esophageal mucosal biopsy. Endoscopy is indicated if a structural abnormality is seen on the barium study. Biopsy of the mucosa also may provide information that is not evident by radiography or endoscopy. Endoscopic punch biopsies or suction biopsies of the esophagus may show inflammation, thinning of the epithelium, hypertrophy of the basal regenerative layer, prolongation of the papillae of lamina propria that project into the epithelium, or presence of eosinophils, all of which have been correlated with gastroesophageal reflux (see Chapter 20).

    c. Esophageal motility studies (see Chapter 8).

        i. Manometric examination of the esophagus may be crucial in the diagnosis of an esophageal motility disorder. However, correlation of manometric findings with clinical symptoms may be difficult. Because symptoms and manometric abnormalities are usually intermittent, a normal motility tracing does not exclude a motility disorder. Manometric abnormalities in the absence of symptoms are also difficult to interpret.

It is only when chest pain occurs at the time a motor abnormality is recorded that there is reasonable certainty that the patient's chest pain is caused by the motor disorder.

Several intravenous provocative agents have been used during esophageal manometry to stimulate motor abnormalities and reproduce pain. Ergonovine maleate is the most potent provocative agent, but it also is dangerous; it has been associated with irreversible coronary spasm in a few reported cases when used during coronary arteriography. Currently, ergonovine maleate is regarded as unsafe for clinical use as an esophageal provocative agent unless the patient can be monitored in a cardiac catheterization laboratory. Other agents include pentagastrin, bethanechol chloride, and edrophonium chloride (Tensilon). Of these, edrophonium chloride intravenous (IV), 80 µg/kg, is the most successful in producing a positive response, that is, reproduction of the clinical chest pain in association with development of manometric abnormalities. Edrophonium also appears to be safe.

- ii. **Esophageal motility disorders.** As indicated in Table 22-1, several esophageal motility disorders may be associated with chest pain.
    - a) Classic **diffuse esophageal spasm (DES)** causes substernal pain and is characterized by high-amplitude, broad-based, simultaneous and repetitive contractions. However, DES accounts for only a minority of esophageal motility disturbances (Fig. 22-1).
    - b) Much more frequent are **nonspecific esophageal motility disorders (NEMD),** which include a hypertensive lower esophageal sphincter (LES), in which the resting LES pressure exceeds 45 mmHg in the presence of normal peristalsis in the body of the esophagus; decreased or absent amplitude of esophageal peristalsis with normal LES pressure and relaxation; and other abnormalities of peristaltic sequence, such as abnormal waveforms, isolated simultaneous contractions, and isolated spontaneous contractions.
    - c) The term **nutcracker esophagus** describes an esophagus in which the peristaltic contractions squeeze too tightly. Peristalsis is propagated normally, but the mean amplitude of contractions exceeds 120 mmHg (normal peristaltic contractions are usually in the range of 50 to 100 mmHg), and contractions are often prolonged more than 5.5 seconds.
    - d) **Achalasia** accounts for a small minority of esophageal motor disorders associated with chest pain. Sometimes patients have so-called vigorous achalasia. Their LES is hypercontracting and fails to relax completely on swallowing, as in classic achalasia; instead of absence of peristalsis, however, they have evidence of diffuse spasm or another motility disorder in the body of the esophagus.
- d. The **Bernstein test,** although rarely used in the clinical setting, has been a time-honored study for determining whether or not a patient's chest pain is caused by acid irritation of the esophagus. A tube is positioned in the mid esophagus and saline and 0.1N hydrogen chloride (HCl) are alternately infused at 120 drops per minute in a sequence unknown to the patient. If the patient experiences pain during acid infusion that is identical to the clinical pain, it is presumed that the pain is a result of acid reflux. Measurement of esophageal peristalsis during acid infusion can document a motility disorder that may be responsible for the chest pain. The reliability of the Bernstein test is diminished by its dependence on the subjective interpretations of the patient and the physician.
- e. **Ambulatory pH monitoring** (see Chapter 8) by documenting the frequency and duration of gastroesophageal reflux, may provide evidence for the correlation of chest pain with episodes of reflux.

    In medical centers which specialize in esophageal **motility disorders,** the 24-hour pH monitoring may also be combined with **esophageal** impedance

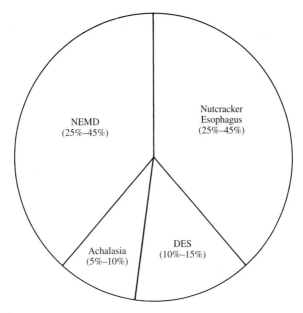

Figure 22-1. Manometric diagnoses of esophageal motility disorders in patients with chest pain of esophageal origin. NEMD, nonspecific esophageal motility disorder; DES, diffuse esophageal spasm. (From data compiled from several reports. See Benjamin DS, Castell DO. Esophageal causes of chest pain. In: Castell DO, Johnson LF, eds. *Esophageal Function in Health and Disease.* New York: Elsevier; 1983.)

studies. There is a drop in impedance with each GER regardless of a change in pH. Thus, impedance measurements allow the measurement and documentation of reflux episodes which may not be detected by pH monitoring as in alkaline or neutral pH GER.

   3. Other diagnostic studies. In most patients with noncardiac chest pain, it is wise to look for gallstone disease by abdominal ultrasonography. Peptic disease can be evaluated during the barium swallow radiographic study by extending the examination to the stomach and duodenum. Similarly, endoscopy during evaluation of esophageal disease should include examination of the stomach and duodenum. In some patients, computed tomography (CT) scanning is necessary to evaluate the pancreas and other abdominal organs.

III. TREATMENT
A. Esophageal motility disorders

   1. With the exception of achalasia, all the esophageal motility disorders are treated in roughly the same manner if they are associated with chest pain. Specific foods or hot or cold beverages associated with symptoms should be avoided. Agents to relax the esophageal smooth muscle have been used. Sublingual nitroglycerin may be sufficient for intermittent symptoms, and long-acting nitrates have been effective in some patients. The calcium channel blocking agents (nifedipine, diltiazem, verapamil) have received much attention, but double-blind, placebo-controlled studies have not shown clear benefit.

   2. Differentiation from angina pectoris. The perceptive reader already has discerned that the pharmacologic treatment of chest pain caused by an esophageal motor disorder is similar to the treatment of angina pectoris. Thus, one may ask whether it makes much difference to distinguish between the two. Although the treatment may be similar, the prognosis and the patient's peace of mind certainly are different when the diagnosis is coronary artery disease.

3. **Esophageal dilatation.** One medical treatment of esophageal motor disorders that does not apply to cardiac disease is esophageal dilatation. Simple passive dilatation of the esophagus with a 30 French (F) to 40 F Maloney dilator has been shown to provide temporary, sometimes long-standing, relief in some patients.

4. **Myotomy.** An occasional patient with a well-documented motility disorder and severe pain unresponsive to medical treatment may benefit from a long surgical myotomy of the esophageal muscle coat.

5. **Achalasia.** The treatment of achalasia traditionally has been either forceful dilatation or rupture of the hypercontracting LES with a balloon dilator or surgical myotomy. Recently, long-acting nitrates and calcium channel blocking agents have been successful in some patients.

B. **Gastroesophageal reflux.** The treatment of gastroesophageal reflux (GER) is described in Chapter 20. A small minority of patients with GER also has an esophageal motility disorder that is stimulated by GER. Treatment of the GER treats the motility disorder in these patients.

C. **Nonmotility esophageal disorders.** The treatments of caustic ingestions, esophageal infections, and esophageal cancer are reviewed in Chapters 16, 19, and 23, respectively.

D. **Nonesophageal disorders.** Identification of a nonesophageal disorder, such as gallstones or peptic ulcer, in a patient complaining of chest pain does not necessarily implicate that disorder as a cause of the chest pain. However, it is reasonable to treat the disorder appropriately. If pain persists after successful treatment, additional esophageal or cardiac diagnostic studies may be indicated.

Selected Readings

Charbel S, et al. The role of esophageal pH monitoring in symptomatic patients on PPI therapy. *Am J Gastroenterol.* 2005;1100:283–289.

Hobson AR, et al. Neurophysiologic assessment of esophageal sensory processing in noncardiac chest pain. *Gastroenterology.* 2006;130:80–88.

Jones H, et al. Treatment of noncardiac chest pain; a controlled trial of hypastherapy. *Gut.* 2006;55:1403–1408.

Liuzzo JP, et al. Chest pain from gastroesophageal reflux disease in patients with coronary artery disease. *Cardiol Rev.* 2005;13:167–173.

Rodriguez-Stanley S, et al. Effect of tegaserod on esophageal pain threshold, regurgitation, and symptom relief in patients with functional heartburn and mechanical sensitivity. *Clin. Gastroenteral Hepatol.* 2006;4:442–450.

Schey R, et al. Noncardiac chest pain: current treatment. *Gastroenterol Hepatol.* 2007;3:255–262.

ESOPHAGEAL CANCER

I. EPIDEMIOLOGY. Esophageal cancer is the sixth leading cause of cancer death worldwide. The incidence varies substantially in different countries. The highest rates are seen in China, Singapore, Iran, South Africa, France, and Puerto Rico.

In the United States, the incidence of esophageal cancer for the year 2006 was 14,550 new cases and 13,770 deaths. It is the seventh leading cause of cancer death in American men. In the last 25 years, there has been a significant increase in the incidence of adenocarcinomas of the distal esophagus and gastroesophageal junction. Also, in the last 30 years, the incidence of **adenocarcinoma of the esophagus** has increased in men and the incidence of **squamous carcinoma of the esophagus** has declined.

The incidence of esophageal carcinoma increases with age. The median age of onset is 69 years. Males are 2 to 4 times more likely to develop esophageal cancer compared to females. Squamous cell carcinoma is more common in African Americans and adenocarcinoma is more common among Caucasians. The incidence rates within the United States are higher in the Northeast and urban areas.

Approximately 10% to 15% squamous cancers originate in the upper third, 35% to 40% in the middle third, and 40% to 50% in the distal third of the esophagus. Adenocarcinomas arise predominately in the distal esophagus and are commonly associated with Barrett's esophagus.

Esophageal cancers may develop as second primary tumors in patients with other primary tumors of the upper aerodigestive tract. Between 5% and 12% of patients with esophageal cancer are found to have synchronous or metachronous aerodigestive tract cancer.

Other **less common tumors of the esophagus** include lymphoma, carcinosarcoma, pseudosarcoma, squamous adenocarcinoma, melanoma, mucoepidermoid carcinoma, squamous cell papilloma, primary small cell carcinoma, verrucous carcinoma, and malignant carcinoid tumor the esophagus. Local spread from the lung and thyroid and metastasis from distant cancers may occur but are rare.

II. PREDISPOSING FACTORS. Chronic use of alcohol and smoking are associated with esophageal carcinoma. This may be due to chronic irritation of the esophageal mucosa with these agents. Other conditions with increased prevalence of esophageal carcinoma are lye strictures, achalasia, previous exposure to ionizing radiation, head and neck cancer, Plummer-Vinson syndrome, tylosis, celiac sprue, and Barrett's epithelium.

Squamous cell carcinoma accounts for less than one half of esophageal carcinomas. Adenocarcinomas of the esophagus, which used to account for less than 10% of esophageal cancers, now account for greater than two thirds of all esophageal malignancies in the United States. Adenocarcinoma usually arises from metaplastic columnar epithelium (Barrett's epithelium) and rarely from esophageal glands. Adenocarcinoma of the stomach may spread to the esophagus by extension.

Gastroesophageal reflux disease (GERD) is thought to be the major risk factor for esophageal adenocarcinoma. Recurrent symptoms of GERD seem to increase the risk of esophageal adenocarcinoma by eightfold. The annual incidence of cancer in Barrett's epithelium is approximately 0.8%. Anticholinergic calcium channel blockers, nitrates, and theophyllines, by decreasing the lower esophageal sphincter tone, are thought to increase the risk of adenocarcinomas of the esophagus. In addition, obesity, which increases intraabdominal pressure and GERD, is an added risk factor.

III. PROGNOSIS. The 5-year survival rate for all patients is approximately 16%. The 5-year survival even with the earliest stages of cancer is only 50% to 80% and with lymph node involvement it drops to below 25%. With locally advanced esophageal cancer the survival drops to 5% to 10% (with radiation or surgery alone) and with chemoradiation and surgery, it may be 25% to 27%.

Esophageal cancers grow extensively locally and invade adjacent structures. The tumor has the propensity to spread longitudinally via lymphatic channels within the esophageal wall to mediastinal cervical and celiac lymph nodes. There may also be hematogenous spread to lungs, liver, and other organs. Esophagobronchial or esophagopleural fistulas may form and manifest as recurrent pneumonia or abscess. Erosion into the aorta may result in exsanguination.

IV. CLINICAL FEATURES. Progressive dysphagia for less than a year, first with solids then with semisolids and liquids, is the most common symptom. Substernal pain, usually steady, radiating to the back may also be present and may suggest periesophageous spread of the tumor. Most patients complain of anorexia and profound weight loss. Patients may have iron-deficiency anemia from blood loss from the lesion, but brisk bleeding is rare. Hoarseness may result from involvement of the recurrent laryngeal nerve. If the lesion is obstructive, patients may aspirate esophageal contents and may present with aspiration pneumonia and pleural effusion. Horner's syndrome, cervical adenopathy, hpeatoroegalys, boney pain, and paraneoplastic syndromes including hypercalcemia, inappropriate ACTH, and gonadotropins may be present.

V. DIAGNOSIS

    A. A **barium swallow** is usually the first noninvasive test ordered to establish the diagnosis of esophageal carcinoma. A double-contrast study may be helpful in identifying small, plaquelike lesions. The usual finding is an irregular luminal narrowing. There may be a ridge or shelf at the superior portion of the tumor. However, the differentiation of the tumor from a benign peptic stricture can be extremely difficult by radiography.

    B. **Endoscopy.** Fiberoptic endoscopy allows direct localization and inspection of the lesion. Retroflexion of the endoscope in the fundus of the stomach allows visualization of lesions at the esophagogastric junction and cardia, which could not be done by rigid scopes. Direct biopsies and brushings provide tissue for histologic and cytologic examination.

    C. **Computed tomography (CT)** is very helpful in determining the extent and spread of extramucosal tumor.

    D. **Endoscopic ultrasonography (EUS).** EUS, with its unique ability to define the anatomy of the gut wall in detail, offers the most accurate method for evaluating the depth of esophageal cancer invasion and detecting abnormal regional lymph nodes. Because esophageal carcinoma originates in the mucosa and progressively invades deeper layers of the esophageal wall, the TNM classification recommended by the International Union Against Cancer and the American Joint Committee on Cancer lends itself to accurate staging with EUS. T indicates depth of primary tumor invasion, N indicates spread of cancer to regional lymph nodes, and M indicates distant metastases.

    E. **Magnetic resonance imaging (MRI)** is a technique in longitudinal and cross-sectional body imaging. Currently, it offers no advantage over CT in detecting infiltrating growth.

    F. **PET scan** may improve the detection of stage IV disease.

    G. **Preoperative thoracoscopy and laparoscopy** may help assess extent of local disease as well as the involvement of regional lymph nodes and celiac and perigastric nodes.

    H. **Staging and prognosis.** Pathologic stage is the most important factor in prognosis. Recurrence and survival are strongly related to depth of tumor invasion, metastases to adjacent lymph nodes and distant organs. TNM system has been revised and used in prognosis. **T1-2, NOMO** are potentially curable with surgery alone.

Tumor invasion into serosa **(T3)** or regional or distant lymph node metastases **(T4)** are associated with significant reduction in survival.

VI. TREATMENT. The therapy for carcinoma of the esophagus is determined by the stage of the disease. The mainstay of therapy has been surgery, with or without radiotherapy and chemotherapy. Inoperable tumors have been treated by radiotherapy because squamous carcinoma of the esophagus is relatively radiosensitive. Chemotherapy alone has not been very successful. Treatment protocols combining chemotherapy and radiation therapy before and after surgery offer somewhat better results than single-modality therapy. Most successful chemotherapeutic agents are the combination of cisplatin, 5-fluorouracil, paclitaxel, irinotecan hydrochloride, vinorelbine tartrate, and gemcitabine hydrochloride preoperatively and as neoadjuvant chemotherapy.

A. Surgery. Total esophagectomy is the surgical procedure of choice. Patients with lesions of the lower third that are less than 5 cm seem to do better. Because the cure rate has been so dismally low with "curative" surgery, palliative resection has been used to alleviate symptoms and allow patients to swallow.

The morbidity and mortality with a large thoracotomy are still very high in these patients. The esophageal resection and esophagogastric anastomosis may be done with a combined abdominal incision and a right thoracotomy. If the lesion is low enough, an abdominal approach may suffice. For most lesions, it is preferred to resect the involved portion of the esophagus with wide margins, bring the stomach into the chest, and create an anastomosis with the remaining esophagus. Colonic or jejunal segment interposition carries a high complication rate. For purposes of palliation, the stomach may be anastomosed to the esophagus in a side-to-side fashion to bypass the obstructed area.

B. Radiation therapy

1. Radiation therapy for **squamous cell carcinoma** of the esophagus has been used for attempted cure with unsatisfactory results. It is used in protocols before or after surgery and for palliation.

2. Presurgical radiation therapy alone has not been found to increase the cure rate.

3. Adenocarcinomas are resistant to radiation therapy.

C. Other palliative measures

1. Mechanical dilatation. When surgery and radiation therapy are contraindicated, or when these treatments have failed, mechanical dilatation of the esophageal lumen may be attempted with Savary or balloon dilators under endoscopic guidance. Because the risk of esophageal perforation is high in these patients, the dilatation should be done slowly and with great care.

2. Tube placement. If it becomes difficult to maintain a lumen at the area of the tumor, a stent (plastic or metal) may be placed in the lumen endoscopically. These tubes may also be used to close off, at least temporarily, a tracheoesophageal fistula. These tubes may erode into the esophageal wall, causing ulceration, bleeding, and perforation.

3. YAG-laser therapy has been found to be quite effective in palliation of patients with advanced obstructing esophageal tumors. These masses may be "pared down" by the laser to open the lumen. Lasers may also be useful in the treatment of very early lesions. Additional controlled studies need to be done using this technique.

4. Injection necrosis of fungating esophageal cancer can be accomplished with intratumoral injection of absolute alcohol or ethylene glycol with endoscopic visualization. In instances of luminal narrowing, malignant strictures may be dilated first, and then injected concentrically to additionally "open up" the lumen.

5. These palliative measures are usually repeated as needed with progressive, repeated growth of the tumor.

D. Selection of therapy. Presently, the optimal therapy for esophageal cancer is unclear. A strong case can be made for establishing comparable diagnostic staging criteria and treating newly diagnosed patients according to well-designed, established research protocols whenever possible. If the use of research protocols is not feasible, a reasonable approach is to use resectional surgery for "resectable" tumors in the distal third of the esophagus (T_{1-3} N_1) with pre- and neoadjuvant chemoradiation therapy. For patients who are poor candidates for surgery or who have obstructing tumors, one or more of the listed palliative measures may be used.

E. Prevention and surveillance. Patients with recurrent symptoms of GERD are recommended to have endoscopy and biopsies for the diagnosis of Barrett's esophagus. Endoscopic surveillance will allow the diagnosis of earlier stage tumors and allow for improved survival. Patients should be advised to stop smoking and use alcohol in moderation. Current recommendations for patients with Barrett's esophagus are still debated, but most centers offer biannual endoscopic surveillance and annually if there is low-grade dysplasia. Patients with high-grade dysplasia are recommended to substantiate the diagnosis by two different pathologists, and then consider undergoing esophagectomy or mucosal ablation with photodynamic therapy.

Selected Readings

Bowrey DJ, et al. Use of alarm symptoms to select dyspeptics for endoscopy causes patients with curable esophagogastric cancer to be overlooked. *Surg. Endosc.* 2006;20:1725–8.

Dar M, et al. Can extent of high-grade dysplasia predict the presence of adenocarcinoma at esophagectomy? *Gut.* 2003;52:486–489.

Fountoulakis A, et al. Effect of surveillance of Barrett's esophagus on the clinical outcome of oesophageal cancer. *Br J Surg.* 2004;91:997–1003.

Lagergren J, et al. Association between medications that relax the lower esophageal sphincter and risk for esophageal adenocarcinoma. *Ann Int Med.* 2000;133:165.

Lagergren J, et al. Symptomatic gastroesophageal reflux as a risk factor for esophageal adenocarcinoma. *N Engl J Med.* 1999;340:825–831.

Largi A, et al. EUS followed by EMR for staging of high grade dysplasia and early cancer in Barrett's esophagus. *Gastrointest Endosc.* 2005;62:16.

May A, et al. Accuracy of staging in early esophageal cancer using high resolution endoscopy and high resolution endosonography: A comparative, prospective trial. *Gut.* 2004;53:634–640.

Papachritou GI, et al. Use of stents in benign and malignant esophageal disease. *Rev. Gastroenterol. Disord.* 2007;7(2):75–88.

Pech O, et al. Long-term results of photodynamic therapy with 5-aminoevulinic acid for superficial Barrett's cancer and high-grade intraepithelial neoplasia. *Gastrointest Endosc.* 2005;62:24–30.

Playford RJ. New British Society of Gastroenterology (BSG) guidelines for the diagnosis and management of Barrett's esophagus. *Gut.* 2006;55:442–443.

Portale G, et al. Comparison of the clinical and histological characteristics and survival of the distal esophageal–gastroesophageal junction adenocarcinoma in patients with and without Barrett's mucosa. *Arch Surg.* 2005;140:570–575.

Ross WA, et al. Evolving role of self-expanding metal stents in the treatment of malignant dysphagia and fistulas. *Gastrointest Endosc.* 2007;65:70–76.

Sharma P. Low-grade dysplasia in Barrett's esophagus. *Gastroenterology.* 2004;127: 1233–1238.

Wang KK, et al. American Gastroenterological Association medical position statement: Role of the gastroenterologist in the management of esophageal carcinoma. *Gastroenterology.* 2005;128:1468–1470.

Wong A, et al. Epidemiologic risk factors for Barrett's esophagus and associated adenocarcinoma. *Clin Gastroenterol Hepatol.* 2005;3:1–10.

24   PEPTIC ULCER DISEASE

$\mathcal{T}$he term **peptic ulcer disease (PUD)** refers to disorders of the upper gastrointestinal tract caused by the action of acid and pepsin. These agents not only cause injury themselves, but also typically augment the injury initiated by other agents. The spectrum of peptic ulcer disease is broad, including undetectable mucosal injury, erythema, erosions, and frank ulceration. The correlation of severity of symptoms to objective evidence of disease is poor. Some patients with pain suggesting peptic ulcer disease have no diagnostic evidence of mucosal injury, whereas some patients with large ulcers are asymptomatic.

I. **PATHOGENESIS.** Gastroduodenal mucosal injury results from an imbalance between the factors that damage the mucosa and those that protect it (Fig. 24-1). Therefore, injurious factors may predominate and cause injury not only when they are excessive, but also when the protective mechanisms fail. Although we have learned much in recent years about the mechanisms of injury and protection of the mucosa of the upper gastrointestinal tract, we still have an imperfect understanding of why discrete ulcers develop and why peptic disease develops in one person and not in another.

A. **Injurious factors.** The mucosa of the upper gastrointestinal tract is susceptible to injury from a variety of agents and conditions. Endogenous agents include acid, pepsin, bile acids, and other small-intestinal contents. Exogenous agents include ethanol, aspirin, other nonsteroidal antiinflammatory drugs, and *Helicobacter pylori* infection.

Acid appears to be essential for benign peptic injury to occur. A pH of 1 to 2 maximizes the activity of pepsin. Furthermore, mucosal injury from aspirin, other nonsteroidal antiinflammatory agents, and bile acids is augmented in the presence of acid. On the other hand, ethanol causes mucosal injury with or without acid. Corticosteroids, smoking, and psychological and physiologic stress appear to predispose or to exacerbate to mucosal injury in some people by mechanisms that are incompletely understood.

B. **Protective factors.** A number of mechanisms work together to protect the mucosa from injury (Table 24-1).

1. **Concepts**

a. **Gastric mucosal barrier.** In the early 1960s, Horace Davenport identified the so-called gastric mucosal barrier, which describes the ability of the gastric mucosa to resist the back diffusion of hydrogen (H⁺) ions and thus to contain a high concentration of hydrochloric acid within the gastric lumen. When the barrier is broken by an injurious agent, such as aspirin, H⁺ diffuses rapidly back into the mucosa, which results in mucosal injury.

b. **Cytoprotection.** More recently, the concept of **cytoprotection** has been developed to explain further the ability of the mucosa to protect itself. The term *cytoprotection* is somewhat of a misnomer in that it does not refer to the protection of individual cells but rather to protection of the deeper layers of the mucosa against injury. The classic experiments of Andre Robert illustrate the phenomenon of cytoprotection. When he introduced 100% ethanol into the stomachs of rats, large hemorrhagic erosions developed. However, when he first instilled 20% ethanol, a concentration by itself that did not cause gross injury, and subsequently administered 100% ethanol, no hemorrhagic erosions developed. Clearly, some endogenous protective mechanism had been elicited by the preliminary exposure to a low concentration

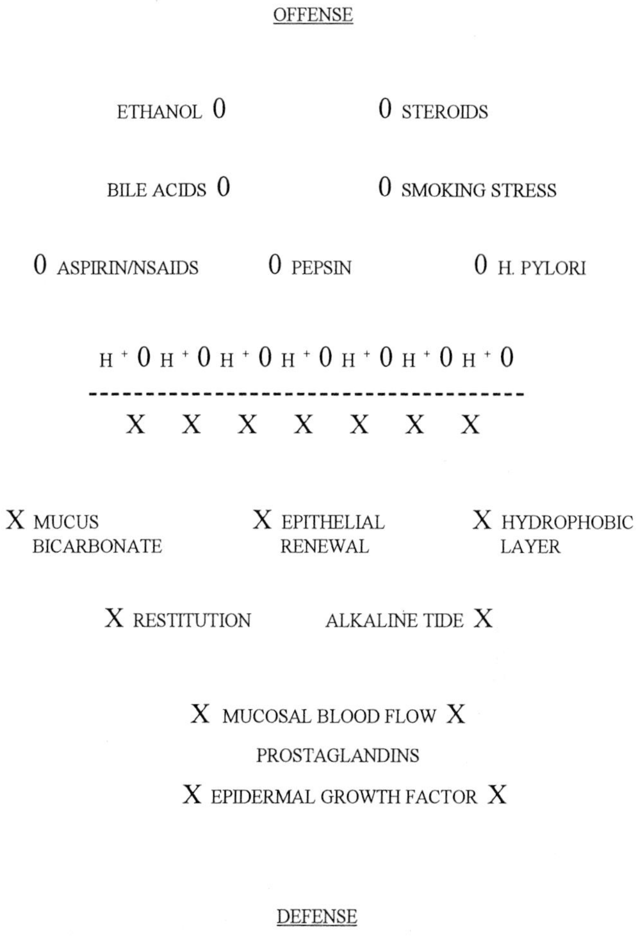

OFFENSE

ETHANOL 0   0 STEROIDS

BILE ACIDS 0   0 SMOKING STRESS

0 ASPIRIN/NSAIDS   0 PEPSIN   0 H. PYLORI

$H^+ 0 H^+ 0 H^+ 0 H^+ 0 H^+ 0 H^+ 0 H^+ 0$

X X X X X X X

X MUCUS   X EPITHELIAL   X HYDROPHOBIC
  BICARBONATE   RENEWAL   LAYER

X RESTITUTION   ALKALINE TIDE X

X MUCOSAL BLOOD FLOW X

PROSTAGLANDINS

X EPIDERMAL GROWTH FACTOR X

DEFENSE

Figure 24-1. Diagram of factors that promote mucosal injury (Offense) versus those that protect the mucosa (Defense). On the offensive side, hydrochloric acid (H^+) is essential for the action of pepsin and many ulcerogenic factors. For example, aspirin, bile acids, and the nonsteroidal antiinflammatory drugs cause much more mucosal injury in an acid milieu. The roles of corticosteroids, smoking, and stress are less clear, but these factors probably contribute to mucosal injury. Alcohol can cause mucosal injury without the assistance of acid. The defense of the mucosa is a complex phenomenon that involves the interaction of a number of protective mechanisms indicated in the figure. (See Table 24-1 and text.)

of the injurious agent. This protective effect was abolished by pretreatment with indomethacin at the time of instillation of 20% ethanol. Because indomethacin is a potent inhibitor of prostaglandin synthesis, this observation suggested that cytoprotection was mediated by endogenous prostaglandins. In fact, application of exogenous prostaglandins has been shown to protect the gastric mucosa. Prostaglandins do inhibit gastric acid secretion, but their cytoprotective effects can be demonstrated at doses below those necessary to inhibit acid.

2. **Mediators of mucosal protection**
   a. **Mucus** is secreted by surface epithelial cells. It forms a gel that covers the mucosal surface and physically protects the mucosa from abrasion. It also

TABLE 24-1	Gastroduodenal Mucosal Protective Factors

Concepts	Mediators
Gastric mucosal barrier Cytoprotection	Mucus Surface bicarbonate Hydrophobic layer Mucosal blood flow Alkaline tide Epithelial renewal Restitution Prostaglandins Epidermal growth factor

resists the passage of large molecules, such as pepsin; however, H⁺, other small particles, and ethanol seem to have little difficulty in penetrating mucus to reach the mucosal surface.

b. Bicarbonate is produced in small amounts by surface epithelial cells and diffuses up from the mucosa to accumulate beneath the mucous layer, creating a thin (several micrometers) layer of alkalinity between the mucus and the epithelial surface.

c. The **hydrophobic layer** of phospholipid that coats the luminal membrane of surface epithelial cells is believed to help prevent the back diffusion of hydrophilic agents such as hydrochloric acid.

d. Mucosal blood flow is important not only in maintaining oxygenation and a supply of nutrients, but also as a means of disposing of absorbed acid and noxious agents.

e. The **alkaline tide** refers to the mild alkalinization of the blood and mucosa that result from the secretion of a molecule of bicarbonate (HCO_3^-) by the parietal cell into the adjacent mucosa for every H⁺ ion that is secreted into the gastric lumen. This slight alkalinity may contribute to the neutralization of acid that diffuses back into the mucosa and may augment the effects of mucosal blood flow.

f. Epithelial renewal, which involves the proliferation of new cells and subsequent differentiation and migration to replace old cells, but which requires several days, is necessary in the healing of deeper lesions, such as erosions and ulcers.

g. Restitution refers to the phenomenon of rapid migration, within minutes, of cells deep within the mucosa to cover a denuded surface epithelium. This process probably accounts for the rapid healing of small areas of superficial injury.

h. Prostaglandins, particularly of the E and I series, are synthesized abundantly in the mucosa of the stomach and duodenum. They are known to stimulate secretion of both mucus and bicarbonate and to maintain mucosal blood flow. Prostaglandins also may have beneficial protective effects directly on epithelial cells.

i. Epidermal growth factor (EGF) is secreted in saliva and by the duodenal mucosa and may exert topical protective effects on the gastroduodenal mucosa.

C. Relation of *Helicobacter pylori* to peptic disease. Since 1983, evidence has accumulated to implicate a bacterium, *H. pylori*, in the pathogenesis of some forms of peptic disease. The organism is found adherent to the gastric mucosal surface and, when looked for, has been identified in more than 90% of patients with duodenal ulcer. Its presence has also been correlated with gastritis, gastric ulcer, and gastric erosions and with chronic infection, gastric mucosal atrophy, intestinal metaplasia, and in a minority of patients, gastric adenocarcinoma and MALT lymphoma. Some patients with *H. pylori* are asymptomatic and may even have normal-appearing gastric mucosa by endoscopy, but identification of the organism is associated with histologic gastritis in nearly 100% of patients.

1. The **mechanisms** by which *H. pylori* are involved in the pathogenesis of peptic conditions are unclear. *H. pylori* produce ammonia and elaborate other toxins that may directly damage the mucosa and initiate an inflammatory response. The organism can be treated by bismuth-containing compounds (e.g., bismuth subsalicylate [Pepto-Bismol]), PPI, and some antibiotics, which appear to facilitate the treatment of the associated peptic condition. For example, patients with *H. pylori*-associated duodenal ulcer have a longer period of remission when they receive treatment for both the ulcer and the organism than when they are treated for the ulcer alone.

2. **Treatment.** Several studies have shown that duodenal ulcers may be curable by eradication of *H. pylori* with so-called triple therapy (e.g., bismuth subsalicylate q.i.d., tetracycline (or ampicillin) 500 mg q.i.d., and metronidazole 250 mg q.i.d. for 2 weeks, plus omeprazole (Prilosec) 20 mg b.i.d. until healing. Other studies have shown eradication rates higher than 90% **with omeprazole (Prilosec)** 40 mg b.i.d. or **lansoprazole (Prevacid)** 30 mg b.i.d. or **Pantoprazole** 40 mg q.d. or **Esomeprazole** 40 mg q.d., or Rabeprazole 20 mg b.i.d., plus **amoxicillin** 1 g b.i.d. and **clarithromycin (Biaxin)** 500 mg b.i.d. for 7 to 14 days. In penicillin-allergic patients, **metronidazole (Flagyl)** 500 mg b.i.d. may be used instead of Amoxicillin. *H. pylori* eradication clearly reduces peptic ulcer recurrence rates and is recommended for all patients with peptic ulcer disease who are infected with *H. pylori*.

D. **Relation of aspirin and other nonsteroidal antiinflammatory drugs to peptic disease.** Aspirin and other nonsteroidal antiinflammatory drugs (NSAIDs) cause mucosal injury and ulceration throughout the entire gastrointestinal tract, especially in the esophagus, stomach, and duodenum. The mechanisms of injury are multifactorial and include both direct mucosal injury and inhibition of prostaglandins that are protective to the mucosa. The risk for mucosal damage related to aspirin and NSAID ingestion is related to a previous history of peptic ulcer disease, high and frequent doses of the drugs, and concomitant use of corticosteroids or use of more than one NSAID. The mucosal injury may be diffuse, and ulcers may be multiple. Patients may be asymptomatic or may have frank bleeding, anemia, or strictures. There is some clinical evidence that the gastric infection, *H. pylori*, may contribute to enhance mucosal damage from NSAIDs. Treatment is to discontinue the offending agents and, if necessary, begin histamine-2 (H_2) blocker or PPI therapy. If NSAID treatment must be continued, therapy with the synthetic prostaglandin E_1 derivative, misoprostol 100 to 200 µg q.i.d. or a proton-pump inhibitor (PPI) (e.g., omeprazole 20–40 mg daily) has been shown to heal the mucosal lesions. Prostaglandins are produced in the gastric mucosa by the progressive enzymatic action of cycloxygeranase I and II (COX) on arachidonic acid released from membrane phospholipids. NSAIDS inhibit COX I and COX II enzymes. Specific COX II inhibitors have been developed to allow the selective inhibition of those prostaglandins that are proinflammatory (e.g., in the joints). **COX II inhibitors (e.g., celecoxib [Celebrex])** inhibit prostaglandins that are effective in gastroduodenal mucosal protection to a much lesser degree, and thus are thought to be safer to use in patients with history of peptic ulcer disease.

II. COMPLICATIONS OF PEPTIC ULCER DISEASE

A. **Bleeding/hemorrhage.** It is estimated that PUD is responsible for greater than 50% of all cases of UGI tract hemorrhage. Ulcers may erode into blood vessels and may result in life-threatening hemorrhage. If bleeding is slower or intermittent, iron-deficiency anemia may result. Some patients may also present with occult GI bleeding.

1. **Patients with brisk bleeding from PUD** usually present with hematemesis, melena, and/or with hematochezia with clots and hypotension.

2. **Risk factors for bleeding from PUD** include ingestion of aspirin, NSAIDS, platelet inhibitory drugs, coagulopathy, older age, and the presence of *H. pylori* infection.

3. **Treatment** of GI bleeding from PUD is discussed in Chapter 14.

B. Perforation. Duodenal or gastric ulcers may perforate into the peritoneal cavity. In 10% of patients, perforation is accompanied by hemorrhage. Initially, patients feel an abrupt onset of intense abdominal pain which is then followed by hypotension and shock as the peritoneal cavity is flooded by gastric juice and contents and peritonitis develops. Mortality is imminent if appropriate therapy is not initiated immediately.

The risk of perforation is increased in patients with PUD who smoke, use NSAIDs, and who are elderly. Use of crack cocaine has been associated with perforated ulcers in the younger patients, most likely as a result of cocaine-induced vasoconstriction and ischemia of the gastric or duodenal wall.

Diagnosis is clinical; however, free air is noted within the abdominal cavity on plain and upright x-rays of the abdomen in approximately 75% of patients. CT scan offers confirmatory information. Endoscopy should be avoided. Patients should receive intravenous broad spectrum antibiotics and immediate surgery is recommended to close the perforation and irrigate the peritoneal cavity.

C. Penetration occurs when PUD burrows through the gut wall into an adjacent organ (i.e., pancreas, liver, or colon). Occasionally fistulas may develop. Pancreatitis, hemorrhage, or peritonitis may develop. Diagnosis is usually by CT scan. Treatment should be tailored to pathology and may include surgery.

D. Obstruction. PUD of the antrum, pyloric channel, and duodenum may result in gastric outlet obstruction. Patients may present with early satiety, nausea, vomiting, epigastric pain, and bloating. Dehydration and electrolyte abnormalities may occur.

Diagnosis may be made by plain x-rays, CT scan, and more definitely by UGI endoscopy. The narrowed segment may be dilated endoscopically. Some cases require surgery.

III. DIAGNOSIS
A. Clinical presentation
    1. History. The classic symptoms of peptic ulcer disease—epigastric burning pain on an empty stomach that is relieved by food or antacids—are familiar to most physicians and laypeople. Sometimes the pain radiates to the back, suggesting an ulcer of the posterior aspect of the duodenal bulb that may have penetrated into the pancreas. However, many patients with peptic disease experience non-specific abdominal discomfort, which broadens the differential diagnostic considerations to include gastroesophageal reflux disease (GERD); gallbladder disease; pancreatic disorders; cancer of the stomach, pancreas, or biliary system; mesenteric vascular insufficiency; and irritable bowel syndrome. A minority of patients has gastrointestinal bleeding, weight loss, or vomiting; the vomiting may be caused by partial or complete gastric outlet obstruction.

    Over the past three decades, the yearly incidence of discrete peptic ulcer disease appears to have decreased, but peptic disease of other types, such as gastritis and duodenitis, sometimes related to ingestion of aspirin, nonsteroidal antiinflammatory drugs, corticosteroids, or ethanol have increased in incidence. Thus, important historical information includes a record of drug and alcohol use and a history of smoking, and previous diagnosis of peptic disease.

    2. Physical examination. The physical examination of a patient with peptic disease may be normal. Some patients have upper abdominal tenderness and guarding. Rigidity of the abdomen and absent bowel sounds suggests perforation. Stool should be tested for occult blood.

B. Diagnostic studies
    1. Most patients with dyspepsia or uncomplicated peptic disease may initially require no diagnostic study. It may be sufficient to begin empiric treatment H_2 blockers or PPIs to control acid secretion. Patients also should be advised regarding diet, smoking, and lifestyle, as described in section IV. If they do not respond to treatment within a reasonable time, usually 2 to 4 weeks, endoscopy should be considered, during which biopsies can be obtained to test for *H. pylori* and, in the case of a gastric ulcer, to evaluate for a cancerous lesion.

    2. Patients with potential complications. A minority of patients present initially with signs or symptoms that should act as "red flags" to alert the physician to the increased possibility of complications of peptic disease or cancer.

These warnings are clinically significant weight loss, evidence of gastrointestinal bleeding, repeated vomiting, and intractable abdominal pain. If one of these circumstances is present, prompt diagnostic evaluation rather than empiric therapy is recommended. The diagnostic procedure preferred is upper gastrointestinal (GI) endoscopy because of its superior diagnostic accuracy over upper GI series. The upper GI series is often ambiguous or nondiagnostic and patients have to undergo subsequent endoscopy to clarify the questions that remain. In general, judicious use of endoscopy as the initial diagnostic study in selected patients with peptic complaints probably is the most cost-effective approach.

3. **Laboratory studies.** Most patients with uncomplicated peptic disease require no laboratory studies except for the determination of *H. pylori* status by serologic testing. However, a complete blood count and serum electrolytes are indicated in the evaluation of patients who have bleeding or vomiting. A serum amylase is helpful in evaluating patients with persistent pain that radiates to the back. If peptic disease is persistent or there is a strong family history of peptic disease, the patient should be evaluated for a hypersecretory syndrome (see section III.C).

4. **Serum gastrin** levels may be elevated in conditions in which gastric acid secretion is very low or absent or in conditions in which there is gastric acid hypersecretion (Table 24-2). Because acid is the major inhibitory influence on antral gastrin release, hypo- or achlorhydric conditions predispose to hypergastrinemia. However, in these conditions there is no known adverse consequence of the hypergastrinemia because the major end organ for gastrin, the parietal cell mass, is absent.

   In hypersecretory conditions associated with hypergastrinemia, the source of gastrin either is independent of normal physiologic control (e.g., **Zollinger–Ellison syndrome [ZES]** and retained antrum syndrome), is an unusual physiologic variant that results in too many G cells (antral G-cell hyperplasia), is a consequence of antral stimulation (e.g., gastric outlet obstruction), is a result of unopposed action of gastrin (e.g., hypersecretion after small-bowel resection), or develops because of poor renal excretion of gastrin caused by renal disease.

   Serum for gastrin determination should be drawn in the fasting state. Because some patients with ZES may have intermittent secretion of gastrin, repeated fasting serum gastrin determinations may be indicated.

5. **The secretin stimulation test** takes advantage of the peculiar response of gastrinomas to secretin. Normally, intravenous secretin inhibits the release of gastrin from antral G cells, and serum gastrin either falls or remains unchanged after secretin injection. In patients with a gastrinoma, however, secretin stimulates release of gastrin from the tumor, causing a prompt rise in serum gastrin.

   To perform the test, give secretin-kai 2 U/kg of body weight by rapid intravenous push. Draw blood for serum gastrin 15 minutes and 1 minute before the secretin injection, and at 2, 5, 10, 20, and 30 minutes after injection. In patients with gastrinoma, the serum gastrin levels should rise rapidly within 5 to 10 minutes of secretin administration. The increase usually is greater than 400 pg/mL. With other causes of hypergastrinemia that are associated with hypersecretion of gastric acid,

TABLE 24-2	Hypergastrinemic Conditions
Hypergastrinemia without gastric acid hypersecretion	**Hypergastrinemia with gastric acid hypersecretion**
Pernicious anemia	Zollinger–Ellison syndrome (gastrinoma)
Gastric atrophy	Retained antrum syndrome
	Antral G-cell hyperplasia
	Gastric outlet obstruction
	Partial small-bowel resection
	Renal insufficiency

such as the retained antrum syndrome (observed occasionally after an antrectomy and gastrojejunostomy), gastric outlet obstruction, small-bowel resection, and renal insufficiency, the serum gastrin level should decline or remain unchanged.

IV. TREATMENT. If peptic disease is complicated by bleeding, obstruction, or perforation, the usual initial treatment includes intravenous fluids and nothing by mouth, and intravenous administration of H_2 blockers or PPIs. For the patients with uncomplicated peptic ulcer disease, in addition to medical therapy, recommendations regarding diet and lifestyle **modifications are given.**

A. Diet

    1. Food. Several controlled trials have indicated that rigid dietary restrictions are of little or no benefit in healing peptic ulcers that are not accompanied by bleeding, obstruction, or perforation. Thus, patients are advised to eat what they want. Because food intolerances are unique to each person, patients should be advised to avoid foods that they know cause discomfort. Alcoholic beverages and coffee are restricted because of their ability to irritate the mucosa and stimulate gastric acid. Frequent small feedings are unnecessary. Although food does buffer acid, it also stimulates acid secretion. Because there are very effective methods for controlling acid secretion pharmacologically, there is no need to rely on intragastric food to buffer acid. Thus, patients are advised to eat three nutritionally balanced meals a day. For the same reason, milk, which in the past achieved almost medicinal status, should be used in moderation. Although milk does dilute and buffer acid, the calcium and peptides it contains are strong stimulants of acid secretion, which may overwhelm any initial benefit of milk.

    2. Drugs and lifestyle modifications. Patients are recommended to stop smoking, decrease or eliminate drinking alcohol, and not use aspirin and other NSAIDS (prescribed or over-the-counter). In special circumstances when patients have to take these drugs for cardiovascular, neurologic, or rheumatologic reasons, concomitant use of PPIs are recommended.

B. Control of smoking. Cigarette smoking appears to be a risk factor for the development, maintenance, and recurrence of peptic ulcer disease. Several epidemiologic observations support this relation. First, smokers are more likely than nonsmokers to have peptic ulcers. Second, peptic ulcers in smokers are more difficult to heal; they may require longer periods of treatment, may require higher doses of antiulcer medications, or may be refractory to healing. Finally, after healing has been accomplished in smokers, relapse occurs sooner and more frequently than in nonsmokers. Clinical trials suggest that, if smokers with healed ulcers stop smoking, the rate of ulcer recurrence approximates that of nonsmokers.

    Smoking has a number of effects on the function of the upper gastrointestinal tract that may be relevant to the pathogenesis of peptic disease, including the following:

    1. Increased gastric acid secretion.

    2. Interference with the action of H_2 antagonists.

    3. Increased gastric emptying of liquids.

    4. Increased duodenogastric reflux.

    5. Inhibition of pancreatic bicarbonate secretion.

    6. Diminished mucosal blood flow.

    7. Inhibition of mucosal prostaglandin production.

    The increased gastric emptying may present higher concentrations of acid to the duodenum, whereas the inhibition of pancreatic bicarbonate secretion interferes with the neutralization of acid within the duodenum. The adverse effects on mucosal blood flow and prostaglandin synthesis would be expected to decrease the mucosal resistance to injury.

    All available evidence indicates that the adverse effects of smoking on gastric emptying, duodenogastric reflux, pancreatic bicarbonate secretion, mucosal blood flow, and mucosal prostaglandin production are related directly to the act of smoking, and cessation of smoking is associated with recovery of these functions within minutes to hours.

C. Drug therapy

1. Agents that control acid

a. Antacids neutralize gastric acid within the lumen of the esophagus, stomach, and duodenum. They have been used for many years and are effective in relieving peptic symptoms.

i. Composition. The magnesium-containing antacids are more potent than those that do not contain magnesium, but they tend to cause diarrhea. Magnesium-free antacids tend to cause constipation. Sometimes the two types are alternated to provide adequate acid control and regulate tolerable bowel habits. Calcium-containing antacids offer the initial acid neutralization and stimulate gastric acid secretion. Another consideration is the sodium content of an antacid when prescribing for a patient who is on a sodium-restricted diet.

ii. Dosage. Most patients take antacids for amelioration of symptoms only. To treat peptic conditions with a full antacid regimen, about 30 mL should be taken 1 and 3 hours after a meal and at bedtime. This regimen requires a daily antacid intake of more than 200 mL, resulting in a monthly cost in excess of $50. Because few patients are likely to adhere to such a program and because of the expense, other medications, described in the following sections, are preferred.

b. H$_2$ antagonists. Histamine is a potent stimulant of gastric acid secretion. For this reason, agents that block the histamine receptor on the parietal cell, so-called H$_2$ antagonists, are effective inhibitors of acid secretion. Interestingly, the H$_2$ antagonists inhibit not only histamine-stimulated acid secretion, but also acid that is stimulated by the vagus nerve (acetylcholine) and by gastrin. This phenomenon suggests an interrelation among these three receptors. The commercially available H$_2$ antagonists are cimetidine **(Tagamet), ranitidine (Zantac), famotidine (Pepcid), and nizatidine (Axid).**

i. Dosage. Typical full therapeutic doses of these agents are cimetidine, 300 mg q.i.d. or 400 mg b.i.d.; ranitidine, 150 mg b.i.d.; famotidine, 20 mg b.i.d. or 40 mg once before bed; and nizatidine, 300 mg once before bed. Alternate regimens also have been used, such as cimetidine, 800 mg at bedtime; and ranitidine, 300 mg at bedtime.

ii. Side effects. The H$_2$ antagonists are remarkably safe, although side effects have been reported. These reports include rare instances of leukopenia and the occasional occurrence of elevated liver enzymes, skin rash, constipation, and diarrhea. Long-term use of cimetidine has been associated with gynecomastia. Ranitidine appears to offer some advantage over cimetidine in that it appears to cause less feminization in men and fewer central nervous system effects, and it has lesser affinity for the cytochrome-P450 system in the liver than does cimetidine, resulting in fewer drug interactions. Both cimetidine and ranitidine interfere with gastric mucosal alcohol dehydrogenase and, if taken before ingestion of alcohol, may increase serum alcohol levels. This effect on alcohol dehydrogenase does not occur with famotidine. Famotidine appears to offer many of the advantages of ranitidine and is slightly longer acting. Nizatidine has a similar profile to ranitidine.

c. Prostaglandins. Prostaglandins are attractive on theoretical grounds because they affect both sides of the mucosal injury-protection balance. They inhibit acid secretion and exert a cytoprotective effect on the mucosa. However, the dose required to elicit the cytoprotective effect is much lower than the acid-inhibitory dose. When prostaglandins are administered in the lower, cytoprotective dose, there is little evidence that they have any clinical benefit.

Prostaglandin analogs (e.g., misoprostol [Cytotec]) have been used to treat peptic conditions in clinical trials and appear to be as effective as H$_2$ antagonists in healing ulcers when administered in doses that inhibit acid secretion. However, there is little evidence that synthetic prostaglandins are clinically effective when given in the lower, purely cytoprotective doses that have no effect on acid secretion. Whether the synthetic prostaglandins offer any practical advantages over current therapy is debatable, although one analog that is commercially available, **misoprostol,** appears to be useful in the prevention and treatment of NSAID-induced gastric ulcers or erosions (see section I.D). Side effects of prostaglandins are diarrhea and abdominal cramping related to the stimulatory effects of prostaglandins on intestinal smooth muscle and secretion. The contractile effect of prostaglandins on uterine smooth muscle could lead to abortion in pregnant women. For this reason, prostaglandins are not recommended for pregnant women or women of childbearing age who are not using a method of contraception.

   d. **Proton-pump inhibitors (PPIs).** Currently there are six commercially available PPIs in the United States: **omeprazole (Prilosec) and esomeprazole (Nexium), lansoprazole (Prevacid), rabeprazole (Protonix), and omeprazole sodium bicarbonate (Zegerid).** PPIs inhibit gastric acid secretion nearly completely by covalently bonding to the H^+-K^+–ATPase or the proton pump in the luminal aspect of the cell membrane of the parietal cells. These drugs have been shown to be superior to H_2 antagonists in healing erosive esophagitis and duodenal and gastric ulcers. Omeprazole was approved by the Food and Drug Administration in 1989, lansoprazole in 1995, rabeprazole in 1999, pantoprazole in 2000, and esomeprazole sodium in 2001. Pantoprazole, esomeprazole, and lansoprazole are also available in the intravenous formulation in the United States.

   PPIs produce faster healing of duodenal ulcers than H_2 antagonists, typically healing ulcers in 2 weeks rather than 4 weeks. PPIs also heal ulcers that were resistant to therapy with H_2 antagonists. Similarly, PPIs heal gastric ulcers faster than H_2 antagonists and heal gastric ulcers that are resistant to H_2 antagonist therapy. Clinical studies have shown that PPIs heal gastric and duodenal ulcers better than H_2 antagonists in patients who continue to take NSAIDs. Furthermore, PPIs provide better prophylaxis against NSAID damage in the duodenum and stomach than H_2 antagonists. All PPIs have been shown to be highly effective as part of an anti–*H. pylori* regimen when used along with clarithromycin and either amoxicillin or metronidazole.

   PPIs are the drugs of choice for the treatment of patients with the ZES. Extensive studies with omeprazole, lansoprazole, rabeprazole, pantoprazole, and esomeprazole sodium confirmed their efficacy and long-term safety. Because PPIs are safe, have minimal side effects, and heal peptic ulcers faster than H_2 blockers, they are the drugs of choice in the treatment of peptic diseases.

2. **Other drugs. Sucralfate (Carafate)** is a substituted disaccharide related to sucrose that appears to act, at least in part, by stimulating endogenous cytoprotection. The drug disperses rapidly in gastric juice of any pH and adheres to tissue protein. In addition to its cytoprotective effects, therefore, sucralfate may temporarily cover ulcers and erosions to help protect them from gastric contents, acid, and pepsin as they heal.

   Sucralfate (1 g q.i.d.; or 2 g b.i.d.) is as effective as H_2 antagonists in healing peptic ulcers. It also has been used to treat gastritis associated with NSAIDs and erosive esophagitis. The drug may cause constipation but has no serious side effects.

3. **Perspective on drug therapy**
   a. **Choice of drugs.** A wide variety of antiulcer drugs are available to the practitioner. There is little difference in efficacy among treatment regimens using an antacid, an H_2 antagonist, a prostaglandin, or sucralfate.

   However, PPIs offer advantages in terms of acceleration of healing and are preferred in the treatment of esophageal, gastric, and duodenal ulcers as well as refractory peptic ulcer disease and gastric hypersecretory syndromes (e.g., ZES). All of the drugs are remarkably safe, and the choice of a drug regimen depends largely on patient or physician preference, cost, and ease of administration. All patients with peptic ulcer disease should be tested for *H. pylori* either by serologic testing, breath test, or by endoscopic biopsy techniques and treated for the cure of *H. pylori* infection.

b. **Long-term treatment.** Peptic ulcer disease in most patients is a chronic relapsing condition. Numerous studies have shown that maintenance therapy with a dose of medication that is lower than the dose used to treat acute disease markedly reduces the risk of ulcer recurrence. For example, treatment of patients who have a healed duodenal ulcer with either cimetidine 400 mg at bedtime, ranitidine 150 mg at bedtime, famotidine 20 mg at bedtime, or sucralfate 1 g b.i.d. for 1 year reduces the ulcer recurrence rate to about 25% compared to a 75% recurrence rate in placebo-treated patients.

This experience raises some issues. On one hand, one must consider the costs and risks of the drugs over the long-term; on the other hand, one must also consider the cost and morbidity of ulcer recurrence. In some patients, because of frequent symptoms or complications such as recurrent ulcer bleeding, it is clear that a long-term treatment program is indicated. Other patients have symptoms at predictable times and benefit from therapy that is limited to several weeks to months. Still other patients have such infrequent or mild symptoms that short, intermittent courses of antiulcer drugs are sufficient.

In patients who have *H. pylori* infection and peptic ulceration, eradication of *H. pylori* has been shown to reduce the recurrence rate of duodenal and gastric ulcers. In patients with recurrent ulcers, *H. pylori* eradication may result in permanent cure. See Chapter 26.

c. **Treatment of *H. pylori*** can be accomplished by various regimens including bismuth based or PPI regimens that include two antibiotics. Since effective treatment requires patient compliance, the simpler regimens are preferred. These oral regimens included a PPI b.i.d., clarithromycin 500 mg b.i.d., and amoxicillin 1 g b.i.d. or metronidazole 500 mg b.i.d. for 7 to 14 days or Pylera, a new combination tablet that contains bismuth, tetracyclene, and metronidazole as perscribed at does of 3 tablets t.i.d. Plus a PPI b.i.d. In resistant cases, Rifampin may be used as an additional antibiotic.

D. **Surgery** for the treatment of peptic disease has decreased drastically over the past two decades, probably because of the increased effectiveness of medical treatment and the decline in prevalence of peptic ulcer in westernized countries. Surgery may be performed because of hemorrhage, obstruction, perforation, or intractability. Intractability means that medical management has failed to relieve pain or heal an ulcer that has caused obstruction or recurrent bleeding.

Most operations for peptic disease fall into the following categories:

1. **Truncal vagotomy and pyloroplasty.** In truncal vagotomy the vagi are cut as they enter the abdomen adjacent to the esophagus. This not only deprives the parietal cell mass of its vagal innervation, but also obliterates the vagal innervation to the muscle of the stomach, intestine, and gallbladder. A major consequence is impairment in gastric emptying, which results in gastric stasis. To counteract this effect, a gastric-emptying procedure, usually a pyloroplasty, must be performed to allow adequate emptying of the stomach.

2. **Highly selective vagotomy.** Sometimes called a **parietal cell vagotomy or proximal gastric vagotomy,** this operation selectively denervates the parietal cell mass in the body and fundus while leaving intact the vagal innervation to the antrum, thereby preserving antral motility and gastric emptying. This procedure obviates the need for a pyloroplasty.

The operation usually takes longer than a standard vagotomy and pyloroplasty because each neurovascular bundle that comes off the major branch of the vagus along the lesser curve (the nerve of Latarjet) to supply the parietal cell mass must be ligated and sectioned.

3. **Billroth I and Billroth II.** Billroth I operation is an antrectomy with reanastomosis between the stomach remnant and the proximal duodenum; a Billroth II procedure is an antrectomy with reanastomosis between the stomach remnant and a loop of proximal jejunum. Both operations are usually coupled with a truncal vagotomy. Thus, the cephalic (vagal) and gastric (gastrin) phases of acid secretion are markedly attenuated. A Billroth procedure is more physiologic because food traverses the same alimentary pathway as it did before surgery

except that the antrum has been removed. In a Billroth II procedure, the food bypasses a large portion of the proximal intestine, resulting in suboptimal stimulation of bile and pancreatic secretion and poor mixing of food with these secretions (see Chapter 28). Whether a Billroth I or Billroth II is performed depends largely on technical considerations at the time of surgery.

E. Treatment of hypersecretory states

1. Gastrinoma. Current management of gastrinoma, or ZES, includes treatment with H_2 antagonists or PPIs, such as omeprazole, often in high doses. For example, ranitidine 1,200 mg per day in divided doses is a typical regimen, but some patients may require up to 6 g per day. Omeprazole 60 to 80 mg a day, or any other PPI, effectively inhibits acid secretion in most patients who have ZES. Some evidence indicates that highly selective vagotomy lessens the requirement for H_2 antagonists in many of these patients, but the use of PPI has decreased the need for this operation.

2. Antral G-cell hyperplasia. Patients with antral G-cell hyperplasia have increased numbers of antral G cells, which results in excessive gastrin secretion. Whether antral G-cell hyperplasia is a distinct entity or is merely the extreme end of a range of quantitatively different G-cell populations remains conjectural. The secretin test (see section III.B.5) does not result in a rise in serum gastrin, as it does in ZES. Most patients respond well to H_2 antagonists. Because antrectomy removes the source of gastrin in these patients, the operation should be considered in patients with refractory illness.

3. Retained antrum syndrome. Retained antrum syndrome develops only in patients who have had an antrectomy and gastrojejunostomy (Billroth II). At the time of surgery, deformity of the antroduodenal area may make identification of the demarcation between antral and duodenal mucosa difficult.

Inadvertently, a small portion of antral mucosa may remain behind and become incorporated into the duodenal stump after the antrum has been resected and the proximal duodenal stump has been oversewn. The G cells of the retained antrum are bathed constantly in an alkaline milieu, which promotes constant, uninhibited secretion of gastrin. Serum gastrin levels may rise to the range of the ZES. However, the secretin tests (see section III.B.5) should not produce a rise in serum gastrin as it does in ZES. Patients may respond to H_2 antagonists or omeprazole, but the definitive treatment is reoperation to remove the small portion of retained antrum.

Selected Readings

Barrison AF, et al. Patterns of proton pump inhibitors in clinical practice. *Am J Med.* 2001; 111:469–473.

Chan FKL, et al. Celecoxib versus diclofenac and omeprazole in reducing the recurrent ulcer bleeding in patients with arthritis. *N Engl J Med.* 2002;347:2104–2110.

Johnson JH. Endoscopic risk factors for bleeding peptic ulcers. *Gastrointest Endosc.* 2002;56:1–6.

Kahi CJ, et al. Endoscopic therapy versus medical therapy for bleeding peptic ulcers with adherent clot—a meta analysis. *Gastroenterology.* 2005;129:855–863.

Law JYW, et al. Effect of intravenous omeprazole on recurrent bleeding after endoscopic treatment of bleeding peptic ulcers. *New Engl J Med.* 2000;343:310–316.

Leontiadis G, et al. Proton pump inhibitor therapy for peptic ulcer bleeding: Cochrane collaboration meta-analysis of randomized controlled trials. *Mayo Clin Proc.* 2007; 82(3):286–296.

Leontiadis GI, et al. Systematic review and meta-analysis of proton pump inhibitor therapy in peptic ulcer bleeding. *BMJ.* 2005;330:568–570.

Rostom A, et al. Gastrointestinal safety of cyclooxygenase-2 inhibitors: A Cochrane Collaboration systematic review. *Clin. Gastroenterol Hepatol.* 2007;7(5):818.

Sridhar S, et al. Hydrogen peroxide (H_2O_2), *H. pylori*, NSAIDS, and clot stability: Do they matter? American College of Gastroenterology Annual Mtg P-37, 2005.

Talley NJ, et al. Practice Parameters Committee of the American College of Gastroenterology. Guidelines for the management of dyspepsia. *Am J Gastroenteral.* 2005;I00:2324–37.

Zargar SA, et al. Pantoprazole infusion as adjuvant therapy to endoscopic treatment in patients with peptic ulcer bleeding: prospective randomized controlled trial. *J Gasteroenterol Hepatol.* 2006; 21:716–721.

$\mathcal{S}$**tress ulcer** refers to an ulcer or, more often, multiple ulcers that develop during the severe physiologic stress of serious illness.

I. The pathogenesis of stress ulcer is unclear but probably is related to a reduction in mucosal blood flow or a breakdown in other normal mucosal defense mechanisms (see Chapter 24) in conjunction with the injurious effects of acid and pepsin on the gastroduodenal mucosa.

A. The ulcerations may be superficial and confined to the mucosa, in which case they are more appropriately called erosions, or they may penetrate deeper into the submucosa. The former may cause diffuse mucosal oozing of blood, whereas the latter may erode into a submucosal vessel and produce frank hemorrhage.

B. Location. Stress ulcerations may develop anywhere within the stomach and proximal duodenum but are more likely to occur in fundic mucosa, which lines the body and fundus of the stomach. This is in contradistinction to the location of ordinary peptic ulcers, which typically are found in the gastric antrum and the duodenum.

C. The clinical setting is usually one of severe and often multisystem illness. For example, elderly patients in a surgical intensive care unit (ICU) with heart and lung disease have a high postoperative prevalence of stress ulcers. Similarly, patients in a medical ICU, particularly those who require respirators, are at high risk of development of stress ulcers. Although not proved, it is possible that poor mucosal oxygenation, differences in acid–base balance, and elevated circulating corticosteroids may contribute to the formation of these ulcers.

II. DIAGNOSIS. Upper gastrointestinal bleeding is the usual clinical manifestation of stress ulceration. In the appropriate clinical setting, the onset of bleeding makes the diagnosis likely. The diagnosis can be confirmed and the extent of involvement documented by upper gastrointestinal endoscopy after the initial management of gastrointestinal bleeding has been started (see Chapter 14).

III. Treatment of stress ulceration usually begins with prevention. Careful attention to respiratory status, acid–base balance, and treatment of other illnesses helps prevent the conditions under which stress ulcers occur.

Patients who develop stress ulcers typically do not secrete large quantities of gastric acid; however, acid does appear to be involved in the pathogenesis of the lesions. Thus, it is reasonable either to neutralize acid or to inhibit its secretion in patients at high risk. In patients admitted to surgical ICUs, hourly antacid titration to keep the intragastric pH above 4 has been shown to reduce markedly the frequency of acute bleeding. Because gastric-acid suppression with PPIs is much more profound, allowing the gastric pH to rise to 5 or 6, PPI infusion IV is more effective in the prevention of stress ulcers and stress ulcer bleeding.

Not all patients in an ICU require acid suppressive prophylaxis. Patients who should be considered for a prophylactic regimen include those who are on respirators and have multisystem disorders and those with a history of peptic ulcer or upper gastrointestinal bleeding. Once bleeding has occurred, however, intravenous acid suppressive therapy with a PPI to keep intragastric pH above 5 remains the most appropriate therapy (see Chapter 14).

Selected Readings

Chak A, et al. Effectiveness of endoscopy in patients admitted to the intensive care unit with upper G.I. hemorrhage. *Gastrointest Endosc.* 2001;53:6.

Dore MP, et al. Ulcers and gastritis. *Endoscopy.* 2004;36:42–47.

James YW, et al. Effect of intravenous omeprazole on recurrent bleeding after endoscopic treatment of bleeding peptic ulcers. *N Engl J Med.* 2000;343:310–316.

Klebl FH, et al. Therapy insight: prophylaxis of stress-induced gastrointestinal bleeding in critically ill patients. *Nat Clin Pract Gastroenterol Hepatol.* 2007;4(10):562–570.

Martindale RG, et al. Contemporary strategies for the prevention of stress-related mucosal bleeding. *Am J Hosp Pract.* 2005;62(suppl):S511–S517.

Wolfe MM, et al. Acid suppression: Optimizing therapy for gastroduodenal ulcer healing, gastroesophageal reflux disease and stress-related erosive syndrome. *Gastroenterology.* 2000;118(suppl 2):S9.

I. EPIDEMIOLOGY. *Helicobacter pylori* (*H. pylori* **or HP**) is a microaerophilic, flagellated, highly motile, gram-negative spiral bacteria that was first isolated from mucosal biopsies of patients with chronic active gastritis by two Australian investigators, Warren and Marshall, who subsequently received the Nobel Prize in 2005 for their discovery. The organism was first named *"Campylobacter pyloris,"* then the name was changed to *Helicobacter pylori* when it was shown genetically that it was not a member of the *Campylobacter* genus. HP is one of the most common human infectious agents and is causally linked with neutrophilic gastritis, chronic active gastritis, atrophic gastritis, peptic ulcer disease, gastric intestinal metaplasia, gastric adenocarcinoma, gastric mucosa-associated lymphoid tissue (MALT) lymphoma, and gastric B-cell lymphoma.

HP infection occurs primarily during childhood and usually persists for life unless the infection is adequately treated. The major risk factor for infection is the socioeconomic status of the family during childhood. The prevalence of HP in the United States has decreased in the white middle- and upper-class population 50 years of age and younger, but the infection is still common among older persons (infected at a younger age), the socially disadvantaged, and the immigrant populations.

HP has been found in water, stool, dental plaque, and saliva. There is strong epidemiologic evidence for waterborne transmission in Peru and Colombia. Primary mode of transmission is person to person, but oral, gastro-oral, and fecal spread is likely.

II. VIRULENCE FACTORS OF HP ARE NUMEROUS AND INCLUDE

  A. Motility. HP with its spiral shape and unipolar flagella is able to move from the gastric lumen with low pH to gastric mucosal surface where pH is neutral, as well as to other parts of the gastric surface where its growth potential is optimal.

  B. Adherence factors. HP binds to gastric-type epithelium. This tissue tropism and binding prevents the organism from being easily shed during cell and mucus turnover. HP has several adhesion proteins that bind to the gastric mucosal cell receptors (which are genetically controlled) which increases successful HP infection and spread.

  C. Urease. HP produces urease, an enzyme which hydrolyzes urea to produce ammonia (NH_3) to protect itself from gastric acid. Ammonia neutralizes the acid surrounding HP as well as provides an essential basis for the "CLO" test used for testing mucosal biopsies for the presence or absence of HP.

  D. Toxins. HP possesses and/or elaborates various toxins that cause tissue injury of the gastric mucosa in infected individuals. These include lipopolysaccharide (endotoxin bound to HP), neutrophil activating protein (NAPA), vacuolating cytotoxin (VacA), cytotoxin-associated antigen (CagA-A), and outer membrane inflammatory protein (OipA). Not all strains of HP possess all these toxins. Those strains of HP which possess CagA and OipA seem to be exceptionally virulent and are associated with more severe disease activity, PUD, and cancer.

III. INFECTION. Acute infection has been demonstrated dramatically by Warren and Marshall, who voluntarily ingested a culture of HP and developed acute HP disease. It is not known how often infection with HP spontaneously clears. In most cases, infection is lifelong. Most infected persons develop chronic active gastritis. Gastritis may be confined mostly to the gastric antrum and/or involve the entire stomach. In persons with predominately antral involvement, gastric acid secretion may be normal or increased. In such persons, duodenal ulcer and esophagitis secondary to GER may occur. In persons with diffuse HP infection of the entire stomach, gastric atrophy may develop and acid secretion may diminish; in fact, these persons may develop hypo- and achlordria and even vitamin B_{12} deficiency. In advanced cases, intestinal metaplasia and gastric adenocarcinoma may develop. Once patients develop severe atrophy, intestinal HP metaplasia or gastric adenocarcinoma may not be present in these tissues where there is no acid secretion.

Interestingly, in persons treated with proton pump inhibitors (PPIs) chronically, there is usually a shift of HP infection from the antrum to the corpus and accelerated atrophic changes. Thus some experts advise eradication of HP before long-term PPI therapy is instituted in HP-infected individuals.

In some patients, HP infection arouses a robust induction of lymphocytic infiltration of gastric mucosa with lymphocytic follicle formation and in some cases **MALT lymphoma.** These have been seen to regress after appropriate HP eradication therapy. However, **B-cell lymphomas** that develop in association with HP infection may not regress after HP eradication and may need oncologic intervention.

IV. DIAGNOSIS

A. Endoscopy and biopsy is the gold standard for the diagnosis of HP. Biopsies should be obtained from all parts of the stomach since the colonization of HP is spotty and is affected by the mode of infection, patients' medications, and whether patients are on acid-suppressive therapy. Histology not only confirms the presence of HP, but also gives information on the presence or absence of gastritis, gastric atrophy, intestinal metaplasia, MALT lymphoma, and cancer. Sensitivity ranges from 90% to 95% and specificity 95% to 100%. False negative results occur in the sections of recent GI bleeding, use of Bismuth-containing medications, antibiotics, sucralfate, and acid-suppressive medications.

CLO test, PyloriTek test uses a biopsy in a medium containing urea which undergoes color change if HP is present with urease activity.

HP may be **cultured** from gastric biopsies. This should be considered in patients who have failed two courses of appropriate antibiotic treatment regimens and are thought to have resistant HP.

B. Breath tests. Breath testing in patients infected with HP utilizes their ingesting C_{14} (radioactive) or C_{13} containing urea, then blowing into a container to measure the tagged CO_2 released by HP degradation of urea ($CONH_3$) by its urease which releases CO_2 and NH_3. Sensitivity of breath testing ranges from 85% to 95% and is operator-dependent. False negative results can occur in patients with history of recent antibiotic, bismuth, sucralfate and antisecretionary therapy and in those with advanced histologic changes such as atrophy and intestinal metaplasia.

C. Stool antigen test. A monoclonal and polyclonal antibody test is available to test for HP antigen in stool samples. This has a similar sensitivity and specificity as compared to breath tests. False negative tests are seen as in breath tests as well as in patients with a history of recent GI bleeding.

Both the breath test and stool antigen test should not be done for at least 4 weeks after HP eradication therapy.

D. Serology. HP antibody may be detected in persons who have been infected with HP. However, in many persons the IgG HP antibody persists in the plasma even after proper eradication (at least for 18 months) and thus it is not a good measure of current infection.

Salivary and urinary assay have similar sensitivity and specificity to serology.

E. When and whom to test. HP testing is recommended for patients who are to be treated for the eradication of HP infection. In patients with history of PUD and dyspepsia, if endoscopy is indicated, biopsies should be obtained from multiple sites. In patients with gastric ulcer, biopsies should also be obtained from the ulcer to check for cancer.

After eradication therapy, testing for presence of HP is not routinely practiced. In patients with PUD-related GI hemorrhage or those with recurrent dyspeptic, symptoms may be tested for HP after at least 4 weeks have elapsed from eradication, antibiotic, and acid antisecretory therapy. Stool antigen test, breath test and, in indicated cases, endoscopy and biopsy may be used.

V. THERAPY. Combination therapy is required for successful HP eradication. The current preferred therapy in the United States is twice daily **PPI plus clarithromycin** 500 mg b.i.d. and **amoxicillin** 1 g b.i.d. for 7 to 14 days.

   Dual therapy with PPI and amoxicillin or clarithromycin is **not** recommended.

   In patients with penicillin allergy, metronidazole 500 mg b.i.d. may be used.

   In the United States there is documented resistance to metronidazole (25%), clarithromycin (15%), and amoxicillin (1%).

   Treatment failure may be attributed to patient noncompliance, smoking, concurrent use of sucralfate, and the presence of bacterial resistance to antibiotics.

   Patients who fail the above therapy may be offered **quadruple therapy** recommended by the European *Helicobacter pylori* Study Group. Quadruple therapy consists of metronidazole 500 mg q.i.d., tetracycline 500 mg q.i.d., Bismuth subsalicylate (Pepto-Bismol) tablets q.i.d., and a PPI b.i.d. for 2 weeks. To simplify this regimen, a combination tablet **(Pylera)** is available. It contains Tetracyclene, metronidazole, and bismuth salicate. The dose is 3 tablets t.i.d. plus twice daily PPI.

   In patients who are allergic or wish another regimen, a 10-day course of levofloxacin 500 mg q.d. or 250 mg b.i.d., amoxicillin 1g b.i.d. and a PPI b.i.d. or rifabutin 300 mg q.d., amoxicillin 1 g b.i.d. and a PPI b.i.d. may be used. Rifabutin may cause bone marrow suppression, leukopenia, hepatitis, uveitis, and a polyarthralgia-like syndrome.

Selected Readings

Delchier JL. Gastric MALT lymphoma, a malignancy potentially curable by eradication of *Helicobacter pylori*. *Gastroenterol Clin Biol.* 2003;27:453–458.

Duck WM, et al. Antimicrobial resistance incidence and risk factors among *Helicobacter pylori*–infected persons, United States. *Emerg Infect Dis.* 2004;10:1088–1094.

Gisbert JP, et al. *Helicobacter pylori* "rescue" therapy after failure of two eradication treatments. *Helicobacter.* 2005;10:363–372.

Gisbert JP, et al. Review article: C-urea breath test in the diagnosis of *Helicobacter pylori* infection—a critical review. *Aliment Pharmacol Ther.* 2004;15:1001–1017.

Gisbert JP, et al. Stool antigen test for the diagnosis of *Helicobacter pylori* infection: A systematic review. *Helicobacter.* 2004;9:347–368.

Janssen MJ, et al. Meta-analysis: The influence of pre-treatment with a proton pump inhibitor on *Helicobacter pylori* eradication. *Aliment Pharmacol Ther.* 2005;21:341–345.

Jarbol D, et al. Proton pump inhibitor or testing for *Helicobacter pylori* as the first step for patients presenting with dyspepsia? A cluster-randomized trial. *Am J Gastroenterol.* 2006;I0I:1200–8.

Laey C, et al. *Helicobacter infection* and gastric cancer. *Gastroenterology.* 2001;120:324.

Laine L, et al. Bismuth-based quadruple therapy using a single capsule of bismuth biskalcitrate, metronidazole and tetracycline given with omeprazole versus omeprazole, amoxicillin, and clarithromycin for eradication of *Helicobacter pylori* in duodenal ulcer patients: A prospective, randomized, multicenter North American trial. *Am J Gastroenterol.* 2003; 98:562–567.

Ohata H, et al. Progression of chronic atrophic gastritis associated with *Helicobacter pylori* infection increases risk of gastric cancer. *Int J Cancer.* 2004;109:138–143.

Qasim, A, et al. Rifabutin- and furazolidone-based *Helicobacter pylori* eradication therapies after failure of standard first- and second-line eradication attempts in dyspepsia patients. *Aliment Pharmacol Ther.* 2005;21:91–96.

Saad RJ, et al. Levofloxacin-based triple therapy versus bismuth-based quadruple therapy for persistent *Helicobacter pylori* infection: A meta-analysis. *Am J Gastroenterol.* 2006;101:488–496.

Sepulveda AR, et al. Role of *Helicobacter pylori* in gastric carcinogenesis. *Gastroenterol Clin North Am.* 2002;31:517–535.

Suzuki T, et al. Smoking increases the treatment failure for *Helicobacter pylori* eradication. *Am J Med.* 2006;119:217–224.

Vakil N. *Helicobacter pylori* treatment: A practical approach. *Am J Gastroenterol.* 2006; 101:497–499.

Vakil N. New guidelines for *Helicobacter pylori:* Applying these to your practice. *Rev. Gastroenterol Disorder.* 2007;7(3):111–114.

*M*ost neoplasms of the stomach are malignant, and most of those are adenocarcinoma. A minority are lymphoma, leiomyosarcoma, and liposarcoma. Benign neoplasms include adenomatous, hyperplastic, and hamartomatous polyps; leiomyomas; and lipomas. Rarely, gastrinomas, carcinoids, vascular tumors, fibromas, and squamous cell carcinomas occur in the stomach.

Adenocarcinoma of the stomach is the second most frequent cause of cancer death worldwide. In East Asia, Latin America, and the former Soviet Union, the incidence is up to eight times higher than in the United States and it remains high among immigrants from those areas. Although screening programs in high-risk areas such as Japan may result in the detection of early lesions, in lower risk areas such as the United States and Western Europe, most cancers are relatively advanced by the time of diagnosis.

I. GASTRIC ADENOCARCINOMA
A. Pathogenesis
1. Pathology
a. **Early gastric cancer (EGC)** is gastric cancer that has not penetrated the major muscle layer of the stomach wall. EGC can be divided into three types based on macroscopic appearance (Fig. 27-1).

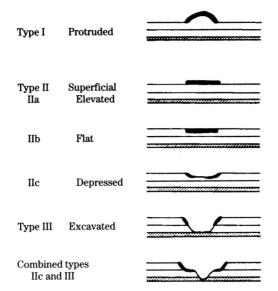

Type I	Protruded
Type II IIa	Superficial Elevated
IIb	Flat
IIc	Depressed
Type III	Excavated
Combined types IIc and III	

Figure 27-1. Classification of early gastric carcinoma according to the Japanese Endoscopy Society. (From Green PHR, et al. Early gastric cancer. *Gastroenterology*. 81;247:1981. Reprinted with permission.)

    b. Advanced gastric cancer is gastric cancer that has penetrated the muscle layer of the stomach. This condition also has been divided into three types:
      i. Polypoid or intestinal
      ii. Diffuse infiltrating or signet ring type
      iii. Ulcerating
2. Risk factors (Table 27-1)
    a. Some **population groups** appear to be at higher risk than others for development of gastric adenocarcinoma. For example, the prevalence of gastric cancer in Japan is about 10 times the prevalence in the United States. Furthermore, in Japan approximately 30% of gastric cancers at the time of diagnosis are EGC, whereas in the United States only 5% can be classified as EGC. Japanese who move away from Japan to a low-risk area have a similar risk to those who remain in Japan. However, second- and third-generation Japanese children of these immigrants have a progressively lower risk that approaches the local population.
    b. Several **dietary factors** have been implicated. Increased consumption of **salt** appears to be a consistent finding. Dietary **nitrates** also may be important. **Cigarette smoking** increases risk. However, a diet rich in fresh fruits and vegetables, daily aspirin use, and COX-II antagonist reduce the risk.
    c. Conditions that predispose to achlorhydria, such as pernicious anemia and atrophic gastritis, carry a higher than average risk of gastric cancer. Whether this is because the reduced acid allows bacteria that have the capacity to nitrosate dietary amines to carcinogenic nitrosamines to grow within the stomach or because of other effects is not clear.
    d. Partial gastrectomy 15 or more years in the past was thought to be associated with a higher risk of development of adenocarcinoma within the gastric remnant. Recent evidence indicates that this increased risk is lower than originally anticipated. Virtually all these patients eventually have chronic gastritis and become hypo- or achlorhydric, which, as indicated previously, may increase the risk of development of cancer.
    e. *Helicobacter pylori* infection has been associated with gastric adenocarcinoma. The cancer is thought to arise from gastric intestinal metaplasia that arises in patients who develop chronic atrophic gastritis with chronic infection with *H. pylori*. Especially those strains that are CagA+ appear to be more carcinogenic than CagA− strains.
B. Diagnosis
1. Clinical presentation
    a. EGC typically is asymptomatic and usually is discovered during endoscopy performed for other complaints. When symptoms have been attributed to EGC, they usually are vague, such as epigastric discomfort and nausea.

TABLE 27-1 **Risk Factors for Adenocarcinoma of the Stomach**

Chronic gastritis with *Helicobacter pylori* infection
National origin (e.g., high risk in Japan, Chile, Finland)
Diet (e.g., high salt consumption, nitrates, smoking)
Achlorhydria
Histologic changes (e.g., atrophic gastritis, intestinal metaplasia)
Gastric adenomatous polyps
Hypertrophic gastropathy (Ménétrièr's disease)
Postgastrectomy
Male vs. female (1.5:1.0)
Blood group A

b. Most patients in North America present with symptoms of advanced gastric cancer.

    i. Symptoms are primarily abdominal pain and weight loss, which may be accompanied by anorexia, weakness, gastrointestinal bleeding, and signs of gastric obstruction, such as early satiety or vomiting.

    ii. Physical examination. An epigastric mass, an enlarged liver due to metastases, or ascites may be evident. An umbilical mass, known as a Sister Joseph's nodule, is unusual. Metastasis to the ovaries has been called a Krukenberg's tumor, although this eponym also has been applied to colonic and other gastrointestinal tumors that metastasize to the ovaries.

2. Diagnostic studies

  a. Upper gastrointestinal x-ray series versus endoscopy. Traditionally, an upper gastrointestinal (GI) x-ray series has been the first diagnostic study. If the patient in fact has gastric cancer and not a benign peptic lesion, the upper GI series may reveal a mass lesion, ulceration, irregularity of the mucosa, lack of distensibility of the stomach, or no definite abnormality. Any of these abnormal findings requires endoscopic confirmation and biopsy.

    Furthermore, because patients with abdominal discomfort plus weight loss, bleeding, or vomiting who have negative or inconclusive findings on upper GI x-ray series still require endoscopy, the most cost-effective approach to such patients may be to begin with endoscopy.

  b. At endoscopy, the appearance of the lesion can be assessed, the lesion can be biopsied and brushed for cytologic study, and the pH of the gastric contents can be determined. In ulcerating lesions, six to eight biopsies of the ulcer edges are necessary to provide a 95% chance of obtaining a positive result if the lesion is indeed cancerous. An acid pH of the gastric aspirate indicates, of course, that the stomach is capable of secreting acid. On the other hand, a neutral pH at endoscopy does not necessarily indicate achlorhydria.

  c. Endoscopic ultrasound is an excellent modality for staging of gastric cancers. The depth of invasion of the tumor can be easily determined, allowing accurate diagnosis of EGC which may be treated by endoscopic mucosal resection (EMR).

  d. Serum carcinoembryonic antigen (CEA) levels are elevated in about one third of patients with advanced gastric cancer but are not helpful in making the diagnosis. As with colon cancer, serial CEA determinations may be useful in the postoperative follow-up of patients to indicate recurrences or to estimate metastatic tumor burden.

  e. Hematocrit and hemoglobin levels may be normal but typically are decreased in advanced gastric cancer due to bleeding and the extent of chronic disease. If the patient has pernicious anemia (as a predisposing cause of gastric cancer), the anemia may be macrocytic.

  f. An **elevated alkaline phosphatase level** may indicate metastases to the liver. An elevated 5′-nucleotidase level confirms that the liver is the origin of the abnormality in alkaline phosphatase.

  g. Computed tomography (CT) of the abdomen should be performed to survey for liver metastases, lymph node enlargement, and the extent of the primary tumor. If endoscopic biopsy fails to make a histologic diagnosis, CT- or ultrasound-guided needle aspiration of a mass lesion or a percutaneous liver biopsy in patients with elevated alkaline phosphatase may provide diagnostic tissue.

C. Treatment

  1. The prognosis for gastric cancer is poor. The overall 5-year survival rate is 18.6%. Untreated, the median life expectancy in advanced disease with liver metastases is 4–6 months and in patients with peritoneal carcinomatosis 4–6 weeks. However, if the tumor is confined to the mucosa and submucosa (EGC) and there are no metastases or lymph node involvement, the 5-year survival rate exceeds 90%. Unfortunately, most patients with gastric cancer in the

United States already have metastases or involvement of contiguous structures or lymph nodes at the time of diagnosis.

2. **Surgery** currently is the only hope of cure. About 20% of patients are deemed inoperable because of the extent of disease or high operative risk. Of the remaining 80% who undergo surgery, about half undergo a curative resection, and the other half are given palliative treatment for bleeding or obstruction. However, only about 20% of patients who have had a curative resection survive 5 years. Results might be better with extensive lymph node dissection and lymphadenectomy.

3. **Chemotherapy and radiotherapy.** Both chemotherapy and radiotherapy alone for gastric cancer have been disappointing. If the patient's condition is operable, the initial resection of as much tumor mass as possible seems to improve the efficacy of chemotherapy and radiotherapy. Adjuvant chemotherapy using 5-fluororacil, mitomycin, doxorubicin, Cisplatin, and irinotecan seems to improve survival. Adjuvant radiotherapy alone has no effect on long-term survival. However, combined chemotherapy and radiation in the adjuvant setting improves overall survival.

4. **Other treatment measures.** Patients with gastric cancer require careful attention to nutritional needs. Partial or complete gastric resection imposes additional nutritional consequences (see Chapter 28). These patients may require supplemental vitamins, particularly vitamin B_{12}, and minerals such as calcium and iron.

5. **Follow-up.** Patients who have been operated on for cure should be examined by the physician every several months for clinical and laboratory evidence of recurrence. Weight loss, gastrointestinal bleeding, and obstruction—all the signs of original disease—may signify recurrence. It is reasonable to check a complete blood count, routine liver tests, and CEA level every 3 to 6 months for the first 1 to 2 years after surgery and every 6 to 12 months thereafter. Yearly upper GI endoscopy to look for local recurrence also is appropriate during the first 5 years.

II. OTHER GASTRIC TUMORS

A. **Malignant tumors.** Other malignant tumors include lymphoma, leiomyosarcoma, liposarcoma, and carcinoid. Of these, primary gastric lymphomas account for most of the noncarcinomatous gastric malignancies. The stomach can also be involved secondarily by disseminated lymphoma or by metastatic cancer from other sites.

1. **Clinical presentation and diagnosis.** Patients with other gastric neoplasms present clinically with abdominal pain, weight loss, anorexia, and vomiting, signs and symptoms that are similar to those observed in patients with adenocarcinoma of the stomach. The methods of diagnosis are also similar.

2. **Prognosis and treatment.** Because lymphoma responds better than adenocarcinoma to radiation and chemotherapy, the prognosis is better. The 5-year survival rate of patients with gastric lymphoma is about 50%. If the lymphoma is confined to the stomach, surgical treatment is indicated. If regional nodes or distant sites are involved, radiotherapy or chemotherapy with or without surgery may be indicated.

B. **MALT lymphoma.** Low-grade B-cell lymphomas of mucosa-associated lymphoid tissue (MALT) are thought to arise within organized lymphoid tissue in the gastric mucosa that is most frequently acquired in response to *H. pylori* infection. Long-term remissions can be induced in the low-grade MALT lymphomas in 70% to 80% of cases by the successful eradication of the *H. pylori* infection. The lymphomas that are most likely to respond to the *H. pylori* eradication are those that are located superficially within the gastric mucosa. Recurrences of low-grade lymphoma are encountered in patients treated by *H. pylori* eradication, but these appear to be infrequent and may be self-limiting and spontaneously regress without surgery. Deeper and higher grade lesions need to be treated as B-cell lymphomas.

C. Polypoid lesions and benign tumors. The term **polyp** refers to any protrusion into the lumen of a viscus and thus does not necessarily connote benign or malignant histopathology. In common medical usage, however, the term *polyp* usually refers to a lesion of epithelial origin.

1. **Histologic types.** Gastric polyps are adenomatous, hyperplastic, or hamartomatous. Of these, only adenomatous polyps and carcinoids appear to have malignant potential. Other benign lesions that may resemble gastric polyps grossly are leiomyomas and lipomas. Small polyps normally seen in the gastric corpus are usually fundic gland polyps that contain dilated gastric glands.

2. **Diagnosis.** Often, benign polypoid lesions are discovered incidentally during upper GI x-ray series or endoscopy. The studies may have been performed for complaints of nausea, abdominal pain, or weight loss, but whether the polyps are responsible for those complaints is conjectural.

   Regardless of how the polypoid lesion has been identified, endoscopy should be performed to clarify the appearance of the lesion, to obtain biopsies, and to survey for other lesions. If possible, adenomatous polyps should be removed endoscopically. Polyps that cannot be removed should be biopsied and brushed for cytologic study.

3. **Treatment.** The diagnosis of frank carcinoma, lymphoma, or other malignancy leads to appropriate treatment of that condition. Removal of an adenomatous polyp removes the risk of malignant degeneration. The diagnosis of a benign, nonadenomatous polypoid lesion is reassuring in that the lesion is not cancerous and will not become cancerous.

Selected Readings

Chan AO, et al. Synchronous gastric adenocarcinoma and mucosa-associated lymphoid tissue lymphoma in association with *Helicobacter* infection: Comparing reported cases between the East and the West. *Am J Gastroenterol.* 2001;96:1922–1924.

Chung DC, et al. A woman with a family history of gastric and breast cancer. *N Eng J Med.* 2007;357:283–291.

Delchier JC. Gastric MALT lymphoma: A malignancy potentially curable by eradication of *Helicobacter pylori. Gastroenterol Clin Biol.* 2003;27:453–458.

El-Serag HB, et al. Epidemiologic differences between adenocarcinoma of the oesophagus and adenocarcinoma of the gastric cardia in the USA. *Gut.* 2002;50:368–372.

El-Zahabi N, et al. The value of EUS in predicting the response of gastric mucosa-associated lymphoid tissue lymphoma to *Helicobacter pylori* eradication. *Gastrointest Endosc.* 2007;65:89–96.

El-Zimaity HM, et al. Patterns of gastric atrophy in intestinal type gastric carcinoma. *Cancer.* 2002;94:1428–1436.

Hwang JH, et al. A prospective study comparing endoscopy and EUS in the evaluation of GI subepithelial masses. *Gastrointest Endos.* 2005;62:202–208.

Kurtz RC, et al. Gastric cardia cancer and dietary fiber. *Gastroenterology.* 2001;120:568.

Laey C, et al. *Helicobacter pylori* infection and gastric cancer. *Gastroenterology.* 2001; 20:324–330.

Lynch HT, et al. Gastric cancer: new genetic developments. *J Surg Oncol.* 2005;90:114–133.

MacDonald JS. Gastric cancer: New therapeutic options. *N Engl J Med.* 2006;355:76–77.

Meining A, et al. Atrophy-metaplasia-dysplasia-carcinoma sequence in the stomach: A reality or merely a hypothesis? *Best Pract Res Clin Gastroenterol.* 2001;15:983–998.

Morita D, et al. Analysis of Sentinel Node involvement in gastric cancer. *Clin Gastroenterol Hepatol.* 2007;5:1046–1052.

Noffsinger A, et al. Preinvasive neoplasia in the stomach: Diagnosis and treatment. *Clin Gastroenterol Heptatol.* 2007;5:1018–1023.

Sakuramoto S, et al. Adjuvant chemotherapy for gastric cancer with S-1. *N Eng J Med.* 2007;357:1810–1820.

Usui S. Laparoscopy-assisted total gastroectomy for early gastric cancer: comparison with conventional open toal gastrectomy. *Surg Laparosc Endosc Percutan Tech.* 2005;15:309–314.

Wagner AD, et al. Chemotherapy for advanced gastric cancer. *Cochrane Database Syst Rev.* 2005;2:CD004064.

28 POSTGASTRECTOMY DISORDERS

$\mathcal{G}$astrectomy usually means removal of part of the stomach and anastomosis of the gastric remnant with either the duodenum (Billroth I) or a loop of proximal jejunum (Billroth II) (see Chapter 24). These operations typically are performed as surgical treatment of peptic ulcer disease or cancer of the stomach. Rarely, the entire stomach is removed.

Removal of part or all of the stomach can be associated with a variety of consequences and complications (Table 28-1). These may range in severity from a simple inability to eat large meals, due to loss of the reservoir function of the stomach, to more serious complications, such as severe dumping and profound nutritional sequelae.

I. DUMPING SYNDROME

A. Pathogenesis. The dumping syndrome develops as a result of the loss of pyloric regulation of gastric emptying. Thus, strictly speaking, a portion of the stomach does not necessarily have to be removed; a pyloroplasty alone can lead to the dumping syndrome. After a pyloroplasty or an antrectomy, hyperosmolar food is "dumped" rapidly into the proximal small intestine.

1. During the **early phase** of the dumping syndrome, the hyperosmolar small-bowel contents draw water into the lumen, stimulate bowel motility, and release vasoactive agents, such as serotonin, bradykinin, neurotensin, substance P, and vasoactive intestinal peptide from the bowel wall. Patients experience abdominal cramps, diarrhea, sweating, tachycardia, palpitations, hypotension, and light-headedness. These effects typically occur within 1 hour after eating.

2. In the **late phase,** because of the absorption of a large amount of glucose after the meal, plasma insulin rises excessively and blood sugar may plummet. Consequently, the patient may experience tachycardia, light-headedness, and sweatiness 1 to 3 hours after a meal.

B. Diagnosis. The typical symptoms and signs in the setting of gastric surgery usually are sufficient to make the diagnosis of dumping syndrome. A blood sugar

---

TABLE 28-1   Complications of Gastric Surgery

I. Dumping syndrome
II. Recurrent ulcer
III. Nutritional and metabolic sequelae
    A. Loss of weight
       1. Poor food intake
       2. Dumping syndrome
       3. Malabsorption
    B. Malabsorption, with or without weight loss
       1. Malabsorption of iron, calcium, folate, vitamin B_{12}
       2. Malabsorption of fat, protein, carbohydrate
IV. **Afferent loop syndrome**
V. **(?)** Carcinoma in the gastric remnant

determination several hours after a meal when symptoms are at their worst may be helpful in confirming the late phase.

C. Treatment. Patients are advised to eat small meals six to eight times a day. Carbohydrates are restricted to minimize glucose absorption. Medications to reduce bowel motility, such as diphenoxylate or loperamide, may be helpful. In rare instances, surgical revision with anastomosis of the gastric remnant to an antiperistaltic segment of jejunum may be necessary.

II. RECURRENT ULCER

A. Pathogenesis. About 1% to 3% of patients who have undergone partial gastrectomy for ulcer disease develop a recurrent ulcer. Recurrent ulcers nearly always occur in small intestinal mucosa adjacent to the anastomosis (duodenal mucosa in a Billroth I, jejunal mucosa in a Billroth II). The factors that contribute to the development of a recurrent ulcer are similar to those that contributed to the original ulcer disease (see Chapter 24). A recurrent ulcer after surgery raises the question of the adequacy of the operation. Also, the possibility of an acid hypersecretory syndrome (e.g., gastrinoma or retained antrum) must be considered.

B. Diagnosis. Patients with recurrent ulcers usually experience abdominal pain that may or may not be similar to their original ulcer pain. Typically, the pain is relieved by food, although in some patients the pain is aggravated by eating. As in ordinary ulcer disease, bleeding, obstruction, and perforation can occur. The diagnosis is established by endoscopy. Because of the surgical deformity at the anastomosis, the endoscopist must be especially attentive to examining the folds and crevices in the vicinity of the anastomosis.

The documentation of a recurrent ulcer is an indication for at least a fasting serum gastrin determination. Formal acid secretory testing (see Chapter 24) may not be reliable because of the loss of acid through the widely patent anastomosis. If the ratio of basal acid output to maximal acid output exceeds 60%, that is suggestive of a gastrinoma or another acid hypersecretory syndrome, but a low ratio does not exclude such a syndrome. If suspicion is high for a Zollinger–Ellison-like syndrome, a secretin stimulation test should be performed (see Chapter 24).

C. Treatment. Conventional ulcer therapy (see Chapter 24) may be sufficient. Some patients require chronic treatment with acid-suppressive drugs. Those in whom such therapy fails may benefit from more extensive surgery. A demonstrated acid hypersecretory condition may require more specific treatment (see Chapter 24).

III. NUTRITIONAL AND METABOLIC SEQUELAE

A. Pathogenesis

1. The **weight loss** that commonly occurs after gastric surgery is multifactorial. First, the storage capacity of the postsurgical stomach is limited, thereby restricting the amount of food that can be consumed at one meal. Second, if the dumping syndrome is present, the patient may reduce food intake to avoid unpleasant consequences. Thus, malabsorption may contribute to weight loss due to failure to absorb adequate calories and nutrients.

2. **The causes of malabsorption are numerous**

   a. The reduction in gastric acid contributes to the **malabsorption of dietary iron.** If the patient has a gastrojejunal anastomosis (Billroth II), bypass of the duodenum also results in poor absorption of iron, calcium, and folate. Thus, iron- or folate-deficiency anemia or a manifestation of calcium deficiency, such as osteoporosis, may develop.

   b. Bypass of the duodenum also means that food-stimulated secretin and cholecystokinin release is diminished, resulting in **delayed and attenuated bile and pancreatic secretions.** Furthermore, the digestive enzymes mix poorly with the food as they "chase" it down the small intestine.

      Rarely, **bacterial overgrowth** develops within the afferent loop after Billroth II surgery, causing deconjugation of bile acids and contributing to the **fat malabsorption.** The dumping syndrome, if present, adds to poor mixing, even in patients with a gastroduodenal anastomosis (Billroth I).

    c. Malabsorption of vitamin B$_{12}$ may occur. Normally, intrinsic factor (IF) is secreted by gastric parietal cells in excess of what is needed to complex with dietary vitamin B$_{12}$. An acid-reducing operation by itself is not sufficient to compromise vitamin B$_{12}$ absorption. However, most patients who have undergone partial gastrectomy have chronic gastritis, presumably because of reflux of small-intestinal contents, which can result in gastric atrophy and loss of parietal cells over several years. Secretion of IF diminishes, and the neurologic or hematologic consequences of pernicious anemia may develop.

B. Diagnosis. Many of the nutritional and metabolic manifestations of the postgastrectomy state are self-evident. Routine hematologic studies plus serum iron, ferritin, and vitamin B$_{12}$ levels help in determining the cause of anemia and in planning appropriate treatment. Because of normal homeostatic mechanisms, serum calcium usually remains normal.

    A quantitative stool fat determination may document the severity of malabsorption. However, even patients who do well after gastric surgery typically have mild elevations in stool fat in the range of 5 to 10 g per day. An abnormal vitamin B$_{12}$ absorption test (Schilling test) without IF, which normalizes with added IF, can document the lack of IF in patients with macrocytic or mixed anemia. Endoscopic biopsy showing atrophic gastritis lacking parietal cells confirms the diagnosis.

C. Treatment. The patient is advised to consume frequent small feedings to accommodate the small gastric remnant. Antidiarrheal agents may be helpful. If fat malabsorption is a prominent feature, a low-fat diet, perhaps supplemented with medium-chain triglycerides (which do not require bile acids for absorption) should be prescribed. In patients with fat malabsorption, an empiric trial of tetracycline, 250 mg four times daily for 7 to 10 days, is justified because documentation of bacterial overgrowth in the afferent loop is difficult.

IV. AFFERENT LOOP SYNDROME

A. Pathogenesis. The afferent loop syndrome may occur in patients with a gastrojejunostomy. This term does not refer to the blind loop syndrome. Occasionally this is a point of some confusion. The blind loop syndrome, which means bacterial overgrowth in a blind or stagnant loop of bowel or within a diverticulum with consequent bile acid deconjugation and fat malabsorption, certainly can occur in the afferent loop.

    The afferent loop syndrome develops because of a stricture or kinking of the afferent, or proximal, loop of a Billroth II anastomosis. This defect impairs the egress of fluid from the duodenum. When the patient eats, biliary, pancreatic, and duodenal secretions enter the duodenum. If these secretions cannot pass easily to the gastrojejunal anastomosis, the afferent loop becomes distended, causing severe epigastric pain. As the pressure within the loop increases, the obstruction is suddenly overcome, culminating in vomiting and prompt relief of pain.

B. Diagnosis. The clinical story of severe abdominal pain developing during or shortly after eating and relieved promptly by vomiting in a patient with a Billroth II anastomosis is highly suggestive. Documentation by objective testing is difficult. HIDA scanning may help confirm the diagnosis if isotope is seen to fill and distend the afferent loop during development of typical pain, without entry into the stomach or distal jejunum. The patient should undergo endoscopy to look for an anastomotic ulcer or a constriction within the afferent loop. However, kinking of the loop is difficult to determine by endoscopy. Although an upper gastrointestinal x-ray series usually is not helpful, it may suggest kinking of the loop and can indicate the length of the afferent loop and its position in the abdomen.

    The diagnosis of afferent loop syndrome is made after much deliberation in patients who have symptoms consistent with the diagnosis and in whom another cause for the symptoms cannot be found.

C. Treatment. Medical management of the afferent loop syndrome usually is unsatisfactory. Sometimes frequent small feedings prevent symptoms. If an anastomotic ulcer is discovered, that can be treated. An occasional patient improves with the passage of time. The definitive treatment is surgical and consists of either relieving adhesive bands or shortening the afferent loop and reforming the anastomosis.

V. CHRONIC GASTRITIS AND CARCINOMA IN THE GASTRIC REMNANT

A. Pathogenesis. In some studies, patients who have undergone partial gastrectomy appear to be at increased risk to develop adenocarcinoma within the remnant 15 years or more after surgery. The first estimates of the prevalence of this complication were about 5%, but subsequent evidence indicates that the risk may be much lower. Postgastrectomy adenocarcinoma usually occurs in the gastric mucosa at the anastomosis. The pathogenesis is thought to be related to the chronic gastritis that invariably develops and is most severe at the anastomosis.

B. Diagnosis. In view of the evidence that the risk of adenocarcinoma arising in the gastric remnant may be considerably less than originally estimated, routine surveillance endoscopy in asymptomatic patients does not appear to be cost effective and thus is not recommended. However, the physician should be attentive to changes in symptoms or clinical status in postgastrectomy patients that may indicate the development of neoplasia. These include the development of new or different abdominal symptoms, anorexia, vomiting, weight loss, and gross or occult gastrointestinal bleeding. The appropriate diagnostic study is endoscopy with biopsy of the anastomosis.

C. The treatment of gastric cancer is discussed in Chapter 27, section I.C.

Selected Readings

Dulucq JL, et. al. A completely laparoscopic total and partial gastrectomy for benign and malignant diseases: a single institute's prospective analysis. *J Am Coll Surg.* 2005; 200:191–197.

Madura JA. Postgastrectomy problems: remedial operations and therapy. In: Camperon JL, ed. Current surgical therapy. St. Louis:Mosby;2001:89–94.

Tersmette AC, et al. Long-term prognosis after partial gastrectomy for benign conditions: survival and smoking-related death of 2633 Amsterdam postgastrectomy patients followed up since surgery between 1931 and 1960. *Gastroenterology.* 1991;101:148.

29   DIARRHEA

$\mathcal{D}$iarrhea can be defined as an increase in the fluidity, frequency, and volume of daily stool output. The daily stool weight is usually increased over the normal average of 200 g due to an increase in the stool water above the normal content of 60% to 75%. There may also be a change in the stool solids.

I. NORMAL INTESTINAL FLUID BALANCE. During fasting, the intestine contains very little fluid. On a normal diet of three meals a day, about 9 L of fluid is delivered to the small intestine. Oral intake accounts for 2,000 mL, and the remainder is secreted from various parts of the gastrointestinal tract into the lumen (Table 29-1). Of this, 90% is absorbed in the small intestine. One to two liters is presented to the colon, and approximately 90% is absorbed. The colon has the capacity to absorb all of the fluid presented to it, but the presence of unabsorbed osmotically active solutes from the diet (e.g., some carbohydrates) and from bacterial action prevents complete fluid absorption and desiccation of the fecal material. This results in 100 to 200 mL of fluid in the stool. Thus, approximately 98% of the fluid presented to the intestine each day is absorbed by the small and large intestines.

Feces on the average contain 100 mL of water, 40 mEq/L of sodium (Na^+), 90 mEq/L of potassium (K^+), 16 mEq/L of chloride (Cl^-), and 30 mEq/L of bicarbonate (HCO_3^-). The remaining anions are organic and result from bacterial fermentation of unabsorbed carbohydrates. The gastrointestinal tract does not have diluting mechanisms; thus, osmolality of the fecal fluid is never less than the osmolality of plasma. In fact, osmolality of fecal fluid is usually greater than that of plasma due to continuing bacterial fermentation of unabsorbed carbohydrates into osmotically active particles after defecation.

Water transport across the intestinal epithelium is passive. It is secondary to osmotic gradients generated by active transport of electrolytes such as Na^+ and Cl^- or other solutes, such as sugars and amino acids. Intestinal ion absorption occurs mainly across epithelial cells that reside at the tips of the villi. Crypt cells are involved in ion secretion: Na^+ is the major ion actively absorbed, and Cl^- is the major ion secreted.

Na^+ is actively absorbed throughout the intestinal tract empowered by the Na^+ pump in the form of Na^+-K^-–ATPase located in the basolateral plasma membrane of intestinal epithelial cells. Thus water is absorbed along with Na^+.

TABLE 29-1	Normal Daily Intestinal Water Input

Source	Volume (mL)
Oral	2,000
Secretions	
Salivary	1,500
Gastric	2,500
Pancreatic	1,500
Biliary	500
Small intestinal	1,000
Total	9,000

Active intraluminal secretion in the intestine is accomplished by active secretion of Cl^-. This process is also powered by Na^+-K^--ATPase located in basolateral membranes of the crypt cells. Cl^- secretion is also followed by water secretion into the intestinal lumen.

Any process that either impairs absorption of Na^+ and water or causes Cl^- and water to be secreted into the intestinal lumen can result in diarrhea.

II. PATHOPHYSIOLOGY OF DIARRHEA. There are four major mechanisms of diarrhea.

A. Osmotic diarrhea, in which there is increased amounts of poorly absorbable, osmotically active solutes in the gut lumen.

B. Secretory diarrhea, in which there is, increased Cl^- and water secretion with or without inhibition of normal active Na^+ and water absorption.

C. Exudation of mucus, blood, and protein from sites of active inflammation into the bowel lumen.

D. Abnormal intestinal motility, with increased or decreased contact between luminal contents and mucosal surface.

III. OSMOTIC DIARRHEA

A. Causes. Osmotic diarrhea is caused by ingestion of a poorly absorbable solute, usually a carbohydrate or a divalent ion (e.g., magnesium [Mg^{2+}] or sulfate [SO_4^{2-}]) (Table 29-2). The higher osmolality of the luminal contents causes water influx into the intestinal lumen across the duodenal and jejunal epithelium to dilute the solute, in an attempt to make the chyme isotonic. Due to the leakiness of this epithelium, Na^+ follows the influx of water from the plasma to the gut lumen due to the difference in the Na^+ concentration gradient. This Na^+ influx causes further influx of water even after the osmolality of the luminal contents and plasma is identical. In contrast, the epithelium of the ileum and colon has a low permeability to Na^+ and to the solute. It also has an efficient active ion transport mechanism that allows it to reabsorb Na^+ and water even against a steep electrochemical gradient. Thus, water is absorbed as it traverses the ileum and colon, and the severity of the osmotic diarrhea is reduced. This has been called "colon salvage." Since the fluid volume entering the colon still exceeds the ability of the colon to absorb, diarrhea results.

In lactase deficiency, lactose from the diet cannot be absorbed in the small intestine, remains in the lumen, and reaches the colon, where it is broken down by the endogenous bacteria into additional osmotically active solute particles, which increase the osmotic load and cause diarrhea.

B. Clinically, osmotic diarrhea stops when the patient fasts. The stool osmolality ($[Na^+]+[K^+]$) × 2 (to account for anions) is less than the osmolality of the stool fluid measured by freezing point depression. This osmotic anion gap accounts for the presence of the poorly absorbable solutes in fecal fluid. Anion gaps greater

---

TABLE 29-2 **Causes of Osmotic Diarrhea**

I. Carbohydrate malabsorption
   A. Disaccharidase deficiency in the small-intestinal mucosa
      1. Primary (e.g., idiopathic lactase, sucrase–maltase deficiency)
      2. Secondary (e.g., after infectious gastroenteritis and with mucosal inflammation)
   B. Ingestion of mannitol, sorbitol (diet candy, soda, chewing gum)
   C. Lactulose therapy
II. General malabsorption
   A. Sprue (idiopathic gluten enteropathy, tropical)
   B. Postradiation, postischemic enteritis
III. Ingestion of sodium sulfate (Glauber's salt), sodium phosphate, magnesium sulfate (Epsom salts), milk of magnesia, magnesium-containing antacids

than 50 are considered clinically significant. Determination of the stool pH may be helpful in the diagnosis of osmotic diarrhea. Carbohydrates in stool yield an acid pH; milk of magnesia, an alkaline pH; and poorly absorbable salts containing Mg^{2+} or SO_4^{2-}, a neutral pH.

IV. SECRETORY DIARRHEA

A. CAUSES. Diarrhea of 1 L or more per day results from secretion of fluid across the intestinal mucosa. In most cases, a pathophysiologic event causes small intestinal secretion by simultaneously stimulating active secretion and partial inhibition of intestinal absorption. Often, the intestinal mucosa is intact and has normal histologic findings. Some causes of secretory diarrhea are listed in Table 29-3.

B. Clinically, there are five features that characterize secretory diarrhea.

1. Stool volume is usually large (>1 L per day).

2. Stools are watery in consistency.

3. Stools do not contain pus or blood.

4. Diarrhea typically continues while the patient fasts for 24 to 48 hours. However, secretory diarrhea from fatty acid malabsorption or from laxative abuse will stop when these agents are not ingested.

5. The osmolality of the stool is close to the osmolality of plasma, and there is no anion gap.

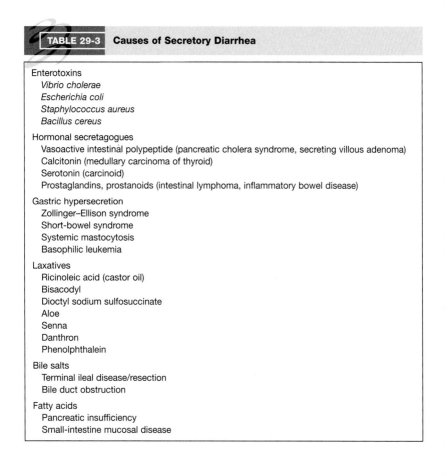

TABLE 29-3 **Causes of Secretory Diarrhea**

Enterotoxins
  Vibrio cholerae
  Escherichia coli
  Staphylococcus aureus
  Bacillus cereus
Hormonal secretagogues
  Vasoactive intestinal polypeptide (pancreatic cholera syndrome, secreting villous adenoma)
  Calcitonin (medullary carcinoma of thyroid)
  Serotonin (carcinoid)
  Prostaglandins, prostanoids (intestinal lymphoma, inflammatory bowel disease)
Gastric hypersecretion
  Zollinger–Ellison syndrome
  Short-bowel syndrome
  Systemic mastocytosis
  Basophilic leukemia
Laxatives
  Ricinoleic acid (castor oil)
  Bisacodyl
  Dioctyl sodium sulfosuccinate
  Aloe
  Senna
  Danthron
  Phenolphthalein
Bile salts
  Terminal ileal disease/resection
  Bile duct obstruction
Fatty acids
  Pancreatic insufficiency
  Small-intestine mucosal disease

V. EXUDATIVE DIARRHEA. If the intestinal mucosa is inflamed and ulcerated, mucus, blood, and pus leak into the lumen and are discharged as stool. This may also create an increased osmotic load. If a large surface area of the bowel lumen is involved, absorption of ions, solutes, and water will also be impaired, and patients may have large-volume diarrhea. Inflammation may generate prostaglandins, which stimulate secretion and may increase bowel motility, thus compounding the diarrhea. The severity of the diarrhea and the systemic signs and symptoms depends on the extent of bowel involvement.

Inflammatory states may be

A. Idiopathic (e.g., Crohn's disease, ulcerative colitis)
B. Infectious (e.g., from invasive organisms or cytotoxins: *Shigella, Salmonella, Campylobacter, Yersinia, tuberculosis, amebae*, and *Clostridium difficile*)
C. Ischemic
D. Vasculitic
E. Due to radiation injury
F. Caused by abscess formation (e.g., diverticulitis, infected carcinoma)

VI. MOTILITY DISTURBANCES. Both reduced and increased motility of the intestine may result in diarrhea.

A. **Increased motility of the small intestine** results in decreased contact time of chyme with absorptive surfaces. Large amounts of fluid delivered to the colon may overwhelm its absorptive capacity and result in diarrhea. The reduced contact time in the small intestine may interfere with absorption of fatty acids and bile salts, allowing them to reach the colon where they induce a secretory diarrhea. Diarrhea associated with hyperthyroidism, carcinoid, and postgastrectomy dumping syndrome are examples.

B. **Decreased motility of the small intestine** may allow colonization of the small intestine with colonic-type bacteria. The digestion and absorption of fats, carbohydrates, and bile salts may be affected, resulting in osmotic or secretory diarrhea. This mechanism is involved in the diarrhea seen with diabetes, hypothyroidism, scleroderma, amyloidosis, and postvagotomy states.

C. **Increased colonic motility** with premature emptying of colonic contents is the major cause of diarrhea in the irritable bowel syndrome.

D. **Anal sphincter dysfunction** caused by neuromuscular disease, inflammation, scarring, and postsurgical states may result in fecal incontinence, which may be interpreted by the patient as diarrhea.

VII. CLINICAL APPROACH. It is helpful to classify diarrhea into clinical categories, taking into consideration the duration, setting, and sexual preference of the patient. Diarrhea of abrupt onset of less than 2 to 3 weeks' duration is called **acute diarrhea.** If the diarrheal illness lasts longer than 3 weeks, it is called **chronic diarrhea.** The causes of acute and chronic diarrhea are listed in Tables 29-4 and 29-5. If diarrhea occurs in the setting of antibiotic therapy or after a course of antibiotics, antibiotic-associated diarrhea and pseudomembranous colitis due to *C. difficile* cytotoxin should be considered.

A. **Acute diarrhea.** The most common cause of acute diarrhea is infection.

1. **Food poisoning** is produced by a preformed bacterial toxin that contaminates the food. Bacterial replication in the host is not necessary for the development of disease. The resultant illness usually has an acute onset and short duration and occurs in small, well-defined epidemics, without evidence of secondary spread.

2. Diarrhea resulting from **multiplication of organisms in the intestine** may be divided into **inflammatory–invasive versus noninflammatory–noninvasive** categories, as seen in Table 29-4. Most of these types of diarrhea result from ingestion of contaminated food or water after 1 to 2 days of incubation. Animal reservoirs may exist for some common pathogens, including *Salmonella, Campylobacter, Yersinia, Giardia, Cryptosporidium,* and *Vibrio parahaemolyticus.* Waterborne disease in which the pathogens are spread from animals or water to humans is

TABLE 29-4	Causes of Acute Diarrhea

Causes	Characteristics	Organisms
Viral Infections		
Small intestine	Mucosal invasion absent	Rotavirus (children, adults)
	Noninflammatory	
	Watery diarrhea	Norwalk virus
	Fecal leukocyte absent	Enteric adenovirus
Bacterial infections		
Small intestine	Mucosal invasion absent	*Vibrio cholerae*
	Noninflammatory	Toxigenic *Escherichia coli*
	Watery diarrhea	
	Fecal leukocytes absent	
Colon	Mucosal invasion present	*Salmonella*
	Inflammatory	*Shigella*
	Bloody diarrhea	*Campylobacter*
	Fecal leukocytes present	*Yersinia enterocolitica*
		Invasive *E. coli*
		E. coli O157:H7
		Staphylococcus aureu (toxin)
		Vibrio parahaemolyticus (toxin)
		Clostridium difficile (toxin)
Parasitic infections		
Small intestine	Mucosal invasion absent	*Giardia lamblia*
	Noninflammatory	*Cryptosporidium*
	Watery diarrhea	
	Fecal leukocytes absent	
Colon	Mucosal invasion present	*Entamoeba histolytica*
	Inflammatory	
	Bloody diarrhea	
	Fecal leukocytes present	
Food poisoning		
Small intestine	Toxin induced	*Staphylococcus aureus*
	Mucosal invasion absent	*Bacillus cereus*
	Noninflammatory	*Clostridium perfringens*
	Watery diarrhea	*Clostridium botulinum*
Drugs		
Laxatives		
Sorbitol		
Antacids (Mg^{2+}, Ca^{2+} salts)		
Lactulose		
Colchicine		
Quinidine		
Diuretics		
Digitalis		
Propranolol		
Theophylline		
Aspirin		
Nonsteroidal antiinflammatory drugs		
Chemotherapeutic agents		
Antibiotics		

(continued)

TABLE 29-4   Causes of Acute Diarrhea *(Continued)*

Heavy metals (Hg, Pb)
Cholinergic agents

Miscellaneous
Fecal impaction
Diverticulitis
Ischemic bowel disease

TABLE 29-5   Causes of Chronic Diarrhea

Type	Agent
Infection	*Giardia lamblia*
	Entamoeba histolytica
	Tubercle bacillus
	Clostridium difficile
Inflammation	Ulcerative colitis
	Microscopic colitis
	Collagenous colitis
	Crohn's disease
	Ischemic colitis/enteritis
	Solitary rectal ulcer
	Diverticulitis/abscess
Drugs	Laxatives
	Antibiotics
	Antacids
	Diuretics
	Alcohol
	Theophyllines
	Nonsteroidal antiinflammatory drugs
Malabsorption	Small-bowel mucosal disease
	Disaccharidase deficiency
	Pancreatic insufficiency
	Ischemic/radiation enteritis
	Short-bowel syndrome
	Bacterial overgrowth
Endocrine	Zollinger–Ellison syndrome
	Hyperthyroidism
	Carcinoid
	Non-β-cell pancreatic tumor
	Villous adenoma
Motility disorders	Irritable bowel syndrome
	Postvagotomy syndrome
	Postgastric surgery dumping syndrome
	Tumor/fecal impaction overflow diarrhea
	Narcotic bowel

caused by *Salmonella, Campylobacter, Shigella,* Norwalk virus, *Giardia, Vibrio cholerae,* toxigenic *Escherichia coli,* and *E. coli:* H7.

3. Diarrhea developing in individuals during or just after traveling is commonly infectious. The most likely organisms are enterotoxigenic *E. coli, Salmonella, Giardia,* and amebae.

4. **Homosexual individuals** are at a higher risk of exposure to infectious agents. In this setting, it is important to consider amebiasis, giardiasis, shigellosis, rectal syphilis, rectal gonorrhea, and lymphogranuloma venereum caused by *Chlamydia trachomatis* and herpes simplex infections of the rectum and perianal area. In patients with acquired immunodeficiency syndrome (AIDS), infectious agents could include cytomegalovirus, *Cryptosporidium,* and *Candida* as well as all of the organisms noted in homosexual persons and immunocompetent individuals. (See Chapters 42 and 43.)

B. **Chronic and recurrent diarrhea.** Any diarrheal illness lasting longer than 3 weeks should be clinically investigated.

1. **Infections.** Most viral and bacterial diarrheas are self-limiting and abate within 3 weeks. Diarrhea from *Campylobacter* and *Yersinia* may last a few months but rarely becomes chronic. Bowel infections with tuberculosis, amebae, and *Giardia* may become chronic.

2. **Inflammatory bowel disease.** Ulcerative colitis and **Crohn's disease** may result in diarrhea of varying severity, depending on the extent and degree of bowel involvement. Diarrhea in Crohn's disease of the small bowel may be compounded by concomitant bile salt and fat malabsorption.

3. **Malabsorption syndromes**

   a. **Diseases of the small intestine** may cause chronic diarrhea of varying severity. The mechanism of the diarrhea is usually multifactorial and complex. These diseases include:

      i. Sprue (nontropical, tropical)
      ii. Amyloidosis
      iii. Whipple's disease
      iv. Lymphoma
      v. Carcinoid
      vi. Radiation enteritis
      vii. Lymphangiectasia
      viii. Bowel resection/bypass

   b. **Pancreatic insufficiency** from chronic pancreatitis and cystic fibrosis may cause severe fat malabsorption, resulting in chronic diarrhea.

   c. **Zollinger-Ellison syndrome** resulting from a gastrin-secreting tumor causes increased gastric acid output that overwhelms the absorptive capacity of the proximal small intestine, neutralizes the bicarbonate, and inactivates the pancreatic enzymes secreted into the duodenum. The resulting diarrhea is complicated by malabsorption and bile salt—and fatty acid—stimulated colonic secretion.

   d. **Postgastrectomy, enterostomy** states may result in diarrhea due to decreased mucosal–chyme exposure as well as poor mixing of digestive juices with luminal contents, resulting in malabsorption.

   e. **Bacterial overgrowth** of the small intestine may occur in patients with diabetes mellitus, scleroderma, amyloidosis, blind loop syndrome, and large and multiple diverticula of the small bowel. Bacterial degradation of carbohydrates, fatty acids, and bile salts results in diarrhea.

   f. **Disaccharidase deficiency.** Lactase is deficient to a variable degree in many adult populations, especially in blacks, Asians, southern Europeans, and those of Jewish descent. Even small amounts of dairy products may cause intermittent diarrhea in these individuals.

4. **Endocrine disorders**

   a. Hyperthyroidism
   b. Diabetes mellitus
   c. Adrenal insufficiency

d. Carcinoid

e. Medullary thyroid cancer

f. Hormone-secreting pancreatic tumors

g. Tumors secreting vasoactive intestinal polypeptide

h. Gastrinoma

5. Neoplasms. Villous adenoma, colon cancer with obstruction, and fecal impaction may present with diarrhea.

6. Drugs and laxatives. Surreptitious use of laxatives and drugs, including those listed in Table 29-4, should always be considered in the evaluation of chronic diarrhea.

7. Irritable bowel syndrome is very common and may present with only chronic intermittent diarrhea, constipation, or a combination of both. Most patients also complain of abdominal cramps, gas, belching, and mucous stools.

8. Incontinence of stool. Anal sphincter dysfunction due to the presence of fissures, fistulas, perianal inflammation, tears from childbirth, anal intercourse or other trauma, diabetic neuropathy, or neuromuscular disease may result in frequent stools, which may be interpreted by the patient as diarrhea.

VIII. DIAGNOSIS

A. History. The physician should find out from the patient an accurate description of the nature of the diarrhea: the duration, frequency, consistency, volume, color, and relation to meals. Also, it is important to determine the presence of any underlying illnesses or systemic symptoms and to establish the patient's recent travel history, use of medications or drugs, and sexual preferences.

1. The history can help determine whether the pathology is in the **small or large bowel.** If the stools are large, watery, soupy, or greasy, possibly containing undigested food particles, the disorder is most likely in the small intestine. There may be accompanying periumbilical or right lower quadrant pain or intermittent, crampy abdominal pain.

2. If the disease is in the **descending colon or rectum,** the patient usually passes small quantities of stool or mucus frequently. The stools are usually mushy and brown, and sometimes mixed with mucus and blood. There may be a sense of urgency and tenesmus. If there is pain, it is usually achy and located in the lower abdomen, pelvis, or sacral region. The passage of stool or gas may provide temporary relief of the pain.

3. Blood in the stool suggests inflammatory, vascular, infectious, or neoplastic disease. The presence of fecal leukocytes indicates mucosal inflammation.

4. Diarrhea that stops with fasting suggests osmotic diarrhea, except that secretory diarrhea due to fatty acids and bile salt malabsorption may also stop with fasting. Large-volume diarrhea that continues during fasting is most likely secretory. Persistence of diarrhea at night suggests the presence of an organic cause rather than irritable bowel syndrome. Fecal incontinence may be due to anal disease or sphincter dysfunction.

5. Diet. The correlation of patients' symptoms with ingestion of milk, other dairy products, or sorbitol-containing artificially sweetened diet drinks, candy, and chewing gum should also be noted.

B. Physical examination of the patient should focus on the general condition of the patient, degree of hydration, presence of fever, and other systemic origins of toxicity. A variety of physical findings can be sought in a patient with chronic diarrhea and may give clues to the etiology of the diarrheal process. These include goiter, skin rash, arthritis, peripheral neuropathy, postural hypotension, abdominal bruit, perianal abscess, fistula, and rectal mass or impaction.

C. Diagnostic tests. The initial laboratory evaluation of the patient should include a complete blood count with differential, serum electrolytes, blood urea nitrogen, and creatinine. A chemistry profile and urinalysis may also help to assess the systemic involvement with the diarrheal state.

1. Examination of the stool is the most important diagnostic test in the evaluation of a patient with acute or chronic diarrhea. A fresh sample of stool should be examined for the presence of pus (white cells), blood, and bacterial and parasitic organisms. Best yield is obtained if the examination is repeated on three fresh stool samples obtained on three separate days.

   a. Presence of white blood cells. Wright or methylene blue stain of the stool smeared on a glass slide will demonstrate the white cells if they are present. The presence of fecal leukocytes suggests intestinal inflammation as a result of a mucosal invasion with bacteria, parasite, or toxin (Table 29-4). Inflammatory bowel disease and ischemic colitis may also result in white blood cells in the stool.

   b. The absence of fecal leukocytes suggests a noninflammatory noninvasive process (e.g., viral infection, giardiasis, drug-related); however, it is never diagnostic because a false-negative result may occur in inflammatory states.

   c. Occult or gross blood in the stool suggests the presence of a colonic neoplasm, an acute ischemic process, radiation enteritis, amebiasis, or severe mucosal inflammation.

   d. Bacterial and parasitic organisms. Fresh stool samples must be examined for the presence of ova and parasites. Organisms that colonize the upper small intestine (Table 29-4) may not be found in stool samples and duodenal or jejunal aspirates or biopsies or the string test may be required. Stool cultures will help determine the bacterial pathogen in most cases. However, special techniques may sometimes be necessary, such as for *Yersinia, Campylobacter, Neisseria gonorrhoeae, C. difficile,* and *E. coli:* H7.

   e. Fat and phenolphthalein. In the evaluation of chronic or recurrent diarrhea, stool should also be examined for the presence of fat (qualitative and quantitative) and phenolphthalein. Phenolphthalein is found in many laxative preparations and gives a red color when alkali is added to the stool filtrate.

2. **Sigmoidoscopy or colonoscopy** or both should be performed without cleansing enemas. Stool samples may be obtained with a suction catheter for microscopic examination and cultures. Most patients with acute or traveler's diarrhea do not need proctosigmoidoscopic examination. Sigmoidoscopy is especially helpful in the evaluation of:

   a. Bloody diarrhea

   b. Diarrhea of uncertain etiology

   c. Inflammatory bowel disease, pseudomembranous colitis, pancreatic disease, or laxative abuse (*melanosis coli*)

3. **Radiologic studies.** Most causes of diarrhea become apparent after the preceding tests. However, in chronic or recurrent diarrhea, barium studies of the large and small intestine may demonstrate the location and extent of the disease. It should be remembered that once barium is introduced into the bowel, examination of the stool for ova and parasites and cultures may be fruitless for several weeks because barium alters the gut ecology.

4. **Other tests.** In cases of chronic diarrhea, other specialized tests may be necessary to assess for malabsorption, bacterial overgrowth, or abnormal hormonal states. These are discussed in appropriate chapters.

IX. TREATMENT. Acute diarrhea with fluid and electrolyte depletion is a major cause of mortality, especially in children in developing countries of the world. Fluid repletion by intravenous or oral routes can prevent death. Oral rehydration therapy can be accomplished with a simply prepared oral rehydration solution. Physiologically, water absorption follows the absorption of glucose-coupled sodium transport in the small intestine, which remains intact even in the severest of diarrheal illnesses.

   Oral rehydration solution can be prepared by adding 3.5 g of sodium chloride (or three fourths of a teaspoon or 3.5 g of table salt), 2.5 g of sodium bicarbonate (or 2.9 g of sodium citrate or 1 teaspoon of baking soda), 1.5 g of potassium chloride (or 1 cup of orange juice or 2 bananas), and 20 g of glucose (or 40 g of sucrose or 4 tablespoons of sugar) to a liter (1.05 qt) of clean water. This makes a solution of approximately 90 mmol of sodium, 20 mmol of potassium, 80 mmol of chloride, 30 mmol of bicarbonate, and 111 mmol of glucose per liter. Not only is this solution lifesaving in severe diarrhea, but also it is less painful, safer, less costly, and superior to intravenous fluids because the patient's thirst protects against overhydration. It should therefore be the preferred route of rehydration in conscious adult and pediatric patients in tertiary and intensive care units. Furthermore, the output of stool can be reduced with food-based oral rehydration therapy. With the additional sodium-coupled absorption of neutral amino acids and glutamine (a key mucosal nutrient in the small bowel, analogous to short-chain fatty acids in the colon), oral rehydration therapy can also be used to speed recovery from small-bowel injury.

The composition of **cereal-based oral rehydration solution** is like that of standard oral rehydration solution (3.5 g of sodium chloride, 2.5 g of sodium bicarbonate, and 1.5 g of potassium chloride), except that the 20 g of glucose is replaced by 50 to 60 g of cereal flour (rice, maize, millet, wheat, or sorghum) or 200 g of mashed, boiled potato; stirred into 1.1 L of water; and brought to a boil. Not only can oral rehydration therapy (especially with cereal and continued feeding) reverse the loss of fluid, but also it can prevent the fatal hypoglycemia seen with failure of gluconeogenesis, a major cause of death in children with diarrhea in developing areas. Furthermore, simple oral rehydration therapy can be started early in the home and can prevent most complications of dehydration and malnutrition.

Attention should also be directed at reduction of the patient's symptoms and discomfort to reduce absenteeism from work or school as well as to improve the sense of well-being of the patient. Available drugs can be divided into groups based on their mechanisms of action: absorbents, antisecretory agents, opiate derivatives, anticholinergic agents, and antimicrobial agents.

A. Absorbents (e.g., Kaopectate, aluminum hydroxide) do not influence the course of the disease but help produce solid stools. This effect may allow the patient to alter the timing of stooling and permit a more voluntary control of defecation.

B. Antisecretory agents. In most cases of diarrhea, regardless of etiology, invasive or noninvasive, intestinal secretion contributes greatly to the stool volume. Antisecretory drugs, including prostaglandin synthesis inhibitors, have been used to diminish bowel secretion.

Bismuth subsalicylate (Pepto-Bismol) has been shown to block the secretory effects of *V. cholerae*, enterotoxigenic *E. coli*, and *Shigella* as well as to prevent intestinal infection by these agents if given prophylactically. The usual therapeutic dosage of Pepto-Bismol is 30 mL every 30 minutes for eight doses. The prophylactic dosage is 60 mL or two tablets q.i.d. for the duration of the prophylaxis (e.g., for travelers). Pepto-Bismol tablets are as effective as the liquid preparation.

C. Opiate derivatives are widely used in both acute and chronic diarrhea. By diminishing peristalsis, they delay gut transit of fluid and allow more time for fluid absorption. They may be used in patients with moderate symptoms (3–5 stools per day) but should not be used in patients with fever, systemic toxicity, or bloody diarrhea. Their use should be discontinued in patients who have not shown improvement or whose condition has worsened on therapy.

Opiate derivatives include paregoric (tincture of opium), diphenoxylate with atropine (Lomotil), and loperamide (Imodium). Imodium has two advantages over Lomotil in that it does not contain atropine and it has fewer central opiate effects.

D. Anticholinergic agents do not appear to be useful in the treatment of most diarrheal disorders. Some patients with irritable bowel syndrome may benefit from use of dicyclomine hydrochloride (Bentyl).

E. Antimicrobial agents. When the diarrhea is severe and the patient has systemic signs of toxicity, stool cultures should be performed to identify the pathogenic organism. The most effective antimicrobial agent for the particular pathogen should be used. In selected cases of severe diarrhea, if a laboratory is not available, empiric antibiotics with activity against both *Shigella* and *Campylobacter* strains may be administered (e.g., ciprofloxacin or trimethoprim/sulfamethoxazole or erythromycin). Recently, rifaximin (Xifaxan), a nonabsorbable (gut specific) antibiotic has become available for the treatment of traveler's diarrhea. Table 29-6 lists common pathogens and recommended therapeutic agents. Table 29-7 summarizes an approach to therapy of acute diarrhea.

TABLE 29-6	Antimicrobial Therapy of Infectious Diarrhea

Pathogen	Clinical disease	Therapy
Shigella	Dysentery	Trimethoprim/sulfamethoxazole 160/800 mg p.o. b.i.d. for 5 d **or** tetracycline 500 mg p.o. q.i.d. for 5 d **or** ciprofloxacin 500 mg p.o. b.i.d. for 5 d
Salmonella	Enteric	No antimicrobial therapy
	Bacteremia	Ampicillin **or** amoxicillin 1 g p.o. t.i.d. **or** q.i.d. for 14 d **or** chloramphenicol 1 g p.o. **or** IV q8h for 14 d **or** trimethoprim/sulfamethoxazole 160/800 mg p.o. b.i.d. for 10 d **or** a third-generation cephalosporin **or** ciprofloxacin 500 mg p.o. b.i.d. for 5 d
Campylobacter	Dysentery	Erythromycin 250 mg p.o. q.i.d. for 5–10 d **or** ciprofloxacin 500 mg p.o. b.i.d. for 5–7 d
Clostridium difficile	Watery diarrhea; pseudomembranous colitis	Cholestyramine 4 g p.o. t.i.d. for 7 d **or** metronidazole 250 mg p.o. t.i.d. for 7 d **or** vancomycin 125–500 mg p.o. q.i.d. for 7 d rifaximin 200 mg p.o. b.i.d. for 3 d
Enterotoxigenic *Escherichia coli,* *E. coli* O157:H7, and traveler's diarrhea	Watery diarrhea; bloody diarrhea	Trimethoprim/sulfamethoxazole 160/800 mg p.o. for 5 d **or** ciprofloxacin 500 mg p.o. b.i.d. for 5 d **or** ofloxacin 300 mg p.o. b.i.d. for 5 d **or** norfloxacin 400 mg p.o. b.i.d. for 5 d **or** rifaximin (Xifaxan) 200 mg p.o. t.i.d. for 3 day
Entamoeba histolytica	Asymptomatic carrier; colitis	Diloxanide furoate 500 mg p.o. t.i.d. for 10 d plus diiodohydroxyquin 650 mg p.o. t.i.d. for 20 d **or** metronidazole 750 mg p.o. t.i.d. for 10 d
Giardia lamblia	Watery diarrhea	Quinacrine hydrochloride 100 mg p.o. t.i.d. for 7 d **or** metronidazole 250 mg p.o. t.i.d. for 7 d **or** furazolidone 100 mg q.i.d. **or** 7 d

p.o., by mouth; b.i.d., twice a day; q.i.d., four times a day; t.i.d., three times a day.

TABLE 29-7	An Approach to Therapy of Acute Diarrhea	

Severity of illness	No. of diarrheal stools/day	Therapy
Mild	1–3	Fluids only
Moderate	3–5	Fluids, nonspecific therapy (e.g., Pepto-Bismol, Lomotil, Imodium)
Severe ($\pm$ fever)	>6	Fluids, antimicrobial agent; if laboratory not available, trimethoprim/sulfamethoxazole, erythromycin, ciprofloxacin, or norfloxacin

Treatment of *E. coli* O157:H7 with a systemically absorbed antimicrobial agent is controversial since there is some inconclusive data that suggests complications with hemolytic uremic syndrome may be higher with antimicrobial therapy. However, in patients with severe diarrhea, antimicrobial therapy (e.g., ciprofloxacin hydrochloride 500 mg twice daily, by mouth) may be used with caution.

F. Chemoprophylaxis of traveler's diarrhea. Bismuth subsalicylate, doxycycline, and trimethoprim/sulfamethoxazole, norfloxacin, and ciprofloxacin hydrochloride have been shown to be effective in preventing most causes of traveler's diarrhea. Doxycycline resistance among enteric bacterial pathogens does occur in some regions. Starting on the first day of travel, the dosage of each drug is as follows: bismuth subsalicylate, 60 mL q.i.d.; doxycycline, 100 mg daily; trimethoprim/sulfamethoxazole, 160/800 mg daily; ciprofloxacin hydrochloride, 500 mg daily; norfloxacin, 400 mg daily. Aztreonam, 100 mg daily, has also been shown to be effective. Each drug should be continued for 1 to 2 days after returning home. No drug should be taken for more than 3 weeks.

Recently, **rifaximin (Xifaxan)**, a nonabsorbable, gut specific antibiotic, has been approved by the FDA for the treatment of traveler's diarrhea at a dose of 200 mg one tablet t.i.d. for 3 days.

The use of antimicrobial chemoprophylaxis should be discouraged for most travelers. Each drug has its side and adverse effects and will confer antimicrobial resistance to the gut flora of the individual. This may present a therapeutic problem if another infection (e.g., a urinary tract infection) develops. Antimicrobial chemoprophylaxis should be restricted to 2 to 5 days in persons who are on a special "business" trip and who accept the risks of side and adverse effects.

Rifaximin (Xifaxan) is an exception to the above statements. This gut-specific, nonabsorbable antibiotic has been shown to be effective in preventing traveler's diarrhea if it is taken daily as prophylaxis during the travel period. It is recommended for persons traveling to areas of the world with high risk of GI infections with *E. coli* and other fecal pathogens, at a dose of 200 mg p.o. t.i.d.

G. Chronic or recurrent diarrhea. The therapy of chronic and recurrent diarrhea should be based on the etiology and pathophysiology of the disease process. Occasionally, when a diagnosis cannot be made, an empiric trial of diet restriction (e.g., lactose, gluten, and long-chain fatty acids), pancreatic enzyme supplements along with histamine-2 (H_2) blockers, cholestyramine, clonidine, and antimicrobial (e.g., metronidazole) therapy may be use. When all fails, the judicious use of antidiarrheal opiate derivatives may result in symptom relief.

Selected Readings

Al Ghamdi MY, et al. Causation: Recurrent collagenous colitis following repeated use of NSAIDs. *Can J Gastroenterol.* 2002;16:861–862.

Alaedini A, et al. Narrative review—celiac disease: Understanding a complex autoimmune disorder. *Ann Intern Med.* 2005;142:289–298.

AUS, et al. *Giardia intestinalis. Curr Opin Infect Dis.* 2003;16:453–460.

Aziz B, et al. 25-year-old man with abdominal pain, nausea and fatigue. *Mayo Clin Proc.* 2007;82(3):359–362.

Bardhan PK, et al. Screening of patients with acute infectious diarrhoea: Evaluation of clinical features, faecal microscopy, and faecal occult blood testing. *Scand J Gastroenterol.* 2000; 35:54–60.

Bengmark S, et al. Prebiotics and synbiotics in clinical medicine. *Nutr Clin Pract.* 2005; 20:244–261.

Butler T, et al. New developments in the understanding of cholera. *Curr Gastroenterol Rep.* 2001;3:315.

Chermesh I, et al. Probiotics and the gastrointestinal tract: Where are we in 2005? *World Gastroenterol.* 2006;12:853–857.

Erim TD, et al. Collagenous colitis associated with *Clostridium difficile*: A cause effect? *Dig Dis Sci.* 2003;48:1374–1375.

Guarner F. Enteric flora in health and disease. *Digestion.* 2006;73(suppl 1):5–12.

Headstrom PD, et al. Chronic diarrhea. *Clin Gastroenterol Hepatol.* 2005;3:734–737.

Jaskiewicz K, et al. Microscopic colitis in routine colonoscopies. *Dig Dis Sci.* 2006; 51:241–244.

Lo W, et al. Changing presentation of adult celiac disease. *Dig Dis Sci.* 2003;4:395–398.

Nyhlin N, Bohr J, Eriksson S, Tysk C. Systematic review: microscopic colitis. *Ailment Pharmacol Ther.* 2006;23:1525–1534.

Quigley EMM, et al. Small intestinal bacterial overgrowth: Roles of antibiotics, prebiotics and probiotics. *Gastroenterology.* 2006;130:S78–S90.

Sanders JW, et al. Diarrhea in the returned traveler. *Curr Gastroenterol Rep.* 2001;3:304.

Saulsbury FT. Clinical update: Henoch-Schonlein purpura. *Lancet.* 2007;669:976–978.

Schiller JR. Chronic diarrhea. *Gastroenterology.* 2004;127:287–293.

Snelling AM. Effects of probiotics on the gastrointestinal tract. *Curr Opin Infect Dis.* 2005;18:420–426.

Thomas, PD, et al. Guidelines for the investigation of chronic diarrhea, 2nd. Edition. *Gut.* 2003;53(supp 1):v1–v15.

Wong CS, et al. The risk of hemolytic uremic syndrome after antibiotic treatment of *Escherichia coli* O157:H7 infections. *N Engl J Med.* 2000;342:1930.

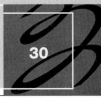
*V*arious microorganisms infect the gastrointestinal tract and cause gastroenteritis. This chapter reviews pathogens that affect immunocompetent patients. A discussion of opportunistic infections in immunocompromised patients is found in Chapter 43.

I. VIRAL GASTROENTERITIS. It is estimated that 30% to 40% of instances of infectious diarrhea in the United States are caused by viruses; these infections far outnumber the documented instances of bacterial and parasitic diarrhea.

Five major categories of viruses that cause gastroenteritis in humans have been identified: **rotavirus, enteric adenovirus, calcii virus, astrovirus,** and **Norwalk** and **Norwalk-like viruses.** The first four viruses cause diarrhea in infants and young children but may also infect adults. Norwalk-group viruses, however, produce epidemics of gastroenteritis in adults and school-age children.

A. Rotavirus

   1. Epidemiology. Human rotavirus is an RNA virus. It has been classified into three genetically and antigenically distinct groups: **A, B,** and **C.** Groups A and C have been associated with diarrheal epidemics around the world, and group B has caused epidemics of diarrheal disease in adults in China. Rotavirus is the most important cause of dehydrating diarrheal illness throughout the world, accounting for 40% to 70% of all episodes requiring hospitalization of children under the age of 2. In industrially developing countries, rotavirus causes approximately 125 million cases of diarrhea annually, 18 million of the cases severe, with an estimated death rate of 800,000 to 900,000 per year. Severe rotavirus infection is seen most frequently in children 3 to 15 months of age. After age 3, the infections are usually asymptomatic. The illness is rare in adults except among those in close contact with infected children, in travelers, and in geriatric populations; it is also found in epidemic form after exposure to contaminated water. The virus is shed in great numbers in feces and is transmitted by the fecal–oral route. In North America and northern Europe, the infection occurs seasonally, especially in the winter months. In countries within 10 degrees of the equator, the infection occurs year-round.

   2. Pathology and pathophysiology. Rotavirus infection spreads from the proximal small intestine to the ileum over 1 to 2 days. The virus infects the mature enterocytes at the tips of intestinal villi and causes cell lysis resulting in shortening of villi, hyperplasia of crypts, and round-celled lamina propria. It is associated with decreased microvillous enzyme activity (e.g., sucrose, lactose), net intestinal secretion, and increased gut mucosal permeability.

   3. Clinical disease and complications. Rotavirus infection is frequently asymptomatic. In symptomatic infection, the incubation period is 1 to 3 days, and the illness lasts 5 to 7 days. The gastroenteritis is characterized by frequent vomiting, fever, watery diarrhea, and dehydration. Necrotizing enterocolitis, Henoch-Schönlein purpura, and hemolytic-uremic syndrome have been associated with rotavirus infections.

   4. Diagnosis. Fecal leukocytes may be present in 20% of patients. Viral antigens may be demonstrated from stool specimens by a variety of assays such as the **Rotazyme test.** The virus can also be visualized with electromicroscopy.

   5. Treatment and prevention. Treatment of rotavirus infection is symptomatic and supportive. Fluid and electrolyte replacement is essential. Oral rehydration solutions (e.g., Rehydralylate, Pedialyte, and Rosol) are highly effective, even in the presence of vomiting. Breastfeeding and transplacentally transmitted maternal antibodies have been found to prevent rotavirus infections. Progress is being made toward the development of a vaccine.

B. Enteric adenovirus

1. **Epidemiology.** Adenovirus serotypes 40 and 41 are enteric adenoviruses that cause gastroenteritis without nasopharyngitis and keratoconjunctivitis. Infection is transmitted from person to person. Enteric adenovirus is second to rotavirus as the cause of pediatric viral gastroenteritis, especially in children under the age of 2. Nosocomial outbreaks occur, but spread to adults is uncommon.

2. **Clinical disease.** Endemic enteric adenovirus gastroenteritis may occur year-round without seasonal preference. The incubation period is 8 to 10 days. The onset is with low-grade fever and watery diarrhea, followed by 1 to 2 days of vomiting. Illness typically lasts 1 to 2 weeks but occasionally lasts longer.

3. **Diagnosis.** There are no fecal leukocytes in stool. Diagnosis may require demonstration of the virus by electron-microscopy in stool samples, use of nucleic acid hybridization, and radioimmunoassays using monoclonal antibodies specific for adenovirus 40 and 41.

4. **Treatment** is supportive and symptomatic.

C. Norwalk virus and Norwalk-like viruses

1. **Epidemiology.** Norwalk virus is the prototype of the Norwalk-like group of viruses that, unlike rotavirus and enteric adenoviruses, are small and round and resemble the other small gastroenteritis viruses (e.g., calcii viruses, astroviruses, and small featureless viruses). These viruses are refractory to in vitro cultivation and purification. Norwalk virus possesses a single-stranded RNA, which has been detected in diarrheal stools by immune electromicroscopy. The Norwalk virus family causes approximately 40% of epidemics of gastroenteritis that occurs in recreational camps; on cruise ships; in schools, colleges, nursing homes, hospital wards, cafeterias, and community centers; and among sports teams and families by the ingestion of contaminated foods such as salad and cake frosting. Epidemics occur year-round, affecting older children and adults but not infants and young children. Infection spreads rapidly by the fecal–oral route, with an incubation period of 12 to 48 hours. In food-borne outbreaks, infectious virus may be excreted in the feces for at least 48 hours after the patients have recovered. Airborne transmission by means of droplets of vomit or through the movement of contaminated laundry also occurs.

2. **Histopathology.** The infection affects the small intestine, sparing the stomach and the colonic mucosa. There is blunting of villi and microvilli and cellular infiltration in the lamina propria, especially in the jejunum. Malabsorption of d-xylose, lactose, and fat occurs, but absorption returns to normal within 1 to 2 weeks after recovery. It is thought that gastric emptying is delayed, which would explain the nausea and vomiting that accompanies the watery diarrhea.

3. **Clinical disease.** The onset is rapid with abdominal pain, low-grade fever, vomiting, and diarrhea that usually last 48 to 72 hours.

4. **Diagnosis.** There are no fecal leukocytes. Specific diagnostic techniques are restricted to a few research laboratories that use both a radioimmunoassay (RIA) and an enzyme-linked immunosorbent assay (ELISA); the tests may be used to measure Norwalk viral antigens in stool and antibody in serum.

5. **Treatment** is supportive.

D. Calcii virus

1. **Epidemiology.** Human calcii viruses are poorly understood agents that are related to the Norwalk virus group. They affect mostly infants and young children but may also infect adults in epidemics.

2. **Clinical disease.** The incubation period is 1 to 3 days. The clinical presentation resembles that of rotavirus or Norwalk viral gastroenteritis. The diarrhea is accompanied by vomiting, abdominal pain, and low-grade fever.

3. **Diagnosis.** Calcii virus can be detected in stool by electron-microscopy and by RIA from serum. Serum antibody may be protective against reinfection.

4. **Treatment.** The treatment is supportive.

E. Astrovirus
   1. **Epidemiology.** The virus can be cultivated in cell cultures. Astrovirus is a single-stranded RNA virus with five human serotypes. It causes outbreaks of diarrhea in children 1 to 7 years of age; in the elderly, especially in nursing homes; and rarely in young adults, suggesting that adults may be protected by previously acquired antibodies.
   2. **Clinical disease.** The incubation period is 1 to 2 days. Watery diarrhea may be accompanied by vomiting.
   3. **The diagnosis** is by stool electron-microscopy and ELISA.
   4. **Treatment** is supportive.
F. Other viruses associated with gastroenteritis. Several other groups of viruses known to cause diarrhea in animals are associated with gastroenteritis in humans, but their causative relation to disease is unclear. **Coronaviruses** are detected by electron-microscopy in stools of persons living under poor sanitary conditions. It has been associated with outbreaks in nurseries and with necrotizing enterocolitis in newborns. **Echoviruses** and picornaviruses also have been implicated in diarrheal disease of the young. **Enteroviruses** have been shown in controlled epidemiologic studies not to be important causes of acute gastroenteritis.

II. BACTERIAL INFECTIONS OF THE BOWEL. Bacterial gastroenteritis may result from the ingestion of a preformed bacterial toxin present in the food at the time of ingestion, by the production of a toxin or toxins in vivo, or by invasion and infection of the bowel mucosa by the bacterial pathogen. In this chapter, the most common bacterial pathogens affecting immunocompetent hosts are discussed. Enteric bacterial infections in HIV-infected and other immunocompromised patients are discussed in Chapter 44.
A. Toxigenic bacteria. In general, toxigenic bacteria produce watery diarrhea without systemic illness. There may be low-grade fever in some patients. Some microorganisms can produce other toxins in addition to an enterotoxin, for example, neurotoxins that can cause extraintestinal manifestations. The stools contain no blood or fecal leukocytes, which helps to distinguish these diseases from diarrheas caused by tissue-invasive organisms. Table 30-1 lists some of the common causes of toxigenic diarrhea.
   1. *Staphylococcus aureus*
      a. **Epidemiology.** Staphylococcal food poisoning is the most frequent cause of toxin-mediated vomiting and diarrhea encountered in clinical practice. All coagulase-positive staphylococci can produce enterotoxins. Staphylococci are introduced into food by the hands of food-handlers. The organisms multiply and produce the toxin if the food is kept at room temperature. The foods most commonly implicated are coleslaw, potato salad, salad dressings, milk products, and cream pastries. Food contaminated with staphylococci is normal in odor, taste, and appearance.
      b. **Clinical disease.** Staphylococcal food poisoning is manifested by an abrupt onset of vomiting within 2 to 6 hours after ingestion of the contaminated food. The diarrhea is usually explosive and may be accompanied by abdominal pain. Fever is usually absent.

TABLE 30-1 **Some Etiologic Agents for Toxigenic Diarrhea**

Staphylococcus aureus	Other toxigenic diarrheas
Bacillus cereus	Scrombrotoxin poisoning
Vibrio cholerae	Paralytic shellfish poisoning
Enterotoxigenic *Escherichia coli*	Neurotoxic shellfish poisoning
Vibrio parahaemolyticus	Ciguatoxin poisoning
Clostridium perfringens	Tetrodotoxin poisoning
Clostridium botulinum	

    c. The diagnosis is usually suspected from the history. In most instances, the organism can be cultured from the contaminated food.

    d. Treatment. Gastroenteritis resolves with supportive care within 12 to 24 hours. Antimicrobial therapy is not indicated.

2. *Bacillus cereus*

    a. Epidemiology. *Bacillus cereus* is a common gram-positive, spore-forming organism found in soil. Contamination of food occurs before cooking. Vegetative growth continues at temperatures of 30° to 50°C, and spores can survive extreme temperatures. The spores of the organism germinate and produce toxins during the vegetative stage.

       B. cereus is a frequent cause of food poisoning from many sources, but is usually associated with contaminated rice or meat from Chinese restaurants.

    b. Clinical disease. *B. cereus* intoxication manifests as two distinct clinical syndromes. The "emesis syndrome" is caused by the thermostable toxin and mimics staphylococcal food poisoning. Within 2 to 6 hours after ingestion of the contaminated food, the patient has severe vomiting and abdominal pain with or without diarrhea. There is no accompanying fever or systemic manifestations. Illness is self-limited and lasts 8 to 10 hours. The "diarrhea syndrome" is caused by the thermolabile enterotoxin and occurs after 8 to 16 hours of ingestion of the contaminated food. It is characterized by a foul-smelling, profuse watery diarrhea, usually accompanied by nausea, abdominal pain, and tenesmus. Most of the symptoms resolve in 12 to 24 hours.

    c. Diagnosis is made by history and stool cultures demonstrating the organism.

    d. Treatment is supportive.

3. *Vibrio cholerae*

    a. Epidemiology. *V. cholerae* is a mobile, gram-negative bacterium with a single flagellum and is easily recognizable by a fecal Gram's stain. It produces a thermostable enterotoxin, which stimulates the adenylate cyclase in small-intestinal crypt cells, especially in the jejunum, resulting in profuse secretory diarrhea. *V. cholerae* is seen occasionally in the United States, especially along the Gulf coast. Any fecal contaminated water or food has the potential to cause cholera, but contaminated saltwater crabs and freshwater shrimp are responsible for most instances seen in the United States.

    b. Clinical disease. The incubation period is 1 to 3 days after ingestion. Cholera is characterized by an abrupt onset of profuse, large-volume, watery diarrhea. The stools are isotonic and do not contain blood or mucus. There is usually no associated fever, abdominal pain, vomiting, or tenesmus. Hypotension, shock, and death may result if volume depletion is not adequately treated.

    c. Diagnosis. Organisms may be demonstrated by dark-field microscopy of the stool and by stool cultures.

    d. Treatment. The mainstay of therapy is volume repletion intravenously or orally with fluids that contain glucose and electrolytes. If dehydration is adequately reversed, patients recover in 7 to 10 days without antimicrobial therapy. The duration of the disease may be shortened to 2 to 3 days with oral tetracycline 500 mg q.i.d. or doxycycline 300 mg in a single dose. In resistant instances, alternative antimicrobials are furazolidone 100 mg q.i.d., erythromycin 250 mg q.i.d., or trimethoprim/sulfamethoxazole 160/800 mg b.i.d. for 3 days.

4. Enterotoxigenic *Escherichia coli*

    a. Epidemiology. Enterotoxigenic *E. coli* (ETEC) can cause diarrhea by tissue invasion or via its enterotoxin. The enterotoxin is thermolabile and produces diarrhea by the same mechanism as the cholera enterotoxin. The organism is transmitted from contaminated water and food by the fecal oral route. Even though it may cause outbreaks in the United States, ETEC is the most common traveler's pathogen. A large inoculum is required for disease. The incubation period is 1 to 3 days.

    b. The clinical disease is similar to cholera. The watery diarrhea is profuse and lasts 3 to 5 days. There may be accompanying mild abdominal pain.

c. **The diagnosis** is by history and clinical observation. Serotyping of *E. coli* is available only in research settings.

d. **Treatment.** Most patients require no antimicrobial therapy. Intravenous or oral volume replacement with glucose–electrolyte solutions is usually adequate. Severe instances may be treated with tetracycline, trimethoprim/sulfamethoxazole, or ciprofloxacin.

5. ***Vibrio parahaemolyticus***

   a. **Epidemiology.** *V. parahaemolyticus* is a gram-negative bacillus that survives in water with a high salt content. It is recognized as an important pathogen in the Far East and more recently in the United States. It is most common in the summer and least common in the winter months because the bacterial populations in the ocean are temperature-dependent. It is associated with acute diarrheal disease after the ingestion of contaminated raw or cooked fish or shellfish. The organism produces a variety of toxins. The incubation period is 12 to 48 hours after ingestion.

   b. **Clinical disease.** The illness is characterized by explosive watery diarrhea. Headaches, vomiting, and abdominal cramps are common. Low-grade fever and chills occur in 25% of the patients. Bloody diarrhea may occur in some instances. The stools are not as profuse as in *V. cholerae*, but hypotension and shock have been seen. The illness is usually self-limiting and resolves within 1 to 7 days.

   c. **Diagnosis.** The diagnosis is by stool culture on thiosulfate–citrate–bile salt–sucrose agar.

   d. **Treatment** is supportive with fluid repletion. Complicated instances may be treated with oral tetracycline.

6. ***Clostridium perfringens***

   a. **Epidemiology.** *Clostridium perfringens* is a gram-positive, spore-forming obligate anaerobe found in soil and in the gastrointestinal tract of humans and animals. It produces 12 toxins. The thermolabile exotoxin is an important cause of toxigenic diarrhea. The toxin is a structural component of the spore's coat and is formed during sporulation. Most of the toxin is synthesized before ingestion. Additional toxin is produced in the gastrointestinal tract after ingestion of contaminated beef, beef products, or poultry. The pathogenesis of infection requires the food to be inadequately precooked and then reheated before it is served. The toxin has its maximal activities in the ileum. It inhibits glucose transport and activates adenylate cyclase of small-intestinal crypt cells stimulating intestinal secretion. Outbreaks may occur in institutions or after large gatherings.

   b. **Clinical disease.** Watery diarrhea with severe, crampy abdominal pain usually occurs 8 to 24 hours after the ingestion of contaminated food. Vomiting, fever, chills, and headaches are not seen. The stools are usually foul smelling. The disorder is self-limited and resolves within 24 to 36 hours.

   c. **The diagnosis** is by history.

   d. **Treatment** is supportive.

7. ***Clostridium botulinum***

   a. **Epidemiology.** *C. botulinum* is a gram-positive, anaerobic, spore-forming bacillus. Three exotoxin types, **A**, **B**, and **E**, have been associated with *C. botulinum* intoxication. Types A and B are associated with improperly prepared home-canned fruits and vegetables. Type E outbreaks are associated with smoked freshwater fish and are most frequent in the Great Lakes region. The contaminated foods may not appear, taste, or smell spoiled, thereby inciting no suspicion of their contamination. The exotoxin is neurotoxic and thermolabile. It can be inactivated by boiling in water for 15 minutes.

   b. **Clinical disease.** *C. botulinum* is responsible for one third of the deaths from food-borne diseases. The intoxication results in acute cranial nerve dysfunction, dysarthria, diplopia, blurred vision, dysphagia, and a symmetric descending weakness without a sensory component. Dilated pupils occur in 15% of patients. Respiratory muscle insufficiency may occur. The neurologic disease may last for months and can result in death.

TABLE 30-2	Infectious Organisms That Result in Watery Diarrhea

Viruses
Rotavirus
Norwalk and related viruses
Adenovirus
Bacteria
Vibrio cholerae
Escherichia coli (enterotoxigenic)
All bacteria listed in Table 30-3
Protozoa
Giardia lamblia
Cryptosporidium

     c. The diagnosis is made by history and culture or toxin assay from the contaminated food or the patient's blood or stool. Electromyography may be used to differentiate the disease from Guillain–Barré syndrome.

     d. Therapy. When intoxication is suspected, therapy should be started immediately with administration of the polyvalent antitoxin and penicillin. Gastrointestinal lavage with orally administered solutions (e.g., GoLYTELY or Colyte) may help eliminate the toxin from the gastrointestinal tract. Guanidine hydrochloride may be used to reverse the motor weakness. Some patients may require ventilatory support.

B. Bacteria causing "enteric" infection. The resulting diarrhea may be watery or bloody. Although watery diarrhea is often associated with infections with viruses, protozoa, and toxin-producing bacteria such as *Vibrio cholerae* and enterotoxigenic *E. coli,* invasive bacteria can also cause watery diarrhea (Table 30-2). The diarrhea is usually greater than 1 L/day. Systemic symptoms such as fever, headache, myalgia, and arthralgias are usually absent.

     Bloody diarrhea, or dysentery, is usually accompanied by abdominal pain, tenesmus, nausea, vomiting, and systemic symptoms such as fever and malaise. Bacteria that result in bloody diarrhea are listed in Table 30-3. These enteric infections cannot be distinguished easily from one another clinically. Diagnosis must be based on the identification of the infectious agent by appropriate cultures.

1. *Campylobacter jejuni* and *Campylobacter fetus*

     a. Epidemiology. *C. jejuni* is the most common bacterial pathogen that causes bloody diarrhea in the United States. It is implicated in infections in underdeveloped countries also. The organism is a microaerophilic, gram-negative curved rod transmitted to humans from contaminated pork, lamb, beef,

TABLE 30-3	Infectious Organisms That Result in Bloody Diarrhea

Campylobacter
Escherichia coli (enteropathogenic and invasive)
Shigella
Salmonella
Escherichia coli O157:H7
Yersinia
Vibrio parahaemolyticus
Clostridium difficile
Entamoeba histolytica

milk and milk products, and water, and from exposure to infected household pets. The organism is destroyed by appropriate cooking, pasteurization, and water purification. The incubation period is 1 to 7 days.

b. **Histopathology.** The bacterial endotoxin causes mucosal inflammation in the small and large intestine that resembles the lesions seen in ulcerative colitis and Crohn's disease and those seen with *Salmonella* and *Shigella* infections. The infection is usually more severe in the colon than in the small bowel.

c. **Clinical disease**

   i. **Enterocolitis.** Bowel infections with *C. jejuni* and rarely *C. fetus* cause a diarrheal illness resembling enteritis from *Salmonella* and *Shigella*. Occasionally there is a prodrome of headache, myalgia, and malaise for 12 to 24 hours, followed by severe abdominal pain, high fever, and profuse watery and then bloody diarrhea. The diarrhea is usually self-limited and in most instances resolves in 7 to 10 days; however, in one fifth of the instances, the diarrhea has a protracted or a relapsing course.

   ii. **Systemic infection.** *C. fetus* and rarely *C. jejuni* may cause a systemic infection, especially in elderly, debilitated patients, and in those with alcoholism, diabetes mellitus, and malignancies. Bacteremia may be transient or may lead to localized infection such as endocarditis, meningitis, cholecystitis, and thrombophlebitis. There may or may not be clinically evident enterocolitis.

d. **Complications.** *Campylobacter* infection may be complicated by Reiter's syndrome, mesenteric adenitis, terminal ileitis (resembling Crohn's ileitis), and rarely an enteric fever like illness.

e. **Diagnosis** is made by stool and blood cultures. Stool Gram's stain may show the organism with its characteristic "gull wings." In dark-field/phase-contrast microscopy, the organism shows "darting motility." Fecal leukocytes are present in 75% of instances.

f. **Treatment.** In mild cases, supportive therapy is given. In cases with bloody diarrhea, erythromycin 250 mg p.o. q.i.d. for 5 to 7 days or ciprofloxacin 500 mg p.o. b.i.d. for 3 to 7 days is effective.

2. *Salmonella*

a. **Epidemiology.** The three primary species of *Salmonella* (*Salmonella typhi*, *Salmonella choleraesuis*, and *Salmonella enteritidis*) may cause disease in humans. *S. enteritidis* is a common cause of infectious diarrhea. There are 1,700 serotypes and variants of *Salmonella*, which are classified into 40 groups. Ninety percent of *Salmonella* organisms that are pathogenic for human beings are in groups B, C, and D. The organism is transmitted from fecally contaminated foods and water with fecal–oral contact. Poultry and poultry products constitute the major reservoir for the bacteria. A large inoculum (>105 organisms) is required to produce infection. Thus, the incidence is relatively low despite the widespread contamination of commonly ingested foods.

b. **Pathology.** *Salmonella* elaborates an enterotoxin, which is responsible for the watery diarrhea. The organism also adheres to the mucosal surface and invades the epithelium, resulting in colitis and bloody diarrhea.

c. **Clinical disease.** *Salmonella* invades the mucosa of the small and large intestine and produces an enterotoxin that causes a secretory diarrhea. Watery diarrhea is more common, but bloody diarrhea may occur. Patients complain of headache, malaise, nausea, vomiting, and abdominal pain within 6 to 48 hours after ingesting the contaminated food. The disease is usually self-limited and resolves in 7 days. Fever and bacteremia occur in less than 10% of patients. Immunosuppression, malignancy, hemolytic states, liver disease, achlorhydria, and chronic granulomatous disease of children predispose patients to progressive salmonellosis with bacteremia, with localized infection in joints, bones, meninges, and other sites. In 5% of patients, the bacteria may localize in the reticuloendothelial system and may cause an enteric fever (especially *S. typhi*). A carrier state also exists in some patients, with bacteria carried in the gallbladder or in the urinary tract.

    d. The diagnosis is made by history and stool and blood cultures. A fourfold rise in serum O and H agglutinin titers 3 to 4 weeks after infection confirms the diagnosis.

    e. Treatment is supportive in most instances. Antimicrobial therapy is contraindicated for most patients because it can increase the carrier state. However, antimicrobial agents such as ampicillin, chloramphenicol, trimethoprim/sulfamethoxazole, ciprofloxacin hydrochloride, or third-generation cephalosporins can be used in young children or in patients who are susceptible to bacteremia and prolonged salmonellosis (Table 30-4). Patients with bacteremia, enteric fever, and metastatic infection should be treated with antimicrobial therapy. Also, patients with underlying acquired immunodeficiency syndrome (AIDS), hemolytic states, lymphoma, and leukemia, and neonates, the elderly and chronic carriers should receive antimicrobials. Anticholinergic agents and opiates should not be used because they can prolong the excretion of the bacteria.

3. Shigella

    a. Epidemiology. There are four major groups: *Shigella dysenteriae, Shigella flexneri, Shigella boydii,* and *Shigella sonnei. S. dysenteriae* causes the severest form of dysentery. In the United States, 60% to 80% of instances of bacillary dysentery are caused by *S. sonnei* with a seasonal preference for winter. In tropical countries, *S. flexneri* dysentery is more common especially in the late summer months. It is transmitted by the fecal–oral route. Human beings

---

TABLE 30-4   **Treatment of Common Acute Enteric Infections**

Organism	Antimicrobial therapy
Campylobacter	Erythromycin 250 mg p.o. q.i.d. for 5–10 d **or** ciprofloxacin 500 mg p.o. b.i.d. for 5 d
Shigella	Trimethoprim/sulfamethoxazole DS p.o. b.i.d. for 5 d **or** tetracycline 500 mg p.o. q.i.d. for 5 d **or** ciprofloxacin 500 mg p.o. b.i.d. for 5 d
Salmonella (severe disease)	Ampicillin **or** amoxicillin 1 gm p.o. t.i.d. **or** q.i.d. for 14 d **or** chloramphenicol 1 gm p.o. **or** IV q8h for 14 d **or** trimethoprim/sulfamethoxazole DS p.o. b.i.d. for 10 d **or** a third-generation cephalosporin **or** ciprofloxacin 500 mg p.o. b.i.d. for 5 d Rifaximin 200 mg p.o. t.i.d.
Enterotoxigenic *Escherichia coli, E. coli* O157:H7, and traveler's diarrhea	Trimethoprim/sulfamethoxazole DS p.o. b.i.d. for 5 d **or** ciprofloxacin 500 mg p.o. b.i.d. for 5 d **or** ofloxacin 300 mg p.o. b.i.d. for 5 d **or** norfloxacin 400 mg p.o. b.i.d. for 5 d
Giardia lamblia	Quinacrine hydrochloride 100 mg p.o. t.i.d. for 7 d **or** metronidazole 250 mg p.o. t.i.d. for 7 d **or** furazolidone 100 mg q.i.d. for 7 d
Entamoeba histolytica	Diloxanide furoate 500 mg p.o. t.i.d. for 10 d plus diiodohydroxyquin 650 mg p.o. t.i.d. for 20 d
Yersinia enterocolitica	Trimethoprim/sulfamethoxazole DS p.o. b.i.d. for 7 d **or** tetracycline 250–500 mg p.o. for 7 d
Vibrio cholerae	Tetracycline 500 mg p.o. q.i.d. for 3 d **or** trimethoprim/sulfamethoxazole DS p.o. b.i.d. for 3 d
Noncholera *Vibrio*	Tetracycline 250 mg p.o. q.i.d. for 7 d
Clostridium difficile Mild disease	Cholestyramine 4 gm p.o. t.i.d. for 7 d **or** metronidazole 250 mg p.o. t.i.d. for 7 d
Severe disease	Metronidazole 250 mg p.o. t.i.d. for 7 d **or** vancomycin 125–500 mg p.o. q.i.d. for 7 d

Trimethoprim/sulfamethoxazole DS, trimethoprim 160 mg/sulfamethoxazole 800 mg; p.o., by mouth; q.i.d., four times a day; b.i.d., twice a day; t.i.d., three times a day.

are the only natural host for this organism. Enteric infections with *Shigella* are most commonly seen in children 6 months to 5 years old, although persons of all ages can become infected. Clinical shigellosis is highly contagious and can be caused by a very small inoculum: fewer than 200 organisms. Food, water, and milk can be contaminated, which can result in epidemics. Incidence of the disease increases in crowded, unsanitary conditions.

b. **Pathophysiology.** Shigella elaborates an enterotoxin that is responsible for the watery diarrhea. The organism also adheres to the mucosal surface and invades the epithelium, resulting in colitis and bloody diarrhea.

c. **Clinical disease.** The incubation period is 1 to 3 days. In most individuals, the disease starts as lower abdominal pain and diarrhea. Fever is present in less than half of the patients. In many patients, there is a biphasic illness that begins as fever, abdominal pain, and watery diarrhea. In 3 to 5 days, rectal burning, tenesmus, and small-volume bloody diarrhea characteristic of severe colitis develop. Toxic megacolon and colonic perforation may recur. Extraintestinal complications include conjunctivitis, seizures, meningismus, Reiter's syndrome, thrombocytopenia, and hemolytic uremic syndrome.

The course of shigellosis is variable. In children, it may resolve in 1 to 3 days and in most adults in 1 to 7 days. In severe instances, it may last longer than 3 to 4 weeks with associated relapses. It may be confused with idiopathic ulcerative colitis. A minority of patients become chronic carriers.

d. **The diagnosis** of shigellosis is made by identification of the gram-negative bacillus in the stool. Sigmoidoscopic findings are identical to those of idiopathic inflammatory bowel disease.

e. **Treatment.** Patients should receive supportive therapy with antipyretics and fluids. Antiperistaltic agents such as diphenoxylate hydrochloride (Lomotil) or loperamide hydrochloride (Imodium) should be avoided. Antimicrobial therapy decreases the duration of fever, diarrhea, and excretion of the organisms in the stool. Trimethoprim/sulfamethoxazole, tetracycline, and ampicillin (but not amoxicillin) are all effective; however, resistance has been demonstrated. Ciprofloxacin and norfloxacin are also effective.

4. ***Escherichia coli.*** In addition to ETEC, other serotypes of *E. coli* also cause diarrhea. These include enteroinvasive *E. coli* (EIEC), enteropathogenic *E. coli* (EPEC), enterohemorrhagic *E. coli* (EHEC), diffuse adherence *E. coli* (DAEC), and enteroaggregating *E. coli* (E AGGEC). All of these bacteria possess plasmid-encoded virulence factors. They make specific interactions with the intestinal mucosa by way of bacterially derived adhesions. Some produce enterotoxins and cytotoxins. Transmission is fecal–oral.

a. **Enteroinvasive *E. coli***

i. **Epidemiology.** EIEC is a traveler's pathogen. Epidemics have been described resulting from imported cheese. The organism also causes epidemics in young children, 1 to 4 years of age.

ii. **Clinical disease.** Similar to *Shigella*, EIEC invades and destroys the colonic mucosal cells and causes, first, watery diarrhea followed by a dysentery like syndrome. The incubation period is 1 to 3 days. The fever and diarrhea last 1 to 2 days.

iii. **Diagnosis.** Fecal leukocytes are present. Serotyping and ELISA are available only in research settings.

iv. **Treatment** is supportive. Bismuth subsalicylate, by decreasing colonic secretions, seems to decrease the diarrhea and other symptoms in all infections with *E. coli* species. The antimicrobials used in shigellosis are effective, as well as rifaximin 200 mg p.o. t.i.d.

b. **Enteropathogenic *E. coli***

i. **Epidemiology.** EPEC is a major cause of diarrhea in both economically developed and underdeveloped countries. It commonly causes outbreaks in nurseries affecting children up to 12 months of age. It may also cause sporadic diarrhea in adults. The bacteria adhere closely to the enterocyte membrane via an adherence factor with destruction of microvilli.

ii. **Clinical disease.** Disease onset is with fever, vomiting, and watery diarrhea. Symptoms may continue for longer than 2 weeks and patients may relapse.

iii. **Diagnosis** is by serotype analysis

iv. **Treatment.** Nonabsorbable antibiotics such as neomycin, colistin, and polymyxin have been recommended. Ciprofloxacin hydrochloride, norfloxacin, and aztreonam are also effective and preferred.

c. **Enterohemorrhagic *E. coli***

i. **Epidemiology.** EHEC or *E. coli* O157:07, and rarely *E. coli* O26:H11 have been detected in contaminated hamburger meat; outbreaks have occurred in nursing homes, daycare centers, and schools.

ii. **Pathogenesis and clinical disease.** EHEC elaborates a *Shigella*-like toxin (verotoxin 1) that is identical to the neuroenterocytotoxin of *S. dysenteriae* and to verotoxin 2 and an adherence factor encoded by a plasmid. Transmission is fecal–oral. Although the disease is more common in children, several outbreaks have occurred in adults from contaminated beef. The bloody diarrhea may be copious but may show no fecal leukocytes. It usually lasts 7 to 10 days but may be complicated by hemolytic uremia syndrome.

iii. **Diagnosis.** Stool cultures and serotyping sorbitol-negative *E. coli* isolates may yield the organism.

iv. **Treatment.** Symptomatic treatment and ciprofloxacin or norfloxacin may be used in severe illness. Supportive measures are recommended.

d. **Diffuse adherence *E. coli* (DAEC)** affects young children, especially in economically underdeveloped countries. Diarrhea is usually watery, lasts less than 2 weeks, and may become persistent.

e. **Enteroaggregating *E. coli* (EAGGEC)** has been recognized recently as a pathogen especially affecting the ileum and the terminal ileum. The aggregating bacteria gather around the villi and cause epithelial destruction. The pathogenesis is transferred by a plasmid via fimbriae. It causes persistent diarrhea in children and is more common in economically underdeveloped countries. The management of the diarrheal illness is similar to that of other *E. coli* species strains.

5. ***Yersinia enterocolitica***

a. **Epidemiology.** *Y. enterocolitica* can be found in stream and lake water and has been isolated from many animals, including dogs, cats, chickens, cows, and horses. It is transmitted to humans via contaminated food or water, or from human or animal carriers. It most commonly affects children and rarely causes disease in adults. It is found worldwide, especially in Scandinavia and Europe, and may result in epidemics.

b. **Pathogenesis and clinical disease.** *Yersinia* causes a spectrum of diseases ranging from gastroenteritis to invasive ileitis and colitis. The organism is invasive and elaborates a heat-stable toxin. These properties allow its invasion into and through the distal small-bowel mucosa and subsequent infection of the mesenteric lymph nodes. The incubation period is 4 to 10 days. The disease normally lasts several weeks but can be prolonged for many months.

The manifestation of *Yersinia* infection is variable. In infants and young children less than 5 years, it may be febrile gastroenteritis lasting 1 to 3 weeks. In older children, it may mimic acute terminal ileitis, mesenteric adenitis, or ileocolitis. It may be confused with acute appendicitis. The enterocolitis presents with bloody diarrhea, fever, and abdominal pain accompanied by anorexia, nausea, and fatigue. The diarrhea usually lasts 1 to 3 weeks but may be protracted (>3 months). Polyarthritis, erythema multiforme, and erythema nodosum occasionally develop 1 to 3 weeks after the onset of diarrhea. Bacteremia is rare but may be seen in immunosuppressed patients and may result in hepatosplenic abscess, meningitis, and infections of other organs. Metastatic foci may occur in joints, lungs, and bones.

   c. **Diagnosis** can be made by stool and blood cultures using special media and culture conditions. The laboratory should be notified. Serologic tests have been useful in Europe and Canada. The serotypes found in the United States do not give reliable serologic results.

   d. **Treatment** in most instances is supportive. Antimicrobials such as tetracycline, chloramphenicol, and trimethoprim/sulfamethoxazole may be used in severe illness.

6. *Aeromonas hydrophila*

   a. **Epidemiology.** *A. hydrophila* is a member of the *Vibrionaceae* family.

      It is transmitted from contaminated food and water, especially in the summer months.

   b. **Pathogenesis and clinical disease.** *Aeromonas* produces several toxins. The heat-labile enterotoxin and the cytotoxin are implicated in the intestinal infection. The disease commonly follows ingestion of untreated water just before the onset of symptoms and consists of fever, abdominal pain, watery diarrhea, and vomiting lasting about 1 to 3 weeks in children and 6 weeks or longer in adults. In 10% of instances, diarrhea is bloody and mucoid. Chronic diarrhea and choleralike presentation have also been described. In immunocompromised patients and patients with hepatobiliary disease, bacteremia may occur.

   c. **Diagnosis.** Stool cultures are diagnostic. Fecal leukocytes may be present in one third of instances.

   d. **Treatment** is supportive in mild instances. In severe illness and with chronic diarrhea, antibiotics may shorten the duration of the disease. *Aeromonas* is resistant to beta-lactam antibiotics. Trimethoprim/sulfamethoxazole, tetracycline, and chloramphenicol have been effective.

7. *Plesiomonas shigelloides*

   a. **Epidemiology.** *Plesiomonas* is another member of the *Vibrionaceae* family that causes sporadic diarrheal disease affecting travelers to Mexico, Central America, and the Far East after ingestion of raw shellfish. It produces a choleralike toxin but also has invasive potential.

   b. **Clinical disease.** Diarrhea is usually watery, but in one third of the patients it is bloody. Abdominal pain is usually severe. Vomiting and fever may be present. Although the disease is usually over in 1 week, it may last longer than 4 weeks.

   c. **Diagnosis** is by stool culture. Fecal leukocytes may be present.

   d. **Treatment** is supportive. The organism has the same microbial sensitivity as *Aeromonas.*

8. *Clostridium difficile*

   a. **Epidemiology.** *C. difficile* is a spore-forming obligate anaerobe. It is found as "normal flora" in 3% of adults, 15% of hospitalized patients, and 70% of infants in pediatric wards. It may cause disease in people of all ages, but it most frequently affects elderly and debilitated patients. The transmission is usually fecal–oral; however, it may be transmitted environmentally by spores carried on fomites or on contaminated hands of health care workers. The disease usually follows antibiotic use with disruption of the normal colonic flora. All antimicrobial agents with the exception of vancomycin and parenterally administered aminoglycosides have been linked with *C. difficile* enterocolitis. In most instances, the ingestion of the antimicrobial agent is within 6 weeks of the onset of the diarrhea. Case reports of *C. difficile* disease in patients who have not received antibiotics include patients with neutropenia or uremia, those undergoing cancer chemotherapy, and homosexual males.

   b. **Pathogenesis and clinical disease.** *C. difficile* produces two major toxins. Toxin A is an enterotoxin, and toxin B is a cytotoxin used in commercial latex agglutination testing for detection of the infection. Toxin A binds to receptors on the colonic mucosal surface and causes severe inflammatory changes. The toxigenic effect is catalyzed by previously present trauma or injury to the mucosal cells. The severity of the disease varies from watery diarrhea to severe pseudomembranous colitis with bloody diarrhea, fever, and systemic toxicity.

c. Diagnosis is made by stool cultures or by the demonstration of the presence of the associated cytopathic toxin produced by *C. difficile* in stool samples. Fecal leukocytes may be absent in 50% of instances. Toxin assay may be negative in 10% to 20% of instances. Sigmoidoscopy, colonoscopy, and histologic examination of the mucosal biopsies support the diagnosis. Pseudomembranes, if present, are most common in the rectum and distal colon. Occasionally, however, they are present only in the transverse colon or cecum.

d. Treatment. The strategies for treatment vary according to the severity of the symptoms. Unnecessary antibiotics should be stopped. Corticosteroids and antiperistaltic agents should be avoided because they may prolong *C. difficile* carriage and exacerbate the diarrhea. Patients with colitis may be treated with oral vancomycin 125 mg q.i.d. for 10 days or oral metronidazole 250 mg q.i.d. for 10 days. Cholestyramine may be used in mild disease to aid in binding the elaborated toxins. Relapse after antimicrobial therapy occurs in 20% of patients within 1 week after therapy. In such patients, the eradication of *C. difficile* may require vancomycin 250 to 500 mg q.i.d. for 1 month or pulsed doses of therapy for 5 days each time as long as necessary. Combining rifampin 600 mg with vancomycin produces a synergistic effect.

Probiotics or bacterial therapeutic agents such as *Lactobacillus* or *Saccharomyces boulardii* may add additional benefit. Over-the-counter yogurt varities containing probiotics may be beneficial when ingested daily over several weeks.

III. PARASITIC INFECTIONS OF THE BOWEL. Numerous parasites infect the human bowel and cause disease. This chapter discusses only the most common parasitic infections, namely, protozoan pathogens seen in the United States in normal, immunocompetent people.

In recent years, there has been an increase in protozoan infections of the bowel caused by increases in international travel to tropical and subtropical areas of the world, in male homosexuality, and in AIDS. The protozoan infections seen in AIDS are discussed in Chapter 43. The antimicrobial therapy is summarized in Table 30-4 (page 204).

A. Giardia lamblia

1. Epidemiology. *Giardia* is a flagellated protozoan seen worldwide. It is transmitted by the fecal–oral route from fecally contaminated water and food. It is also a traveler's pathogen and affects children and adults, especially people with IgA deficiency, hypochlorhydria, and malnutrition.

2. Pathogenesis and clinical disease. After ingestion of the cysts, excystation releases the organism in the upper small intestine. *Giardia* adheres to the brush border membrane of the enterocytes. Histologically, it may cause a celiac sprue-like lesion, resulting in lactose deficiency and malabsorption. Incubation after ingestion of the organisms is 1 week. Most infections produce mild, self-limiting enteritis with watery diarrhea, abdominal bloating, cramps, and flatulence lasting 1 to 3 weeks. The stools may be bulky and foul smelling. In a minority of the patients, the infection persists and results in a chronic or recurrent disease with weight loss and malabsorption.

3. Diagnosis is made by multiple stool examinations because the shedding of the protozoan is episodic. In difficult illnesses, duodenal aspirates and touch preparations made by duodenal biopsy specimens can be used.

4. Treatment is with quinacrine hydrochloride (Atabrine), metronidazole (Flagyl), or furazolidone (Furoxone). In recurrent illness, combination drug therapy may be more efficacious.

B. Cryptosporidium

1. Epidemiology. *Cryptosporidium* is an important coccidian protozoan in veterinary medicine. It is also a ubiquitous human pathogen affecting both immunocompetent and immunosuppressed patients. There is a high rate of infection among homosexual men, children in daycare facilities, and immigrants arriving from economically underdeveloped countries. It accounts for 1% to 4% of instances of infectious diarrhea in the economically developed world. The incidence of infection is greater in the summer and fall. The organism may be transmitted by a variety of routes including fecal–oral, hand–to-mouth, and person-to-person via contaminated food, water, and pets (especially cats).

2. **Clinical disease.** In normal hosts, profuse watery diarrhea, anorexia, and low-grade fever occur approximately 5 days after ingestion of the oocysts. In most instances, it is a self-limited disease lasting 5 to 20 days. In immunodeficient hosts, it can be a chronic, relentless disease with watery diarrhea of up to 17 L per day. The organism infects the jejunum most heavily but has been found in the pharynx, esophagus, duodenum, ileum, pancreatic ducts, gallbladder, bile ducts, appendix, colon, and rectum.

3. **Diagnosis** may be established by the demonstration of the oocysts in the stool specimens or the organisms in biopsy specimens obtained at endoscopy. Giemsa, acid-fast, and silver stains increase the diagnostic yield.

4. **Treatment** is supportive with fluid and electrolytes. Octreotide, the synthetic somatostatin analog, may reduce the volume of watery diarrhea. Spiramycin and puromycin have been used with limited efficacy.

C. *Entamoeba histolytica*

1. **Epidemiology.** *E. histolytica* is an endemic and travel-associated, tissue-invasive protozoan transmitted via the fecal–oral route. It is common in institutionalized patients and homosexual males. In the United States, the prevalence is about 5%.

2. **Pathology.** The infection starts with ingestion of the cysts. The excystation occurs in the colon with the release of trophozoites, which invade the mucosa and lead to mucosal inflammation and ulceration similar to that seen in idio-pathic inflammatory bowel disease. The classic lesions of amebiasis are the "flask-shaped ulcers" that may extend to the submucosa.

3. **Clinical disease.** The infection manifests in a spectrum of disease with varying severity. In the mild form, patients have crampy abdominal pain, intermittent diarrhea, and tenesmus. In the more severe form, there is bloody diarrhea with abdominal pain, tenesmus, and fever.

Acute abdomen secondary to perforation or peritonitis may be seen. The infection may encompass the entire colon but may be in the form of amebomas, which are single or multiple annular inflammatory lesions more often seen in the cecum or the ascending colon.

4. **Diagnosis** is made by the demonstration of the organism in the stool. In mildly affected patients and in carriers, cysts are usually present in the stool. Trophozoites may be demonstrated in stool or biopsy specimens obtained from ulcer margins at sigmoidoscopy or colonoscopy. In amebic colitis, the serology by indirect hemagglutination test is positive in greater than 90% of patients.

5. **Therapy** is variable depending on the severity of the symptoms and disease. Asymptomatic intestinal infection is treated with diiodohydroxyquin (iodoquinol [Diquinol]) 650 mg t.i.d. for 20 days or diloxanide furoate (Furamide) 500 mg t.i.d. for 10 days. Patients with moderate-to-severe intestinal disease are treated with metronidazole (Flagyl) 750 mg t.i.d. for 10 days plus diiodohydroxyquin 650 mg t.i.d. for 20 days. The alternative treatment is paromomycin 25 to 35 mg/kg t.i.d. for 7 days plus diiodohydroxyquin 650 mg t.i.d. for 20 days.

Selected Readings

Ali S, et al. *Giardia intestinalis. Curr Opin Infect Dis.* 2004;16:453–460.

Bardham PK, et al. Screening of patients with acute infectious diarrhea; evaluation of clinical features, faecal microscopy and faecal occult blood testing. *Scand J Gastroenterol.* 2000;35:55–60.

Basnyat B, et al. Enteric (typhoid) fever in travelers. *Clin Infect Dis.* 2005;41:1467–1472.

Gahatsatos P, et al. Meta-analysis of outcome of cytomegalovirus colitis in immuno-competent hosts. *Dig Dis Sci.* 2005;50:609–616.

Issa M, et al. Impact of Clostridium difficile on inflammatory bowel disease. *Clin Gastroenterol Hepatol.* 2007 Mar;5:345–351.

Levwohl MV, et al. Giardiasis. *Gastrointest Endosc.* 2003;7:906–913.

Poutanen SM, et al. Clostridium difficile-associated diarrhea in adults. *CMAJ.* 2004; 171:51–58.

Reid G, et al. Selecting, testing and understanding probiotic microorganisms. *FEMS Immunol Med Microbiol.* 2006;46:149–157.

Rossignol JF, Infectious diarrhea. Etiology, diagnosis and treatment. *US Gastroenterol Rev.* 2007;1:76–80.

Sanders JW, et al. Diarrhea in the returned traveler. *Curr Gastroenterol Rep.* 2001;3:315.

Stanley SL, Jr., Amoebiasis. *Lancet.* 2003;361:1025–1034.

Sunenshine RH, et al. Clostridium difficile-associated disease: new challenge from established pathogen. *Cleveland Cin J Med.* 2006;73(2):187–197.

Surawicz CM. Treatment of recurrent *ostridium difficile*-associated disease. *Nat Clin Pract Gastroenterol Hepatol.* 2004;1:32–38.

MALABSORPTION 31

$\mathcal{T}$he term **malabsorption** connotes the failure to absorb or digest normally one or more dietary constituents. Patients with malabsorption often complain of diarrhea, and sometimes the distinction between malabsorption and diarrhea of other causes (see Chapter 29) initially is difficult. For example, patients with primary lactase deficiency fail to absorb a specific dietary constituent, lactose, and a watery, osmotic diarrhea develops. However, most patients with malabsorption present with a syndrome characterized by large, loose, foul-smelling stools and loss of weight. On additional study, it is found that they cannot absorb fat and often carbohydrate, protein, and other nutrients also. Table 31-1 indicates that a wide variety of disorders of the organs of digestion can cause malabsorption or maldigestion.

I. DIAGNOSTIC STUDIES. Before discussing the disorders that may cause malabsorption, it is useful to review several of the diagnostic studies that are available to aid in evaluating patients with this condition. The number and order of diagnostic studies used depends on the clinical signs and symptoms of the patient.

A. Blood tests. The hemoglobin and hematocrit levels may identify an anemia that accompanies malabsorption. A low mean cell volume (MCV) may be found in iron deficiency, whereas a high MCV may result from malabsorption of folate or

TABLE 31-1 Disorders That May Cause Malabsorption or Maldigestion of One or More Dietary Constituents

Digestive disorder	Examples
Pancreatic exocrine insufficiency	Chronic pancreatitis
	Pancreatic carcinoma
Bile acid insufficiency	Small-bowel bacterial overgrowth
	Crohn's disease of the terminal ileum
Small-bowel disease	
Mucosal disorders	Celiac sprue
	Collagenous sprue
	Tropical sprue
	Whipple's disease
	Radiation enteritis
	Ischemic disease
	Intestinal lymphoma
	Regional enteritis
	(Crohn's disease)
	Amyloidosis
Specific absorptive defects	Primary lactase deficiency
	Abetalipoproteinemia
Lymphatic disorders	Intestinal lymphangiectasia
Mixed defects in absorption	Zollinger-Ellison syndrome
	Postgastrectomy disorders

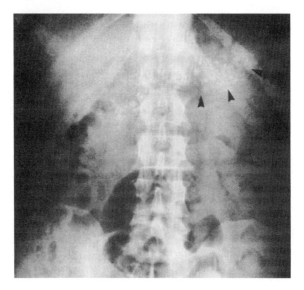

Figure 31-1. Plain x-ray film of the abdomen in a patient with extensive calcification of the pancreas (*arrows*) and pancreatic insufficiency.

vitamin B_{12}. Serum levels of liver enzymes, protein, amylase, calcium, folate, and vitamin B_{12} may be abnormal and should be ordered.

B. Radiographic studies

1. **Plain films or computed tomography scan of the abdomen** may show calcification within the pancreas, which indicates chronic pancreatic insufficiency (Fig. 31-1).

2. **A barium examination of the upper gastrointestinal tract,** including the small bowel, usually is one of the first diagnostic studies in the evaluation of malabsorption syndrome. Often the findings are nonspecific. The bowel may be dilated and the barium diluted because of increased intraluminal fluid. A more specific finding is thickening of the intestinal folds caused by an infiltrative process, such as lymphoma, Whipple's disease, or amyloidosis. The narrowed, irregular terminal ileum in Crohn's disease is virtually diagnostic (Fig. 31-2), although lymphoma and other infiltrative disorders also must be considered. Diverticula, fistulas, and surgical alterations in bowel anatomy also may be evident.

C. Fecal fat determination. Malabsorption of fat (steatorrhea) is common to most malabsorptive conditions (Table 31-2). Patients should ingest at least 80 g of fat per day to obtain reliable interpretation of qualitative or quantitative fat determination. Mineral oil and oil-containing cathartics should be avoided.

1. **Qualitative screening test.** The Sudan stain for fecal fat is easy to perform and reasonably sensitive and specific when interpreted by an experienced person. A small amount of fresh stool is mixed thoroughly with normal saline or water on a glass slide. A drop of glacial acetic acid is added, and the slide is heated to hydrolyze the fatty acids from the triglycerides in the stool. The Sudan stain is then added. Increased stool fat is indicated by abnormally large or increased numbers (>100/40 × field) of fat droplets.

2. **The quantitative determination** of **stool fat** is more accurate than qualitative screening, but the collection of stool often is disagreeable to patients, family, and nursing personnel. The stool is collected over 72 hours in a large sealed container, which can be enclosed in a plastic bag and refrigerated to contain unpleasant odors. Most normal people excrete up to 6 g of fat per 24 hours on a diet that contains 80 to 100 g of fat. Stool fat in excess of 6 g per 24 hours can result from a

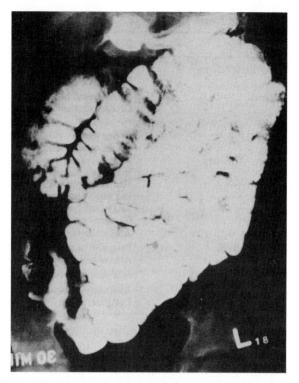

Figure 31-2. Small-bowel x-ray series in a patient with Crohn's disease. Note the narrowed, irregular contour of the terminal ileum and cecum (*arrow*). (From Eastwood GL. *Core Textbook of Gastroenterology*. Philadelphia: Lippincott Williams & Wilkins; 1984:102. Reprinted with permission.)

disorder of fat digestion at any stage, including pancreatic insufficiency (decreased lipase), bile acid insufficiency, mucosal disease, or lymphatic obstruction.

D. Pancreatic function tests

1. **Collection of pancreatic secretions from the duodenum.** The volume of pancreatic secretion and the content of bicarbonate and enzymes can be measured by collecting pancreatic secretions from the duodenum after stimulation of the pancreas with secretin or with a test meal. Pancreatic insufficiency or carcinoma of the head of the pancreas, which partially obstructs the pancreatic duct, may be detected by this means. For example, bicarbonate concentrations less than 90 mmol/L suggest pancreatic insufficiency. However, pancreatic secretory tests are performed so infrequently in most gastrointestinal laboratories that the results may be unreliable.

2. The **bentiromide test** is a test of pancreatic exocrine function that does not require duodenal intubation. The chemical name of bentiromide is N-benzoyl-L-tyrosyl-P-aminobenzoic acid. The test is performed by administering a single oral dose of 500 mg of bentiromide after an overnight fast and the urine is then collected for 6 hours. The pancreatic enzyme chymotrypsin cleaves the molecule within the lumen of the small intestine, releasing paraaminobenzoic acid (PABA). The PABA is absorbed and excreted in the urine. Less than 60% excretion of PABA suggests pancreatic insufficiency, although mucosal disorders, renal disease, severe liver disease, and diabetes also can cause low PABA excretion.

3. **Radiographic studies.** Although computed tomography of the abdomen (see Chapter 9) and endoscopic retrograde cholangiopancreatography (ERCP) (see Chapter 5) do not measure pancreatic function directly, abnormalities such as

TABLE 31-2 Expected Diagnostic Findings According to Cause of Malabsorption

Disorder	Diagnostic Test				
	Small-bowel x-ray	Fecal fat	Xylose tolerance test	Schilling test	Small-bowel biopsy
Pancreatic exocrine insufficiency	Abnormal	Severe steatorrhea	Normal	May be abnormal	Normal
Bile acid insufficiency	Normal[a]	Mild-to-moderate steatorrhea	Normal[a]	Normal[a]	Normal[a]
Small-bowel mucosal disease	Abnormal	Mild-to-severe steatorrhea	Abnormal	Usually normal[b]	Abnormal
Lymphatic disease	May be abnormal	Mild steatorrhea	Normal	Normal	Abnormal

[a]May be abnormal in bacterial overgrowth.
[b]Abnormal if terminal lieum is involved.

dilated or strictured ducts, calcification, and pancreatic masses can imply pancreatic disease.

E. Bile acid breath test. Conjugated bile acids that are secreted into the duodenum are resorbed with about 95% efficiency in the terminal ileum. If radiolabeled $[^{14}C]$-glycocholate is given orally to a healthy person, about 5% of it enters the colon and undergoes bacterial deconjugation. The carbon dioxide $(^{14}CO_2)$ derived from the glycine is absorbed and excreted by the lungs and can be measured in expired air. Bacterial overgrowth in the small intestine promotes earlier bacterial deconjugation of the $[^{14}C]$-glycocholate, and consequently, a larger amount of $^{14}CO_2$ is measured in the breath. Similarly, disease or resection of the terminal ileum allows more bile acids to pass into the colon and undergo bacterial deconjugation, resulting in an increase in expired carbon dioxide.

F. Xylose tolerance test. D-Xylose is a five-carbon sugar that remains intact when it is absorbed across intestinal mucosa. Consequently, measurement of xylose absorption can be used as a screening test for diffuse disease of the small-intestinal mucosa. The patient drinks 25 g of xylose dissolved in 500 mL of water, and the urine is collected for the next 5 hours. A healthy person absorbs enough xylose to excrete more than 5 g of xylose. Because low xylose excretion can result from inadequate hydration, the patient is encouraged to drink an additional 1,000 mL of water during the 5 hours of urine collection. In addition to mucosal disease, a low urinary xylose excretion can result from small-bowel bacterial overgrowth, decreased circulatory volume, massive ascites, and renal disease. To avoid the problem of urine collection in patients with renal disease or who are unable to collect the urine accurately, a blood xylose level at 2 hours after ingestion of the xylose can be determined. The normal 2-hour blood xylose level is above 40 mg/dL.

G. Lactose absorption tests. The lactose tolerance test is an indirect measurement of the activity of intestinal lactase, a brush border enzyme that hydrolyzes lactose to glucose and galactose. To perform the lactose tolerance test, a fasting blood glucose level is drawn, and the patient swallows 50 g of lactose mixed in 500 mL of water. The blood glucose level is determined 15, 30, 60, and 90 minutes after ingestion of lactose. If the patient is lactase deficient, the blood glucose level fails to rise more than 20 mg/dL above the fasting level (Fig. 31-3).

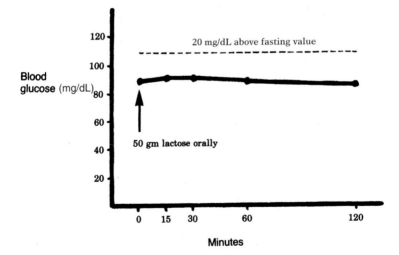

Figure 31-3. Serial blood glucose levels during a lactose tolerance test in a patient with primary lactase deficiency. The blood glucose failed to rise more than 20 mg/dL above the fasting value. (From Eastwood GL. *Core Textbook of Gastroenterology.* Philadelphia: Lippincott Williams & Wilkins; 1984:113. Reprinted with permission.)

Lactose absorption also can be assessed by measuring breath hydrogen (H_2) after oral administration of 25 g of lactose. If lactose absorption in the small bowel is impaired, an abnormally large amount of lactose reaches the colon, where bacteria ferment it, forming excessive amounts of H_2. The H_2 is absorbed and excreted by the lungs.

H. Vitamin B_{12} absorption (Schilling) test. The standard Schilling test measures the 24-hour urinary excretion of orally administered cobalt-labeled vitamin B_{12} and has been used to diagnose conditions in which intrinsic factor (IF) may be absent, such as pernicious anemia or gastric atrophy. When IF is given with vitamin B_{12}, the test becomes a measure of terminal ileal or pancreatic function, because dietary vitamin B_{12} is bound in the stomach to an endogenous protein called R protein. Pancreatic enzymes degrade the R protein in the proximal small bowel and lower its affinity for vitamin B_{12}, resulting in the rapid transfer of B_{12} to IF. The IF-B_{12} complex continues to the terminal ileum, where it binds to specific receptors on the surface of the epithelial cells. Thus lack of sufficient pancreatic enzymes or of terminal ileal mucosa may result in abnormal vitamin B_{12} excretion. Normally, more than 10% of the labeled dose is excreted within 24 hours. Other conditions that predispose to a low urinary excretion include poor hydration, decreased circulatory volume, renal disease, small-bowel bacterial overgrowth, and infestation with the tapeworm *Diphyllobothrium latum.*

1. Small-bowel biopsy. The specific diagnosis of several mucosal diseases can be made by small-bowel biopsy, and the diagnosis of other disorders can be inferred on the basis of nonspecific findings (see Chapter 5).

Photomicrographs of normal human small-intestinal mucosa and of the mucosa from a patient with celiac sprue are shown in Figs. 31-4 and 31-5, respectively.

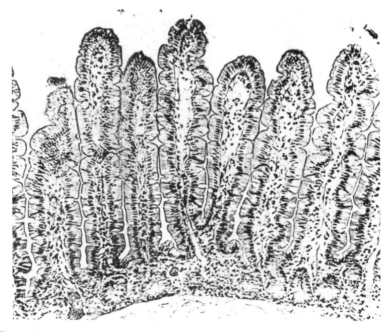

Figure 31-4. Photomicrograph of a normal human small-intestinal mucosal biopsy taken from the distal duodenum. The villi are tall and straight and the villus-to-crypt ratio is about 5:1. (From Eastwood GL. *Core Textbook of Gastroenterology.* Philadelphia: Lippincott Williams & Wilkins; 1984:105. Reprinted with permission.)

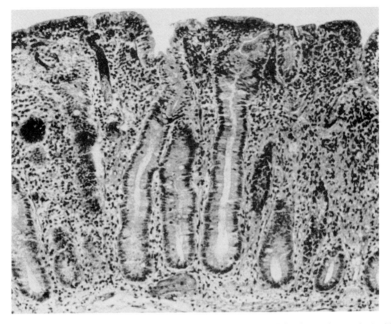

Figure 31-5. Photomicrograph of a mucosal biopsy from the distal duodenum in a patient with celiac sprue. The villi are severely blunted, the crypts are elongated, the surface epithelial cells are flattened, and the lamina propria contains a dense inflammatory cell infiltration.

II. PANCREATIC EXOCRINE INSUFFICIENCY

A. Pathogenesis. Pancreatic insufficiency usually is the result of chronic inflammatory disease of the pancreas. Most often, this is caused by alcohol abuse, but it may result from traumatic pancreatitis, familial pancreatitis, or chronic hypercalcemic pancreatitis. Rarely, pancreatic carcinoma presents as pancreatic insufficiency before jaundice and pain develop. Because pancreatic enzymes are necessary for the digestion of fat, protein, and carbohydrate, pancreatic insufficiency leads to panmalabsorption.

B. The **diagnosis** of pancreatic insufficiency is suspected on clinical grounds in a person with chronic relapsing pancreatitis. Abdominal pain may or may not be a feature, but loss of weight is common. Calcification evident on abdominal plain x-ray films is a sure sign of pancreatic exocrine insufficiency, although insufficiency certainly can exist in the absence of calcification.

Table 31-2 outlines the expected findings of several diagnostic studies that may be applied to the evaluation of patients with malabsorption. Not all of the studies listed are necessarily performed in patients with suspected pancreatic insufficiency. The small-bowel x-ray series in pancreatic insufficiency may be abnormal in a nonspecific manner; that is, the barium may be diluted and segmented because of the increased intraluminal contents. Because pancreatic lipase is essential for fat digestion, the 24-hour quantitative fecal fat determination is elevated, sometimes in the range of 30 to 40 g.

The xylose tolerance test and small-bowel biopsy usually are not performed in patients with pancreatic insufficiency. If performed, they are normal. If the Schilling test is performed, it may indicate mild malabsorption of vitamin B_{12} because of the role the pancreas plays in facilitating vitamin B_{12} absorption (see section I.H). The bentiromide test is usually abnormal in patients with moderate-to-severe pancreatic insufficiency.

C. Treatment. Pancreatic enzyme preparations can be given orally to augment or replace endogenous enzymes. Because these tablets are inactivated rapidly by gastric acid, two to three tablets must be taken before, during, and after each meal. Supplemental acid-suppressive medications may prolong the activity of these preparations. Specially designed sustained-release pancreatic enzyme preparations, which are unaffected by gastric acid, are also available. A low-fat diet may be useful in the control of severe steatorrhea. Some patients require supplemental calcium, vitamin D, and other fat-soluble vitamins.

III. BILE ACID INSUFFICIENCY

A. Pathogenesis. Insufficient bile acids can result from a disorder at any step in the enterohepatic circulation of bile acids. In severe intrinsic liver disease, the liver may not produce enough bile acids; in partial biliary obstruction, the bile acids do not reach the intestinal lumen in sufficient concentration; in bacterial overgrowth of the small intestine, bile acids are deconjugated before they can participate in fat absorption; and in disorders of the terminal ileum, bile acids are not reabsorbed adequately to maintain the bile acid pool. Because bile acids facilitate the absorption of dietary fat by the formation of intraluminal micelles, a deficiency in bile acids results in malabsorption of fat. Absorption of protein and carbohydrate is normal.

B. Diagnosis. The upper gastrointestinal and small-bowel x-ray series usually are normal in bile acid insufficiency, unless the results suggest a lesion that obstructs the common bile duct; small-bowel stasis or diverticula, which may allow bacterial overgrowth; or terminal ileal disease.

Because bile acids facilitate but are not necessary for fat absorption, steatorrhea usually does not exceed 20 g per 24 hours. The bile acid breath test is abnormal if bacterial overgrowth or terminal ileal disease is present. A normal xylose tolerance test and a normal small-bowel biopsy are expected unless there is bacterial overgrowth. Bacterial overgrowth and disease of the terminal ileum also may cause abnormal results on the Schilling test.

C. The **treatment** of bile acid insufficiency varies with the cause. Improvement in the liver disease or relief of the biliary obstruction may be adequate.

1. **Small-bowel bacterial overgrowth.** Patients who have small-bowel bacterial overgrowth may respond to the administration of metronidazole or tetracycline or another broad-spectrum antibiotic or rifaximin (Xifaxan) 400 mg p.o. t.i.d. for 10 days more. If bile acid deficiency is not correctable, a reduction in dietary long-chain triglycerides is indicated. Medium-chain triglycerides, which do not require bile acids for absorption, can be used to supplement dietary fat. Additional fat-soluble vitamins may be indicated.

2. **Terminal ileal disorders.** Patients who have disorders of the terminal ileum may have malabsorption of vitamin B_{12} and of bile acids. An abnormal Schilling test in these patients indicates that they should receive monthly injections of vitamin B_{12}. When disease of the terminal ileum impairs bile acid absorption, the bile acids pass into the colon, where unconjugated dihydroxy bile acids inhibit the absorption of water and electrolytes. Thus, these patients may have both steatorrhea as a result of bile acid deficiency and watery diarrhea from the effects of bile acids on the colon. More extensive disease or resection of the terminal ileum predisposes to greater reductions in the bile acid pool, and steatorrhea predominates. In patients with lesser involvement, watery diarrhea is prominent, and steatorrhea may not be clinically evident.

Cholestyramine, which binds bile acids, may be taken orally to treat the watery diarrhea in patients who have less extensive disease or small resections. The dosage ranges from one-half packet (2 g) once or twice a day to several packets a day with meals. Because bound bile acids do not participate in fat absorption, the steatorrhea may actually worsen. In patients with little involvement of the terminal ileum, however, the net effect may be an improvement in the diarrhea. In patients with more extensive involvement in whom steatorrhea is aggravated by cholestyramine, supplemental medium-chain triglycerides may be necessary. Nearly all patients benefit from restriction of long-chain triglycerides (i.e., ordinary dietary fat).

If Crohn's disease is responsible for the terminal ileal dysfunction, treatment with mesalamines, sulfasalazine, immune modulating drugs, or steroids may be necessary (see Chapter 37).

IV. SMALL-BOWEL DISEASE

A. Mucosal disorders

1. **Pathogenesis.** A number of disorders of varying etiology affect the mucosa of the small intestine (see Chapter 5, section IV.C.3). Because all ingested foodstuffs are assimilated across the small-bowel mucosa, disorders that affect the mucosa have the potential for causing malabsorption of fat, protein, carbohydrate, vitamins, and minerals. Whether malabsorption is clinically significant depends on the site and extent of involvement. For example, in celiac sprue (gluten-sensitive enteropathy), the lesion begins first in the proximal intestine and extends distally. Because iron, calcium, and folate are absorbed preferentially in the proximal small bowel, these nutrients may not be absorbed normally in patients with celiac sprue. On the other hand, because Crohn's disease most often affects the distal ileum, which is the site of vitamin B_{12} and bile acid absorption, patients with Crohn's disease may have vitamin B_{12} and bile acid deficiency.

2. **Diagnosis**

   a. The **small-bowel x-ray series** usually is abnormal in small-bowel mucosal disease. It may be nonspecifically abnormal, showing dilatation of the bowel and dilution of the barium, such as in celiac sprue. In contrast, infiltrative disorders, such as Whipple's disease, lymphoma, or amyloidosis, cause thickening of the mucosal folds. Irregular mucosal contour and narrowed loops may suggest Crohn's disease.

   b. **Small-bowel biopsy.** When small-bowel mucosal disease is suspected, the question often is when to perform the small-bowel biopsy. Some physicians proceed directly to biopsy in the clinical setting of apparent panmalabsorption and an abnormal small-bowel x-ray series without clinical suspicion of pancreatic disease. Others first order a xylose tolerance test to confirm mucosal disease and obtain a 72-hour stool fat collection to quantitate the steatorrhea. A Schilling test usually is not performed. The small-bowel biopsy may or may not be diagnostic (see Chapter 5, section IV).

      i. **Celiac sprue (CS) (celiac disease/gluten-sensitive enteropathy)** is a chronic disorder. Classical presentation is with malabsorption, diarrhea, bloating, flatulence and weight loss. However, it can also present with anemia, chronic fatigue, fibromyalgia, short stature, infertility, seizures, osteopenia, and osteoporosis. It may coexist with autoimmune and connective tissue disorders (see Table 31-3). Patients with dermatitis herpetiformis (DH) often have the intestinal pathology; however, not all patients with CS have DH.

      Celiac sprue is most prevalent in non-Hispanic Caucasians, especially in persons of western European and Irish descent. The prevalence may be as high as 1:125 to 1:300 in the Western world. There is a 70% concordance rate in identical twins and a prevalence of 10% in first-degree relatives. HLA studies indicate that most celiacs possess DR3-DQ2 or DR5/7-DQ2 and some celiacs have DR-4-DQ8.

      Patients with celiac sprue have inappropriate mucosal T-cell response to ingested gluten or prolamines from dietary grains resulting in intestinal mucosal injury. The putative prolamines include gliadin in wheat, secalin in rye, and **hordein** in barley. **Avenin** in oats does not induce immunoreactivity.

      It is thought that **prolamines such as gliadin** form an immunogenic complex with tissue transglutaminase (tTG). This gliadia-tTG complex forms the substrate for antigliadin antiendomysial and anti-tTG antibodies. The resulting T-cell response mediates small intestinal mucosal damage.

      Diagnosis is confirmed with combination of clinical, serologic and histopathologic findings. **IgA and IgG antigliadin antibodies (AGA)** are sensitive but nonspecific. **Endomysial IgA antibody (EMA)** and **IgA tTG** have 95% sensitivity and specificity, especially in classic cases of CS. Both have lower sensitivity in patients with lesser degrees of villous atrophy.

TABLE 31-3	Conditions Associated with Celiac Disease

Disorder	Examples
Anemia	
Iron deficiency	Primary biliary cirrhosis
Folate deficiency	Primary sclerosing cholangitis
Vitamin B_{12} deficiency	
Prolonged prothrombin time	
Osteopenic bone disease	Autoimmune cholangitis
Short stature	
Idiopathic hepatits	
and cirrhosis	
Infertility	
Neuropsychiatric disorders	
Peripheral neuropathy	Lymphocytic gastritis
Ataxia	Lymphocytic colitis
Seizures	
Cognitive deficits	
Hyperactivity-attention deficit disorder	
IgA deficiency	Non-Hodgkin's lymphoma
IgA nephrolpathy	Intestinal T-cell lymphoma
	Intestinal adenocarcinoma
Type I diabetes mellitus	
Oropharyngeal and esophageal squamous	
cell carcinoma	
Autoimmune thyroid disease	
Autoimmune adrenal disease	
Sjögren's syndrome	
Systemic lupus erythematosis	
Rheumatoid arthritis	

To ascertain the diagnosis of celiac sprue, small-bowel biopsy is recommended since the mucosal involvement may be patchy. At least six distal duodenal sites should be biopsied during endoscopy. Biopsies should not be obtained from the duodenal bulb or the immediate post-bulbar duodenum since the presence of submucosal mucous glands in these areas may influence epithelial and mucosal histology. Diagnostic features include villous blunting; deepening of crypts; and increased intraepithelial lymphocytes (IEL), monocytes, and plasma cells.

Serologic tests should not replace small-intestinal biopsy findings for making the diagnosis of celiac sprue. However, if small-intestinal biopsies are unavailable, the presence of high titer EMA or IgA tTG is most suggestive of CS. Because IgA deficiency is common in patients with celiac sprue, IgA levels should be determined. In patients with IgA deficiency, IgG tTG may have value in diagnosing celiac sprue.

ii. **Other mucosal disorders.** The mucosal lesion of **Whipple's disease** is characterized by blunted villi that are distended by dense accumulations of periodic acid—Schiff (PAS)—positive macrophages. These PAS-positive macrophages contain the etiologic agent of Whipple's disease: *Tropheryma Whippelii*, a gram-positive actinomycete. *T. Whippelii* has also been isolated from pleural fluid, vitrous sample, and peripheral blood mononuclear cells by polymerase chain reaction.

Whipple's disease is a systemic disorder that usually presents with weight loss, cough, fever, diarrhea, hypotension, abdominal swelling, anemia, and mental status changes. PAS-positive macrophages may be found in the small bowel, pericardium, endocardium, synovia, lymph nodes, lung, brain, meninges, uvea, retina, and optic nerves. The disease in some instances may present as a sarcoidlike syndrome and involve the mediastinal nodes.

Other small-bowel mucosal disorders include abetalipoproteinemia, which is identified by villous epithelial cells that contain large fat vacuoles. The absence of plasma cells suggests agammaglobulinemia. Other disorders may or may not be evident on mucosal biopsy (see Chapter 5, section IV.C.3).

3. **Treatment.** A discussion of the clinical management of all the small-bowel mucosal disorders is beyond the scope of this book. The reader is referred to standard textbooks of medicine and gastroenterology.

a. **Celiac sprue.** The treatment of celiac sprue is primarily the rigorous restriction of all dietary gluten. The patient must avoid all wheat, barley, and rye. Rice, corn, soy, and the flours of these grains are acceptable. Sprue patients must also avoid many commercially prepared foods, such as some brands of ice cream, some desserts, and meats that contain wheat fillers. Even some vitamin and drug preparations are enclosed in capsules that contain small amounts of gluten, which may be sufficient to produce mucosal injury in some patients. Adjunctive treatment of sprue may include vitamin, calcium, and iron supplements.

b. **Whipple's disease.** Patients with Whipple's disease should receive procaine penicillin G, 1.2 million units per day intramuscular (IM) injection or intravenously, plus streptomycin 1 g per day IM for 2 weeks, followed by trimethoprim/sulfamethoxazole double-strength twice daily for 1 year.

c. The **mucosal lesion in other disorders,** such as intestinal lymphoma, parasitic infestations, and Crohn's disease, responds to treatment directed at the underlying disease. If clinically significant steatorrhea persists, restriction of dietary fat is indicated. Supplemental vitamins and minerals may be necessary.

B. **Specific absorptive defects**
1. **Lactase deficiency**
a. **Pathogenesis.** Primary lactase deficiency is an example of a defect in a specific brush border enzyme, lactase, which causes the malabsorption of the disaccharide lactose. Infants and young children in all populations and most white adults of North America and Europe normally have sufficient lactase to hydrolyze milk lactose to its constituents, glucose and galactose.

However, most of the adult populations of the world, including blacks, Asians, South and Central Americans, and Inuits, are typically "lactase-deficient." On a worldwide scale, therefore, whether the presence or lack of lactase is normal or abnormal depends on the population under consideration.

b. **Diagnosis.** People with lactase deficiency typically experience abdominal cramps and watery diarrhea within minutes after ingesting milk. These symptoms develop because the unhydrolyzed lactose is not absorbed and remains within the intestinal lumen, where it acts as an osmotic cathartic.

As the lactose passes into the lower bowel, bacterial action converts it to lactic acid and carbon dioxide, which contribute to the catharsis and cramping. The clinical history of abdominal cramps and diarrhea after milk ingestion usually is sufficient evidence of lactase deficiency. If the diagnosis is uncertain, however, a lactose tolerance test can be performed (see section I.G).

c. **Treatment** consists of restricting milk and milk products. Some milk is available commercially in which the lactose has been hydrolyzed.

2. **Abetalipoproteinemia**
a. **Pathogenesis.** Because lipoproteins are necessary for the formation of the apoprotein that combines with triglycerides, cholesterol, and phospholipids within the intestinal absorptive cells to form chylomicrons, the lack of beta-lipoproteins results in an accumulation of fat within the enterocyte and consequent fat malabsorption.

    b. Diagnosis. Stool fat is increased, but the small-bowel x-ray series and the xylose tolerance test are normal. Serum cholesterol and triglycerides are low, and beta-lipoproteins are absent. A small-bowel biopsy is diagnostic, showing villous epithelial cells distended with fat, but the appearance is otherwise normal.

    c. Treatment. There is no specific treatment of the underlying disease. The fat malabsorption improves with restriction of dietary long-chain triglycerides and substitution of medium-chain triglycerides, which do not require chylomicron formation but rather are absorbed directly from the villous epithelial cells into the blood. Fat-soluble vitamins also are indicated.

V. LYMPHATIC DISORDERS

  A. Pathogenesis. Obstruction of lymphatic drainage from the gut causes dilatation of the lymphatics (lymphangiectasia) and loss of fat and protein in the stool. In some patients, the disorder appears to be congenital or idiopathic. In others, there is an association with Whipple's disease, congestive heart failure, right-heart valvular disease, or frankly obstructive lesions, such as abdominal lymphoma, retroperitoneal fibrosis, retractile mesenteritis, mesenteric tuberculosis, and metastatic cancer.

  B. Diagnosis. Patients commonly seek treatment for weight loss, diarrhea, and edema caused by the decrease in plasma proteins. Some patients have chylous ascites. Barium examination of the small intestine may be normal, may have an appearance of nonspecific malabsorption, or may indicate a nodular mucosal pattern caused by distended or infiltrated villi. Steatorrhea usually is mild. The xylose tolerance test should be normal unless the underlying disease (e.g., lymphoma) has infiltrated the mucosa. Small-bowel biopsy should confirm the diagnosis by identifying dilated lymphatics within the cores of the villi.

  C. Treatment. In addition to undergoing treatment of any associated disorder that may be responsible for the lymphatic obstruction, patients with lymphatic disease should receive medium-chain triglycerides, limit their intake of long-chain triglycerides, and take supplemental fat-soluble vitamins.

VI. MIXED DEFECTS IN ABSORPTION

  A. Gastric acid hypersecretory states

    1. Pathogenesis. Malabsorption may accompany the Zollinger-Ellison syndrome and other gastric acid hypersecretory conditions. The large amounts of acid that reach the duodenum and proximal small intestine may have several adverse effects. First, there may be villous blunting and mucosal inflammation. These conditions may impair absorption in the proximal bowel. Second, the mucosal lesion may predispose to the inadequate release of cholecystokinin and secretin with consequent poor stimulation of gallbladder contraction and pancreatic secretion. Third, the acid environment in the duodenum also inactivates pancreatic enzymes and may precipitate glycine-conjugated bile acids, additionally impairing the digestion of fat, protein, and carbohydrate. Finally, in hypergastrinemic conditions, gastrin itself may inhibit absorption of water and electrolytes in the small bowel, which contributes to the diarrhea that occurs in some patients.

    2. Diagnosis and treatment. The upper gastrointestinal and small-bowel x-ray series may show peptic ulcerations in the stomach, duodenum, or proximal small intestine and may have a nonspecific malabsorption pattern. Other tests of malabsorption may or may not be abnormal, depending on the severity of the disease. The diagnosis and treatment of the Zollinger-Ellison syndrome and other hypersecretory conditions are discussed in Chapter 24.

  B. Postgastrectomy disorders. The multiple causes of malabsorption and maldigestion in patients after gastric surgery, and their diagnosis and treatment, are discussed in Chapter 28.

Selected Readings

Buchman AL, et al. AGA technical review on short bowel syndrome and intestinal transplantation. *Gastroenterology*. 2003;124:1111–1134.

Catassi C, et al. Association of celiac disease and intestinal lymphomas and other cancers. *Gastroenterology.* 2005;128:S79–S86.

Chitkara DK, et al. Gastrointestinal complications of cystic fibrosis. *Clin Perspect Gastroenterol.* July/August 2000:201.

Cureton P, The gluten-free diet: can your patient afford it? *Pract Gastroenterol.* 2007; xxxi(4):75–84.

Desai AA, et al. Bacterial overgrowth syndrome. *Curr Treatment Options Infect Dis.* 2003;5:189–196.

Dewar DH, et al. Clinical features and diagnosis of celiac disease. *Gastroenterology.* 2005;128:S19–S24.

Ginsburg PM, et al. Malabsorption testing: A review. *Curr Gastroenterol Rep.* 2000;2:370.

Graham DY, et al. Visible small intestinal mucosal injury in chronic NSAID users. *Clin Gastroenterol Hepatol.* 2005;3:55–59.

Kagnoff MF. Overview and pathogenesis of celiac disease. *Gastroenterology.* 2005;128: S10–S18.

Kupper C. Dietary guidelines and implementation for celiac disease. *Gastroenterology.* 2005;128:S121–S127.

Leung WK, et al. Small bowel enteropathy associated with chronic low-dose aspirin therapy. *Lancet.* 2007;369:614.

Rostom A, et al. The diagnostic accuracy of serologic tests for celiac disease: A systemic review. *Gastroenterology.* 2005;128:S38–S46.

Snow CF. Laboratory diagnosis of vitamin B_{12} and folate deficiency: A guide for the primary care physician. *Arch Intern Med.* 1999;159:1289.

Southerland JC, et al. Osteopenia and osteoporosis in gastrointestinal diseases: Diagnosis and treatment. *Curr Gastroenterol Rep.* 2001;3:399.

Sundaram A, et al. Nutritional management of the short bowel syndrome in adults. *J Clin Gastroenterol.* 2003;34:207–210.

Swartz MN. Whipple's disease—past, present, and future. *N Engl J Med.* 2000;342:647.

32 SMALL-INTESTINAL NEOPLASMS AND CARCINOID TUMORS

Neoplasms of the small intestine, either benign or malignant (Table 32-1), are unusual but not rare, comprising less than 5% of all gastrointestinal tumors. Because they are uncommon and relatively inaccessible to standard diagnostic studies, the diagnosis of small-bowel tumors is sometimes delayed.

I. DIAGNOSIS

A. Clinical presentation. Small-intestinal (SI) tumors usually occur in people over age 50. The presenting signs and symptoms are similar whether the tumors are benign or malignant. Small-bowel obstruction, either partial or complete, manifested by abdominal pain or vomiting or both, is a frequent presentation. Chronic partial obstruction may predispose to stasis and bacterial overgrowth, leading to bile acid deconjugation and malabsorption (see Chapter 31). Bleeding from the tumor or ulceration in association with the tumor also is common. Perforation of the bowel is rare. If a duodenal tumor is located in the vicinity of the ampulla of Vater, obstruction of the common bile duct may develop, resulting in biliary stasis and jaundice. Weight loss commonly accompanies malignant tumors.

The physical examination usually is nondiagnostic. Signs of small-bowel obstruction may be evident, such as a distended, tympanic abdomen and high-pitched bowel sounds. Occasionally malignant small-bowel tumors can be palpated. Stool may be positive for occult blood.

B. Laboratory and other diagnostic studies

1. Blood studies. Anemia may develop because of blood loss or malabsorption. Hypoalbuminemia can result from malabsorption, extensive metastatic liver disease, or chronic illness. Evaluation of serum alkaline phosphatase or bilirubin levels may indicate biliary obstruction or metastatic liver disease.

2. An upright plain x-ray film of the abdomen may show air-fluid levels in patients with small-bowel obstruction. If the obstruction is acute and does not resolve with nasogastric suction and intravenous fluids, surgery may be required without additional diagnostic testing.

3. Barium-contrast x-ray studies. The patient who has a small-bowel tumor without frank obstruction but perhaps with colicky pain or bleeding typically undergoes

---

TABLE 32-1 Neoplasms of the Small Intestine

Malignant	Benign
Adenocarcinoma	Adenoma
Lymphoma	Leiomyoma
Leiomyosarcoma	Lipoma
Carcinoid	Hamartoma
Metastatic tumors	Neurogenic tumors
Melanoma	Endometrioma
Kaposi's sarcoma	Inflammatory polyp

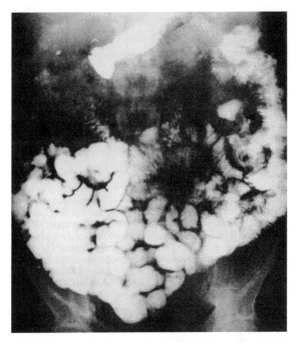

Figure 32-1. Small-bowel x-ray series showing a polypoid filling defect in the proximal small intestine (*arrow*). At surgical resection, the lesion was found to be a histiocytic lymphoma.

barium-contrast x-ray studies. The small-bowel series may show a polypoid lesion (Fig. 32-1) or the typical "napkin ring" deformity of adenocarcinoma encircling the bowel. Often the routine upper gastrointestinal x-ray series with small-bowel follow-through is nondiagnostic because the lesion is obscured by the large amount of barium in the small intestine. In these instances, a small-bowel enema, or enteroclysis, may delineate the lesion. This procedure is performed by passing a small tube into the proximal duodenum and instilling a small amount of barium with air. This provides excellent air–barium contrast of the small intestine and enhances the diagnostic capability. For example, a diffuse nodular appearance of the mucosa on barium-contrast study may suggest lymphoma.

4. **Endoscopy and biopsy.** If a lesion is within the duodenum, endoscopic examination and biopsy are indicated.
5. **Capsule endoscopy** may be used to directly visualize SI tumors. There is risk of the capsule being retained if the tumor is large.
6. **Ultrasound and computed tomography scan.** In patients with biliary obstruction, abdominal ultrasound may help define the lesion and identify dilated bile ducts. These patients also should undergo endoscopic retrograde cholangiopancreatography (ERCP) or percutaneous transhepatic cholangiography (PTC). Computed tomography (CT) scanning of the abdomen is useful in delineating mass lesions and surveying for metastatic disease to the liver, lymph nodes, and mesentery.
7. **Selective arteriography** of the celiac axis and superior mesenteric artery may be helpful to the surgeon in planning appropriate surgery.

II. TREATMENT
A. **Surgery.** The treatment of most small-bowel tumors, benign or malignant, is surgical. Even malignant tumors that have metastasized may require surgical palliation

for obstruction or bleeding. In patients with small-intestinal lymphoma, surgery may be required to make the diagnosis. The role of surgery in treating lymphoma depends on the extent of involvement and on local institutional protocols, which may include surgical resection in addition to radiotherapy and chemotherapy.

B. Radiation therapy and chemotherapy of other malignant small-bowel tumors have been largely ineffective.

C. Nutritional therapy. Patients who have undergone partial resection of the small intestine for a small-bowel tumor typically lose only a small portion of the bowel and thus do not suffer nutritionally as a consequence of the surgery. However, nutrition may be a clinical issue if the patient has extensive metastatic disease, the duodenum has been bypassed, or the terminal ileum has been resected. Bypass of the proximal small intestine leads to malabsorption of iron, calcium, and folate and to ineffective stimulation of pancreatic and biliary secretions. Terminal ileal resection may result in vitamin B_{12} and bile acid malabsorption, the latter leading to fat and fat-soluble vitamin malabsorption.

III. CARCINOID TUMORS. In the United States, the incidence of carcinoid tumors is approximately 8 per 100,000. Since most cases are asymptomatic and follow an indolent course, the true incidence may be higher.

Carcinoid tumors are most commonly found in the appendix, ileum, rectum, stomach, and lungs.

Carcinoid tumors are commonly classified according to their derivation from the embryonic gut: **foregut** (bronchial and gastric), **midgut** (small intestine [SI] and appendiceal), and **hindgut** (rectal). The clinical presentation and management of these tumors varies according to their site of origin.

Of the **foregut carcinoids, gastric carcinoids** are usually asymptomatic and are found incidentally; however, patients with **bronchial carcinoids** may present with cough, hemoptysis, postobstructive pneumonia, Cushing's syndrome, or carcinoid syndrome.

Midgut carcinoids, especially **small-intestinal carcinoids,** may cause intermittent SI obstruction or mesenteric ischemia. **Appendiceal carcinoids** are usually found incidentally. If there are metastases, carcinoid syndrome may occur.

Hindgut or rectal carcinoids are usually found incidentally, but may cause constipation and rectal bleeding. Carcinoid syndrome is rarely seen even if there are metastases.

A. Bronchial carcinoid tumors comprise about 2% of primary lung tumors. They usually present in the fifth decade of life and are rarely associated with carcinoid syndrome; however, they have been associated with ectopic ACTH secretion resulting in Cushing's syndrome. One third of patients, especially smokers, may present with atypical carcinoids which are much more aggressive and usually metastasize to the mediastinal lymph nodes. Surgery may be indicated.

B. Gastric carcinoid tumors make up less than 1% of gastric neoplasms. They are classified into three distinct groups:

   1. Type I: Associated with chronic atrophic gastritis

   2. Type II: Associated with the Zollinger-Ellison syndrome and ectopic gastric secretion

   3. Type III: Sporadic gastric carcinoids

     Both **type I and type II gastric carcinoids** are associated with achlorhydria and hypergastrinemia, which is thought to result in hyperplasia of the enterochromaffin cells in the stomach, leading to small, multiple carcinoid tumors. These tumors generally follow an indolent course and are rarely invasive. The small tumors may be resected endoscopically. Larger or recurrent tumors may require more extensive surgery. In patients with atrophic gastritis, antrectomy has been used to eliminate the source of the gastrin production to achieve tumor regression. In patients with Zollinger-Ellison syndrome, the use of somatostatin analogs has resulted in tumor regression.

     Between 15% and 25% of **gastric carcinoids** are sporadic and develop in the absence of hypergastrinemia. These are usually solitary and greater than 1 cm in size. They are frequently invasive, metastatic, and tend to pursue an aggressive clinical course. Sporadic gastric carcinoids have been associated with an atypical carcinoid syndrome which is primarily manifested by flushing through and thought to be mediated by histamine. Most of these tumors are treated with total gastrectomy.

C. **Small-intestinal carcinoid** tumors make up one third of all SI tumors and generally present in the sixth or seventh decade of life with abdominal pain and/or small-bowel obstruction (SBO). Between 5% and 7% may present with carcinoid syndrome and have liver metastases. These tumors are usually multicentric and grow into the SI wall. Detection is often difficult with SI barium x-rays or CT scan; however, their detection may be increased by the use of capsule endoscopy. Most SI carcinoid tumors are found in the distal ileum. The tumor size is an unreliable predictor of metastatic disease, since metastases have been reported from tumors smaller than 0.5 cm. Mesenteric fibrosis and mesenteric ischemia are often present with SI carcinoids. These tumors are also frequently associated with "buckling" or tethering of the SI due to extensive mesenteric involvement. Surgical resection of the SI primary tumor along with the mesenteric metastases leads to significant reduction in tumor-related obstruction and pain, and is therefore recommended even in patients with known metastatic disease.

D. **Appendiceal carcinoid tumors** are thought to arise from the subepithelial neuroendocrine cells and are more commonly diagnosed in younger patients, mostly during appendectomy. About 95% of appendiceal carcinoid tumors are smaller than 2 cm in diameter at the time of diagnosis and rarely associated with metastases. Tumors greater than 2 cm in diameter often have nodal or distant metastases. For this reason, simple appendectomy is the treatment of choice for smaller tumors; however, complete right colectomy is recommended for tumors larger than 2 cm. In elderly patients or patients with other comorbid conditions, simple appendectomy may be tried.

E. **Rectal carcinoid tumors** comprise only 1% to 2% of all rectal tumors and are usually found in the sixth decade of life. Fifty percent are asymptomatic and are usually found at colonoscopy. When symptoms occur, patients complain of rectal pain, constipation, and bleeding.

Rectal carcinoids of less than 1 cm in size are rarely metastatic and are successfully treated with local excision. The management of tumors larger than 1–2 cm is controversial. Endoscopic ultrasound is useful in examining extent of rectal wall invasion and those without invasion of the muscularis propria, local resection may suffice. Tumors larger than 2 cm, or those with invasion of the muscularis propria, may require low anterior resection or abdominoperineal resection.

F. **Metastatic carcinoid tumors**
   1. **Diagnosis.** Patients in whom metastases are suspected should be evaluated with **abdominal CT scan** to rule out liver metastases. Liver chemistry tests may be normal and are unreliable. Since carcinoid liver metastases are often hypervascular and may become isodense relative to the liver and may be missed with the administration of intravenous (IV) contrast, CT scan should be performed both with and without IV contrast administration.

   Somatostatin receptor scintography with IV administration of radiolabeled octreotide also provides a useful imaging modality for the detection of metastatic disease. Over 90% of neuroendocrine carcinoid tumors contain high concentrations of somatostatin receptors. The uptake of radiolabeled octreotide is also predictive of a clinical response to therapy with somatostatin analogs.

   Twenty-four-hour urinary serotonin metabolite **5-hydroxyndoleacetic acid (HIAA) levels** are elevated in about 75% of patients with metastatic carcinoid tumors of the midgut and not useful in patients with foregut (gastric and bronchial) and hindgut (rectal) carcinoid tumors.

   Chromogranin A (CGA) is a protein contained in the neurosecretory vesicles of neuroendocrine tumor cells. CGA concentrations in the blood are a more sensitive marker than urinary 5-HIAA levels in patients with carcinoid tumors. CGA levels greater than 5,000 mg/mL are associated with poor prognosis.

2. Treatment

a. Surgical resection of the involved liver segment(s), when possible, may provide long-term symptomatic relief and prolonged survival times.

b. Liver transplantation may be offered to patients with liver-isolated metastatic disease; however, the role of OLT in such patients is unclear.

c. Hepatic artery embolization may be used as a palliative procedure in patients with liver metastases who are not candidates for surgical resection. However, the duration of response may be brief, ranging from 4 to 24 months. Side effects may include renal failure, hepatic necrosis, and sepsis.

d. Radiofrequency ablation and cryoablation (either alone or in tandem with surgical resection) may be offered as less invasive procedure; however, efficacy, especially in patients with extensive hepatic metastases, has not been well studied.

e. Systemic therapy

i. Somatostatin analogs (i.e., **octreotide**) at a dose of 150 µg t.i.d. improves the symptoms of carcinoid syndrome in nearly 90% of patients. **Long-acting octreotide** at a dose of 20 mg intramuscularly may be administered once monthly with gradual increase in dose as needed to control symptoms. Patients may also use additional short-acting octreotide for breakthrough symptoms. **Lanreotide** (another somatostatin analog) has similar clinical efficacy. These drugs are well tolerated by patients; however, possible side effects include injection-site reactions, stearrhea, and hyperglycemia.

ii. Interferon-α (IFN) may be used alone or in combination with somatostatin analogs. The addition of IFN-α therapy to somatostatin analogs has been reported to be effective in controlling symptoms in patients with carcinoid syndrome who may be resistant to somatostatin analogs alone. The combination of these drugs may also significantly slow the rate of tumor progression in the majority of patients. Side effects of IFN-α therapy include bone marrow suppression (especially myelosuppression), autoimmune thyroid disease, fatigue, and depression.

iii. Chemotherapy. Streptozocin combined with fluorouracil (5-FU), cyclophosphamide, or doxorubicin have been used in patients with metastatic carcinoid disease with poor results. Even though there may be slight survival benefit with streptozocin and 5-FU, the renal toxicity, myelosuppression, nausea, vomiting, and fatigue limits the use of these drugs as first-line therapy.

iv. Newer agents in the treatment of metastatic carcinoid include radiolabeled somatostatin analog drugs, inhibiting binding of proangiogenic growth factor **(vascular endothelial growth factor, or VEGF)** to its receptor **(vascular endolethial growth factor receptor, or VEGFR)** with blocking antibodies such as **bevacizumab (Avastin)** and **sunitinib (Sutent).**

Selected Readings

Eamonn MM, et al. Small intestinal transplantation. *Curr Gastroenterol Rep.* 2001;3:408.

Gill SS, et al. Small intestinal neoplasms. *J Clin Gastroenterol.* 2001;33:267–282.

O'Neil BH. Management of carcinoid tumors and the carcinoid syndrome. *Clin Perspect Gastroenterol.* 2001;4:279.

IRRITABLE BOWEL SYNDROME 33

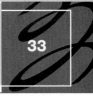

$\mathcal{T}$he **irritable bowel syndrome (IBS)** is the most common of all digestive disorders, affecting nearly everyone at one time or another and accounting for up to 50% of patients referred to a gastroenterology practice. Although characterized as a disorder of bowel motility, in many patients it usually is an exaggeration of normal physiologic responses and possibly heightened perception of pain.

Numerous terms have been used to describe the syndrome (Table 33-1). **Irritable bowel syndrome** seems to be the most appropriate. Terms that include the words *colon* or *colitis* are inaccurate because the condition is not limited to the colon, and inflammation is not a feature. Furthermore, use of the term *colitis* leads to confusion with ulcerative colitis and conveys an inaccurate impression to the patient.

In many patients IBS may be characterized as **diarrhea predominant (IBS-D), constipation predominant (IBS-C),** and for some patients, an **alternation of diarrhea with constipation (alternators).**

I. **PATHOGENESIS.** The causes and pathogenesis of IBS remain obscure. Nevertheless, clinical and laboratory evidence indicate that it most likely is a disorder of bowel motility and increased sensory perception of pain. Constipation and abdominal cramps are prominent complaints of many patients with **IBS-C.** These symptoms could be explained on the basis of hypertonic segmental contractions, which would slow transit by increasing the resistance to passage of feces. On the other hand, it is possible that patients with diarrhea **(IBS-D)** have a hypomotile bowel, which would decrease resistance to passage of feces, or that they simply have an increase in peristaltic contractions.

A. **Myoelectric activity of the colon** is composed of slow waves and spike potentials superimposed on the slow waves. In healthy individuals, slow-wave frequency ranges from 6 to 10 cycles per minute, although rates of 3 cycles per minute occur some of the time. The superimposed spike potentials take the form of short spike bursts and long spike bursts. The short spike bursts are less than 5 seconds and occur at the same time as the slow waves, resulting in muscular contractions of the same frequency as the slow waves. On the other hand, long spike bursts last from 15 seconds to several minutes and produce sustained contractions. Abnormalities in colonic myoelectric activity have been described in patients with IBS, but the findings have been inconsistent and, thus far, of no practical clinical use.

B. **Intestinal motor activity.** In patients with IBS the increase in colonic motor activity that normally occurs after eating is blunted but continues longer than in

TABLE 33-1	**Synonyms for Irritable Bowel Syndrome**
Irritable colon syndrome	Splenic flexure syndrome
Spastic bowel syndrome	Functional bowel disease
Spastic colitis	Psychophysiologic bowel disease
Mucous colitis	Nervous bowel

asymptomatic individuals and may even become stronger. Emotional stress also induces colonic motor activity, both in healthy individuals and in patients with IBS, but it is possible that symptoms are perceived to a greater degree in patients with IBS. Balloon distention of the rectosigmoid colon in patients with IBS causes spastic contractions of greater amplitude than in asymptomatic subjects. Furthermore, there is evidence that patients with IBS who complain of gaseous distention and abdominal cramps cannot tolerate quantities of small-bowel intraluminal gas that are easily tolerated by healthy individuals (see Chapter 34).

II. DIAGNOSIS
A. Clinical presentation
  1. Symptoms. Patients with IBS typically complain of crampy abdominal pain, diarrhea, or constipation. In some patients, chronic constipation is punctuated by brief episodes of diarrhea. A minority of patients have only diarrhea. Symptoms usually have been present for months to years, and it is common for patients with IBS to have consulted several physicians about their complaints and to have undergone one or more gastrointestinal evaluations.

  2. Timing of symptoms. The patient may be able to correlate symptoms with emotional stress, but often such a relation is not evident or becomes apparent only after careful questioning as the physician becomes acquainted with the patient. If abdominal cramps are a feature, they often are relieved temporarily by defecation. Bowel movements may be clustered in the morning or may occur throughout the day, but rarely is the patient awakened at night. Stools may be accompanied by an excessive amount of mucus, but blood is not present unless there is incidental bleeding from hemorrhoids.

  3. The differential diagnosis is broad, including most disorders that cause diarrhea and constipation (see Chapters 28, 29, 30, and 35). However, there are several features that suggest the diagnosis of IBS (Table 33-2). Several organic disorders may mimic IBS and, in fact, may be unrecognized for years in patients who mistakenly have been diagnosed as having IBS. Patients with **lactose intolerance** typically have postprandial diarrhea associated with crampy pain (see Chapter 31). They are healthy in all other respects. A careful history and a trial of a lactose-free diet usually are sufficient to make a diagnosis. **Celiac sprue, Crohn's disease,** and **endometriosis** also can masquerade as IBS because of the vagueness of the symptoms in many patients. A clinical history of postprandial abdominal pain suggests the possibility of **gallbladder, pancreatic, or peptic disease.** Because IBS may affect the entire digestive tract, belching and symptoms of gastroesophageal reflux and dyspepsia are common in patients with IBS.

  Anorexia, weight loss, fever, rectal bleeding, and **nocturnal diarrhea** all suggest a cause other than IBS for the patient's symptoms. The physician

---

TABLE 33-2 **Features Suggestive of Irritable Bowel Syndrome**

Characteristic	Uncharacteristic
Constipation or diarrhea or both	Anorexia
Crampy abdominal pain	Weight loss
Mucus in stools	Rectal bleeding
Symptoms related to stress	Fever
Weight stable or increasing	Nocturnal diarrhea
Appearance of health	Recent onset of symptoms
Chronic symptoms	

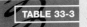

| TABLE 33-3 | Clinical and Laboratory Evaluation of Patients with Suspected Irritable Bowel Syndrome |

All patients	Selected patients

Stool for occult blood
If diarrhea, stool for leukocytes, ova,
    parasites, bacterial pathogens
	Ultrasound of gallbladder
	Abdominal and pelvic CT scan
	Serum amylase level
	Lactose tolerance test
	UGI endoscopy, colonoscopy and mucosal
	    biopsy of small bowel and colon

CT, computed tomography; UGI, upper gastrointestinal.

should remember, however, that other gastrointestinal disorders can develop in patients with IBS, thus one should be alert to a change in the patient's complaints.

4. **Physical examination.** Patients generally appear healthy, although they may be somewhat tense or anxious. If abdominal pain is a prominent symptom, voluntary guarding may be evident, and sometimes a tender, firm sigmoid colon is palpable. A thorough physical examination, including a rectal examination, is important in the evaluation for a non-IBS disorder.

B. **Diagnostic studies.** Because the diagnosis of IBS is largely one of exclusion, a number of clinical and laboratory studies should be performed to rule out other treatable disorders (Table 33-3). The extent of the evaluation depends on the age of the patient, nature of the patient's symptoms, and the adequacy of previous evaluations.

Again, it is important to note that patients with IBS are not immune to the development of other gastrointestinal disorders. Thus, the length of time that has elapsed since the last evaluation and the character of the current symptoms affect the decision of whether to proceed again with further diagnostic studies.

1. **Routine tests** such as a complete blood count, an erythrocyte sedimentation rate, and a stool test for occult blood are appropriate for all patients. If the patient complains of diarrhea, the stool should be examined for leukocytes, ova, parasites, and bacterial pathogens.

2. Whether **additional diagnostic studies** are indicated is a matter of judgment. If the postprandial pain is predominantly in the upper abdomen, ultrasonography of the gallbladder may be indicated to rule out gallstones. Postprandial pain also raises the possibility of pancreatic disease. If the clinical context is suggestive of a pancreatic disorder, a **serum amylase** level and perhaps a **computed tomography (CT) scan** of the abdomen are indicated. A **lactose tolerance test** may be necessary to confirm lactase deficiency in some patients. If there is blood in the stool, **colonoscopy** and an **upper-GI endoscopy** may be indicated. Lymphocytic and collagenous colitis can be diagnosed only by colonic mucosal biopsies. **Small-bowel biopsy** may be indicated to rule out small-intestinal mucosal disease (e.g., celiac sprue, Whipple's disease, Crohn's disease, and others). Because Crohn's disease can be confused with IBS, an upper gastrointestinal series with a small-bowel follow-through should be performed in patients with persistent abdominal pain, particularly if they have had some weight loss. In selected patients, capsule endoscopy may be helpful.

III. TREATMENT (TABLE 33-4)

A. **Emotional support.** Making the diagnosis of IBS is sufficient in some patients to alleviate anxiety about their symptoms. In particular, patients who suffer from cancer phobia are relieved to learn that they are cancer-free. However, most

TABLE 33-4	Treatment of Irritable Bowel Syndrome

All patients	Anticholinergics–antispasmodics
Reassurance and emotional support	(e.g., dicyclomine hydrochloride
Stress reduction	[Bentyl], 10–20 mg b.i.d.–q.i.d.)
Judicious use of tricyclic	Patients with diarrhea
antidepressants and serotonin	Antidiarrheal agents (e.g.,
reuptake inhibitors	diphenoxylate hydrochloride
Patients with abdominal pain and	[Lomotil], 2.5–5.0 mg, or loperamide
constipation	hydrochloride [Imodium], 2 mg q6h
Increase dietary fiber	p.r.n.)
Stool softeners (e.g., Colace)	Increase dietary fiber
Laxatives (e.g., lactulose, MiraLax,	Tricyclic antidepressants
and Senokot)	

b.i.d., twice a day; q.i.d., four times a day; p.r.n., as needed.

patients with IBS experience no relief merely from reassurance. Many have carried the diagnosis of IBS for years and continue to experience distressful symptoms despite supportive reassurance and diet and drug therapy. Although these patients often understand that they have a "nervous bowel," that understanding does little to alleviate symptoms, and they continue to seek treatment. Stress reduction programs may be helpful.

B. Diet and fiber therapy. The commonsense approach to diet therapy is the most appropriate. There is no need for bland or highly restrictive diets in the treatment of IBS. Patients should avoid foods that they find cause symptoms. If lactose-containing foods produce cramps and diarrhea, these should be eliminated from the diet.

The role of fiber in the treatment of IBS has been controversial. However, clinical experience suggests that a high-fiber diet and/or fiber supplements provide symptomatic relief in some patients. Patients with crampy abdominal pain and constipation seem most likely to benefit, although sometimes patients with watery diarrhea also experience a firming of their stools after the fiber content of the diet has been increased. However, fiber supplements may result in increased gas and bloating due to bacterial fiber.

C. Drug therapy

  1. Antispasmodics. Unfortunately, drug therapy of IBS often is empiric. Patients with diarrhea and abdominal pain may benefit from a so-called antispasmodic. These drugs are anticholinergic in their mode of action, but whether they actually relieve spasm is conjectural. A reasonable choice is **dicyclomine hydrochloride, 10 to 20 mg three to four times daily** because it is less likely than others to cause unpleasant nongastrointestinal anticholinergic side effects. Regardless of what preparation is used, patients should be cautioned about the possibility of the development of dry mouth, blurred vision, and urinary retention.

  2. Laxatives should be used judiciously in the treatment of the IBS with constipation (IBS-C). However, many patients with constipation become dependent on the long-term use of laxatives and may need to be withdrawn from these agents.

  3. Tegaserod (Zelnorm), a partial 5-HT$_4$ agonist, has clinical efficacy in the treatment of IBS-C in female patients up to age 65. It facilitates the secretion of serotonin within the intestinal wall and thus enhances peristalsis through the GI tract. It is contraindicated in patients with cardiovascular risk factors. (Zelnorm has been removed from the U.S. market by the manufacturer for further evaluation of its safety in long-term use.)

4. **Lubiprostone (Amitiza)** is indicated in the treatment of chronic constipation in both male and female adults of all ages. It increases small- and large-intestinal stool transit by increasing the stool fluid content and volume. Its mode of action is stimulation of chloride channels of the intestinal mucosal and facilitation of chloride and water secretion into the small-intestinal lumen. Since excess water and eletrolytes are reabsorbed in the colon it does not result in systemic electrolyte or water imbalance.

5. **Diphenoxylate hydrochloride (Lomotil) and loperamidehydrochloride (Imodium).** The diarrhea of IBS often responds to low doses of diphenoxylate or loperamide hydrochloride (see Table 33-4). These drugs are synthetic opioids with low potential for abuse. They control diarrhea by reducing gastrointestinal motility and by inhibiting watery secretion. **Loperamide hydrochloride (Imodium)** may be preferred for long-term use because of its longer duration of action. Also, it does not cross the blood–brain barrier and thus is less likely to cause addiction.

6. **Tranquilizers and antidepressants** may be useful in selected patients for the short-term management of situational anxiety and depression. Low-dose tricyclic antidepressants such as **amitriptyline hydrochloride (Elavil)** or **desipramine hydrochloride (Norpramin)** may be helpful in some patients with diarrhea-predominant IBS. **Serotonin uptake inhibitors (SSRIs)** such as fluoxetine hydrochloride (Prozac), sertraline hydrochloride (Zoloft), and paroxetine (Paxil) may help some patients with IBS. **Cymbalta,** a newer psychotropic agent, may also be useful.

Selected Readings

Cash BD, et al. Fresh perspectives in chronic constipation and other functional bowel disorders. *Rev. Gastroenterol Disord.* 2007;7(3):116–133.

Hammer J, et al. Disturbed bowel habits in patients with non-ulcer dyspepsia. *Ailment Pharmacol Ther.* 2006;24:405–I0.

Henningsen P, et al. Management of functional somatic syndromes. *Lancet.* 2007;369:946–955.

Johanson JF, et al. A dose-ranging, double-blind, placebo-controlled study of lubiprostone in subjects with irritable bowel syndrome and constipation (c-IBS). *Gastroenterology.* 2006;130(4 suppl 2):A-131.

Longstreth GF, et al. Functional bowel disorders. *Gastroenterology.* 2006;130:1480–1491.

Marshall JK, et al. Post-infectious irritable bowel syndrome (IBS) after the Walkerton outbreak of waterborne gastroenteritis (GE). *Gastroenterology.* 2006;130(4 suppl 2): A-T1160.

Pimentel M, et al. A 10 day course of rifaximin, a nonabsorbable antibiotic, produces a durable improvement in all symptoms of irritable bowel syndrome: A double-blind, randomized controlled study. *Gastroenterology.* 2006;130(4 suppl 2):A-134.

Quigley EMM. The use of probiotics in functional bowel disease. *Gastroenterol Clin North Am.* 2005;34:533–545.

Saier MH Jr, et al. Priobiotics and prebiotics in human health. *J Mol Microbiol Biotechnol.* 2005;10:22–25.

Sander DS, et al. Association of adult coeliac disease with irritable bowel syndrome: A case-controlled study in patients fulfilling ROME II criteria referred to secondary care. *Lancet.* 2001;358:1504–1508.

Spiller R. Clinical update: irritable bowel syndrome. *Lancet.* 2007;369:1586–1588.

Tack J, et al. A randomized controlled trial assessing the efficacy and safety or repeated tegaserod therapy in women with irritable bowel syndrome with constipation. *Gut.* 2005;54(12):1707–1713.

Tack J, et al. Functional gastroduodenal disorders. *Gastroenterology.* 2006;I30:I466–79.

34   INTESTINAL GAS AND BLOATING

$\mathcal{G}$as occurs normally within the gastrointestinal tract, yet many patients complain of excessive gas. The complaint of gas has no uniform connotation. Some patients mean that they belch too much, others experience abdominal discomfort and attribute it to gas, whereas still others regard the amount of flatus passed as being excessive.

I. COMPOSITION AND SOURCES OF INTESTINAL GAS

A. Composition. Nitrogen, oxygen, carbon dioxide, hydrogen, and methane make up more than 99% of the volume of intestinal gas. Their proportions vary widely in healthy people (Table 34-1). These five gases are odorless; the characteristic odor of flatus is conferred by a combination of trace gases that together constitute no more than 1% of the total volume of intestinal gas. The odoriferous trace gases include ammonia, hydrogen sulfide, volatile amino acids, and short-chain fatty acids.

B. Sources. All people swallow air in variable amounts. Swallowed air is the major source of nitrogen and oxygen (Fig. 34-1). Nitrogen and oxygen also diffuse from the blood into the intestinal lumen. Oxygen is largely consumed by intestinal aerobic bacteria.

Large amounts of carbon dioxide are generated by neutralization of gastric acid, fatty acids, and amino acids within the upper gastrointestinal tract. Carbonated drinks also provide an exogenous source of carbon dioxide. Most carbon dioxide within the upper gastrointestinal tract is absorbed and excreted by the lungs. Carbon dioxide in flatus is derived largely from the action of bacteria on intestinal substrates. Bacterial action on intestinal substrates also produces hydrogen and, in about one third of adults, methane.

TABLE 34-1   **Composition and Sources of Intestinal Gas**

Gas	Amount (%)	Sources
Nitrogen	25–80	Swallowed air, diffusion from blood
Oxygen	0.1–2.5	Swallowed air, diffusion from blood
Carbon dioxide	4.5–30.0	Neutralization of gastric acid, fatty
acids, and		amino acids by bicarbonate
		Ingestion of carbonated beverages
		Bacterial action on intestinal substrates
Hydrogen	0.5–50.0	Bacterial action on intestinal substrates
Methane	0–25	Bacterial action on intestinal substrates
Trace gases (ammonia,	<1	Bacterial and digestive action on
hydrogen sulfide,		intestinal substrates
volatile amino acids,		
short-chain fatty acids)		

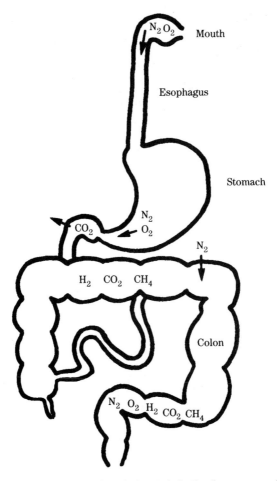

Figure 34-1. Diagram of the gastrointestinal tract, indicating the sources and composition of intestinal gas. (From Eastwood GL. *Core Textbook of Gastroenterology.* Philadelphia: Lippincott Williams & Wilkins; 1984:188. Reprinted with permission.)

II. PATHOGENESIS. Patients with gaseous symptoms may complain of belching, abdominal pain and bloating, or of excessive flatus. The pathogenesis of each condition is different. Also, there is considerable overlap in the patients who complain of gas and bloating and those with irritable bowel syndrome (see Chapter 33).

    A. Belching is caused by the eructation of swallowed air. If the normal volume of swallowed air cannot be passed into the proximal small bowel because of a motility disorder, gastroparesis or gastric outlet obstruction, or due to an incompetent lower esophageal sphincter (LES), belching may develop. Thus, patients with gastroesophageal reflux disease (GERD), gastric carcinoma, peptic ulcer disease, or uremia may complain of belching.

    Patients with gallbladder disease often belch for unknown reasons. Sometimes belching is a nervous habit, and the swallowed air may not even reach the stomach before eructation takes place. Rarely, belching of feculent-smelling gas indicates chronic gastric stasis or a gastrocolic fistula.

B. Abdominal pain and bloating are often attributed to an excess of gas. In some instances, failure to adequately digest a component of food (e.g., lactase deficiency) with consequent bacterial degradation and gas production is responsible for the abdominal pain and bloating. In other patients, the cause of symptoms is unclear. When patients with abdominal pain and bloating who did not have specific food intolerance were compared to healthy people, they did not differ with respect to volume or content of intestinal gas, either under fasting conditions or after a meal. However, patients with gaseous complaints seem to have more reflux of gas from the duodenum into the stomach and experience painful symptoms after infusion of gas into the proximal small bowel in volumes that are well tolerated by healthy people. Thus, patients who complain of bloating and abdominal gas may be suffering from a defect in gut motility and a decreased threshold to pain rather than from too much gas. As indicated previously, some of these patients may suffer from irritable bowel syndrome.

C. Excessive flatulence may result from a disorder of intestinal motility but usually is a consequence of increased amounts of gas produced by the action of bacteria on dietary substrates. Lactase deficiency is a good example, although the list of dietary substrates that could be implicated is virtually endless. Bacterial degradation of undigested carbohydrates and simple sugars also cause gas and bloating.

III. DIAGNOSIS

A. Belching. A careful history may identify nervous air swallowing or ingestion of excessive quantities of carbonated beverages. An abdominal ultrasound examination to evaluate the gallbladder and either an upper gastrointestinal (GI) x-ray series or endoscopy to evaluate the proximal gastrointestinal tract may be indicated.

B. Abdominal pain and bloating. Patients who complain of abdominal pain and bloating present a different diagnostic problem. Some have intolerance for a specific dietary component, such as lactose. Other organic diseases must be considered, such as celiac sprue, regional enteritis, recurrent partial small-bowel obstruction, or even giardiasis. The evaluation of such patients usually includes ultrasound of the abdomen, Esophagogastroduodenoscopy (EGD), biopsy, upper GI and small-bowel x-ray series, and, if stools are loose, stool examination for ova, parasites, and bacterial pathogens and possibly colonoscopy and biopsy.

C. Excessive flatus. Complaints of excessive flatus should be evaluated by a search for a specific food or group of foods that may be causing symptoms.

IV. TREATMENT.

Unless a specific diagnosis such as gallstones, peptic ulcer, or lactase deficiency is made, the treatment of patients who complain of gas is often unrewarding. Patients with nervous air swallowing may improve simply by becoming aware of their air swallowing. Elimination of milk, legumes, cabbage, and similar foods, and white-sugar- and flour-containing foods may be effective in patients who complain of abdominal pain, gas, bloating, or flatus. Extensive elimination diets are helpful in occasional patients who have the perseverance to eliminate one dietary constituent at a time each week for several weeks.

In patients who do not have a demonstrable, treatable disorder or in whom a specific food has not been implicated, so-called antispasmodic agents, such as dicyclomine hydrochloride, or bulking agents sometimes are useful. However, bulking agents, because they contain nondigestible substrates, have the potential for increasing flatus. Some patients have responded to stress-reduction techniques or psychological counseling.

Selected Readings

Camilleri M. Treating irritable bowel syndrome: Overview, perspective and future therapies. *Br J Pharmacol.* 2004;141:1237–1248.

Comilleri M. Diabetic gastroparesis. *New Engl J Med.* 2007;356:820–829.

Floch MH. Use of diet and probiotic therapy in the irritable bowel syndrome: Analysis of the literature. *J Clin Gastroenterol.* 2005;39(4 suppl 3):S243–S246.

Levitt MD, et al. The relation of passage of gas and abdominal bloating to colonic gas production. *Ann Intern Med.* 1996;124:422.

Levitt MD, et al. Evaluation of an extremely flatulent patient, case report and proposed diagnostic and therapeutic approach. *Am J Gastroenterol.* 1998;93:2276.

Pimentel M, et al. Eradication of small intestinal bacterial overgrowth reduces symptoms of irritable bowel syndrome. *Am J Gastroenterol.* 2000;95(12):3503–3506.

Poredenoord AJ, et al. Physiologic and pathologic belching. *Clin Gastroenterol Hepatol.* 2007;5(7):772–775.

Reddymason S, et al. New methodology in assessing gastric emptyizing and gastrointestinal transit. *US Gastroenterol Rev.* 2007;1:19–22.

Reid G. Porbiotics in gastrointestinal management—what's new. *US Gastroenterol Rev.* 2007;1:66–75.

Serra J, et al. Intestinal gas dynamics and tolerance in humans. *Gastroenterology.* 1998; 115:542.

Spiller R. Clinical update: irritable bowel syndrome. *Lancet.* 2007;369:1586–1588.

Spiller RC. Postinfectious irritable bowel syndrome. *Gastroenterology.* 2003;124:1662–1671.

Suarez FL, et al. An understanding of excessive intestinal gas. *Curr Gastroenterol Rep.* 2000;2:413.

Suarez FL, et al. Intestinal gas. *Clin Perspect Gastroenterol.* July/August 2000:209.

35   DIVERTICULAR DISEASE

$\mathcal{T}$he term **diverticular disease** generally refers to diverticulosis of the colon and its complications. However, diverticula can occur throughout the gastrointestinal tract. In the esophagus, diverticula may be associated with dysphagia (see Chapter 21). Diverticula of the stomach usually are asymptomatic. In the small intestine, they can predispose to bacterial overgrowth and malabsorption (see Chapter 31). In this chapter, we confine the discussion to diverticula of the colon.

Colonic diverticulosis is exceedingly common in westernized countries. The prevalence of diverticula increases with age: About 30% of the general population at age 60 and about 80% at age 80 have colonic diverticula. Although 90% of people with diverticula remain asymptomatic, because of the high prevalence of the condition, symptomatic diverticular disease occurs frequently.

I. **DEFINITIONS.** Several of the terms used to describe colonic diverticula and their complications have caused confusion or have been misused. Thus, it is important to review some terminology (Table 35-1).

A single outpocketing from the bowel wall is called a **diverticulum.** Because *diverticulum* is a Latin neuter word, it ends in *um,* and its plural form ends in *a.* Thus several outpocketings are referred to as **diverticula,** not *diverticuli* or *diverticulae.*

The presence of a diverticulum or diverticula is called **diverticulosis.** Diverticulosis does not imply a pathologic condition or set of symptoms. Diverticulitis means inflammation in one or more diverticula. Sometimes the diagnosis of diverticulitis is assumed on the basis of clinical symptoms (see section IV.A.1) that may overlap with the symptoms of irritable bowel syndrome (see Chapter 33) and gaseousness (see Chapter 34). In the absence of firm evidence for diverticulitis, perhaps a more general term should be used, such as *diverticular disease* or *symptomatic diverticulosis.*

II. **PATHOGENESIS.** True diverticula, that is, those in which the walls contain all layers of the bowel, are found occasionally in the colon. However, the most prevalent colonic diverticula are pseudodiverticula. These are herniations of mucosa and submucosa through the muscularis propria at the sites of penetration of the nutrient arteries. The development of diverticula seems to be related to increased pressure within the lumen of the bowel, which over time causes the herniations. Most diverticula occur in the sigmoid and descending colons, although they also may be found more proximally.

Epidemiologically, the prevalence of colonic diverticulosis is related to age and diet. The condition is much more frequent in populations in which dietary fiber has been replaced by refined carbohydrates.

TABLE 35-1   Terminology of Diverticulosis
Diverticulum—singular
Diverticula—plural
Diverticulosis—the presence of one or more diverticula
Diverticulitis—inflammation in one or more diverticula
Diverticular disease—any complication of diverticulosis

III. SYMPTOMATIC DIVERTICULOSIS
A. Diagnosis

1. **Clinical presentation.** Most people with colonic diverticula are asymptomatic. However, some patients complain of chronic or intermittent left lower abdominal pain. Typically, these patients also report infrequent bowel movements or constipation. Flatulence and dyspepsia may accompany the lower abdominal pain. In many patients, symptoms of irritable bowel syndrome and of diverticular disease are indistinguishable.

   The physical examination may reveal tenderness and a firm, feces-filled sigmoid colon in the left lower abdomen. By rectal examination, the stool may be firm, and tests for occult blood are usually negative.

2. **Diagnostic studies.** It is a matter of clinical judgment whether patients with mild symptoms of diverticular disease require diagnostic studies if they are otherwise healthy. However, patients who consult a physician for a particular complaint usually are concerned enough that additional investigation is warranted. Certainly, diagnostic studies are indicated if the patient is anorectic or has lost weight or if there is blood in the stool.

   A complete blood count and urinalysis are appropriate initial laboratory studies. These should be followed by CT scan of abdomen and pelvis, sigmoidoscopy, and barium enema x-ray or colonoscopic examination (Fig. 35-1). In many patients with symptomatic diverticulosis, the evaluation is similar to that for irritable bowel syndrome (see Chapter 33).

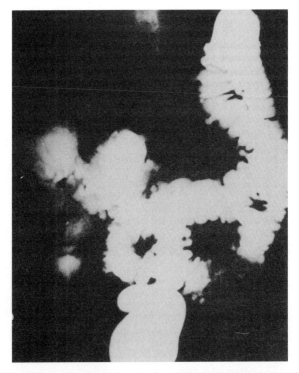

Figure 35-1. Barium enema x-ray examination showing extensive diverticulosis throughout the colon. Note the numerous barium-filled pockets protruding outside the bowel lumen. The distortion of the normal mucosal architecture by diverticulosis sometimes makes it difficult to exclude carcinoma or polyp by barium enema examination.

3. **The differential diagnosis** includes the irritable bowel syndrome, frank diverticulitis (see section IV), carcinoma of the colon, Crohn's disease or proctocolitis, urologic disorders, and gynecologic disorders.

B. **Treatment.** In many respects, the treatment of uncomplicated symptomatic diverticulosis resembles the treatment of irritable bowel syndrome (see Chapter 33). A high-fiber diet has been shown to alleviate the discomfort of diverticular disease. Fiber also can be added in the form of unprocessed bran and other hydrophilic bulk laxatives, such as Metamucil. Antispasmodic–anticholinergic drugs, such as dicyclomine hydrochloride, may be useful in the treatment of crampy abdominal pain. In constipated patients, lubiprostone (Amitiza) may be preferred to induce softer stools. Cathartic laxatives should be avoided.

IV. DIVERTICULITIS
A. Diagnosis
1. **Clinical presentation.** The point at which symptomatic diverticulosis becomes diverticulitis may be difficult to determine in some patients. Fully developed diverticulitis is characterized by acute lower abdominal pain, fever, and tachycardia. The lower abdomen is tender to palpation, and there may be rebound tenderness. The patient may present with an acute abdomen (see Chapter 13); more typically, symptoms evolve over several hours or days. A mass in the lower abdomen may connote an abscess or inflammatory phlegmon. Bowel sounds may be active if partial or complete obstruction has occurred, or they may be hypoactive or absent if peritonitis has developed. A rectal examination may help localize the abscess or inflammatory mass.

   In some patients with chronic diverticulitis, chronic inflammatory changes may develop that resemble inflammatory bowel disease (IBD) or Crohn's disease.

2. **Diagnostic studies**
   a. **Blood studies.** The white blood cell count typically is elevated in acute diverticulitis, with a predominance of immature forms (left shift) in the differential count. Hemoglobin and hematocrit levels may reflect hemoconcentration.
   b. A **urinalysis** may show white blood cells and red blood cells. An unusual complication of diverticulitis is a colonic–urinary bladder (colovesical) fistula; in this condition, the urine contains large numbers of white blood cells and bacteria and possibly feces. Patients with colovesical fistulas frequently complain of pneumaturia.
   c. **Plain abdominal x-ray films,** both supine and upright, should be obtained. Air-fluid levels suggest ileus or obstruction. Free air in the abdomen, indicating a perforated diverticulum, may be evident on lateral decubitus abdominal films or under the diaphragm on the upright chest x-ray film.
   d. **Computed tomography (CT) scan** and/or **ultrasound** of the abdomen and pelvis are helpful in identifying the inflammatory mass or an abscess cavity and by demonstrating other conditions in the differential diagnosis, such as an ovarian cyst.
   e. **Sigmoidoscopy, colonoscopy, and barium enema x-ray examinations.** Sigmoidoscopy or colonoscopy may be performed cautiously if perforation is not suspected. However, it is best to delay these tests until symptoms have subsided. The radiologic diagnosis of diverticulitis by barium enema requires evidence of perforation of a colonic diverticulum by demonstrating either a fistulous tract or an abscess cavity. Although these findings are unequivocal, they are not necessary to make the clinical diagnosis of diverticulitis. Acute lower abdominal pain in association with fever and an elevated white blood cell count in a person with demonstrated diverticula are sufficient.

3. The **differential diagnosis** includes inflammatory bowel disease, infectious *C. difficile* or ischemic colitis, carcinoma of the colon, other causes of bowel obstruction, gynecologic disorders (e.g., ruptured ovarian cyst), and urologic disorders (e.g., renal colic).

B. Treatment

1. **General.** Patients with severe acute diverticulitis are best treated by allowing nothing by mouth and administering intravenous fluids and electrolytes. Intravenous broad-spectrum antibiotics, such as the combination of ampicillin, gentamicin, and ciprofloxacin hydrochloride or second- or third-generation cephalosporin and metronidazole, are indicated and should be continued for 10 to 14 days. If an abscess is identified by ultrasonography or CT scan, percutaneous drainage under ultrasound or CT guidance should be considered. Patients whose symptoms are less severe may be treated with oral antibiotics (e.g., ciprofloxacin hydrochloride 500 mg p.o. b.i.d. or Levaquin 500 mg q.d. and metronidazole 250–500 mg p.o. t.i.d. for 10–14 days).

2. **Surgery.** Few would argue that generalized peritonitis, with or without evidence of free perforation, should be treated surgically. Unresolved obstruction and colovesical fistula also are indications for surgical treatment. Because most patients with uncomplicated diverticulitis recover with medical treatment and do not have recurrences of acute disease, surgery is not recommended routinely. However, failure to improve after several days of medical treatment or recurrence after successful treatment are indications for surgery in a patient whose operative risk is reasonable.

   A one-stage procedure with resection and primary anastomosis is ideal. If active infection is evident, a primary resection with a proximal colostomy, followed several months later by reanastomosis, may be indicated. Alternatively, the surgeon may elect to perform a proximal diverting colostomy as the primary operation, allowing the infection and inflammation to resolve, before proceeding at a later date with the resection and anastomosis.

V. Diverticular bleeding is one of the most common causes of lower gastrointestinal bleeding in older people. The clinical dictum is that diverticular bleeding and acute diverticulitis rarely coexist. However, it is likely that some degree of peridiverticular inflammation is present in patients who bleed from diverticula. (See Chapter 14 for a discussion of the diagnosis and treatment of diverticular bleeding.)

Selected Readings

Anaya DA, et al. Risk of emergency colectomy and colostomy in patients with diverticular disease. *Arch Surg.* 2005;140:681–685.

Chapman JR, et al. Diverticulitis: a progressive disease? Do multiple recurrences predict less favorable outcomes? *Ann Surg.* 2006;243:876–883.

Constantinide VA, et al. Primary resection with anastomosis is Hartman's procedure in nonelectric surgery for acute colonic diverticulitis: a systematic review. *Dis Colon Rectum.* 2006;49:966–981.

Jacobs DO. Diverticulitis. *N Eng J Med.* 2007;357:2057–2066.

Jensen DM, et al. Urgent colonoscopy for diagnosis and treatment of severe diverticular hemorrhage. *N Engl J Med.* 2000;342:78.

Korzenik JR. Case closed? Diverticulitis: epidemiology and fiber. *J Clin Gastroenterol.* 2006;40: Suppl 3:S112–S116.

Kumar RR, et al. Factors affecting the successful management of intraabdominal abcesses with antibiotics and the need for percutaneous drainage. *Dis Colon Rectum.* 2006;49:183–189.

Mueller MH, et al. Long-term outcome of conservative treatment in patients with divrticulitis of the sigmoid colon. *Eur J Gastroenterol Hepatol.* 2005;17:649–654.

Parra-Blanco A. Colonic diverticular disease: pathophysiology and clinical picture. *Digestion.* 2006; 73(suppl)1:47–57.

Rafferty J, et al. Buie and the Standards Committee of the American Society of Colon and Rectal Surgeons. Practice parameters for sigmoid diverticulitis. *Dis. Colon Rectum.* 2006;49:939–944.

Ramirez FC, et al. Successful endoscopic hemostasis of bleeding colonic diverticula with epinephrine injections. *Gastrointest Endosc.* 1996;43:167.

Salzman H, et al. Diveticular disease: diagnosis and treatment. *Am Fam Physician.* 2005;72:1229–1234.

Stollman N, et al. Diverticular disease of the colon. *Lancet.* 2004;363:631–639.

Zaidi E, et al. CT and clinical features of acute diverticultis in an urban U.S. population: rising frequency in young, obese adults. *AJR Am J Roentgenol.* 2006;187:689–694.

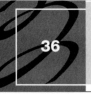

CONSTIPATION AND FECAL IMPACTION

$\mathcal{C}$onstipation, like diarrhea, is difficult to define with precision due to the wide variation in normal bowel habits. However, because 95% of people have at least three bowel movements per week, for practical purposes constipation can be defined as a condition in which fewer than three stools per week are passed. In addition, patients may experience difficulty in passing stools, may use manual maneuvers (i.e., digital disimpaction, pressing on the perineum and/or lower abdomen), and may complain of hard and lumpy stools.

The economic costs of constipation are impressive. In the United States, more than $250 million is spent annually on laxatives. Additional costs of unknown magnitude are incurred in the evaluation of patients for underlying disorders that may predispose to constipation.

I. **ETIOLOGY AND DIFFERENTIAL DIAGNOSIS.** Constipation is a symptom, not a disease. It may develop as a functional condition, in which case it appears to be related to changes in bowel motility or pelvic floor dysfunction; or it may be a secondary condition, such as symptomatic diverticular disease or irritable bowel syndrome; or it may result from a specific abnormality or disorder, such as an obstructing cancer of the colon or hypothyroidism or other causes as listed in Table 36-1.

A. **Diet.** Functional or idiopathic constipation occurs with somewhat greater frequency in women and increases in prevalence with age in both sexes. It appears to be influenced by the composition of the diet, particularly the fiber and fluid content. Normal daily stool weight in the United States ranges from 100 to 200 g, and the stool is composed of about 80% water. Increasing the dietary fiber and fluid intake increases the stool weight, primarily because of retained water, and increases the stool frequency.

Recent evidence also indicates that several grams of dietary carbohydrates and polysaccharides found in fruits and vegetables normally pass undigested to the colon, where they are metabolized by bacteria to osmotically active particles and cathartic agents. Thus, a diet low in fruits and vegetables may contribute to constipation.

B. **Lack of exercise** also is associated with constipation. It's difficult to determine whether this is the major predisposing factor to constipation of bedridden patients and elderly people and if their poor dietary intake of fiber, carbohydrates, and fluids is an additional important factor.

C. **Colonic obstruction.** Some patients with an obstructing lesion, such as a sigmoid carcinoma or a fecal impaction, may have diarrhea (overflow diarrhea), characterized by the frequent passage of small amounts of loose or liquid stool. This is because the stool water proximal to the obstruction is poorly absorbed and seeps around the obstruction. The physician must be attentive in recognizing this condition in such patients to avoid inappropriate treatment with antidiarrheal medications, which would only worsen the underlying disorder.

II. **DIAGNOSIS**
A. **Clinical presentation**
1. **History.** To paraphrase a common saying, "One man's constipation is another man's diarrhea." Thus it is important that the physician determine what the patient means by *constipation.* How frequently are stools passed? What is their

TABLE 36-1	Differential Diagnosis of Constipation

"Functional" constipation
Conditions in which constipation is part of the symptom complex
    Irritable bowel syndrome
    Symptomatic diverticular disease
    Disorders of bowel muscle function (e.g., pseudoobstruction, myotonic dystrophy, systemic sclerosis)
Disorders that can cause constipation
    Endocrine–metabolic conditions (e.g., diabetes, hypokalemia, hypothyroidism, hypercalcemia, pregnancy)
    Bowel obstruction (e.g., neoplasm, benign stricture, ischemic colitis, surgical stenosis)
Disorders causing painful passage of stool (e.g., proctitis, anal fissure)
Neurogenic disorders (e.g., Hirschsprung's disease [aganglionosis], autonomic neuropathy, multiple sclerosis, Parkinson's disease)
Drugs (e.g., calcium channel blockers, nitrates, anticholinergics, antidepressants, opiates)

consistency? Is the condition **acute** or **chronic?** Are there associated signs or symptoms, such as weight loss, abdominal pain, or blood in the stool?

Constipation of long duration accompanied by crampy abdominal pain without weight loss or systemic symptoms suggests functional or idiopathic constipation, irritable bowel syndrome, or symptomatic diverticular disease. On the other hand, constipation of recent onset, blood in the stool, or change in the stool caliber suggests another causative disorder, such as carcinoma of the lower bowel. A history of calcium channel blocker, anticholinergic, or opiate drug intake should be sought as a possible explanation for constipation.

2. The **physical examination** may give a clue to systemic disease, such as hypothyroidism or a neurologic disorder. An abdominal mass may indicate an obstructing lesion or merely firm stool in the colon. The character of the stool itself and the tone of the anal sphincter as well as the possible presence of anal fissures, painful hemorrhoids, and rectal prolapse can also be determined by rectal examination.

B. **Diagnostic studies.** Most patients who have constipation that is severe enough to cause them to consult a physician require some diagnostic evaluation beyond the history, physical examination, and stool testing for occult blood. The extent of the evaluation varies according to the individual circumstances, but in general, a minimal evaluation of constipation may include serum electrolytes, thyroid function studies, blood glucose, serum calcium, and a colonoscopic examination if indicated.

Anorectal manometry (see Chapter 8, section III) is helpful in making the diagnosis of the rare disorder **Hirschsprung's disease** (aganglionosis of the distal colon or rectum). The normal relaxation of the internal anal sphincter is absent in Hirschsprung's disease when the rectum is distended by stool or a balloon. However, some patients with long-standing constipation in whom the rectal vault remains chronically distended may also have an abnormal rectoanal reflex. The barium enema in Hirschsprung's disease characteristically shows a narrow rectum, corresponding to the aganglionic segment. For best results, the barium enema should be performed in an unprepared bowel, that is, with stool in the distal colon. Rectal biopsies are of value only if they show the presence of ganglia, thus ruling out Hirschsprung's disease. Sampling error and failure to obtain deep enough tissue may yield inadequate specimens. The absence of ganglia does not necessarily imply Hirschsprung's disease, however. If the diagnosis remains in question, a full-thickness surgical biopsy of the rectal wall may be necessary.

III. Treatment of constipation involves addressing a number of issues, including lifestyle, diet, and medications. If a specific cause of constipation is identified, therapy of course includes treatment of the cause.

  A. Lifestyle. Some patients literally do not take time to have a bowel movement. Their busy schedules require frequent cortical inhibition of the urge to defecate. Although it may be difficult to put in practice, simply recognizing the urge to defecate and acting on it may be the first step for many patients in achieving normal bowel habits. A program of mild exercise (e.g., walking) for sedentary patients may also be helpful.

  B. Diet. The average daily intake of crude fiber in the United States is about 4 g. This is roughly one fifth of the daily intake of the native populations of some areas in Africa, who typically have four or five bulky stools per day. Because fiber is hydrophilic, increasing the fiber intake should produce large stools that require more frequent passage.

    Dietary fiber can be increased by eating fruits, vegetables, potato skins, and bran-containing foods. Some patients find it easier to consume fiber in the form of raw, unprocessed bran, 1 to 2 tablespoons per day, or a commercial product such as Metamucil. Bran or commercial fiber supplements should be mixed in water or juice before ingestion. Increasing total daily intake of water to 1 to 2 L augments the laxative effects of dietary fiber.

  C. Laxatives. Most patients with chronic constipation have had ample experience with laxatives. Sometimes a vicious cycle develops: Constipation is relieved by laxatives or cathartics; because the bowel has been evacuated, the patient has no urge to pass stool for several days and becomes concerned; the patient perceives constipation again and resumes intake of laxatives.

    The chronic use of laxatives is to be avoided, although from time to time a laxative may be necessary to relieve constipation.

    1. Mineral oil. Virtually any patient with functional constipation responds to mineral oil, provided enough is given. The initial dosage is 1 tablespoon a day, preferably taken in the morning while the patient is upright for several hours after taking it. If that amount is ineffective, the dosage can be increased by 1 tablespoon each day until constipation is relieved, up to a maximum of 4 tablespoons. Mineral oil should be avoided in patients who might aspirate it since lupoid pneumonia may occur. Also, it should not be taken chronically because of its interference with the absorption of fat-soluble vitamins.

    2. Lactulose. If a patient has a genuine need for frequent laxation, a reasonable alternative to the traditional laxatives and cathartics is lactulose. Lactulose is a disaccharide that is not absorbed but is metabolized by colonic bacteria to osmotically active particles. It also acidifies the stool by the production of lactic acid. The usual dosage is 1 to 2 tablespoons one to four times daily. Lactulose may also be given in powder form. (See Chapter 17 for discussion of the use of lactulose in the treatment of hepatic encephalopathy.)

    3. Polyethylene glycol (PEG) laxative, MiraLax, or GlycoLax may be used daily to lubricate the stool and relieve constipation. The usual dose is one to four glasses each day. This agent is indicated only for short-term use.

    4. Tegaserod (Zelnorm) is a partial 5-HT4 agonist that increases gastrointestinal motility by facilitating the release of serotonin in the Auerbach's plexus. It has been shown to increase spontaneous bowel movements when taken 6 mg twice daily. It is indicated in adults up to age 65 and is not recommended for patients who may have intraabdominal adhesions, gallbladder disease or cardiovascular risk factors. However, it has been removed from the market in the U.S.

    5. Lubiprostone (Amitiza) is novel agent approved by the FDA for the treatment of chronic idiopathic constipation in adults, regardless of age and gender. It works intraluminally by enhancing chloride ion and water secretion into the intestinal lumen by stimulating the chloride-2 channels found in crypts in the apical membrane of intestine (especially in the small intestine [SI]). The increased stool water increases stool volume and intestinal transit. The excess water and electrolytes are reabsorbed in the proximal colon. This mechanism of action results in soft stools and predictable bowel function. In the studies, there were no electrolyte or fluid imbalances or drug–drug interactions. Recommended dose is 24 µg p.o. b.i.d. Clinical studies show that it is also effective in the treatment of IBS-C.

IV. FECAL IMPACTION. Impaction of a firm, immovable mass of stool is found most often in the rectum but may occur within the sigmoid or descending colon. Fecal impaction typically develops in elderly, inactive patients, but the differential diagnosis is the same as for ordinary constipation, ranging from functional constipation to hypotonic bowel disorders to distal bowel obstruction (Table 36-1).

Regardless of the underlying cause, the treatment consists of several approaches. First, the impaction may be broken manually during digital rectal examination. If that attempt is not completely successful, the mass can be softened and evacuated by warm water or saline lavage through a sigmoidoscope or rectal tube. Sometimes glycerine suppositories or mineral oil enemas are useful. Oral mineral oil may be administered if there is no risk of aspiration. Occasionally dilatation of the anus under general anesthesia is used to gain access to the fecal impaction. Rarely, surgical removal of the impaction is necessary.

Selected Readings

Brandt LJ, et al. Systematic review on the management of chronic constipation in North America. *Am J Gastroenterol.* 2005;100:S5–S22.

Camilleri M, et al. Effect of a selective chloride activator, lubiprostone, on gastrointestinal transit, gastric sensory and motor functions in healthy volunteers. *Am J Physiol Gastrointest Liver Physiol.* 2006;290:G942–G947.

Cash BD, et al. Fresh perspectives in chronic constipation and other functional bowel disorders. *Rev. Gastroenterol Disord.* 2007;7(3):116–133.

Chiaroni G, et al. Biofeedback is superior to laxatives for normal transit constipation due to pelvic floor dyssynergia. *Gastroenterology.* 2006;130:675–664.

Dukas L, et al. Association between physical activity, fiber intake, and other lifestyle variable and constipation in a study of women. *Am J Gastroenterol.* 2003;98:1790–1796.

Ehrenpreis E. Constipation, colonic inertia and colonic marker studies. *Pract Gastroenterol.* 2001;24:18.

Fernandez-Banares F. Nutritional care of the patient with constipation. *Best Pract Res Clin Gastroenterol.* 2006;20:575–587.

Kamm MA, et al. Tegaserod for the treatment of chronic constipation: A randomized, double-blind placebo-controlled multinational study. *Am J Gastroenterol.* 2005;100: 362–372.

Kamm, MA. Clinical case: Chronic constipation. *Gastroenterology.* 2006;131:233–239.

Lembo A, et al. Chronic constipation. *N Engl J Med.* 2003;349:1360–1368.

Muller-Lissner SA, et al. Myths and misconceptions about chronic constipation. *Am J Gastroenterol.* 2005;100:232–242.

Rao SS. Constipation: Evaluation and treatment. *Gastroenterol Clin North Am.* 2003;32: 659–683.

Talley NJ. Definition, epidemiology, and impact of chronic constipation. *Rev Gastroenterol Disord.* 2004;4(suppl 2):S3–S10.

Ueno R, et al. Evaluation of safety and efficacy in a twelve-month study of lubiprostone for the treatment of chronic idiopathic constipation. *Am J Gastroenterol.* 2006;101:S491. Abstract 1269.

Wald A. Chronic constipation: advances in management. *Neurogastroenterol Motil.* 2007; 19:4–10.

37 INFLAMMATORY BOWEL DISEASE

$\int$**nflammatory bowel disease (IBD)** refers to the idiopathic inflammatory bowel disorders, ulcerative colitis, Crohn's disease, and microscopic or lymphocytic and collagenous colitis. Clearly, a number of other conditions also are associated with inflammation, including bacterial and parasitic infections, ischemic bowel disease, and radiation colitis. Nevertheless, until the causes of ulcerative colitis and Crohn's disease are identified, the term *inflammatory bowel disease* serves a useful purpose in distinguishing these conditions from other bowel disorders.

IBD has a prevalence of 0.3% to 0.5% in the adult U.S. population with a slight female preponderance. It is most commonly seen in young patients between the ages of 15 and 25; however, there is second peak in the incidence of IBD at 40 to 60 years. Approximately 15% of patients with IBD have close relatives who also have IBD.

I. **DISTINGUISHING FEATURES OF ULCERATIVE COLITIS (UC) VERSUS CROHN'S DISEASE (Table 37-1).** Ulcerative colitis is an inflammatory disorder of the mucosa of the rectum and colon. The rectum is virtually always involved, and if any portion of the remaining colon is involved, it is in a contiguous manner extending proximally from the rectum. On the other hand, Crohn's disease typically affects all layers of the bowel wall and may do so usually in a patchy distribution throughout the entire gastrointestinal (GI) tract. Crohn's disease may involve any part of the GI tract from the mouth to the anus, most frequently involves the terminal ileum. Approximately one third of cases involve the small bowel only, one third involve the colon only, and one third involve both the colon and the small bowel. The rectum may be spared. Crohn's disease in the elderly usually involves only the colon. Crohn's disease of the esophagus, stomach, and duodenum is rare, but may present alone or in combination with involvement of the other segments of the GI tract.

Patients with Crohn's disease may have predominantly inflammatory, obstructive, or perianal disease. Chronic inflammation leads to fibrosis and strictures. Fistulas may connect the diseased bowel with another bowel loop (enteroenteric), the bladder (enterovesical), vagina, or skin (enterocutaneous). The presentation of Crohn's disease

TABLE 37-1 **Distinguishing Features of Ulcerative Colitis versus Crohn's Disease**

Ulcerative colitis	Crohn's disease
Pain crampy, lower abdominal, relieved by bowel movement	Pain constant, often in right lower quadrant, not relieved by bowel movement
Bloody stool	Stool usually not grossly bloody
No abdominal mass	Abdominal mass, often in right lower quadrant
Affects only colon	May affect small and large bowel, occasionally esophagus and stomach
Mucosal disease (granulomas are not a feature)	Transmural disease (granulomas found in a minority of patients)
Continuous from rectum	May be discontinuous (skip areas)

| TABLE 37-2 | Extraintestinal Manifestations of Inflammatory Bowel Disease |

Common to both ulcerative colitis and Crohn's disease		Conditions related to Crohn's disease
Area	**Condition**	
Joints	Peripheral arthritis	Gallstones
	Sacroiliitis	Renal oxylate stones
	Ankylosing spondylitis	Vitamin B_{12} deficiency
Skin	Erythema nodosum	Malabsorption
	Pyoderma gangrenosum	Anemia
Eyes	Conjunctivitis	Obstructive hydronephrosis
	Iritis	
	Episcleritis	
Liver	Fatty infiltration	
	Chronic active hepatitis	
	Pericholangitis	
	Sclerosing cholangitis	
	Bile duct carcinoma	
Kidneys	Pyelonephritis	
	Renal stones	
General	Amyloidosis	
	Anemia	

varies with the site and degree of involvement. It may be gradual in onset or may present with recurrent episodes of abdominal pain, diarrhea, and/or low-grade fever. Physical examination may reveal a right lower quadrant mass or tenderness, anal fissures, perianal abscess, or fistulas. Some 10% to 15% of patients with either ulcerative colitis or Crohn's disease have extraintestinal manifestations of the disease (Table 37-2).

In most patients, the two disorders can be distinguished on clinical, radiologic, and pathologic grounds. However, in about 20% of patients with IBD affecting the colon, it is impossible to make a definitive diagnosis **(indeterminate colitis).**

II. ETIOLOGY. Because the causes of IBD are not known, the pathophysiology of the disorders is incompletely understood. An immunologic mechanism in the pathogenesis is assumed, but the inciting causes are incompletely understood. The intestinal flora, various cytokines including tumor necrosis factor (TNF) and some of the interleukins, and other factors are thought to play a role in the ongoing inflammatory process.

Hereditary factors appear to play a role; patients with ulcerative colitis or Crohn's disease have a 10% to 15% chance of having a first- or second-degree relative who also has one or the other type of IBD.

III. DIFFERENTIAL DIAGNOSIS. A variety of conditions can cause intestinal inflammation and present with signs and symptoms similar to those of ulcerative colitis or Crohn's disease. These conditions are summarized in Table 37-3.

The bacterial and parasitic colitides must be considered in all patients with new-onset bloody diarrhea and rectal or colonic mucosal inflammation; also, some infections are associated with exacerbations of known idiopathic IBD. Thus, stool examinations for ova and parasites, bacterial pathogens, and *Clostridium difficile* toxin is indicated. Eosinophilic colitis–enteritis is a variation of IBD of unknown etiology. It may represent an allergic reaction of the mucosa to allergen.

TABLE 37-3	Differential Diagnosis of Inflammatory Bowel Disease

Bacterial colitis	Behçet's colitis
Campylobacter	Sexually transmitted colitis
Shigella	Gonococcus
Salmonella	Chlamydia
Escherichia coli (invasive)	Herpes
Clostridium difficile–associated colitis	Trauma
Parasitic colitis	Crohn's disease look-alikes
Amebiasis	Lymphoma
Schistosomiasis	*Yersinia*
Ischemic colitis	Tuberculosis
Radiation colitis	

Ischemic colitis, which may occur in patients with cardiac arrhythmias or cardiovascular disease, or individuals taking estrogen, birth control pills, or estrogen agonists (SERMs), can be confused with IBD, particularly Crohn's disease, because of its segmental distribution and tendency to produce strictures.

Radiation bowel injury may involve any portion of the GI tract but typically affects the rectum or sigmoid colon in patients who have received pelvic irradiation. Acute radiation injury occurs during or shortly after the radiation treatment, but chronic radiation colitis, which is a form of ischemic bowel disease, may occur months to years later.

Because lymphoma, *Yersinia enterocolitis*, and tuberculosis often involve the distal small intestine and the cecum, they may be confused with Crohn's disease. The diagnosis of lymphoma may be made by biopsy of enlarged lymph glands or other involved organs. Sometimes laparotomy is necessary. *Y. enterocolitis* can be diagnosed by stool cultures or serologic tests. Enteric tuberculosis is rare in the United States but should be suspected in patients from areas of the world in which the disease is endemic.

IV. CLINICAL PRESENTATION
A. History
    1. Signs and symptoms. Patients with ulcerative colitis typically complain of bloody stool. If the inflammation is confined to the rectum, stools may be formed. Patients may even present with constipation. More extensive involvement of the colon is associated with bloody diarrhea caused by the diminution in absorption of water, electrolytes, and oxidation by the affected mucosa. Crampy lower abdominal pain is temporarily relieved by bowel movements.

        Patients with Crohn's disease usually have a history of additional chronic signs and symptoms, such as fatigue, weight loss, and persistent abdominal pain, often in the right lower quadrant. Blood in the stool occurs if there is colonic involvement. Stools are often formed but may be loose if there is extensive involvement of the colon or if there is disease of the terminal ileum. The latter causes diarrhea because of the malabsorption of bile salts and the consequent inhibition of water and electrolyte absorption in the colon. Bile acid malabsorption also may reduce the bile acid pool, which leads not only to fat malabsorption but also to supersaturation of cholesterol in bile in the gallbladder and risk of development of cholesterol gallstones. The fat malabsorption also predisposes to oxalate renal stones. The inflammatory nature of Crohn's disease can be responsible for several complications outside the bowel, including hydronephrosis due to ureteral obstruction and pneumaturia secondary to an enterovesical fistula.

    2. Onset and course of symptoms. Both Crohn's disease and ulcerative colitis typically begin in childhood or early adulthood, although ulcerative colitis may develop in patients of any age; a second peak in incidence of Crohn's disease occurs in the elderly, in whom the illness can be confused with ischemic bowel disease. Most patients with ulcerative colitis experience intermittent exacerbations with nearly complete remissions between attacks.

In ulcerative colitis, about 5% to 10% of patients have one attack without subsequent symptoms for decades. A similar number have continuous symptoms, and some have a fulminating course requiring total proctocolectomy. Patients with Crohn's disease generally have recurrent symptoms of varying frequency.

3. **Growth retardation and failure to develop sexual maturity** are common in children and adolescents with ulcerative colitis or Crohn's disease. In fact, these complications may be the primary reason for the patient to consult a physician. Growth failure is rarely caused by endocrine abnormalities but rather is a consequence of reduced caloric and nutritional intake or utilization. Treatment of the ulcerative colitis or Crohn's disease, with attention to good nutrition, usually results in reestablishment of normal growth and development.

B. **Physical examination.** Patients with IBD often are thin and undernourished. Pallor due to anemia of blood loss or chronic disease may be evident. Tachycardia may result from dehydration and diminished blood volume, and a low-grade fever may be present. Mild-to-moderate abdominal tenderness is characteristic of ulcerative colitis. A tender mass in the right lower quadrant is typical of Crohn's disease. The rectal examination in patients with ulcerative colitis reveals bloody stool or frank blood, whereas in Crohn's disease, perianal scarring or fistulas may be identified. Abdominal distention, rebound tenderness, absence of bowel sounds, and high fever suggest toxic megacolon or abscess (see section VII.A). Extraintestinal manifestations of IBD may be evident (Table 37-2).

V. **DIAGNOSTIC STUDIES.** IBD is diagnosed based on integration of clinical, endoscopic, histopathologic, radiologic, and other imaging data.

A. **Laboratory studies.** A complete blood count (CBC), urinalysis, and serum chemistry tests are appropriate during the initial evaluation of a patient with suspected IBD.

Serologic examination of blood for specific antibodies, such as ANCA, is recommended. Several different serologic markers for IBD have been identified, including perinuclear antineutrophil cytoplasmic antibodies (pANCA), antibodies to Saccharomyces cerevisiae (ASCA), pancreatic antibodies (PAB), antibodies to the outer membrane Porin C of *Escherichia coli* (anti-Omp C), antibodies to a DNA sequence from *Pseudomonas Fluorescens* (anti-12) and anti-C B 1 flagellin.

These antibodies are not sufficiently sensitive to be used to screen for IBD in the general population. However, they may be helpful for predicting the phenotype of IBD. The finding of ASCA+/pANCA− predicted Crohn's disease in 80% to 95%, the finding of pANCA+/ASCA− predicted ulcerative colitis in about 90% of patients tested. Several studies suggest that Crohn's disease patients with more positive serologies and higher titers are more likely to have complications such as strictures, fistulae, perforations, and requirement for surgery.

Several commercial laboratories offer "panels" of the serologic markers using computerized recognition patterns to distinguish subtypes of IBD (CD vs. UC).

B. **Examination of the stool.** Stool from patients suspected of having ulcerative colitis should be examined for leukocytes and ova and parasites, cultured for bacterial pathogens including *Escherichia coli* O157:47, *Campylobacter jejuni*, and *Yersinia enterocolitica* and tested for C. *difficile* toxin titer.

1. **Fecal leukocytes** are common to most inflammatory conditions of the colon but are not common in irritable bowel syndrome or noncolonic diarrhea.

2. Examination for **ova and parasites** may establish the diagnosis of amebiasis, although the sensitivity of stool examination for amebae is lower than 40%. The serum indirect hemagglutination and gel diffusion precipitant tests are more than 90% sensitive for amebic infection. It is particularly important to obtain several fresh stool samples for examination of ova and parasites before barium-contrast studies are performed because the presence of barium in the GI tract can obscure ova and parasites for a week or more.

3. **Bacterial pathogens** may be identified by stool culture. Of particular interest is ***Campylobacter jejuni*** ileocolitis, which may present with acute, colicky lower

abdominal pain, fever, bloody diarrhea with mucus, and many of the endoscopic, radiologic, and histologic features of ulcerative colitis. The disease typically subsides within several days but may run a protracted course, in which case treatment with erythromycin or ciprofluxin may provide relief of symptoms.

Another pathogen that may complicate the diagnosis of ulcerative colitis is **C. difficile,** the bacterial agent that has been implicated in antibiotic-associated pseudomembranous colitis. *C. difficile* may be relevant to ulcerative colitis in two ways. First, antibiotic-associated colitis may be confused with ulcerative colitis. Second, *C. difficile* may be responsible for exacerbations of preexisting ulcerative colitis. When chronic ulcerative colitis is in remission, the demonstration of *C. difficile* toxin in the stool is probably related to recent treatment with sulfasalazine or antibiotics. Colonic infection with enteroinvasive *E. coli,* especially *E. coli* O157:H7, may resemble ulcerative colitis and present with similar findings.

C. **Flexible sigmoidoscopy or colonoscopy** is indicated in the evaluation of rectal bleeding of any cause. The normal rectal and colonic mucosa appears pink and glistening. When the bowel is distended by insufflated air, the submucosal vessels can be seen. Normally, there is no bleeding when the mucosa is stroked with a cotton swab or touched gently with the tip of the sigmoidoscope.

In ulcerative colitis, the mucosal surface becomes irregular and granular. The mucosa is friable, meaning that it bleeds easily when touched. With more severe inflammation, bleeding may be spontaneous. These findings are nonspecific and may be seen in most of the conditions listed in Table 37-3. In some patients with chronic ulcerative colitis, pseudopolyps develop. The rectal mucosa is normal in patients who have Crohn's disease without rectal involvement. If the disease does affect the rectum, the appearance may be similar to that of ulcerative colitis or may include aphthous, deep or linear ulcerations and fissures.

D. **Mucosal biopsy.** Sigmoidoscopic or colonoscopic mucosal biopsies in patients with IBD generally are safe; however, they should not be performed if toxic megacolon is suspected. In ulcerative colitis, the histopathology of the rectal mucosa may show a range of abnormal findings. These include infiltration of the mucosa with inflammatory cells, flattening of the surface epithelial cells, a decrease in goblet cells, thinning of the mucosa, branching of crypts, and crypt abscesses (Fig. 37-1). All of these findings, including crypt abscesses, are nonspecific and may be seen in other colitides, including Crohn's disease, bacterial colitis, and amebiasis. Because endoscopic biopsies include mucosa and a variable proportion of submucosa, the transmural nature of Crohn's disease cannot be appreciated. However, substantial submucosal inflammation or fissuring of the mucosa may suggest Crohn's disease. The finding of noncaseating granulomas also strongly favors a diagnosis of Crohn's disease (Fig. 37-2), but granulomas are identified infrequently in mucosal biopsies from patients with established Crohn's disease and may accompany other conditions, such as tuberculosis and lymphogranuloma venereum. The identification of amebic trophozoites by biopsy confirms that diagnosis. Large numbers of mucosal eosinophils are typical of eosinophilic colitis.

E. **Radiography**
1. The **plain film of the abdomen** usually is normal in patients with mild-to-moderate IBD. Air in the colon may provide sufficient contrast to indicate loss of haustral markings and shortening of the bowel in ulcerative colitis or narrowing of the bowel lumen in Crohn's disease.

In severe colitis of any cause, the transverse colon may become dilated (Fig. 37-3). When this finding is accompanied by fever, elevated white cell count, and abdominal tenderness, toxic megacolon is likely (see section VII.A). The plain film of the abdomen should be repeated once or twice a day in patients with toxic megacolon to follow the course of colonic dilatation.

2. **Computed tomography (CT) of the abdomen and pelvis** may be very informative in patients presenting with chronic or recurrent abdominal pain and suspicion of IBD. Abdominal masses and abscesses, fistulas, and, most commonly, inflammatory thickening of the involved bowel wall may facilitate the diagnosis of IBD.

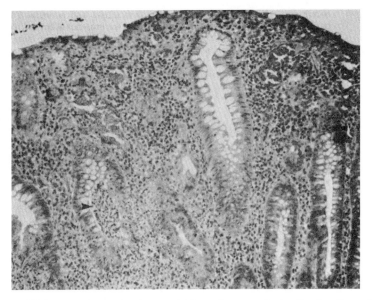

Figure 37-1. Photomicrograph of a rectal biopsy from a patient with ulcerative colitis. Inflammatory cells predominate in the lamina propria. The surface epithelial cells are flattened, and the number of goblet cells appears to be decreased. A crypt abscess is evident (*arrow*).

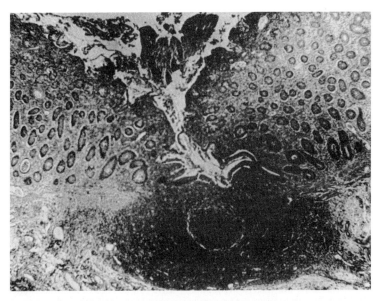

Figure 37-2. Photomicrograph of the mucosa and submucosa within a resected portion of terminal ileum from a patient with Crohn's disease. A fissure extends through the mucosa to the submucosa. At the base of the fissure is a granuloma. (From Eastwood GL. *Core Textbook of Gastroenterology.* Philadelphia: Lippincott Williams & Wilkins; 1984:137. Reprinted with permission.)

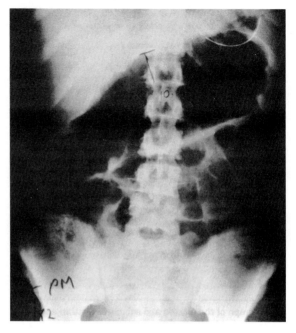

Figure 37-3. Plain abdominal x-ray film of a patient with toxic megacolon showing dilatation of the transverse colon.

3. **CT enterography and colography** are much more sensitive than UGI, SBFT, and barium enema and should be preferred when available.
4. **Barium enema** should not be performed in patients who are acutely ill with colitis because of the possibility that the preparation for barium enema or the procedure itself may precipitate toxic megacolon. Even in patients with mild-to-moderate colitis, vigorous cathartic preparation for barium enema should be avoided. Rather, oral PEG electrolyte solutions are preferable to prepare patients for barium enema or colonoscopy.

   Some patients with early ulcerative colitis have normal findings on barium enema examination. Double-contrast studies, however, usually reveal a diffuse granular appearance of the mucosa. Loss of haustration, ulcerations, pseudopolyps, and shortening of the bowel are later developments (Fig. 37-4). Sometimes an area of narrowing requires differentiating between a benign stricture and carcinoma. Reflux of barium into the terminal ileum may show dilatation and mild mucosal irregularity for several centimeters, the so-called backwash ileitis associated with ulcerative colitis.

   The diagnosis of Crohn's disease can be inferred on the basis of several radiologic findings (Fig. 37-5; see also Fig. 31-2). Narrowing of the bowel from fibrosis or edema and formation of fistulas reflect the transmural nature of the disease. Involvement of the terminal ileum and presence of skip areas in either the large or the small bowel strongly favor a diagnosis of Crohn's disease rather than ulcerative colitis. Finally, mucosal changes of deep ulcers and linear fissures are characteristic of Crohn's disease.
5. **An upper GI and small-bowel series** may be of diagnostic help in the evaluation of Crohn's disease. It is important to remember that, in the radiologic evaluation of a patient with chronic or recurrent abdominal pain, a routine

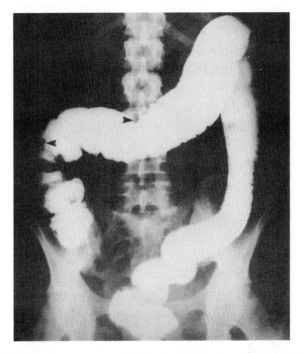

Figure 37-4. Barium enema x-ray examination showing ulcerative colitis involving the entire colon from rectum to cecum. The mucosal pattern is irregular, the haustral markings are absent from the left colon, and several pseudopolyps are evident (*arrows*). (From Eastwood GL. *Core Textbook of Gastroenterology.* Philadelphia: Lippincott Williams & Wilkins; 1984:132. Reprinted with permission.)

upper GI series is not sufficient. It should be accompanied by a small-bowel series to evaluate the small intestine for Crohn's disease, tumors, and strictures. The typical findings of Crohn's disease in UGI and SBFT include stricture formation and fistulous tracts.

As indicated previously, **Crohn's disease** can affect any portion of the digestive tract. However, about 75% of patients with Crohn's disease have, at a minimum, involvement of the **terminal ileum**. In about 5%, Crohn's disease involves the **duodenum**. Sometimes these patients clinically resemble patients with peptic ulcer disease. Although they may improve with a peptic ulcer regimen, symptoms typically recur. Nodularity and narrowing of the proximal duodenum and sometimes involvement of the adjacent antrum are evident by barium-contrast studies. The diagnosis is confirmed by endoscopy and biopsy.

F. **Colonoscopy and upper GI endoscopy.** Colonoscopy with intubation of the terminal ileum is useful in diagnosis of IBD. Periodic colonoscopy also is recommended for screening patients who have IBD for longer than 7 years for cancer and precancerous changes (see section VII.C). Although the diagnosis of Crohn's disease often is made on the basis of clinical and radiologic findings, colonoscopy is useful in obtaining biopsy material from the proximal colon and the terminal ileum to help confirm the diagnosis. As with barium enema examination, colonoscopy may precipitate toxic megacolon in patients with severe colitis, thus should be performed when clinically indicated. The preceding comments regarding preparation for barium enema apply also to colonoscopy.

Upper GI endoscopy may be useful in differentiating Crohn's disease of the duodenum from peptic ulcer disease.

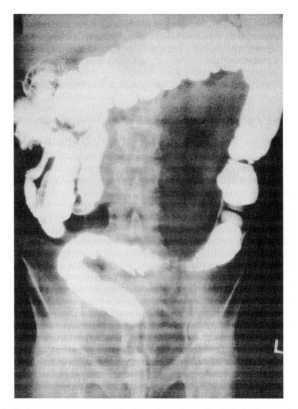

Figure 37-5. Barium enema x-ray examination of a patient with Crohn's disease showing a stricture in the sigmoid colon. Several years before, the patient had undergone resection of the terminal ileum and right colon with an ileum–transverse colon anastomosis. (From Eastwood GL. *Core Textbook of Gastroenterology.* Philadelphia: Lippincott Williams & Wilkins; 1984:143. Reprinted with permission.)

    G. Pill-cam imaging has become a newer useful tool in the diagnosis of small-intestinal Crohn's disease. The pill may become lodged in narrow structures and may require surgical removal. Nonspecific superficial ulcers may signify Crohn's ulcers, or may have resulted from use of aspirin or nonsteroidal anti-inflammatory drugs. Thus, clinical judgement is needed to make the appropriate diagnosis.

VI. TREATMENT
    A. Diet and nutrition. Patients with mild symptomatic IBD usually are able to take food orally. The diet should be nutritious. Traditionally, fiber has been restricted during periods of active symptoms. Some patients cannot tolerate milk, which may or may not be related to lactase deficiency. Patients with Crohn's disease who have terminal ileal involvement and steatorrhea may require supplemental fat-soluble vitamins, medium-chain triglycerides, and parenteral vitamin B_{12}. Replacement iron may be indicated in patients who are iron-deficient. Patients in remission do not require any restriction of fiber or other dietary constituent except as dictated by his or her own experience.

        In severe IBD, an elemental oral diet or nothing by mouth with total parenteral nutrition (TPN) has been recommended when patients are hospitalized. The use of TPN to treat fistulas of Crohn's disease is controversial. Administration of TPN over

TABLE 37-4	Sulfasalazine and 5-ASA (Mesalamine) Preparations	
Drug name	**Formulation**	**Dosage**
Azulfidine	500-mg tablets	1–2 tablets global p.o. q.i.d (1–4 g/d)
Dipentum	500-mg tablets	2 capsules p.o. b.i.d. (1 g/d)
Asacol	400-mg tablets	2–4 tablets p.o. t.i.d (2.4–4.8 g/d)
Pentasa	250-mg capsules	4 capsules p.o. t.i.d. (3–4 g/d)
Colazal	750-mg capsules	3 capsules p.o. t.i.d. (1,250 mg/d)
Rowasa enema	4 g-unit dose/60-mL enema	1–2 daily (preferably at bedtime)
Canasa suppositories	500-mg rectal suppositories	1–2 times daily

ASA, aminosalicylic acid; p.o., orally; q.i.d., four times daily; t.i.d., three times daily.

several weeks has been associated with the closure of a high proportion of fistulas. However, the fistulas commonly recur after reinstitution of oral feedings.

   B. Drugs. Because the etiology of IBD is incompletely understood, drug treatment is aimed at alleviating and reducing inflammation.

   1. Sulfasalazine and aminosalicylates (mesalamines) (Table 37-4). **Sulfasalazine (Azulfidine)** historically has been the most commonly used drug in the treatment of colitis. It has been show to be efficacious in the treatment of UC and Crohn's disease when the colon is involved. The drug consists of sulfapyridine linked to 5-aminosalicylic acid (5-ASA or mesalamine) via an azo bond. Intestinal bacteria break the azo bond and release the two components. The sulfapyridine moiety is systemically absorbed and excreted in the urine and the 5-ASA moiety, the active component, stays in the intestinal lumen in contact with the mucosa and eventually is excreted in the feces.

   a. Side effects. Abdominal discomfort is common and is attributed to the effects of the salicylate portion of the drug on the upper GI tract. This problem is minimized by ingestion of the sulfasalazine after eating. Patients also may become folate-deficient because of competition between folate and sulfasalazine for absorption. Other side effects, such as skin eruptions and bone marrow suppression, are less common and are attributed to the sulfa portion.

   b. Dosage. The initial daily dose is low (1 g) to minimize GI side effects. A therapeutic dose of 3 to 4 g per day is appropriate. A CBC and liver chemistry tests should be obtained before starting therapy, every 1 to 3 months initially, and every 6 to 12 months during long-term treatment.

   c. Maintenance treatment with sulfasalazine has been shown to reduce the frequency of exacerbations of ulcerative colitis. The usual maintenance dosage is 2 to 3 g per day in divided doses, although an occasional patient may benefit from 1 g per day (i.e., 500 mg twice daily).

   2. Other 5-ASA (mesalamine) preparations. Because the serious side effects of sulfasalazine are related to the sulfa portion, there has been much interest in developing similar drugs that retain the salicylate portion but replace the sulfapyridine. Several oral 5-ASA preparations are available (Table 37-4).

   Olsalazine (Dipentum), which consists of two 5-ASA molecules joined by an azo bond such as sulfasalazine, requires bacterial degradation in the colon. It is as effective against active UC and in maintaining remission. High incidence of diarrhea as a side effect of Dipentum limits its use in most patients.

   Asacol is a controlled-release tablet form of 5-ASA, which is encapsulated by an acrylic resin that dissolves at a pH higher than 6.0. It has been shown to be effective in both active and remitted UC and Crohn's disease, especially when the ileum is involved. The usual dose is 2.4–4.8 mg daily in two or three divided doses.

Pentasa is a controlled-release formulation of 5-ASA that is encapsulated in ethylcellulose microgranules. It is effective in active and remitted UC and in active Crohn's disease regardless of disease location. Pentasa appears to help in maintaining remission in both small-bowel and colonic Crohn's disease. The recommended dose is 1 g q.i.d.

Balsalazide disodium (Colazal) is a 5-ASA preparation containing an azo bond. The active 5-ASA moiety is released in the colon by cleavage of the azo bond by colonic bacteria. It is primarily effective in treating IBD involving the entire colon, as well as left-sided colitis and proctitis. The recommended dose is 750 mg three tablets t.i.d. one a day.

Once daily dosing with mesalamine **(Liallda)** has recently been made available. The tablets contain a novel matrix which protects the mesalamine from degredation until it reaches the colon, then allows its gradual release through the entire length of the colon. The recommended dose is 1–2 g 2–4 tablets daily. The topical 5-ASA preparations include **Rowasa** enema and **Canasa** rectal suppositories. These are effective in active and remitted distal UC and ulcerative proctitis.

The 5-ASA preparations are also recommended for patient with Crohn's disease to prevent postoperative recurrence of Crohn's disease, especially in patients with colitis and to some extent in patients with small-bowel involvement. The 5-ASA preparations and sulfasalazine are safe to use in pregnant women.

3. **Corticosteroids.** Historically, corticosteroids have been used in patients with severe UC or Crohn's disease to induce a remission. Intravenous (IV) steroids (i.e., hydrocortisone 100 mg IV q6h or methylprednisolone 10–30 mg IV q6–8h) are usually used in such patients. When patients can take oral medications, prednisone at doses of 40 to 60 mg per day is usually given. If symptoms improve, the drug is tapered and withdrawn over a period of several weeks to months. Steroids are not recommended for maintenance therapy of UC or Crohn's disease, because steroids do not prevent relapse of Crohn's disease or UC and they have major side effects. However, many patients become steroid dependent and experience recurrence of symptoms when the dose of prednisone is reduced to less than 15 mg per day. One strategy is to use **6-mercapopurine (6-MP),** or **azathioprine (Imuran)** for steroid-dependent patients to help taper them off steroids. Biologic agents such as **Remicade** and **Humira** may be used instead of corticosteroids.

Several **corticosteroid enema preparations** are available for the treatment of proctitis and distal colitis. These are usually administered once or twice a day.

Budesonide (Entecort) is an orally administered corticosteroid that is released in the ileum and right colon at a pH of about 5.5. It has low systemic effects due to less than 20% absorption into the systemic circulation and a very efficient first-pass metabolism in the liver. It is effective in treating Crohn's disease involving the ileum and right colon, as well as microscopic (lymphocytic) colitis. The dose is 9 mg daily in active disease. It is usually tapered from 6 to 3 mg daily after 2 to 6 months. It is helpful in inducing remission. The drug is then stopped. Due to its low systemic bioavailability, it has minimal side effects of glucocorticoid steroids. However, bone mineral density may diminish during therapy. Patients receiving glucocorticoid therapy should be offered supplemental calcium and vitamin D.

4. **Antibiotics.** Most patients with mild-to-moderate IBD are successfully maintained on therapy with either sulfasalazine or 5-ASA and occasionally may require systemic or topical steroid therapy to treat disease relapses. However, about 20% to 25% of patients with UC and one third of patients with Crohn's disease require additional therapy for refractory disease, steroid dependency, and fistulas. Bacteria is known to play an important role in the pathogenesis of Crohn's disease and it may play a role in UC. In Crohn's diseases, the indications for the use of antibiotics include perianal disease, localized peritonitis due to microperforation, bacterial overgrowth secondary to a chronic stricture, and as an adjunct to drainage therapy for abscesses and fistulas. Antibiotics should

be considered in patients not responding to 5-ASA preparations prior to initiating of corticosteroid therapy. The antibiotics most commonly used in IBD include metronidazole, ciprofloxacin, Levaquin, and Xifaxan.

- **a. Metronidazole (Flagyl)** has been shown to be effective in patients with Crohn's disease of the colon or combined small-bowel and large-bowel disease as well as patients with perirectal Crohn's disease and fistulas. Some patients with UC or indeterminate colitis also respond successfully to metronidazole. The usual dosage is 250 to 500 mg three times daily. In patients with Crohn's disease, metronidazole therapy has been shown to decrease the severity of early recurrence and clinical recurrence rate at 1 year.

  Major limitations regarding the use of metronidazole include its side effects (peripheral neuropathy, stomatitis, nausea, and headache). Alcohol should be avoided due to its potential Antabuse-like side effects. Its use during pregnancy is controversial due to its potential teratogenic effects.

- **b. Ciprofloxacin hydrochloride** (500 mg twice daily) has been successfully used in patients with Crohn's disease with colonic involvement as well as in patients with perirectal and fistulizing Crohn's disease. The data for the use of ciprofloxacin hydrochloride in patients with UC are controversial; however, there is anecdotal evidence that the drug may be effective in some patients with UC.

- **c. Metronidazole plus ciprofloxacin hydrochloride** in combination has been used in the treatment of active, refractory Crohn's disease. In a comparison trial with steroids, the remission rate was similar. This combination may also be used in UC.

5. Immunomodulators

- **a. Azathioprine (Imuran, AZA)** at 2 to 2.5 mg/kg/d or its active metabolite, 6-MP (1 to 1.5 mg/kg/d), is effective and safe. Indications include refractory Crohn's disease, steroid-dependent Crohn's disease, fistulizing Crohn's disease, Crohn's disease remission maintenance, refractory UC, steroid-dependent UC, UC remission maintenance, and prevention of postoperative Crohn's disease recurrence. Maximum clinical response takes 2 to 3 months. Monthly or bimonthly CBC is recommended to monitor and prevent neutropenia. Data are available for their long-term safety when used longer than 5 years and, based on renal transplant experience, these drugs seem to be safe for use during pregnancy. AZA is metabolized to **6-Thioguanine (6-T6)** which is the active metabolite. The blood level of T6 may be monitored to ensure proper dosing of AZA. **Thiopurine methyltransference (TPMT)** plays a key role in the metabolism of AZA. One in 300 persons are homozygous for a recessive mutation and produce exceedingly high levels of 6-T6 and develop profound leucopenia. **TPMT genotype/phenotype** should be determined in patients prior to initiation of AZA therapy. Allopurinol (a xanthine oxidase inhibitor) competes with AZA for xanthine oxidase and increases levels of AZA metabolites. The dose of AZA should be decreased in patients also taking Allopurinol.

- **b. Methotrexate (1.5–7.5 mg per week by mouth [p.o.] or 25 mg per week intramuscularly [IM])** has been effective in the treatment of refractory and steroid-dependent Crohn's disease but not in UC. Its effect on long-term remission with maintenance therapy is not clear. Clinical response is rapid (2–8 weeks). Liver biopsy may be helpful prior to starting therapy in patients with liver chemistry abnormalities to monitor adverse effects. Monthly monitoring for bone marrow and hepatic toxicity is required. If cytopenias occur, methotrexate should be withheld for 2 to 3 weeks and then restarted at a lower dose. In all patients, liver biopsy should be performed after every 1,500 mg of methotrexate administered. A minority of patients develops pulmonary fibrosis.

- **c. Cyclosporin (Neoral/Sandimmune) (4 mg/kg per day IV; therapeutic range 250–350 mg/mL)** has been used successfully in severe steroid refractory UC as a bridge therapy to either long-term immunomodulatory therapy (i.e., with Imuran or 6-MP) or definitive colectomy (e.g., in pregnant or young patients in whom immediate surgery is not optimal.) However, while the short-term response rates are impressive, over half of these patients must undergo colectomy during 6 months of follow-up. In patients with Crohn's disease, cyclosporin has not been consistently effective.

Oral cyclosporin at low doses ($\leq$5 mg/kg per day) is not efficacious in IBD. Higher doses (8–10 mg/kg per day) of cyclosporin may be more effective; however, the side effect profile (hypertension, and nephro- and bone marrow toxicities) limits its usefulness. Cyclosporin should not be used for the maintenance of remission for UC or Crohn's disease.

Clinical response in patients who respond to cyclosporin therapy is rapid (within 2 weeks). The total duration of therapy should not exceed 4 to 6 months. Monitoring of nephrotoxicity is required. The dose should be adjusted downward whenever the baseline serum creatinine level increases by 30%.

d. Infliximab (Remicade) is a chimeric monoclonal antibody to human tumor necrosis factor-2 (TNF-2), a proinflammatory cytokine that plays an important role in the pathogenesis of Crohn's disease. Controlled trials have demonstrated high efficacy for infliximab in moderate to severely active Crohn's disease, in fistulizing Crohn's disease, and in severe UC with sufficient evidence for its safety. Clinical response is rapid (within 1–2 weeks) and the duration of response ranges from 8 to 12 weeks per infusion. Infliximab has probably supplanted the role of cyclosporin and corticosteroids in Crohn's disease. Infliximab is administered IV (5 mg/kg) over 2 hours. Infusions for active or fistulizing Crohn's disease are given as three doses at 0, 2, and 6 weeks for a starting dose. Infusion reactions may be minimized by pretreatment with an antihistamine and a steroid preparation. To minimize symptomatic disease recurrence, the IV infusions are repeated at 8-week intervals.

Toxicities observed for infliximab therapy include formation of human antichimeric antibodies (HACA), autoantibodies and a serum sickness–like delayed hypersensitivity reaction in some patients 2 to 4 years after initial treatment. There may be activation of dormant tuberculosis (TB). Patients should be tested for TB prior to initiation of therapy with infliximab. The risk of development of lymphoma in treated patients seems to be slightly increased.

e. Adalimumab (Humira) (Human antitumor necrosis factor [TNF] monoclonal antibody) has been approved by the FDA for the treatment of rheumatoid arthritis and Crohn's disease. It has also been shown to be effective in the treatment of Crohn's disease unresponsive to conventional therapies and also to a percentage of patients who have not responded to Remicade or who have lost their response to Remicade. The advantage of adalimumab over Remicade is that it has less immunogenicity and that it is administered subcutaneously (sc) 40 mg every 2 weeks after a starting dose of 80 mg sc. The dose may be increased to weekly in refractory patients.

f. Certolizumab pegol (Cimzia) is a humanized TNF alpha Fab monoclonal antibody fragment linked to polyethylene glycol (PEG). It is waiting for FDA approval for the treatment of moderate to severe Crohn's disease. This biologic drug is administered subcutaneously at weeks 0, 4, and 8 weeks, then once monthly at the same dose (400 mg). It has been shown to be effective in inducing response and remission in adult patients with active Crohn's disease unresponsive to conventional therapy as well as other biologic agents.

g. Thalidomide has shown anti-TNF activity in a subset of patients with Crohn's disease; however, due to its highly teratogenic potential, it is not suitable for routine use.

h. Nicotine given in enema form has shown some benefit in patients with distal UC but due to its side effect profile, it is not widely used.

6. Prebiotics and probiotics. It is believed that luminal bacterial flora influences the development and/or progression of IBD.

Prebiotics are nutrients utilized by specific microorganisms and support the growth of these organisms that interact with the host to improve the host barrier function and impact the innate immune response. Prebiotics include carbohydrates resistant to digestion (i.e., inulin, lactulose, and other oligosaccharides).

Probiotics are live microorganisms that are important for the development of a healthy innate immune system. Commonly used probiotics include *Lactobacillus*, *Bifidobacterium*, and other organisms including yeast such as *Saccharomyces* and combination VSL#3.

The data whether pre- and probiotics are helpful in IBD are controversial. However, probiotics have been shown to be effective in the treatment of pouchitis.

7. **Antidiarrheal medications.** If diarrhea does not improve with the previously described medical therapy in patients with mild-to-moderate IBD, treatment with an antidiarrheal drug may be helpful. **Codeine** is most effective, although **loperamide (Imodium) or diphenoxylate (Lomotil)** may be preferred because of their lower addictive potential. These and other opiate derivatives should not be used in patients with severe IBD because of the possibility of inducing toxic megacolon.

   Nonsteroidal antiinflammatory drugs (NSAIDs) should not be used in patients with IBD. The role of cyclooxygeranase (Cox)-2 NSAIDs in pain control for IBD is not clear.

8. **Bile acid-binding resins and medium-chain triglycerides.** Because many patients with Crohn's disease have involvement of the terminal ileum with consequent bile acid malabsorption, diarrhea, and steatorrhea, treatment with a bile acid-binding resin such as cholestyramine or with medium-chain triglyceride supplements may be indicated (see Chapter 30) in addition to other antidiarrheal drugs.

   In summary, patients with **mild and moderate IBD** are usually started on a **5-ASA,** and clinical response is determined within 2 to 4 weeks. If patients continue to be symptomatic, an **AZA is added** to the treatment. Patients who achieve remission are followed at 1 to 3 months clinically. Those who do not reach remission are then offered **pulse steroid therapy** or **a biologic agent.**

C. **Psychotherapy.** Formal psychotherapy appears to be of little benefit in the primary treatment of IBD. However, emotional support of the patient by the physician, family, clergy, and other concerned people is important. Psychotherapy may be indicated in some patients to help them cope with living with a chronic disease.

D. **Surgery**
   1. **Ulcerative colitis.** The standard noncontroversial indications for surgery in ulcerative colitis include toxic megacolons perforation, abscess, uncontrollable hemorrhage, unrelieved obstruction, fulminating disease, carcinoma, and high-grade dysplasia on colonic biopsies. Usually a total proctocolectomy is performed. Historically, this operation has been accompanied by a permanent ileostomy. Currently rectal sphincter-saving operations are the norm. In this operation, the rectal mucosa is removed, but the muscular wall of the rectum is left intact. The terminal ileum is anastomosed to the anus, usually with the formation of a reservoir pouch. If the operation is performed in an acutely ill patient with severe colitis, it is usually carried out in two steps: the colectomy first and the reanastomosis several months later.

      Despite increased surgical experience and patient appeal, problems with the ileal pouch–anal anastomosis remain. Technical failure occurs in approximately 5% to 8% of patients within the first 5 to 10 years. Pouchitis occurs acutely in 40% to 50% of patients. Most of these patients respond to a course of antibiotic therapy with metronidazole or ciprofloxacin hydrochloride, or both. Xifaxan has also been shown to be effective in some patients. Approximately 5% to 8% will develop chronic pouchitis and require maintenance suppressive therapy or possible pouch takedown and formation of a permanent ileostomy. There are reports of the development of neoplasia in the pouch after a number of years.

   2. **Crohn's disease.** Surgery in Crohn's disease is indicated for perforation, abscess, obstruction, unresponsiveness to treatment, intractable disease, and some fistulas. Because removing a segment of diseased bowel does not "cure" the patient of Crohn's disease as proctocolectomy cures a patient with ulcerative colitis, the dictum is to remove as little bowel as is necessary to correct the

problem. Patients with a single, short segment of Crohn's disease respond the best to surgery. The rectal sphincter-saving operation is not an option in Crohn's patients because of the possibility that anorectal Crohn's disease may develop later. Stricturoplasty may be a surgical option in some patients with stricturing Crohn's disease.

a. The recurrence rate after surgery of Crohn's disease is high: 30% after 5 years, 50% after 10 years, and 70% after 15 years. Whether this is because of some deleterious effect of surgery on the bowel or merely represents the natural history of patients with severe Crohn's disease is difficult to determine. In any event, the aim of surgery is to remove grossly diseased bowel and preserve as much normal-appearing bowel as possible. If the terminal ileum has been removed, the patient should undergo a Schilling test 3 to 6 months after surgery to survey for vitamin B_{12} malabsorption. Most patients will require monthly vitamin B_{12} injections.

b. Fistulas often respond to medical treatment, and even those that persist do not always require surgery. However, enterocutaneous fistulas that are poorly tolerated by the patient and all enterovesical fistulas may require surgical correction. Also, fistulas between loops of bowel should be corrected surgically if clinically significant malabsorption occurs.

VII. SPECIAL ISSUES

A. Toxic megacolon and severe IBD. Toxic megacolon is a condition in which the colon becomes atonic and dilated because of transmural inflammation. It is characteristically associated with severe ulcerative colitis, but it may complicate any severe inflammatory condition of the bowel, including Crohn's disease, bacterial colitis, amebiasis, pseudomembranous colitis, and ischemic colitis. Patients with toxic megacolon are seriously ill. They typically have fever, elevated white blood cell count, bloody diarrhea, and sepsis. Some patients with severe ulcerative colitis do not have toxic megacolon but require similar intensive treatment.

1. Pathogenesis. In most instances of colitis, the inflammatory process is confined to the mucosa and submucosa. Toxic megacolon develops as a result of the extension of the inflammatory process to the muscularis propria and serosa, causing atony and leading to perforation and peritonitis. Several factors appear to predispose to the development of toxic megacolon. These include dosage reduction of medications for IBD; enteric infections; cessation of smoking in patients with UC; hypokalemia; and the administration of NSAIDs, narcotics, anticholinergics, and other agents that diminish bowel motility. Bowel stasis may facilitate extension of the inflammatory process to the deeper layers of the colonic wall with subsequent penetration of bacteria. Barium enema and colonoscopy also have been implicated as causative factors in some patients with toxic megacolon, perhaps for similar pathogenic reasons.

2. Diagnostic features at the onset of the disease are worsening of the diarrhea (more than six stools per day), hematochezia, fever, abdominal tenderness, and abdominal distention. As the disease progresses, the stool frequency may diminish as the colon becomes atonic and dilated.

On **physical examination** the patient appears severely ill. Signs of systemic toxicity include fever, tachycardia, and change in mental status. The abdomen is diffusely tender with diminished-to-absent bowel sounds, and there may be signs of peritoneal inflammation. The rectal examination typically reveals bloody stool.

3. Diagnostic studies

a. Laboratory studies. The CBC may reveal anemia and leukocytosis, often with a left shift. Blood sugar; blood urea nitrogen (BUN); serum electrolytes, albumin, and creatinine; urinalysis; and arterial blood gases should be obtained. Plain chest x-ray films and an electrocardiogram also should be ordered. A CT scan of the abdomen and pelvis will be helpful to exclude perforation, abscess formation, and masses.

b. Stool studies. Stool samples should be examined for ova and parasites, cultured, and tested for C. *difficile* toxin.

c. **Abdominal plain x-ray films.** Measurement of the diameter of the transverse colon on supine films of the abdomen taken every 12 to 24 hours is useful in assessing the status of the illness (see Fig. 37-3). A diameter greater than 6 cm is regarded as abnormal. Perforation is a common complication of toxic megacolon. Thus, upright or lateral decubitus films also should be taken to rule out free air in the abdomen. Because air in the bowel seeks the most superior location, lateral decubitus films may show dilatation of the ascending or descending colon rather than of the transverse colon.

d. **CT scan of the abdomen and pelvis** is more sensitive in the detection of intraabdominal free air and abscesses.

e. **Sigmoidoscopy.** Physicians often wonder whether sigmoidoscopy should be performed in patients with severe colitis or toxic megacolon because of concerns about perforation and worsening of the bowel distention by insufflated air. Limited sigmoidoscopy, by an experienced endoscopist using either a rigid or a flexible instrument, is both safe and indicated in such patients. The examination should be limited to the rectum or distal sigmoid colon. The severity of the mucosal injury can be assessed, and other conditions in the differential diagnosis, such as Crohn's disease, ischemic colitis, and pseudomembranous colitis, may be eliminated.

f. **Colonoscopy and barium enema** are contraindicated in severe colitis or toxic megacolon. One or both of these studies may be indicated later, after recovery has occurred, to document the extent of the colitis and to survey for development of complications, such as stricture, pseudopolyps, dysplasia, and cancer.

4. **Management**

a. **General medical management.** Patients should receive nothing by mouth and IV fluids. Opiates and anticholinergic agents should be stopped. Nasogastric suction is indicated. Careful attention should be paid to correcting electrolyte imbalances. Anemic patients may require blood transfusions. The clinical status is assessed frequently by physical examination, determination of vital signs, and abdominal flat and decubitus x-ray films every 12 to 24 hours.

b. **Antibiotics.** Patients should be treated with a broad-spectrum antibiotic regimen including anaerobic coverage after cultures of stool, blood, and urine have been obtained.

c. **Corticosteroids.** High-dose IV corticosteroids should be administered; for example, hydrocortisone (100 mg q6h) or methylprednisolone (10–15 mg q6–8h).

d. **Cyclosporin** has been shown to be effective in the management of severe and fulminant colitis at doses of 4 mg/kg per day given IV. The role of cyclosporin in toxic megacolon is controversial, but has been used successfully in some cases. Patients who have responded to the IV regimen should then receive oral cyclosporin twice a day at double the IV dose (4 mg/kg twice daily) to maintain trough levels between 200 and 400 kg/mL and azathioprine or 6-MP therapy should also be started. The azathioprine or 6-MP is continued, but the cyclosporin and corticosteroids are tapered over the next 3 months.

e. **Fufliximab (Remicode)** has been used successfully in patients with severe IBD and may be a safer alternative to intravenous Cyclosporin. The dosing is as in 4d.

f. **Surgery.** Patients with severe colitis or toxic megacolon should be evaluated by a surgeon early during the course of the illness. Indications for surgery are perforation, unremitting colonic hemorrhage, and failure of the clinical status to improve despite intensive therapy with IV corticosteroids as described above or in combination with cyclosporin. In most centers, the patients are treated initially with broad-spectrum antibiotics and IV corticosteroids. Patients who fail to improve on this regimen within the first 3 to 7 days should be offered surgery or IV cyclosporin. Cyclosporin therapy does not increase the risk of postsurgical morbidity.

    If surgery is indicated, subtotal colectomy and ileostomy with formation of a Hartmann's pouch is considered the conservative procedure of choice in patients with systemic toxicity. Restorative proctocolectomy and ileal pouch–anal anastomosis is possible for patients with severe colitis without systemic toxicity.

   f. Subsequent medical management. Patients who improve on medical treatment without surgery should be treated with parenteral nutrition. When they are able to take oral fluids, the steroid therapy can be changed to the equivalent of 40 to 60 mg prednisone daily.

B. Management of pregnant patients with IBD. Statistically, a woman with quiescent IBD runs roughly the same risk of having an exacerbation during 9 months of pregnancy as during any other 9 months of her life. In some women, however, the disease appears to be exacerbated by pregnancy, and in others it is improved. Some women experience their first attack of colitis during pregnancy or within a few weeks of delivery. If colectomy is necessary for the treatment of severe colitis early in pregnancy, therapeutic abortion also may be necessary.

   1. Congenital abnormalities and premature births occur no more frequently in women with IBD than in the general population. Women with active disease during pregnancy are often treated with sulfasalazine or other 5-ASA compounds, antibiotics, or steroids, which appear to have no deleterious effects on the fetus. Metronidazole should not be prescribed for pregnant women. Women who become pregnant while on 6-MP or azathioprine and who continue to take it during pregnancy have not been shown to experience deleterious effects on the pregnancy or on the fetus.

      a. What advice should you give a woman with IBD who is contemplating becoming pregnant? Encourage her to become pregnant during a period of remission. Reassure her that exacerbations of the disease most likely can be treated effectively with medications. Inform her that most likely she will do well but that there is a small chance severe symptoms will develop. If blood loss or malabsorption is evident, supplemental iron and vitamins should be administered.

C. Cancer surveillance in IBD

   1. Chronic ulcerative colitis and Crohn's disease predisposes to adenocarcinoma of the colon. The cancers tend to be multifocal, and infiltrating. The risk of cancer is directly related to the extent of colonic involvement and to the duration of the disease. Data from large referral centers originally indicated that the risk of cancer development in patients with pancolitis begins after about 7 to 10 years of disease and that the incidence of cancer thereafter is about 20% per decade. More recent data suggest that the risk may be somewhat lower but still represent a clinical threat. The current recommendation for cancer surveillance in patients with ulcerative colitis and Crohn's disease is to perform colonoscopy yearly after 7 to 10 years of disease in patients with pan colitis and after 10 to 15 years of disease in patients with colitis only in the descending colon. During colonoscopy, multiple biopsies are taken from cecum to rectum. The colonoscopist should biopsy any grossly suspicious lesions. Otherwise, biopsies should be obtained from noninflamed, flat mucosa because inflammation can be associated with dysplasia and thus affect the pathologic findings. Pathologists are encouraged to interpret the biopsies according to published criteria. Each biopsy should be interpreted as normal, indeterminate, or dysplastic. Dysplastic biopsies are to be read as either low-grade dysplasia or high-grade dysplasia. Patients with biopsies showing indeterminate or low-grade dysplasia should undergo colonoscopy again in 1 to 6 months. The response to an interpretation of high-grade dysplasia has been debated, but many experts believe that the diagnosis is grounds for recommending total colectomy.

   2. Microscopic (lymphocytic and collagenous) colitis is diagnosed in patients presenting with watery chronic diarrhea by histologic examination of the colonic biopsies, especially obtained from the right colon. The visual appearance of the mucosa during colonoscopy is usually normal. However, on histologic examination of the mucosa, if there is increased lymphocytic infiltrate in the lamina propria with preserved crypts, the colitis is called **lymphocytic colitis.** However, if there is a collagen band thicker than 10 mm below the epithelium, the condition is called **collagenous colitis.** The etiology of microscopic colitis is not known.

Treatment is usually initiated with a 4- to 8-week trial of bismuth subsalicylate two tablets three to four times a day. If symptoms do not abate, a 5-ASA compound and/or budesonide may be used to achieve remission. Antibiotics such as ciprofloxacin 500 mg b.i.d. or metronidazole 250–500 mg t.i.d. or Xifaxan 200 mg one or two tablets t.i.d. may be used for 1 to 3 months. In some cases, corticosteroids and immunomodulators may be necessary to induce remission.

Selected Readings

Baumgart DC, et al. Inflammatory bowel disease: cause and immunobiology. *Lancet*. 2007;369:1627–1640.

Baumgart DC, et al. Inflammatory bowel disease: clinical aspects and established and evolving therapies. *Lancet*. 2007;369:1641–1658.

Beaugerie L, et al. Drug-induced microscopic colitis: Proposal for a scoring system and review of the literature. *Aliment Pharmacol Ther*. 2005;22:277–284.

Biancone L, et al. Treatment with biologic therapies and the risk of cancer inpatients with IBD. *Nat Clin Pract Gastroenterol Hepatol*. 2007;4:78–79.

Bonderup OK, et al. Budesonide treatment of collagenous colitis: A randomized, double-blind, placebo-controlled trial with morphometric analysis. *Gastroenterology*. 2003;52: 248–251.

Bosch X, et al. Antineutrophilcytoplasmic antibodies. *Lancet*. 2006;368:404–418.

Caprilli R, et al. Current management of severe ulcerative colitis. *Nat Clin Pract Gastroenterol Hepatol*. 2007;4:92–101.

Colombel JF, et al. Adalimumab for maintenance of clinical response and remission in patients with Chrohn's disease: The CHARM trial. *Gastroenterol*. 2007;132:51–65.

Feagon BG, et al. Mesalamine maintenance therapy for Crohn's disease. *Gastroenterology*. 2001;120:585.

Fernandez-Banares F, et al. Collagenous and lymphocytic colitis: Evaluation of clinical and histological features, response to treatment and long term follow-up. *Am J Gastroenterol*. 2003;98:340–347.

Fichera A, et al. Surgical treatment for Crohn's disease. *J Gastroent. Surg*. 2007;11(6): 791–803.

Hanauer SB, et al. Human anti-tumor necrosis factor monoclonal antibody (adalimumab) in Crohn's disease: The CLASSIC-1 trial. *Gastroenterology*. 2006;130(2):323–333.

Itzkowitz SH, et al. Colorectal cancer screening and surveillance in inflammatory bowel disease. *Inflam. Bowel Dis*. 2005;11(3):314–327.

Jarnerot G, et al. Infliximab as rescue therapy in severe to moderately severe ulcerative colitis: A randomized, placebo-controlled study. *Gastroenterology*. 2005;128:1805–1811.

Lemann M, et al. A randomized, double-blind controlled withdrawal trial in Crohn's disease patients in long-term remission on azathioprine. *Gastroenterology*. 2005; 128(7):1812–1818.

Lemann M, et al. Infliximab plus azathioprine for steroid-dependent Crohn's disease patients: A randomized placebo-controlled trial. *Gastroenterology*. 2006;130(4):1054–1061.

Leung WK, et al. Small bowel enteropathy associated with chronic low-dose aspirin therapy. *Lancet*. 2007;369:614.

Lichtenstein GR, et al. American Gastroenterological Association Institute medical position statement on corticosteroids, immunomodulators, and infliximab in inflammatory bowel disease. *Gastroenterology*. 2006;130(3):935–939.

Lichtenstein GR, et al. American Gastroenterological Association Institute technical review on corticosteroids, immunomodulators, and infliximab in inflammatory bowel disease. *Gastroenterology*. 2006;130(3):940–987.

Lichtenstein GR, et al. Infliximab maintenance treatment reduces hospitalization, surgeries and procedures in Chron's disease. *Gastroenterol*. 2005;128:862–869.

Loftus EV, Jr. Clinical epidemiology of inflammatory bowel disease: incidence, prevalence, and environmental influences. *Gastroenterology*. 2004;126:1504–1517.

Marshall JK, et al. Putting rectal 5-aminosalicylic acids in its place: The role in distal ulcerative colitis. *Am J Gastroenterol.* 2000;95:1628.

Robert M. Pathology of microscopic, lymphocytic, and collagenous colitis. *J Clin Gastroenterol.* 2004;38:517–526.

Rodemann JF, et al. Incidence of clostridium difficile infection in inflammatory bowel disease. *Clin Gastroenterol Hepatol.* 2007 Mar;5:339–344.

Rutgeerts P, et al. Infliximab for induction and maintenance therapy for ulcerative colitis. *Nat Clin Pract Gastroenterol Hepatol.* 2007;4:92–101.

Sabery N. Use of serologic markers as a screening tool in inflammatory bowel disease compared with elevated erythrocyte sedimentation rate and anemia. *Pediatrics.* 2007;119:e193–199.

Sandborn WJ, et al. Optimizing anti-TNF treatment in inflammatory bowel disease. *Gastroenterology.* 2004;126:1593–1610.

Sartor RB. Therapeutic manipulation of the enteric microflora in inflammatory bowel diseases: antibiotics, probiotics, and prebiotics. *Gastroenterology.* 2004;126:1620–1633.

Schiller L. The clinical spectrum of microscopic colitis. *J Clin Gastroenterol.* 2004;38: 527–530.

Schreiber S, et al. A randomized placebo-controlled trial of certolizumab pegol (CDP870) for treatment of Crohn's disease. *Gastroenterology.* 2005;129(3):807–818.

Scheibers S, et al. Maintenance therapy with certolizumab pegol for Crohn's disease. *N Eng J Med.* 2007;357:239–350.

Seidman EG. Clinical use and practical application of TPMT enzyme and 6-mercaptopurine metabolic monitoring in IBD. *Rev. Gastroenterol Disorder.* 2003;3(suppl 1):S1–S9.

Xavier RJ, et al. Unraveling the pathogens of inflammatory bowel disease. *Nature.* 2007; 448(7142):427–434.

Yang YX. Methotrexate for the maintenance of remission in Crohn's disease. *Gastroenterology.* 2001;120:1553.

$\mathcal{V}$ ascular disorders of the gastrointestinal (GI) tract typically present as abdominal pain or bleeding, or both. Several of the disorders that cause bleeding, such as ischemic colitis, angiodysplastic lesions, and vascular–enteric fistulas, are mentioned in Chapters 14 and 44, but are discussed more thoroughly here.

I. MESENTERIC VASCULAR INSUFFICIENCY. The clinical spectrum of mesenteric vascular insufficiency is broad, ranging from transient postprandial "abdominal angina" to severe abdominal pain caused by acute occlusion of a mesenteric vessel. Some patients with mild symptomatic vascular insufficiency are otherwise well, whereas acute occlusion of a mesenteric artery can be catastrophic. Occlusion of a mesenteric vessel by a thrombus or an embolus is dramatic, and the pathogenesis is easy to understand. However, nonocclusive mesenteric vascular disease also is recognized and may affect a larger number of patients than the occlusive type does. The latter includes transient ischemia due to inadequate perfusion under some circumstances, such as the high demand for mesenteric blood flow after eating, resulting in "intestinal angina," or the reduction in blood flow during an episode of heart failure or a cardiac arrhythmia, resulting in bleeding and abdominal pain. Vascular disorders of the bowel are more common in older people, and as the elderly population increases, these disorders are becoming more prevalent.

A. Intestinal circulation. The stomach and intestines are supplied by three unpaired arteries: the celiac axis, the superior mesenteric artery, and the inferior mesenteric artery. The gut receives nearly 30% of the resting cardiac output through these three splanchnic arteries. Small vessels, called **arteriae rectae,** derive from the terminal branches of the intestinal arcade in the small intestine and from the marginal artery in the colon and penetrate the muscle layer of the gut to form a rich submucosal plexus. In the small intestine, arterioles arise from the submucosal plexus to supply each villus. A central arteriole runs the length of each villus and branches at the tip to form a capillary network, which is drained by venules that parallel the central arteriole. Oxygen diffuses directly from the arterial to the venous side along the villus, thus creating a countercurrent mechanism that diminishes the oxygen concentration at the tip of the villus. This shunt is accentuated by low-flow states. It also may explain why small-intestinal ischemia is first manifested by destruction of the villous tips and consequently by breakdown of the barrier to bacteria, which predisposes the mucosa to bacterial invasion. In the colon, arterioles and venules also lie in close approximation, creating a similar predisposition to ischemia at the mucosal surface.

B. Occlusive vascular disease

1. Pathophysiology. Occlusion of the celiac axis, superior mesenteric artery, or inferior mesenteric artery, or their branches, can result from thrombosis or embolus, resulting in acute intestinal ischemia. A dissecting aortic aneurysm also can occlude one or more mesenteric vessels. If collateral circulation is inadequate, the bowel becomes ischemic and the patient experiences severe abdominal pain. The most common cause of arterial thrombosis is ordinary atherosclerotic vascular disease. Emboli may accompany acute myocardial infarction, ventricular aneurysm, atrial fibrillation, valvular heart disease, or bacterial endocarditis.

2. **Clinical presentation.** Occlusion of a splanchnic artery by thrombosis or embolus causes acute abdominal pain. Initially, the pain may be colicky, but as transmural infarction and peritonitis develop, the pain becomes constant and more severe. Tachycardia, hypotension, fever, elevated white cell count, and bleeding ensue. A careful examination should be done to evaluate for abdominal aortic aneurysm, abdominal bruits, and changes in peripheral pulses.

3. **Differential diagnosis.** The differential diagnosis includes most causes of abdominal pain, including dissecting aortic aneurysm, bowel obstruction, perforation of a viscus, acute cholecystitis, appendicitis, diverticulitis, peptic ulcer disease, pancreatitis, and pancreatic carcinoma. Patients with a dissecting aortic aneurysm may have severe abdominal pain radiating to the back. During the dissection, occlusion of the mesenteric vessels also may occur. Bowel obstruction and perforation of a viscus are acute events that may be confused with mesenteric vascular thrombosis or embolus. Inflammatory conditions, such as cholecystitis, appendicitis, and diverticulitis, often have localizing signs but may be difficult to distinguish from ischemic bowel disease that is accompanied by fever and elevated white blood cell counts. The signs and symptoms of peptic ulcer disease, pancreatitis, and pancreatic cancer usually are less acute than those of mesenteric vascular disease.

4. **Diagnostic studies.** Patients in whom acute ischemic bowel disease is suspected should have a complete blood count and differential white cell count and levels of serum amylase and electrolytes. The white cell count and amylase level may be increased in intestinal ischemia, but the latter usually is not elevated more than five times above normal level. Higher levels of serum amylase are more typical of acute pancreatitis. A urinalysis also should be performed. A metabolic acidosis may develop as ischemia worsens.

   Plain films of the abdomen may show distended loops of bowel with air-fluid levels. Bowel loops may be separated by edema and blood within the bowel wall. Barium-contrast studies are not indicated during the initial evaluation and treatment of patients with acute ischemic bowel disease. The diagnosis is confirmed by angiography, although in some instances, when the clinical course is rapid and perforation is suspected, immediate surgery is indicated.

5. **Treatment.** The initial treatment of thrombotic or embolic infarction of the bowel consists of nasogastric suction, intravenous fluid and electrolyte replacement, blood transfusions as indicated, broad-spectrum antibiotics, and, if necessary, vasopressors. Definitive treatment is surgical resection of the infarcted bowel.

C. **Nonocclusive vascular disease**

   1. **Abdominal angina**

      a. **Pathophysiology.** Abdominal angina is an uncommon but distinct condition that, if diagnosed correctly, usually can be corrected, providing the patient with remarkable relief of pain. Patients typically have arteriosclerotic disease involving at least two of the three major visceral arteries (celiac axis, superior mesenteric artery, and inferior mesenteric artery). Arteriosclerotic disease of the heart and other blood vessels usually coexists, sometimes complicated by diabetes mellitus. The pain, which occurs several minutes after eating, is caused by mesenteric ischemia. The postprandial blood flow simply is not sufficient to meet the increased energy demands of the intestine during digestion.

      b. **Clinical presentation.** Postprandial mid-abdominal pain, usually severe and incapacitating, is the hallmark. The pain continues for minutes to hours. Patients are reluctant to eat; consequently, losses of 10 to 30 lb (4.5–13.5 kg) are common. This clinical picture is remarkably similar to that of pancreatic cancer, from which abdominal angina must be differentiated. A mild-to-moderate malabsorption also may contribute to the weight loss. Sometimes patients experience nausea, vomiting, and diarrhea. A minority of patients have intestinal infarction after weeks to months of ischemic symptoms.

         On physical examination, the signs of weight loss are evident. An abdominal bruit may be heard but is not diagnostic.

c. **Diagnostic studies and differential diagnosis.** The clinical presentation of abdominal pain and weight loss is nonspecific and raises the possibility of cancer and other disorders of the stomach, small intestine, colon, gallbladder, and pancreas. Thus patients who ultimately are diagnosed as having abdominal angina usually undergo upper GI and small-bowel x-ray series, barium enema, ultrasound of the gallbladder, and abdominal computed tomography (CT) scan.

The diagnosis of abdominal angina depends on a high degree of clinical suspicion coupled with absence of evidence for other common causes of pain and weight loss and an abdominal arteriogram that shows complete or nearly complete occlusion of at least two of the three major splanchnic arteries.

d. **Treatment.** Arterial bypass surgery or surgical endarterectomy has been the treatment of choice. Percutaneous endarterectomy under fluoroscopic guidance may be an alternative in some patients. Rarely, in patients whose operative risk is prohibitive, treatment with an elemental diet or chronic intravenous alimentation may be attempted.

2. **Ischemic colitis**
   a. **Pathophysiology.** Mucosal ischemia in patients with nonocclusive vascular disease of the bowel is thought to result from transient low flow through an inadequate vascular system. Affected patients typically are elderly or have a cardiovascular condition, such as congestive heart failure or an arrhythmia, which predisposes them to a transient reduction in bowel perfusion. The condition may involve any portion of the small or large intestine but usually affects the descending colon, most commonly in the region of the splenic flexure or the sigmoid colon. These areas are the so-called watersheds between the distributions of the superior mesenteric artery and the inferior mesenteric artery in the first instance and between the inferior mesenteric artery and the internal iliac artery in the second.

   Ischemic colitis may occur in up to 10% of patients in the postoperative period after aortic aneurysm repair because of interruption of inferior mesenteric artery blood flow in the absence of adequate collateral circulation. It has also been reported in patients using birth control pills, estrogen supplement therapy, raloxifene (Evista), and pseudoephedrine.

   b. **Clinical presentation.** Patients with ischemic colitis characteristically report an abrupt onset of lower abdominal pain and bloody stool. The physical examination is variable. Low-grade fever may be present. Typically the abdomen is soft, and there is less tenderness than would be expected from the degree of abdominal discomfort. In most patients, the course is self-limited, with spontaneous recovery. However, a minority of patients may initially or eventually have peritoneal signs and absent bowel sounds, indicating bowel infarction and peritonitis, and require surgical treatment.

   c. **Diagnostic studies and differential diagnosis.** Most causes of abdominal pain and rectal bleeding, in particular ulcerative colitis, Crohn's disease, infectious colitis, and diverticular bleeding, are included in the differential diagnosis. Abdominal plain films may show the typical "thumbprints" in the affected area of bowel (Fig. 38-1). These are nodular protrusions into the bowel lumen caused by accumulations of submucosal edema and blood. A cautious sigmoidoscopic examination may identify a range of findings, including nonspecific colitis, ulcerations, and soft bluish nodules, which are the counterparts of the radiologic thumbprints. If the patient remains stable for 24 to 48 hours, colonoscopy or a single-contrast barium enema can reveal the affected bowel by confirming the thumbprint appearance (Fig. 38-2). In most patients, angiography is of little value. However, angiography may be useful to the surgeon for identifying the vascular anatomy if surgical treatment becomes necessary.

   d. **Treatment.** Initial treatment consists of nothing by mouth and intravenous fluids. The patient should be examined several times a day for the development of peritoneal signs. Congestive heart failure and cardiac arrhythmias

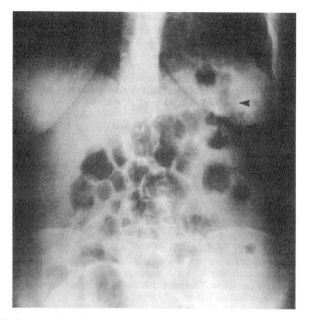

Figure 38-1. Plain x-ray film of the abdomen in an elderly patient with nonocclusive ischemic colitis. Air within the bowel provides a natural contrast medium. The characteristic "thumbprint" indentations are evident in the upper descending colon (*arrows*).

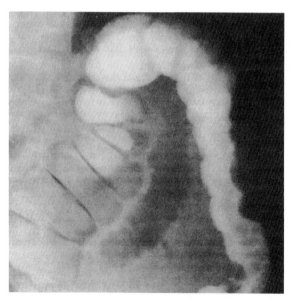

Figure 38-2. Barium enema x-ray film of the region of the splenic flexure in a patient with nonocclusive ischemic colitis. The "thumbprint" pattern is present in the descending colon (*arrows*).

should be treated appropriately. Antibiotics generally are not indicated unless fever persists and peritoneal signs develop. In patients with peritoneal signs, surgical resection of the ischemic segment is indicated, with either primary anastomosis or temporary colostomy. As mentioned previously, most patients with nonocclusive bowel ischemia recover with medical treatment. Some experts recommend a follow-up barium enema examination about 2 months later to determine whether an ischemic stricture has developed.

II. ANGIODYSPLASIA

A. Pathophysiology. Angiodysplasias are ecstatic, vascular lesions within the submucosa consisting of arterial, venous, and capillary elements. They may be found throughout the GI tract but occur most frequently in the cecum and ascending colon. Angiodysplasias are clinically important because they are a cause of acute and chronic GI bleeding, particularly in elderly patients.

Most angiodysplasias are thought to develop as a consequence of normal aging. Aortic stenosis occurs in up to 15% of patients with bleeding angiodysplasias, but pathogenic association is uncertain. In some patients, angiodysplastic lesions may occur throughout the GI tract as part of the hereditary disorder known as Osler-Weber-Rendu disease. In this disease, telangiectatic lesions also are found on the skin, in the nail beds, and in the mucosa of the mouth and nasopharynx.

B. Clinical presentation. Angiodysplasias cause no symptoms until they bleed. In patients who ultimately are diagnosed as having bled from an angiodysplasia, therefore, the only common history is that of GI bleeding. The usual presentation is one of acute lower GI bleeding. Often a cause of bleeding is not found or the bleeding is attributed to another common, coexisting disorder, such as peptic disease or diverticulosis. Patients may experience several bleeding episodes, sometimes over a period of months, before the correct diagnosis is made.

C. Diagnostic studies. The two methods of diagnosing angiodysplasias are colonoscopy and angiography.

   1. Colonoscopy. An angiodysplastic lesion appears as a submucosal red blush resembling a spider angioma of the skin. To optimize the chance of visualizing the lesion by colonoscopy, however, the bowel must be free of blood and debris, which may not be possible during acute bleeding.

   2. Angiography. The lesions may be identified angiographically by the following findings:

   a. An early-filling vein

   b. A vascular tuft of dilated vessels

   c. A slowly emptying vein

D. Treatment. The traditional treatment of a bleeding angiodysplasia has been to resect the segment of bowel that contains the lesion, usually the ascending colon. Up to 30% of patients so treated bleed again, either from a new angiodysplastic lesion or from a lesion that was not resected. An alternative to surgical resection is colonoscopic electrocoagulation if the lesions can be identified by colonoscopy.

III. VASCULAR–ENTERIC FISTULAS

A. Pathophysiology. An unusual cause of GI bleeding is a fistula between a vascular structure and the GI tract. Most commonly, the fistula develops between an aortic graft and the third portion of the duodenum months to years after an aortic aneurysm repair. Fistulas also may develop between an unresected aneurysm and the bowel. Less common sites are the sigmoid colon, the cecum, and the esophagus. Fistulas between aneurysms of the aorta or smaller vessels and virtually every portion of the GI tract have been reported.

B. Clinical presentation. Patients with vascular–enteric fistulas typically have massive hematemesis or hematochezia. A history of an aneurysm or aneurysm repair raises the likelihood. A "herald bleed" is characteristic: Most patients with vascular–enteric fistulas stop bleeding after the initial dramatic hemorrhage, only to rebleed within hours or days.

C. **Diagnostic studies and treatment.** Upper GI endoscopy is useful chiefly in excluding another bleeding lesion but usually does not identify the fistula. Angiography rarely identifies the fistula. Barium studies are not recommended due to the risk of severe bleeding but also are not likely to identify the fistula. CT of the abdomen may show a leaking aneurysm or fistula and therefore is helpful in making the decision to operate. A high index of suspicion for a vascular–enteric fistula in a patient with an aortic aneurysm or a history of an aneurysmectomy is worth more than diagnostic studies because immediate surgery usually is indicated after nondiagnostic upper GI endoscopy is performed.

Selected Readings

Bismar MM, Sinicrope FA. Radiation enteritis. *Curr Gastroenterol Rep.* 2002;4:361–365.

Brandt IJ, et al. AGA technical review on intestinal ischemia. *Gastroenterology.* 2000; 118:195.

Chang L, et al. Incidence of ischemic colitis and serious complications of constipation among patients using alosetron: Systematic review of clinical trials and post-marketing surveillance data. *Am J Gastroenterol.* 2006;101:1069–1079.

Deana DG, et al. Reversible ischemic colitis in young women. Association with oral contraceptive use. *Am J Surg Pathol.* 1995;19:454.

Dowd J, et al. Ischemic colitis associated with pseudoephedrine: Four cases. *Am J Gastroenterol.* 1999;943:2430.

Flobert C, et al. Right colonic involvement is associated with severe forms of ischemic colitis and occurs frequently in patients with chronic renal failure requiring hemodialysis. *Am J Gastroenterol.* 2000;95:195.

Nehme OS, et al. New developments in colonic ischemia. *Curr Gastroenterol Rep.* 2001;3:416.

Noyer CM, et al. Colon ischemia: Unusual aspects. *Clin Perspect Gastroenterol.* November/December 2000:315.

Schuller JG, et al. Cecal necrosis: Infrequent variant of ischemic colitis: Report of five cases. *Dis Colon Rectum.* 2000;43:708.

Shrestha S, et al. Henoch Schonlein purpura with nephritis in adults: adverse prognostic indicators in a UK population. *QJM.* 2006;99:253–265.

Uzoigwe CE, et al. A surgical solution for vasculitis? *Lancet.* 2007;369:1054.

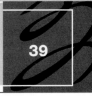

*C*olorectal cancer (CRC) is the second leading cause of cancer mortality in the United States. In men, CRC is second in prevalence only to lung cancer, and in women, it is third behind breast and lung cancer. More than 95% of the cancers are thought to have their origin in adenomatous polyps. In the United States, the prevalence of CRC is 30 to 40 per 100,000 and it increases with age.

I. COLONIC POLYPS

A. Pathogenesis. The term **polyp** refers to any protrusion into the lumen of the gastrointestinal (GI) tract. A **sessile polyp** is a raised protuberance with a broad base. A **pedunculated polyp** is attached to the bowel wall by a stalk that is narrower than the body of the polyp. **Submucosal polyps** are lipomas, leiomyomas, hemangiomas, fibromas, lymphoid tissue, endometriomas, melanomas, or metastatic lesions. Most submucosal polyps are benign; however, many patients with carcinoid metastatic lesions, melanomas, lymphomas, and Kaposi's sarcomas have malignant polyp formation in the colon.

Polyps may be benign or malignant. In the colon, polyps can be described as adenomatous, hamartomatous, hyperplastic, or inflammatory, according to their histopathologic appearance. **Hyperplastic and inflammatory polyps** are usually benign, but are also at risk for carcinoma. **Adenomatous polyps** can be classified as **tubular, villous, or tubulovillous,** depending on whether their histologic appearance is primarily glandular, villous, or mixed, respectively. Although most adenomatous polyps are benign, some may contain carcinoma and others may degenerate later to carcinoma. The risk of a polyp containing carcinoma increases directly with the size of the polyp (Table 39-1). Cancer is more likely to occur in villous adenomas than the other types, and benign adenomatous polyps may coexist with adenocarcinoma elsewhere in the bowel. In short, a colon that has a tendency to produce polyps also is at higher risk of the development of cancer.

B. Clinical presentation. Because colonic polyps are so common—some estimates of prevalence are as high as 50% in people over age 50—they are an important risk factor in the development of CRC in the general population.

Most patients with polyps are asymptomatic. In those instances, the polyps remain undiscovered or are diagnosed during surveillance examination. Sometimes polyps cause occult or gross bleeding. Occasionally patients complain of abdominal

TABLE 39-1	Relation of Polyp Size to Risk of Cancer in the Polyp

Polyp size	Risk of cancer (%)
<1 cm	0–2
1–2 cm	10–20
>2 cm	30–50

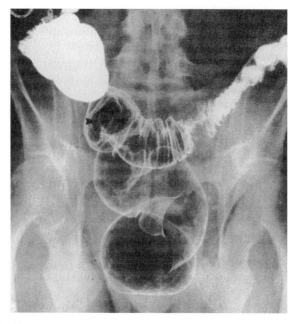

Figure 39-1. Air-contrast barium enema showing a sigmoid polyp on a long stalk (*arrows*).

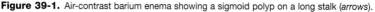

discomfort, which may be caused by tugging on the polyp by peristaltic contractions. If the polyp is large, frank obstruction can occur. Rarely, polyps may cause intussusception of the small or large intestine.

C. Diagnostic and screening. Studies for colonic polyps and CRC include colonoscopy, virtual colonoscopy, CT colography, sigmoidoscopy, and air contrast barium enema x-ray examination (Fig. 39-1). Often the barium enema has been ordered for symptoms that have no relation to the polyp. If the possibility of a polyp is raised by barium enema findings, complete colonoscopy should be performed. Similarly, identification of a polyp by sigmoidoscopy is justification for colonoscopy because the chance that there is a synchronous polyp in the colon above the reach of the sigmoidoscope exceeds 20%. For discussion of cancer surveillance, see section V.

D. Treatment

  1. Polypectomy. Nearly all polyps can be removed during colonoscopy. Polypectomy is performed by encircling the polyp with a wire snare through which an electrocauterizing current is passed. Sessile polyps may be removed in a piecemeal fashion. Injection of saline to the base of sessile lesion before snaring may give better visualization of the polyp and help its complete removal. If a polyp is too large to be removed, it should be adequately biopsied.

  2. Careful histologic examination of resected polyps is essential for formulating appropriate recommendations for the patient. Nonadenomatous polyps are thought to have little or no malignant potential, and removal of those polyps is sufficient treatment. On the other hand, adenomatous polyps not only predispose to the subsequent development of cancer but also may contain cancer at the time of removal. Thus, it is important that all polyps, particularly those larger than 1 cm in diameter, be examined carefully for adenocarcinoma.

  3. Adenocarcinoma may be present in adenomatous polyps in one of four ways (Fig. 39-2, Table 39-2).

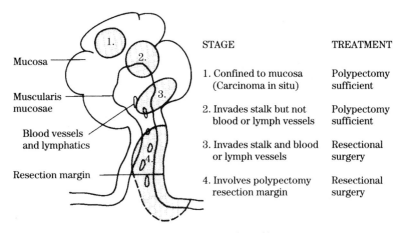

STAGE	TREATMENT
1. Confined to mucosa (Carcinoma in situ)	Polypectomy sufficient
2. Invades stalk but not blood or lymph vessels	Polypectomy sufficient
3. Invades stalk and blood or lymph vessels	Resectional surgery
4. Involves polypectomy resection margin	Resectional surgery

Figure 39-2. Stages of involvement of adenomatous polyps with cancer.

TABLE 39-2 **Diagnosis and Treatment of Cancerous Adenomatous Polyps**

Extent of involvement of polyp by cancer	Implication	Recommendations
Cancer involves only the mucosa without penetration of muscularis mucosae (carcinoma in situ).	The cancer has been cured by polypectomy.	Surgery not indicated; repeat colonoscopy in 1 y.
Cancer (moderately or well differentiated) has penetrated the muscularis mucosae but does not involve blood vessels or lymphatics in the stalk.	The cancer probably has been cured.	Surgery not indicated because the surgical risk outweighs the risk of residual cancer; repeat colonoscopy in 1 y.
Cancer has penetrated the muscularis mucosae and involves blood vessels or lymphatics, or the cancer is poorly differentiated, whether or not it involves blood vessels or lymphatics.	Residual cancer may be present in the colon.	Segmental resection of the colon is indicated if the patient is a good operative risk. If residual cancer is found in the patient at surgery, repeat colonoscopy in 3–6 mo; if no residual cancer, repeat colonoscopy in 6–12 mo.
Cancer involves the resectional margin of the polyp stalk.	Cancer remains in the bowel.	Segmental resection of the colon is indicated if the patient is an operative candidate. Repeat colonoscopy in 3–6 mo.

    a. The **cancerous change involves only the mucosa** and does not penetrate the muscularis mucosa into the stalk of the polyp. This condition is sometimes called **carcinoma in situ** or **high-grade dysplasia.** Colonoscopic resection of the polyp in this instance is regarded as curative. No surgical treatment is indicated. The patient should be scheduled to return in 1 year for follow-up colonoscopy.

    b. The cancer penetrates the muscularis mucosae of the polyp into the stalk but does not involve blood vessels or lymphatics within the resected portion of the stalk, and the cancer is moderately to well differentiated.

        Although a small number of patients with this finding has cancerous involvement of the bowel or local lymph nodes, the mortality (<2%) and morbidity of surgery to resect the portion of the colon that contained the polyp exceeds the risk of residual cancer. Thus, additional surgery for these patients is not recommended. Repeated colonoscopy should be scheduled for 1 year later.

    c. The **cancer** not only penetrates the muscularis mucosae of the polyp but **also has invaded blood vessels or lymphatics within the stalk.** In these patients, cancer also is likely to be present in the bowel or local lymph nodes. Also in this category are patients with poorly differentiated cancers that do not involve blood vessels or lymphatics. If operative risk is not prohibitive, these patients should undergo resection of the segment of colon that contained the polyp. Repeated colonoscopy to examine the anastomosis for recurrent tumor should be scheduled for 3 to 6 months if residual cancer is found at surgery. If no residual cancer is found, colonoscopy should be scheduled for 6 to 12 months.

    d. The cancer involves the resectional margin of the polyp, indicating that residual cancer remains in the patient. If the patient is an operative candidate, segmental resection of the colon is indicated. These patients should undergo follow-up colonoscopy in 3 to 6 months to check for residual tumor at the anastomosis and for other polyps.

II. Polyposis syndromes differ in their clinical manifestations, pathology, patterns of inheritance, and predisposition to carcinoma (Table 39-3).

    A. Familial adenomatous polyposis (FAP) and Gardner's syndrome. These conditions probably are related and expressions of the same genetic syndrome: one that is inherited in an autosomal dominant pattern. The prevalence in the United States is 3 per 100,000 persons. Affected individuals with FAP have hundreds of colorectal polyps in the first three decades of life. Polyps may also occur in the stomach and small intestine. The risk of polyp occurrence in the duodenum is 3% to 5%. Two percent of patients may have pancreatic, thyroid cancer, and hepatoblastoma. If the colon is not resected, virtually 100% of the patients eventually develop cancer. **Gardner's syndrome** is distinguished from FAP by the presence of osteomas, fibromas, and other features (Table 39-3) in addition to the intestinal polyps. Yearly colonoscopy should begin at age 10 in asymptomatic individuals carrying the gene for FAP. Total proctocolectomy with an ileostomy or an anal sphincter–saving procedure is indicated if the diagnosis of FAP is made. Genetic testing is available for family members.

    B. Turcot's syndrome. In this rare disease, colonic polyposis is associated with brain tumors. Both recessive and dominant patterns of genetic transmission have been described. Screening and treatment of affected individuals are the same as for FAP.

    C. In **Peutz-Jeghers syndrome,** intussusception, obstruction, or infarction of the polyps may develop with consequent abdominal pain and bleeding. For these reasons, surgery may be indicated. Because the risk of cancer is less than 3%, prophylactic surgery is not indicated.

    D. The **other polyposis syndromes** are not associated with an increased risk of cancer, although relatives of patients with juvenile polyps may have cancers of the stomach, small intestine, colon, or pancreas. However, patients with these syndromes may have complications of the polyps, such as bleeding and obstruction; if conservative treatment fails, they require surgery.

III. COLON CANCER

    A. Pathogenesis. As mentioned, CRC is the second and third most prevalent cancer in men and women, respectively, in the United States. The lifetime risk of a person in the general population for development of CRC is about 6%. A number of risk factors have been implicated (Table 39-4).

TABLE 39-3 Polyposis Syndromes

Syndrome	Histology of polyps	Location of polyps	Associated abnormalities	Cancer predisposition
Familial polyposis	Adenomas	Colon primarily; also stomach and small bowel	Osteomas of mandible	Yes
Gardner's syndrome	Adenomas	Colon primarily; also stomach and small bowel	Osteomas of mandible, skull, long bones; subcutaneous fibromas, lipomas, epidermoid cysts, exostoses, mesenteric fibromatosis, supernumerary teeth; thyroid and adrenal carcinoma	Yes
Turcot's syndrome	Adenomas	Colon	Brain tumors	Yes
Peutz–Jeghers syndrome	Hamartomas	Small bowel primarily; also stomach and colon	Pigmented plaques of buccal mucosa, hands, feet, perianal skin; bladder and nasal polyps	Yes (low risk, <3%)
Juvenile polyposis	Hamartomas, adenomas	Colon primarily; also stomach and small bowel		Rare
Neurofibromatosis (von Recklinghausen's disease)	Neurofibromas	Stomach and small bowel	Neurofibromas of skin	No
Cronkhite–Canada syndrome	Inflammatory	Small bowel primarily; also stomach and colon	Alopecia, hyperpigmentation, dystrophic nails	No

TABLE 39-4	Conditions That Predispose to Colon Cancer

Advancing age
Family history of colorectal or polyps
High-fat, low-fiber diet
Bowel disorders
   Inflammatory bowel disease (ulcerative colitis, Crohn's disease)
   Adenomatous polyps
   Some polyposis syndromes (see Table 39-3)
   Familial colon cancer syndrome
Genital tract cancer in women

First, merely **growing older** increases the risk. Over age 40, the annual incidence of colon cancer begins to accelerate, doubling every decade. Second, **dietary factors,** such as a high-fat, low-fiber diet, may increase the risk of developing CRC. Third, **bowel conditions** such as ulcerative colitis, Crohn's disease, adenomatous polyps, and some of the polyposis syndromes (see sections I and II) predispose to colon cancer. Finally, there seems to be a **hereditary predisposition** to the development of CRC. The probability of CRC developing in a person who has a first-degree relative with CRC is more than 15%, compared to a 6% risk in the general population. For **hereditary nonpolyposis colon cancer syndrome (HNPCC)** (see section IV), a high risk of development of colon cancer is inherited in an autosomal dominant manner. These patients may have coexisting adenomatous polyps and may also have melanoma or cancer of the uterus or ovaries. Patients with breast cancer may also have increased risk of developing colon cancer.

CRC may develop in any part of the colon. Approximately 45% of CRC is seen in the rectosigmoid and 25% in the ascending colon and cecum. Genetic examination of the tumors shows mutations in K-ras, APC, VCC, and P53 genes.

B. Clinical presentation

   1. History. The most common presenting sign is lower GI bleeding, and the most common symptom is change in bowel habit. Unfortunately, these are both late manifestations of the disease. Bleeding may be gross or occult. Occult bleeding typically is detected on routine rectal examination or stool screening tests. A change in bowel habit may be manifested as a decrease in the caliber of the stool if the lesion is distal and constricts the bowel lumen. Patients may complain of constipation. Sometimes diarrhea develops around a partially obstructing lesion. Mass lesions of the ascending colon, because of the larger diameter of the ascending colon, may grow to a considerable size before symptoms develop. Other possible consequences include anemia, weight loss, anorexia, malaise, abdominal mass, and enterovesical or enterocutaneous fistula. Rarely, the patient may seek treatment initially for symptoms of metastatic disease, such as jaundice or bone pain.

   2. Physical examination may reveal the effects of weight loss, muscle wasting, or anemia. A mass may be evident in the abdomen or by rectal examination. Stool may be positive for gross or occult blood.

C. Diagnostic studies

   1. A complete blood count should be obtained to evaluate for anemia. **Serum iron studies** confirm iron deficiency. An elevated serum alkaline phosphatase level, if confirmed to originate in the liver either by fractionation or by the finding of an elevated 5′-nucleotidase, suggests liver metastases. Sometimes an isolated elevation of serum lactic dehydrogenase or G-glutamyltranspeptidase is the only indicator of liver involvement. Hyperbilirubinemia in conjunction with an elevated alkaline phosphatase level suggests either extensive liver metastases or obstruction of the external bile ducts by metastatic lymph nodes. **Carcinoembryonic antigen (CEA)** may be elevated but is not helpful in making a diagnosis. Its role is largely confined to the follow-up period after primary treatment of the cancer to monitor for recurrence or metastatic spread.

2. Historically, a **barium enema,** preceded by flexible sigmoidoscopy, has been used as the first specific diagnostic study. An irregular filling defect or an encircling "apple core" lesion on the barium enema is highly suggestive of adenocarcinoma.

3. **Colonoscopy** is the gold standard in the evaluation of the colon for the presence of colon polyps or cancer. Polyps amenable for colonoscopic polypectomy are removed and those that are too large or too sessile to remove are biopsied for histopathologic evaluation.

4. **Virtual colonoscopy or CT colography of the colon** may be used for screening of the colon for the presence of polyps and cancer; however, it is not yet widely available. If a polyp is seen or suspected, a colonoscopy needs to be performed to confirm its presence and for its removal.

5. An attempt should be made **to identify metastatic disease. A computed tomography (CT) scan of the chest, abdomen, and pelvis** with intravenous contrast should be obtained. For some patients, **MRI of the liver** may be obtained to assess the number and size of the liver metastases.

D. **Differential diagnosis.** If a patient has weight loss, blood in the stool, and a mass in the colon, the overwhelming likelihood is adenocarcinoma of the colon. Other considerations include other malignant tumors such as leiomyosarcoma and lymphoma. Sometimes an inflammatory mass caused by diverticulitis or amebiasis mimics colon cancer.

Histopathologically, the differentiation between a large, benign polyp and colon cancer is not difficult.

E. **Treatment and prognosis.** Both treatment and prognosis depend largely on how extensively the cancer involves the colon, contiguous structures, and distant sites. The modified Dukes' classification is in common usage to stage colorectal carcinoma and determine prognosis (Table 39-5).

1. **Treatment** for Dukes' A, B, and C lesions is **surgical** unless operative risk is prohibitive. Rectal cancers usually require an abdominoperineal resection. Preoperative chemo radiation therapy of rectal cancers seems to improve surgical and overall outcome. More proximal colon cancers are treated by wide resection of the involved segment. Regional lymph nodes also are removed. Patients with stage D cancers may require palliative resection to control bleeding or to treat or prevent obstruction. Preoperative irradiation, sometimes in conjunction with chemotherapy, has been reported to shift the Dukes' staging to less extensive disease and improve surgical results.

Chemotherapy and radiotherapy in patients with inoperable cancer have been marginally effective. Radiotherapy of bony metastases may relieve bone pain. Adjuvant chemotherapy of metastatic colon cancer involves the administration of 5-fluorouracil, leucovorin, and irinotecan or a combination of oxiplatin and raltitrexed, Avastin and bevacizumab show promise of survival benefit.

2. **Prognosis.** The 5-year survival rate is directly related to the extent of tissue invasion, as indicated by the Dukes' classification (Table 39-5). In addition, prognosis and recurrence are adversely affected when tumors are poorly differentiated. Liver metastases may be resected to increase survival.

IV. **FAMILIAL COLON CANCER SYNDROME.** Hereditary nonpolyposis colorectal cancer (HNPCC) syndrome is a condition that is transmitted in an autosomal dominant fashion with a high degree of penetrance for the development of colorectal carcinoma. Two types are recognized. In type 1, cancers are confined predominantly to the colon. In type 2, cancers occur not only in the colon but also in the female genital tract, breast, brain, small bowel, pancreas, lymph system, and bone marrow. The diagnosis is suspected when CRC occurs in a young person with a family history of CRC.

TABLE 39-5	Modified Dukes' Classification to Stage Colorectal Cancer

Dukes' category	Definition	Five-year survival (%) after treatment
A	Cancer limited to mucosa or submucosa	90
B1	Cancer penetrates into but not through the muscularis propria	80
B2	Cancer penetrates through the muscularis propria or the serosa	70
C1	Same as B1 plus lymph node metastases	50
C2	Same as B2 plus lymph node metastases	50
D	Distant metastases	<30

Surveillance of family members in kindreds that may be affected should begin when members are age 10 with genetic testing. Fecal occult blood should be tested yearly. Total colonoscopy should be performed every 3 years beginning at age 20. Because of the high prevalence of cancers in the proximal colon, flexible sigmoidoscopy is not sufficient. Women with type 2 HNPCC syndrome should undergo yearly pelvic examinations. If colon cancer is detected, total or subtotal colectomy is indicated.

V. RECOMMENDATIONS FOR CANCER SURVEILLANCE AND FOLLOW-UP OF POLYPS AND CANCER

A. Rationale for CRC screening

The overall **5-year** survival rate for patients in the United States is approximately 60%. This correlates almost directly with the stage of diagnosis. Early detection of CRC can improve outcome significantly. The 5-year survival rate for patients with stage I to II disease is 80% to 90%, whereas it is 60% for those with stage III disease and less than 10% for stage IV disease. Studies have shown decreased mortality for CRC when screening is performed and the improved survival is associated with a shift to earlier stages at diagnosis.

The relatively long duration of adenoma-to-cancer sequence provides a period of predisease time during which early detection may be effective. Most sporadic CRCs arise from adenomatous polyps and the progression from normal mucosa through polyp formation and subsequent development of cancer is a process that occurs over a 5- to 15-year period. Consideration of this time frame is important when deciding what intervals are optimal for repeated screening.

B. Tests available for cancer screening

1. Digital rectal examination. Most physicians are able to examine the rectum digitally to a depth of 7 to 9 cm. This should detect about 5% to 10% of polyps. An infiltrating cancer feels hard and irregular, whereas a benign polyp is more likely to be soft and pliable.

2. Test for occult blood in the stool. Because bleeding is the most common sign of CRC, testing for occult blood in the stool is valuable in cancer surveillance. Currently available guaiac-impregnated cards have low false-negative and false-positive rates when used properly. Patients should adhere to a special diet (Table 39-6) for 48 hours before the stool is tested for occult blood. The diet eliminates foods and agents that are likely to give a false-negative or false-positive result but includes "roughage," which is believed to stimulate bleeding from existing bowel lesions. The most reliable method of testing for occult blood is to obtain two smears per day from different parts of the stool for 3 days. A report by Mandel and associates indicates that

TABLE 39-6	Diet for Fecal Occult Blood Testing

Avoid	Include in diet
Red meat	Chicken
Aspirin and nonsteroidal drugs	Tuna fish
Peroxidase-containing foods	Raw or cooked vegetables
(e.g., turnips, horseradish)	Fruit
Vitamin C, citrus juices	Bran cereal
(false-positive)	Peanuts
Iron-containing drugs	Popcorn
(false-positive)	

annual fecal occult blood testing decreased the 13-year cumulative mortality from CRC by 33%.

   3. Colonoscopy, sigmoidoscopy, barium enema x-ray, CT colographic examination. See Chapters 5 and 9.
 C. In the general population. See Figure 39-3.
 D. In patients with colonic polyps. See Figure 39-4.
 E. For people with a family history of CRC. People who have a parent, a sibling, or a second-degree relative with colorectal carcinoma are at higher risk of development of CRC, albeit much less than those who have familial colon cancer syndrome. Such people also are at higher risk of the development of CRC and polyps. People who have one first-degree relative with CRC should undergo CRC screening (preferably with colonoscopy) starting at age 40, or 10 years before the age of the onset in the affected relative. For people with two affected first-degree relatives, or one first-degree relative and one or more second-degree relatives, initial colonoscopy at age 40 may be justified, followed by routine yearly stool occult blood testing and periodic colonoscopy every 3 to 5 years.
 F. For postoperative colonoscopic follow-up of patients with resected CRC. Patients who have had a colorectal carcinoma are at greater risk of the development of another colorectal carcinoma. Patients who have had resection of the colon for cancer should undergo colonoscopy 12 months after surgery to look for recurrence at the anastomosis and elsewhere in the colon. Subsequent colonoscopic examinations should be every 2 to 3 years.
 G. Chemoprevention of prevention of CRC. Compliance to screening programs for CRC remains poor and alternative approaches are being sought. Chemoprevention of CRC involves the long-term use of a variety of oral agents to prevent the development of adenomatous polyps and their subsequent progression to CRC. Molecular analyses of adenomas and CRCs have led to a genetic model of colon carcinogenesis in which the development of cancer results from the accumulation of a number of genetic alterations. By interfering with these molecular events, chemoprevention could inhibit or reverse the development of adenomas or the progression from adenoma to cancer. Recent observations suggest that patients taking inhibitors such as celecoxib, aspirin, NSAIDs, cyclooxygenase-2 (COX-2), supplemental folate, calcium, and estrogen, as seen in postmenopausal women taking hormone replacement therapy, experience a chemopreventive benefit. Other potential chemopreventive agents as ursodiol, eflornithine, and oltipraz are undergoing evaluation in clinical studies.

   Chemoprevention should not replace periodic fecal occult blood tests and endoscopic screening as well as modification in known risk factors of CRC such as reduction in the intake of red meat, appropriate exercise, smoking cessation, and weight control.

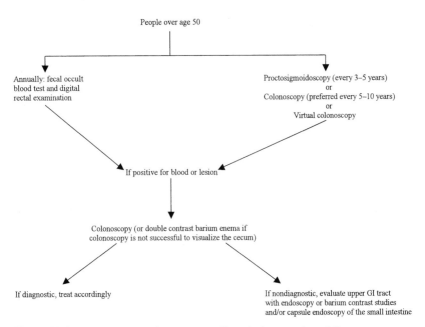

Figure 39-3. Recommendations for cancer surveillance in the general population.

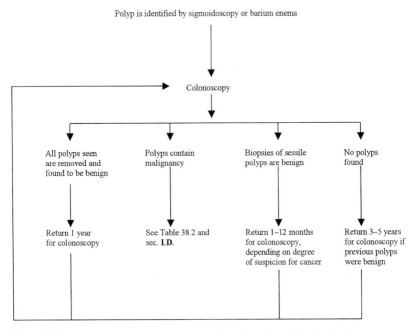

Figure 39-4. Recommendations for cancer surveillance in patients with colonic polyps.

Selected Readings

Anderson JC, et al. Prevalence of colorectal neoplasia in smokers. *Am J Gastroenterol.* 2003;98:2777–2783.

Barclay RL, et al. Colonoscopic withdrawal times and adenoma detection during screening colonoscopy. *N Engl J Med.* 2006;355:2533–2541.

Chan AT, et al. Aspirin and the risk of colorectal cancer in relation to the expression of COX-2. *N Engl J Med.* 2007 May 24;356:2131–2134.

Cho E, et al. Alcohol intake and colorectal cancer: A pooled analysis of 8 cohort studies. *Ann Intern Med.* 2004;140:603–612.

Cole BF, et al. Folic acid for the prevention of colorectal adenomas: A randomized clinical trial. *JAMA.* 2007 June 6;297:2351–2359.

Coluca G, et al. Phase III randomized trial of FOLFIRI versus FOLFAX 4 in the treatment of advanced colorectal cancer. *J Clin Oncol.* 2005;23(22):4866–4875.

DeJong A, et al. Decrease in mortality in Lynch syndrome families because of surveillance. *Gastroenterology.* 2006;130:665–671.

Dove-Edwin I, et al. Prevention of colorectal cancer by colonoscopic surveillance in individuals with a family history of colorectal cancer: A 16 year prospective follow-up. *BMJ.* 2005;331:1047–1052.

Eng C, et al. Impact of quality of life of adding cetuximab to irontecan in patients who have failed prior oxaliplatin-based therapy:the EPIC trial. *J Clin Oncol.* 2007;25:suppl:18s.

Giardiello FM, et al. AGA technical review on hereditary colorectal cancer and genetic testing. *Gastroenterology.* 2001;121:198.

Goldberg RM, et al. A randomized controlled trial of fluoro acid plus leukovour, Irinotecan and oxiplatin combinations in patients with previously untreated metastatic colorectal cancer. *J Clin Oncol.* 2004;22(1):23–30.

Hur C, et al. The management of small polyps found by virtual colonoscopy: results of a decision analysis. *Clin Gastroenterol Hepatol.* 2007;5:237–244.

Kapiteijn E, et al. Preoperative radiotherapy combined with total mesorectal excision for resectable rectal cancer. *N Engl J Med.* 2001;345:638.

King JE, et al. Care of patients and their families with familial adenomatous polyposis. *Mayo Clin Proc.* 2000;75:57.

Latreille MW, et al. Colonoscopy screening for detection of advanced neoplasia. *N Engl J Med.* 2007;356:632–634.

Lierbeman DA, et al. Risk factors for advanced colonic neoplasia and hyperplastic polyps in asymptomatic individuals. *JAMA.* 2003;290:2959–2967.

Offit K, et al. Reducing the risk of gynecologic cancer in the Lynch syndrome. *N Engl J Med.* 2006;354:292–294.

Pickhardt P, et al. Computed tomographic virtual colonoscopy to screen for colorectal neoplasia in asymptomatic adults. *N Engl J Med.* 2003;349:2191–2200.

Poston GJ, et al. Onco Surge: A strategy for improving resectability with curative intent in metastatic colorectal cancer. *J Clin Oncol.* 2005;23(9):2038–2048.

Ratto C, et al. Combined modality therapy in locally advanced primary rectal cancer. *Dis Colon Rectum.* 2003;46:59–67.

Rex DK, et al. ACG colorectal cancer prevention action plan: update on CT-colonography. *Am J Gastroenterol.* 2006;I0I:1410–1403.

Rex DK, et al. Guidelines for colonoscopy surveillance after cancer resection: A consensus update by the American Cancer Society and the U.S. Muti-Society Task Force on Colorectal Cancer. *Gastroenterology.* 2006;130:1865–1871.

Rex DK, Maximizing detection of adenomas and cancers during colonoscopy. *Am J Gastroenterol.* 2006;101:2866–2877.

Tonkef DJ, et al. Cetuximab for the treatment of colorectal cancer. *N Engl J Med.* 2007;357:2040–2048.

Ulrich DM and Potter JD. Folate and cancer—Timing is everything. *JAMA.* 2007 Jun 6; 297:2408–2409.

Winawer S, et al. Colorectal cancer screening and surveillance: Clinical guidelines and rationale-update based on new evidence. *Gastroenterology.* 2003;124:544–560.

Winawer SJ, et al. Guidelines for colonoscopy surveillance after polypectomy: A consensus update by the U.S. Multi-Society Task Force on Colorectal Cancer and the American Cancer Society. *Gastroenterology.* 2006;130:1872–1885.

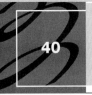

40   OSTOMY CARE

$\mathcal{T}$he word *ostium* means "opening." Thus the words **ileostomy** and **colostomy** refer to openings into the ileum and colon, respectively, which are the subjects of this chapter. Other ostomies include gastrostomies and jejunostomies, which usually are formed for the purpose of alimentation, and ileal loop urostomies, which are formed to replace the urinary bladder.

An ileostomy is usually the end result of a total proctocolectomy. A colostomy may be formed after a partial colon resection, typically for cancer, diverticulitis, or ischemic disease.

I. **FORMATION OF OSTOMIES.** Most ileostomies and colostomies are formed by bringing the bowel out through an incision in the abdominal wall and suturing the mucosa to the skin. Some are "double-barrel," meaning that the bowel leads both to and away from the opening. Two important modifications of ileostomies are available.

    A. The **Kock pouch,** or continent ileostomy, is a pouch fashioned from ileum just proximal to the ostomy and functions as a reservoir for stool. The stoma is formed in the shape of a nipple, which is cannulated for drainage several times a day. Most patients with Kock pouches remain continent and do not require an ostomy bag.

    B. **Ileorectal pull-through.** The second modification is not actually an ileostomy but rather a form of anorectal anastomosis, called an ileorectal pull-through. The entire colon is removed except for the distal rectum. The distal rectum is stripped of mucosa, and the ileum is connected to the anus within the muscular sheath of the rectum, which includes the anal sphincter. To improve continence, a pouch can be formed from the distal ileum.

II. **CONSEQUENCES AND COMPLICATIONS OF OSTOMIES.** Because the colon absorbs water and electrolytes in sufficient amounts to form a firm stool, patients with ileostomies can be expected to lose water and electrolytes more than healthy people do. The normal daily stool of a person whose bowel is intact weighs 100 to 200 g and contains 80% to 85% water. A normally functioning ileostomy discharges 500 to 1,000 g of stool per day, containing 90% to 95% water. Furthermore, whereas healthy people can reduce stool sodium losses to 1 to 2 mEq per day by conserving sodium in the colon, patients with ileostomies have obligatory daily sodium losses of 30 mEq or more.

    If the terminal ileum has been removed in addition to the colon, bile salt and vitamin B_{12} malabsorption may occur (see Chapter 31). The loss of bile salts may predispose to steatorrhea, which worsens the diarrhea.

    Complications of ileostomies and colostomies include irritation of the skin surrounding the ostomy, obstruction of the ostomy, recurrence of inflammatory bowel disease at or proximal to the stoma, and mechanical difficulties with the stoma appliances. Patients also may have psychological and social problems related to the ostomy.

III. **MANAGEMENT OF THE PATIENT WITH AN OSTOMY**

    A. **Preoperative considerations.** Ileostomies and colostomies are performed under elective conditions in most instances. Thus, there should be adequate time to discuss the intended surgery with the patient, explain the necessity for the ostomy, explore the patient's concerns about it, review possible consequences and complications, and reassure the patient that after full recovery from surgery most patients are able to conduct normal lives, including participation in normal physical, sexual, and social activities. The physician, surgeon, and ostomy nurse all play important roles in the preoperative preparation of the patient. Patients almost always benefit from talking with another person who has an ostomy. Such people may be well known to the physician or the ostomy nurse or they may be contacted through the local Ostomy Association, which is listed in the telephone book of most medium-to-large communities. The United Ostomy Association (36 Executive Park, Suite 120, Irvine, CA 92714; telephone 1-800-826-0826) is a source for informational material.

B. Skin care. The skin surrounding an ostomy is at risk for injury. Patients with an ileostomy are likely to have more skin irritation than patients with a colostomy because ileostomy stool is liquid and contains digestive enzymes. Tape and ill-fitting appliances can also contribute to skin excoriation.

Nondetergent soap and water are the most appropriate peristomal skin-cleansing agents. A variety of skin-conditioning agents and seals for appliances are available. However, an improperly fitting appliance will negate the best skin care.

C. Fluids, salt, and diet

   1. Fluids and salt. Because patients with ileostomies may lose up to a liter of water and 30 mEq of sodium in the stool per day, they are encouraged to drink 2 to 3 L of water per day and not to restrict salt. Mild-to-moderate diarrhea may be treated by increasing fluid and sodium intake and by adding bicarbonate of soda and orange juice to provide potassium. More severe diarrhea may require intravenous fluids and electrolytes. Patients with colostomies generally do not have problems with excessive loss of fluid and electrolytes because sufficient colon remains to maintain water- and electrolyte-conserving function.

   2. Diet. Patients should be encouraged to eat a normal diet, with some modification. Gas-producing foods may cause discomfort and embarrassment. Fresh fruits may promote loose stools. Most patients discover through trial and error the diet to which they are best suited.

   3. Vitamin and mineral supplements. Some patients require vitamin and mineral supplements, particularly patients who have steatorrhea or vitamin B_{12} malabsorption.

D. Odors. Disagreeable odors from the ostomy bag can be distressful. The odors are due to gases that are derived from the action of bacteria on intestinal substrates (see Chapter 34). The problem is treated by emptying the bag frequently, avoiding gas-forming foods, and adding a deodorant to the bag, such as chlorine tablets or sodium benzoate.

E. Ostomy dysfunction. Partial obstruction of the ostomy, usually an ileostomy, may result from recurrent disease, impaction of nondigestible material, or kinking of a loop of bowel just proximal to the stoma. Patients experience abdominal cramping pain and increased ostomy effluent.

   1. Diagnosis. Gentle examination of the stoma with the small finger is indicated. This may be followed by endoscopic examination, perhaps with a pediatric sigmoidoscope or fiberoptic gastroscope. Retrograde barium-contrast radiologic studies through the stoma also may be helpful.

   2. Treatment is dictated by the diagnosis. Recurrent inflammatory bowel disease may respond to a course of treatment. Some patients require surgical revision of the stoma.

Selected Readings

Bradley M, et al. Essential elements of ostomy care. *Am J Nurs.* 1997;97:38.

Catanzaro J, et al. High-tech wound and ostomy care in the home setting. *Crit Care Nurs Clin North Am.* 1998;10:327.

Erwin-Toth P. The effect of ostomy surgery between the ages of 6 and 12 years on psychosocial development during childhood, adolescence and young adulthood. *J Wound Ostomy Continence Nurs.* 1999;26:77.

Evans JP, et al. Revising the troublesome stoma: Combined abdominal wall recountering and revision of stomas. *Dis Colon Rectum.* 2003;46:122–126.

Mitchel JV. A clinical pathway for ostomy care in the home: Process and development. *J Wound Ostomy Continence Nurs.* 1998;25:200.

Turnbull GB, et al. Ostomy care: Foundation for teaching and practice. *Ostomy Wound Manage.* 1999;45(suppl 1A):23.

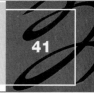

*N*early everyone has experienced anorectal discomfort. Our low-fiber diet, which results in small, hard stools; our lifestyle, which restricts the opportunities for defecation; and our erect posture, which promotes engorgement of the hemorrhoidal plexus all combine to make anorectal problems virtually ubiquitous. The anorectum also is the site of local manifestations of more generalized disorders, such as inflammatory bowel disease. Finally, because the rectum is a sexual organ for some people, sexually transmitted diseases may occur at that site.

I. HEMORRHOIDS

A. Pathogenesis. Hemorrhoids are dilated veins within the anal canal and distal rectum. External hemorrhoids are derived from the external hemorrhoidal plexus below the dentate line and are covered by stratified squamous epithelium. Internal hemorrhoids are derived from the internal hemorrhoidal plexus above the dentate line and are covered by rectal mucosa.

Hemorrhoids are thought to develop in most instances as a consequence of erect posture, straining at stool, heavy lifting, or childbirth. In some patients, portal hypertension predisposes to hemorrhoids; rarely, hemorrhoids develop as a result of an intraabdominal mass.

B. Clinical presentation

1. History. Hemorrhoids typically cause bleeding, which is detected as streaks of red blood on the stool and toilet paper. Patients also may complain of anal itching or pain. However, severe pain is an unusual symptom unless the hemorrhoid is thrombosed.

2. Physical examination. Inspection of the anus may reveal bluish, soft, bulging veins indicative of external hemorrhoids or prolapsed internal hemorrhoids. Nonprolapsed internal hemorrhoids cannot be seen externally and are difficult to distinguish from mucosal folds by digital rectal examination unless they are thrombosed. Thrombosed hemorrhoids usually are exquisitely tender.

C. Diagnostic studies. The anal canal and rectum should be examined by anoscopy and sigmoidoscopy. Symptomatic hemorrhoids usually are accompanied by varying degrees of inflammation within the anal canal. At sigmoidoscopy, the anus and rectum can be evaluated for other conditions in the differential diagnosis of rectal bleeding and discomfort, such as anal fissure and fistula, proctitis and colitis, rectal polyp, and cancer. Barium enema x-ray examination or colonoscopy should be performed in patients over age 50 and in patients of any age whose stool remains positive for occult blood after appropriate treatment for hemorrhoids.

D. Treatment. A high-fiber diet, stool softeners, and avoidance of straining at stool and heavy lifting may be sufficient to treat mild hemorrhoidal symptoms. Warm baths twice a day and anal lubrication with glycerine suppositories provide further comfort. Addition of medicated suppositories, such as Anusol-HC (containing hydrocortisone), may help reduce associated inflammation. However, steroid-containing medications should be limited to 2 weeks of continuous use to avoid atrophy of the anal tissues.

Additional treatment usually requires the expertise of a gastroenterologist or surgeon. Rubber-band ligation is usually the first definitive treatment. The procedure requires no anesthesia and produces excellent results in most patients.

Injection of hemorrhoids with sclerosing solutions, dilatation of the anal sphincter under anesthesia, electrocoagulation, and laser coagulation are alternatives if rubber banding is ineffective. In patients whose hemorrhoids are severe and refractory to these treatments, surgical excision of the hemorrhoidal plexus may be necessary. Rarely, surgical section of the internal anal sphincter is performed.

II. ANAL FISSURES

A. **Pathogenesis.** An anal fissure is a tear in the lining of the anus, usually resulting from the difficult passage of hard stool. Some fissures are a consequence of a more generalized bowel disorder, such as Crohn's disease. Others result from the trauma of anal intercourse or insertion of foreign bodies. Rarely, carcinoma of the anus presents as an anal fissure.

More than 90% of fissures that are not associated with Crohn's disease occur in the posterior midline. The remainder occurs in the anterior midline. Fissures associated with Crohn's disease may occur at any location within the anal canal.

B. **Clinical presentation.** Anal fissures are painful, and the pain is exacerbated by the passing of stool. The pain may lead to a cycle of retention of stool, formation of hard stool, passage of hard stool, and aggravation of the fissure. Bleeding and itching also are common. Anal fissures often coexist with hemorrhoids.

External examination by spreading the patient's buttocks and anal orifice may reveal the fissure. Digital examination usually is quite painful for the patient and thus the rectal examination may be limited. Sometimes the fissure or a mass of granulation tissue can be palpated. Preliminary application of a topical anesthetic decreases the discomfort of the digital rectal examination and subsequent sigmoidoscopic examination.

C. **Diagnostic studies**
1. **Anoscopy and sigmoidoscopy** should be performed to make the definitive diagnosis and to rule out other conditions mentioned in section I, in the discussion of hemorrhoids.
2. **Scraping the fissure.** If the cause of the fissure is suspected to be sexual, a scraping of the fissure should be examined under dark field illumination to consider the possibility of a syphilitic lesion.
3. **Radiologic evaluation.** Patients whose fissures fail to heal or who have fissures that are not in the midline should undergo radiologic evaluation of the large and small bowel for Crohn's disease.
4. The **treatment** of anal fissure is similar to that of hemorrhoids: high-bulk diet, stool softeners, warm baths, and lubricating suppositories. Most fissures heal on this regimen. Chronic anal fissures that are not due to inflammatory bowel disease may require dilatation of the anus, sphincterotomy, or excision of the fissure.

III. FISTULAS AND ABSCESSES

A. **Pathogenesis.** A fistula is a tract lined by inflammatory tissue that usually has an opening through the mucosa of the anus or rectum and another opening in the perianal skin. Sometimes only one opening is evident. Fistulas are always infected with local organisms. An abscess is a collection of pus within the perianal or perirectal tissues, which may or may not be associated with a fistulous tract. Factors that predispose to fistula or abscess formation include local infection of the anal crypts, Crohn's disease, trauma, cancer, and venereal disease.

B. **Clinical presentation and diagnosis.** A fistula or abscess may be painful and cause fever. If the fistula is external, drainage of pus, mucus, or stool may be evident. Physical examination may confirm the external location of the fistula opening. A tender, firm, or fluctuant mass suggests an abscess. Anoscopy, sigmoidoscopy, and barium-contrast studies are indicated as described in section II.C.

C. **Treatment.** Although local treatment with warm baths, high-fiber diet, and stool softeners may be palliative, definitive surgical drainage of the abscess or excision of the fistula usually is indicated. An exception is a fistula associated with Crohn's disease, which may respond to an elemental diet, metronidazole, or steroid therapy. Broad-spectrum antibiotics are indicated for patients with fever, elevated white blood cell count, or signs of systemic toxicity.

IV. PROCTITIS

A. Pathogenesis. Proctitis is an inflammation of the rectal mucosa. It may be idiopathic or related to a specific cause, such as radiation or gonococcal infection.

B. Clinical presentation. Patients with proctitis typically complain of pain and bleeding on defecation. Stools may be loose, but often they are well formed. In fact, some patients move their bowels infrequently to avoid pain and thus become constipated, which aggravates symptoms even more. Digital rectal examination may reveal a small amount of bloody stool or mucus.

Idiopathic proctitis is a chronic, relapsing, localized condition that progresses to ulcerative colitis in some patients. The appearance of an erythematous, friable, sometimes hemorrhagic mucosa, however, is indistinguishable from that of ulcerative colitis. Small ulcerations and pus suggest the possibility of gonococcal proctitis. Ulcers and vesicles of the distal rectum, which may extend to the perianal skin, suggest herpes proctitis.

C. Diagnostic studies. Sigmoidoscopy shows the inflammation to be limited to the rectum, sometimes within several centimeters of the anus. Mucosal biopsy and culture of rectal secretions should be obtained. More extensive bowel involvement may be documented by barium enema or colonoscopy.

D. Treatment

1. Idiopathic proctitis. Treatment of idiopathic proctitis usually consists of mesalamine enemas (i.e., Rowasa) or suppositories (i.e., Canasa) or steroid enemas once or twice daily for 4 to 6 weeks. Patients should be instructed to lie in the left decubitus position and gently insert a suppository or an enema before bedtime and another in the morning after a bowel movement. Some patients require one or two mesalamine or steroid enemas per day for prolonged periods to control symptoms. Patients who have frequent recurrences of proctitis may respond to prophylactic treatment with sulfasalazine (1 to 2 g b.i.d.) or a mesalamine preparation (e.g., Asacol 800 mg t.i.d. or Colazal 2.25 g t.i.d.). Steroid or mesalamine enemas also are somewhat effective in treating radiation proctitis.

2. Infectious proctitis. Treatment of infectious proctitis is directed at the causative agent. For example, gonococcal proctitis typically responds to aqueous procaine penicillin G, 4.8 million units intramuscular (IM), plus 1 g of oral probenecid. For penicillin-allergic patients, tetracycline (orally, 1.5 g followed by 0.5 g q.i.d. for 4 days) is effective.

V. RECTAL PROLAPSE

A. Pathogenesis. Rectal prolapse ranges in severity from prolapse of a small portion of rectal mucosa to protrusion of the entire rectal wall through the anus (procidentia). Straining at stool is thought to be causative, but pelvic surgery, childbearing, and weak pelvic musculature are contributive factors.

B. Clinical presentation and diagnosis. Patients with rectal prolapse complain of bleeding, passage of mucus, and irritation of the exposed mucosa. In some patients, prolapse of the rectal mucosa or of a substantial portion of the rectum may be observed. Other patients must strain to produce the prolapse. Poor anal sphincter tone usually is evident on digital examination. Sigmoidoscopy and, in most patients, barium enema are indicated to define the extent of irritated mucosa and to rule out associated conditions.

C. Treatment. If the prolapse is mild and confined to the mucosa, the treatment regimen is the same as for hemorrhoids. However, frank procidentia requires operative treatment if the surgical risk is good.

VI. PROCTALGIA FUGAX

A. Pathogenesis and clinical presentation. Proctalgia fugax is fleeting pain in the anorectum. The pain is intense, develops suddenly, and typically lasts for seconds to minutes, although occasionally it persists for several hours. There is no known cause. It probably is related to spasm of the musculature of the rectosigmoid or levator muscles. Rarely, it is associated with mucosal inflammatory disease or colonic tumors.

B. The **diagnosis** is made by the typical history of rectal pain and absence of physical findings. Rectal and sigmoidoscopic examinations should be performed to rule out other treatable disorders.

C. **Treatment** is symptomatic, consisting of warm baths and, if symptoms are frequent, analgesics and muscle relaxants. Because of the transient nature of the disorder, however, it is often difficult to determine whether treatment has been effective. The condition usually resolves spontaneously.

VII. PRURITUS ANI

A. **Pathogenesis.** Virtually everyone has experienced perianal itching. When the itching becomes frequent or constant, patients seek medical attention. The causes of pruritus ani are legion, including hemorrhoids, fissures, skin disorders, infections, parasites, neoplasms, excessive moisture, excessive dryness, irritation from soap and other agents, and psychoneurosis.

B. **Clinical presentation.** When patients complain of perianal itching, a careful history of bowel habits, stool-wiping technique, use of cleansing or other local agents, and ingestion of antibiotics should be obtained. Examination may be normal or may reveal erythema, excoriations, or maceration of the perianal skin.

C. **Diagnostic studies.** Rectal and sigmoidoscopic examinations should be performed. Stool culture, examination of the stool for ova and parasites, and examination of the perianal skin for pinworms or *Candida* are performed when clinically indicated.

D. **Treatment** depends on the diagnosis. If no specific cause can be determined, the patient is advised to avoid all topical agents that might irritate the anus and to consume a high-fiber diet. Patients should wipe the anus gently, not vigorously, after defecation, using a moist cotton ball or cotton cloth. Calamine lotion or a steroid cream (not ointment) may be applied to the anus several times a day.

VIII. TUMORS

A. **Pathogenesis.** Tumors of the anus sometimes are confused with other inflammatory and infectious lesions. The most common anal tumor is epidermoid carcinoma, but adenocarcinoma and malignant melanoma also can occur.

B. **Clinical presentation and diagnosis.** Patients complain of anal pain, bleeding, itching, or presence of a mass. They may think that they are having more trouble with their hemorrhoids. The diagnosis of neoplasm is suspected by visual inspection, digital examination, and anoscopy; it is confirmed by biopsy. A search for local extension and metastatic disease is warranted. This typically includes routine liver tests, chest x-ray, and computed tomography of the abdomen and pelvis.

C. **Treatment.** Small anal tumors can be treated by local excision. More extensive lesions require the addition of radiation therapy or chemotherapy, or an abdominoperitoneal resection of the rectum and anus.

IX. SEXUALLY TRANSMITTED ANORECTAL INFECTIONS. See Chapter 42.

Selected Readings

Beets-Tan RGH. Preoperative MR imaging of anal fistulas: Does it really help the surgeon? *Radiology*. 2001;218:75.

Cheung O, et al. The management of pelvic floor disorders. *Ailment Pharmacol Ther*. 2004;19:481–495.

Diamant NE, et al. AGA technical review on anorectal testing techniques. *Gastroenterology*. 1999;116:735.

Dorsky R. Coping with the pain and annoyance of hemorrhoids. *Dis Health Nutr*. January/February 2000:21.

Gosens MJEM, et al. Improvement of staging by combining tumor and treatment parameters: the value for prognostication in rectal cancer. *Clin Gastroenterol Hepatol*. 2007;5(8):997–1003.

Jones MP, Post JP, Crowell MD. High-resolution manometry in the evaluation of anorectal disorders: a simultaneous comparison with water-perfused manometry. *Am J Gastroenterol.* 2007;102:1–6.

Kang YS, et al. Pathology of the rectal wall in solitary ulcer syndrome and complete rectal prolapse. *Gut.* 1996;38:587.

Koslin DB. Anal fistulae. *Rev Gastroenterol Disord.* 2001;1:56.

Madoff RD, et al. AGA technical review on the diagnosis and care of patients with anal fissure. *Gastroenterology.* 2003;124:235–245.

Masderstein EL, et al. Surgical management of rectal prolapse. *Nat Clin Pract Gastroenterol Hepatol.* 2007;4(10):552–561.

Rao SC. How useful are manometric tests of anorectal function in the management of defecation disorders? *Am J Gastroenterol.* 1999;116:735.

Rao SC. Dyssynergic: disorders of the anorectum. *Gastroenterol Clin North Am.* 2001; 31:97–114.

Rao SSC. Diagnosis and management of fecal incontinence. *Am J Gastroenterol.* 2004; 99:1585–16.

Sentovic SM. Fibrin glue for anal fistulas: Long term results. *Dis Colon Rectum.* 2003;46: 498–502.

Sobhani I, et al. Prevalence of high-grade dysplasia and cancer in anal canal in human papilloma virus-infected individuals. *Gastroenterology.* 2001;120:857.

Sotlar K, et al. Human papilloma virus type 16-associated primary squamous cell carcinoma of the rectum. *Gastroenterology.* 2001;120:988.

Wald A, Fecal incontinence in adults. *N Engl J Med.* 2007;356:1648–1655.

42 SEXUALLY TRANSMITTED ENTERIC DISORDERS

$\mathcal{S}$ ubstantial increases in the recognition and prevalence of sexually transmitted enteric disorders have occurred over the past several decades, largely due to increasing freedom of both heterosexual and homosexual expression. The acquired immunodeficiency syndrome (AIDS) has further augmented the diversity and complexity of sexually related enteric disorders. These disorders are summarized in Table 42-1. Gastrointestinal and hepatobiliary disorders that are related to the human immunodeficiency virus (HIV) are discussed in more detail in Chapter 43.

I. **PATHOGENESIS.** Most of the sexually related enteric disorders are infectious (Table 42-1), although trauma may be a clinically significant factor in the pathogenesis of anorectal disease, and neoplasm (Kaposi's sarcoma, lymphoma) can complicate AIDS. The transmission of infectious agents during sexual activity is to be expected, particularly when one considers the variety of means of sexual expression—oral/oral contact, fellatio, cunnilingus, anilingus, and anal intercourse, in addition to ordinary sexual intercourse. Thus, it is no mystery that sexually related diseases occur, particularly in the oropharynx and anorectum, but also elsewhere throughout the digestive system.

II. **DIAGNOSIS.** Knowledge of a patient's sexual practices can be helpful but is not necessary to make an etiologic diagnosis of one of the conditions listed in Table 42-1.

TABLE 42-1   Sexually Related Disorders of the Gastrointestinal Tract

Oropharyngeal disorders	Condylomata acuminata
Gonococcal pharyngitis	(papilloma virus)
Oral syphilis	Traumatic injury
Herpes pharyngitis	Liver disorders
Gastric disorders	Gonococcal perihepatitis
Syphilitic gastritis	Syphilitic hepatitis
Enteric disorders	Hepatitis A; B; non-A, non-B
Campylobacter infections	Cytomegalovirus hepatitis
Salmonellosis	AIDS-related disorders
Shigellosis	Infections with
Giardiasis	*Candida*
Amebiasis	*Cryptosporidium*
Anorectal disorders	*Isospora*
Gonococcal proctitis	*Mycobacterium avium-intracellulare*
Syphilis	Kaposi's sarcoma
Chlamydial infection	Lymphoma
(lymphogranuloma venereum)	
Herpes proctitis	

A. Oropharyngeal disorders

   1. Gonococcal pharyngitis can present with sore throat, exudate of the pharynx and tonsils, and ulcerations of the tongue and buccal mucosa. However, some patients with gonococcal infection of the oropharynx may be asymptomatic but transmit the disease to others. If gonococcal infection is suspected, the lesions should be cultured immediately.

   2. Syphilis. The oral lesions of syphilis are elevated, round, sometimes ulcerated, and usually painless. They occur most frequently on the lips but also may be found on the tongue or tonsils, and elsewhere within the mouth and pharynx. These lesions heal within several weeks but are superseded by the systemic signs and symptoms of secondary syphilis, namely, fever, sore throat, lymphadenopathy, pruritus, and skin lesions. A nonspecific pharyngitis may also be present. The darkfield examination of the primary oral lesions may be confused by the presence of normal oral spirochetes. Serologic tests may not be positive until the secondary form of the disease appears. Aspiration of enlarged lymph nodes for darkfield examination may give an early diagnosis.

   3. Herpes pharyngitis. Patients with herpes pharyngitis have erythema and ulcerations of the mouth, tongue, gingiva, and pharynx. Exudate and lymphadenopathy also may be present. The presence of a herpes infection in the patient's sexual partner makes the diagnosis more likely. Facilities to culture the virus may not be available. The diagnosis can be inferred from serologic tests directed against the herpes simplex virus.

B. Gastric disorders. Although the infectious agents that cause sexually related enteric diseases may pass through the stomach, gastritis per se is not a feature of those diseases. However, secondary syphilis, a rare complication, can involve the stomach. In syphilitic gastritis, the mucosa becomes ulcerated and infiltrated with chronic inflammatory cells. Patients complain of abdominal pain and vomiting. Loss of weight is common. Spirochetes can be identified by darkfield examination of mucosal biopsies. The diagnosis can be confirmed by serologic tests for syphilis. The stomach also can be involved with lymphoma or with Kaposi's sarcoma when these conditions affect AIDS patients.

C. Enteric disorders. Patients with sexually transmitted enteric infections appear similar clinically to those who contract the infection in some other manner. The diagnosis and management of infectious diarrheal conditions are discussed in Chapter 29.

D. Anorectal disorders

   1. Gonococcal proctitis may present with anorectal pain, tenesmus, and a mucopurulent discharge. At sigmoidoscopy, the rectal mucosa appears red and contains pus and small ulcers. Mucosal biopsy shows nonspecific inflammation. The diagnosis is made by Gram's stain and culture of rectal aspirates or mucosal biopsies. Many patients with anorectal gonococcal infection are asymptomatic but are a source of infection to others.

   2. Anorectal syphilis is characterized by a painless chancre, which often is mistaken for an anal fissure. The diagnosis of syphilis is based on a high index of suspicion in a susceptible patient, darkfield examination of the lesion, and serologic follow-up.

   3. *Chlamydia trachomatis* can infect the rectum and intestine with either the lymphogranuloma venereum (LGV) serotype or the non-LGV serotype. The non-LGV infections are similar to infections caused by gonococci. They are usually mildly symptomatic with anorectal discharge, tenesmus, anorectal pain, and mild mucosal inflammation. In contrast, LGV infections typically cause severe proctocolitis. Anorectal pain is severe and is accompanied by bloody purulent discharge, tenesmus, and diarrhea. The rectal mucosa is friable and ulcerated. The histologic appearance may be similar to that in Crohn's disease, with diffuse inflammation and granulomas. Stricturing and fistula formation add to the confusion with Crohn's disease. *C. trachomatis* can be isolated from the rectum. Serologic tests of LGV infection confirm the diagnosis. Response to treatment with tetracycline also is confirmatory of the diagnosis.

TABLE 42-2	Treatment of Sexually Related Gastrointestinal Infections	

Infectious agent	Suggested antibiotic	Alternative antibiotic
Gonococcus		
Oropharyngeal	APPG, 4.8 million units IM + probenecid, 1 g p.o.	TS (80 mg/400 mg), 9 tablets daily × 5 d
Rectal	APPG, 4.8 million units IM + probenecid, 1 g p.o.	Spectinomycin, 2 g IM
Syphilis	Benzathine penicillin G, 2.4 million units IM	Tetracycline, 500 mg p.o. q.i.d. × 15 d
Chlamydia		
LGV	Tetracycline, 500 mg p.o. q.i.d. × 21 d	Erythromycin, 500 mg p.o. q.i.d. × 21 d
Non-LGV	Tetracycline, 500 mg p.o. q.i.d. × 7 d	Erythromycin, 500 mg p.o. q.i.d. × 7 d
Herpes simplex	Acyclovir, 1 tablet 5 times/d × 10 d	Supportive therapy
Papilloma virus (condyloma)	Podophyllin (10%–25%) on lesion every other day	Cryotherapy or surgery
Campylobacter	Erythromycin, 500 mg p.o. q.i.d. × 7 d	Tetracycline, 500 mg p.o. q.i.d. × 7 d
Salmonella	Antibiotic treatment not necessary except for severe cases	Ampicillin, 1 g intravenous q4h × 10 d; TS, 2 tablets p.o. q12h × 10 d
Shigella	TS, 160 mg/800 mg p.o. b.i.d. × 7 d	Ampicillin, 500 mg p.o. q.i.d. × 7 d
Giardia	Metronidazole, 250 mg p.o. t.i.d. × 7 d	Quinacrine hydrochloride, 100 mg t.i.d. × 7 d
Entamoeba	Metronidazole, 750 mg p.o. t.i.d. × 7 d	Diiodohydroxyquin, 650 mg p.o. t.i.d. × 20 d
Candida (esophagitis)	Fluconazole, 50–100 mg × 10 d	Ketoconazole, 200 mg p.o. b.i.d.
Cryptosporidium	Supportive therapy only in immunocompetent patients Spiramycin, 1 g p.o. q.i.d. in patients with AIDS	
Isospora	Supportive therapy only in immunocompetent patients Spiramycin, 1 gm p.o. q.i.d. in patients with AIDS	
Mycobacterium avium-intracellulare	Multidrug antituberculous therapy	

APPG, aqueous procaine penicillin G; TS, trimethoprim/sulfamethoxazole; LGV, lymphogranuloma venereum; IM, intramuscular; p.o., orally; q.i.d., four times daily; t.i.d., three times daily; b.i.d., twice daily; AIDS, autoimmune deficiency syndrome.
Modified from Quinn TC. Clinical approach to intestinal infections in homosexual men. *Med Clin North Am.* 1986;70:611. Reprinted with permission.

4. **Herpes** can involve not only the anus and rectum but also the perianal skin, with the typical herpetic vesicles and ulcerations. Patients complain of pain, rectal discharge, and bloody stool. The diagnosis often can be made on clinical presentation alone. Histologic examination of rectal mucosal biopsies may reveal intranuclear inclusion bodies in addition to focal ulcers and perivascular mononuclear cell infiltrates. Culture of the virus is diagnostic but may not be available. The serologic diagnosis requires seroconversion or a fourfold or greater rise in antibody titer.

5. **Condylomata acuminata, or anal warts,** are caused by the human papilloma virus and are common in people who practice anal intercourse. They appear as small brownish papules around the anus.

6. **Traumatic injury** may have many causes and may take many forms. Dilatation and stretching of the anus from anal intercourse can cause fissures and tearing of the mucosa and underlying structures. The practice of inserting fingers, hands, arms, or foreign objects into the rectum increases the likelihood of anal and rectal trauma. The diagnosis of anorectal trauma is based on historical information unless a foreign object is apparent. Traumatic and infectious disorders can coexist.

E. Liver disorders

1. **Gonococcal perihepatitis** is a consequence of spread of infection from the fallopian tubes in women and through lymphatics or blood in both men and women. The signs and symptoms are similar to those of acute cholecystitis, namely, acute right upper abdominal pain that may radiate to the shoulder, nausea and vomiting, and fever. Although the patient may or may not have symptomatic pelvic gonorrhea, cultures of the uterine cervix for gonococcus typically are positive. The condition must be differentiated from acute cholecystitis and other causes of acute abdominal pain (see Chapter 13).

2. **Syphilitic hepatitis** is an unusual manifestation of secondary syphilis. It is thought to be due to an infiltration of the liver by spirochetes, which arrive through the portal system from primary lesions in the rectum. The clinical picture is one of hepatomegaly and obstructive jaundice. Liver biopsy is diagnostic when it shows granulomas and spirochetes within the liver.

3. **The hepatitis viruses and cytomegalovirus** can be transmitted by sexual contact. The diagnosis and management of these infections are discussed in Chapter 50.

III. TREATMENT. Effective treatment of the infectious causes of sexually related enteric disease depends on the identification of the offending agent or agents and use of the appropriate antibiotic regimen (Table 42-2). Supportive treatment may involve intravenous fluids and nourishment in patients who are unable to swallow or who have severe diarrhea. There is no known effective therapy for Kaposi's sarcoma. Lymphoma may respond to chemotherapy or radiation therapy (see Chapter 32).

Selected Readings

Jones DJ, Goorney BP. ABC of colorectal diseases: Sexually transmitted diseases and anal papillomas. *BMJ*. 1992;305:820.

Laughon BE, et al. Prevalence of enteric pathogens in homosexual men with and without acquired immunodeficiency syndrome. *Gastroenterology*. 1988;94:984.

Owen WF Jr. The clinical approach to the male homosexual patient. *Med Clin North Am*. 1986;70:499.

Quinn TC. Clinical approach to intestinal infections in homosexual men. *Med Clin North Am*. 1986;70:611.

Smith PD, et al. Gastrointestinal infections in AIDS. *Ann Intern Med*. 1992;116:63.

Surawicz CM, et al. Anal dysplasia in homosexual men: Role of anoscopy and biopsy. *Gastroenterology*. 1993;105:658.

Weller ID. The gay bowel. *Gut*. 1985;26:869.

43 GASTROINTESTINAL AND HEPATOBILIARY DISEASES IN PATIENTS WITH HIV AND AIDS

Gastrointestinal Diseases Associated with Human Immunodeficiency Virus (HIV) Infection

The treatment of human immunodeficiency virus (HIV) infection has dramatically improved over the last several years with the use of combination therapy of potent antiretroviral agents including protease inhibitors. With this highly active antiviral therapy (HAART), HIV replication can be profoundly suppressed and in some patients, circulating HIV becomes undetectable. Even patients with advanced HIV disease, the CD4 lymphocyte count rises reflecting a redistribution of CD4 cells. Clinically, with regression of immune suppression, patients become more immunocompetent, the risk for opportunistic infections and processes becomes reduced, and overall survival is improved. Thus, at this time the long-term prognosis is dictated by the severity of the immunodeficiency (absolute number of CD4 cells) and the level of the circulation virus.

Because of HAART, there has been a major change in the management of opportunistic infections (OIs) in HIV and acquired immunodeficiency syndrome (AIDS). When OIs are diagnosed and treated, both the OI and the underlying HIV infection are treated. In fact, in some patients, treatment with HAART alone results in a remission of OI and reduction of relapses. Because of the remarkable success of HAART in reconstitution of the immune system in these patients, the etiology, diagnostic approach, and management of HIV-associated gastrointestinal (GI) diseases learned in the pre-HAART era may not be accurate at this time.

GI complaints and problems are still quite common in HIV-infected patients; however, etiology has shifted toward disorders not associated with HIV-induced immunodeficiency. Also, some of the medications used in HAART regimens have been associated with GI and hepatic side effects. Table 43-1 lists GI pathogens/diseases by location in HIV-infected patients.

I. **DISEASES OF THE ESOPHAGUS.** Before HAART, approximately one third of HIV-infected patients developed esophageal disease. In patients treated with HAART, the frequency of OI of the entire GI tract, including the esophagus, has been dramatically reduced. However, as with other OIs, the incidence of opportunistic disorders increases as the immunodeficiency worsens. The esophagus may often be the site of the first AIDS-defining opportunistic disease. OIs are the most common causes of esophageal disease. However, cytomegalovirus (CMV) and idiopathic esophageal ulceration (IEU) are rarely seen until the CD4 count falls below 100/mL. Almost all esophageal infections in patients with AIDS are treatable. A definitive diagnosis and treatment usually results in better nutrition, weight gain, and a better quality of life for the patient.

A. **Etiologies**

1. **Fungi.** Prior to the use of HAART, Candidiasis was the most common cause of esophageal disease in HIV-infected patients. Esophageal involvement by fungi other than *Candida* is very rare.

2. **Viruses.** CMV is the most common cause of esophagitis in patients with AIDS. In contrast to other immunocompromised states, such as in posttransplant patients, infection with herpes simplex virus (HSV) is uncommon in HIV-infected patients. In a prospective study of 100 patients infected with HIV, HSV esophagitis was found only in 5% of these patients compared to a 50% prevalence of CMV esophagitis.

TABLE 43-1 Gastrointestinal Pathogens in HIV-Infected Patients

Site	Organism
Esophagus	*Candida albicans*
	HSV
	CMV
Stomach	CMV
	MAC
Small intestine	*Salmonella*
	Campylobacter
	MAC
	Cryptosporidium
	Microsporidia (*Enterocytozoon bieneusi*)
	Isospora belli
	Giardia lamblia
Large intestine	CMV
	Adenovirus
	Histoplasma
	Shigella
	Salmonella
	Clostridium difficile
	Campylobacter
	MAC
	Cryptosporidium
	Microsporidia
	Entamoeba histolytica
Anus	HSV, Human papilloma virus

HIV, human immunodeficiency virus; HSV, herpes simplex virus; CMV, cytomegalovirus; MAC, *Mycobacterium avium* complex.

3. **Idiopathic esophageal ulcers (IEUs)** are an important cause of dysphagia and odynophagia in patients with AIDS. IEU is nearly as common as CMV esophagitis, comprising about 40% of esophageal ulcers. The etiology of IEU is unknown and includes disordered immune regulation, increased apoptosis, local HIV infection, and unidentified viruses.

4. **Gastroesophageal reflux disease (GERD),** in the era of HAART, probably represents one of the most common causes of esophageal disease.

5. **Pill-induced esophagitis** is not uncommon in HIV-infected patients on HAART. Medications unique to these patients include **zidovudine (AZT)** and **zalcitabine (ddC).**

B. **Clinical presentation**

1. The **history** is usually helpful in determining the cause and severity of the esophageal disease. Difficulty swallowing (dysphagia), painful swallowing (odynophagia), loss of appetite, and weight loss are the most common complaints. When the pain is unilateral and localized to the neck or hypopharynx, oropharyngeal rather than esophageal disease is likely.

2. **Physical examination.** The presence of oropharyngeal lesions may provide a clue to the underlying cause of esophageal complaints. Approximately two thirds of patients with esophageal candidiasis have concomitant thrush. However, the presence of thrush does not necessarily indicate *Candida* esophagitis. Also, *Candida* esophagitis may coexist with other esophageal diseases in at least 25% of patients. Oropharyngeal ulcers are rarely associated

with esophageal ulcers. Kaposi's sarcoma (KS) lesions may be seen in the oropharynx and are associated with GI KS.

3. **Laboratory tests.** The stage of immunodeficiency determines the differential diagnosis of esophageal disease. The levels of HIV viremia and CD4 lymphocyte count are the two most important laboratory tests. OIs of the esophagus are uncommon until the CD4 count falls below 200/mm^3. IEU and CMV esophagitis are rarely seen until the CD4 count drops below 100/mm^3.

4. **Empiric therapy.** Because candidiasis is the most common cause of esophageal disease in HIV-infected patients, an empiric trial of antifungal therapy is reasonable. Further diagnostic testing is then based on the clinical response. Empirical therapy with **fluconazole** 200 mg per day followed by 100 mg per day for a 7- to 10-day treatment course is recommended. The clinical response of *Candida* esophagitis to the treatment with fluconazole is rapid (within 3 days). If no substantial improvement occurs in 3 to 5 days, endoscopy is recommended. Most patients who fail antifungal therapy do not have candidiasis, but rather esophageal ulcers. Additional empirical trials such as antiviral therapy with acyclovir sodium or ganciclovir sodium are discouraged. In patients with CD4 counts higher than 200/mm^3 and with symptoms typical of GERD, a trial of gastric acid suppressive therapy with high-dose, proton pump inhibiters is recommended.

5. **Barium swallow/upper GI (UGI) series** may document esophageal candidiasis or ulceration in symptomatic patients. However, because there are many causes of esophageal ulcers in AIDS, patients will require endoscopic examination for biopsies.

6. **Endoscopy** is a means of directly visualizing the UGI mucosa as well as for obtaining biopsies for histopathologic examination of the lesions visualized. The endoscopic appearance of a lesion often suggests the diagnosis. Candidiasis appears as cottage cheese–like plaques and coats most of the esophageal mucosa. However, because *Candida* coexists with other lesions at least in 25% of cases, multiple biopsies are required.

   Viral esophagitis may present as diffuse esophagitis or small superficial ulcers with HSV and as one or more large, well-circumscribed ulcers with CMV. Biopsies of the ulcer margins and base are required for histopathologic diagnosis. Immunohistochemical stains of the biopsies will increase the diagnostic accuracy. IEU may resemble CMV ulcers. Multiple biopsies of the ulcer base and margins are required to exclude the presence of CMV. KS appears as elevated blue-violatious nodules.

7. **Treatment** is to be directed to the etiology of the esophageal lesion. Esophageal candidiasis responds well to **fluconazole** or **itraconazole.** Both agents are also available in liquid formulation for patients who cannot swallow tablets or capsules.

   HSV esophagitis is treated with **acyclovir sodium** or **valacyclovir hydrochloride.** For CMV disease, **ganciclovir** sodium is effective. The newer drug, **cidofovir,** may be administered by a once-weekly injection. IEU may be treated with either **prednisone** or **thalidomide:** The response rate is higher than 90%. Patients should be treated or continued on HAART to help expedite healing and to prevent relapse.

II. DISEASES OF THE STOMACH

A. **Gastric lesions.** The most common OI of the stomach is CMV, which usually results in gastric ulceration. Gastric neoplasms include non-Hodgkin's lymphoma and KS. The stomach is the most common site in the GI tract for KS. Patients are usually asymptomatic. Gastric lymphoma may present with epigastric pain, nausea, and vomiting or bleeding. The prevalence of peptic ulcer disease with or without *Helicobacter pylori* and gastric adenocarcinoma is the same as in the general population.

B. **Endoscopy with biopsies** is the preferred diagnostic modality for gastric lesions. The indications for endoscopy include likelihood of an underlying OI, severity of symptoms (nausea, vomiting, early satiety), and the possible need for endoscopic therapy.

C. **Treatment** should be directed to the cause of the problem.

III. DISEASES OF THE SMALL INTESTINE AND COLON

A. Diarrhea is a common complaint in patients with HIV infection especially in patients with CD4 counts of less than 100/mm^3. As with the esophagus, OI of the intestines has decreased in prevalence as a cause of diarrhea in HIV-infected patients. However, the overall incidence of diarrhea has not decreased at the same rate because several of the antiviral agents used in HAART regimens can cause diarrhea. In addition, patients with HIV infections are also susceptible to infection by the same enteric pathogens that cause diarrhea in immunocompetent hosts. As the CD count decreases, however, these patients become more susceptible to a wide variety of OI that affect both the small intestine and the colon.

1. **Etiologic agents.** The most common identifiable causes of diarrhea in HIV-infected patients are enteric bacteria (e.g., *Shigella flexneri, Salmonella enteritidis, Campylobacter jejuni,* and *Clostridium difficile.* When the CD count becomes less than 100/mm^3, CMV, cryptosporidiosis, microsporidia, *Mycobacterium avium* complex (MAC), and other OIs become more commonly seen in these patients.

   CMV is the most common viral agent identified from mucosal biopsy specimens from HIV-infected patients with diarrhea. Other viruses reported to involve the GI tract in patients with AIDS include **adenovirus, rotavirus, astrovirus, pecorino virus, and coronavirus.** The clinical importance of these viruses has not been well established.

   Among the protozoa *Cryptosporidium parvum* and **microsporidia (Enterocytozoon bieneusi** and **Encephalitozoon intestinalis)** are the most potent causes of chronic diarrhea in AIDS patients.

   MAC, which was very commonly seen in patients with AIDS, has become rare in patients undergoing HAART. **Neoplasms** such as KS or lymphoma and other OIs such as histoplasmosis do not lead to diarrhea.

2. **Clinical presentation**

   a. **History.** Diarrhea resulting from enteritis or the involvement of the small intestine is typically manifested by large-volume, watery stools associated with dehydration, electrolyte disturbances, and malabsorption. Abdominal pain and cramps are usually located in the periumbilical area. Associated symptoms include nausea, vomiting, abdominal bloating, and borborygmi.

      Diarrhea arising from colonic involvement and colitis is characterized by frequent, small-volume stools, which often contain mucus, blood, and pus. Symptoms include tenesmus, urgency, and rectoanal pain. Abdominal pain is less likely to be crampy and is usually located in the lower quadrants.

   b. **Physical exam.** Physical findings are nonspecific. Fever usually suggests bacterial or mycobacterial infection. If CMV is suspected, funduscopic examination may reveal retinitis. CMV colitis/ulcers are more common in the ascending colon, thus the abdominal tenderness may be on the right lower quadrant.

3. **Diagnostic studies.** The initial evaluation of the HIV-infected patient with diarrhea must be tailored to the clinical setting, patient's symptoms, physical examination, and the CD4 count.

   a. **Stool studies** should include examination for ova and parasites, culture for bacteria, C. *difficile* toxin assay, and the presence of fecal leukocytes. The positive yield of stool culture increases with repeated stool examination. If fecal leukocytes are absent, additional stool studies should include a modified acid-fast stain to evaluate for *Cryptosporidia*, special stains for microsporidia, and antigen for *Giardia*.

      If MAC is suspected, blood cultures or bone marrow biopsy may be helpful in establishing disseminated MAC, but do not prove active GI involvement. Entamoeba antibody titer is only useful in establishing invasive amebiasis (e.g., liver abscess) and not for colonic infection and colitis with ameba.

   b. **Radiologic studies.** Neither barium enema nor small-bowel follow-through examinations play a role in the evaluation of diarrhea in patients with AIDS. Abdominal and pelvic computed tomography (CT) scan may reveal colonic wall thickening suggesting colitis and the need for colonoscopy.

    c. Endoscopic examination of the UGI tract and the colon are invaluable in the evaluation of diarrhea in patients with AIDS. In addition to direct visualization, biopsies are obtained for histologic examination.

  4. Treatment. Drug-induced diarrhea must always be included in the differential diagnosis of diarrhea in patients undergoing HAART. If diarrhea stops when the retroviral agents are stopped and returns when they are restarted, one or more of these drugs is implicated.

    Even though CMV colitis responds to ganciclovir sodium in over 50% of patients, effective therapy for many of the OIs in AIDS is lacking. So far, there is no effective treatment for microsporidia and *Cryptosporidia* infection. However, improvement of the immune function by HAART is essential and may lead to remission of *Cryptosporidia*- and microsporidia-induced diarrhea.

TABLE 43-2   **Antimicrobial Therapy for Enteric Infections in HIV-Infected Patients**

Organism	Antimicrobial therapy
Bacteria	
Campylobacter	Erythromycin 250–500 mg p.o. q.i.d. for 7 d or ciprofloxacin 500 mg p.o. b.i.d. for 7 d
Salmonella	Amoxicillin 1 g p.o. t.i.d for 3–14 d or trimethoprim/sulfamethoxazole DS p.o. b.i.d. for 14 d or ciprofloxacin 500 mg p.o. b.i.d. for 7 d
Shigella	Trimethoprim/sulfamethoxazole DS p.o. b.i.d. for 5–15 d or ampicillin 500 mg p.o. q.i.d. for 5 d or ciprofloxacin hydrochloride 500 mg p.o. b.i.d. for 7 d
Clostridium difficile	Metronidazole 500 mg p.o. t.i.d. for 7–10 d or vancomycin hydrochloride 125–500 mg p.o. q.i.d. for 7–10 d
Fungi	
Candida	Ketoconazole 100–200 mg b.i.d. for 10–14 d or fluconazole 500–100 mg b.i.d. for 10–14 days for amphotericin B 0.3–0.6 mg/kg/body weight daily
Viruses	
Herpes simplex	Acyclovir 200–800 mg 5 times a day for 7 d or 5–12 mg/kg q8h for 7 d
Cytomegalovirus	Ganciclovir 5 mg/kg IV b.i.d. for 14–21 d or foscarnet sodium 60 mg/kg IV q8h for 14 d, then 90–120 mg/kg daily; maintenance 6 mg/kg IV daily 5 d per week
Protozoa	
Giardia	Metronidazole 250 mg p.o. t.i.d. for 5 d or quinacrine hydrocholoride 100 mg t.i.d. for 5 d
Entamoeba	Metronidazole 750 mg p.o. t.i.d. for 10 d, then iodoquinol 650 mg t.i.d. for 20 d
Isospora	Trimethoprim/sulfamethoxazole DS p.o. t.i.d for 10 d then twice weekly for 3 weeks
Cryptosporidium	Unknown (trials with azithromycin hydrochloride, letrazuril, and paromomycin)
Microsporidia	Unknown (trials with metronidazole and albendazole)
Mycobacteria	
Mycobacterium avium-complex	Unknown (trials with clarithromycin 500–1000 mg p.o. b.i.d. for 2–4 weeks and ethambutin 15–20 mg/kg/d, rifabutin 300–600 mg daily, clofazimine 100–200 mg daily, ciprofloxacin hydrochloride 750 mg daily, and amikacin 7.5 mg/kg daily or b.i.d.)

HIV, human Immunodeficiency virus; p.o., per os; b.i.d., twice daily; q.i.d., four times daily; t.i.d., three times daily; IV, intravenous.

Antimicrobial therapy for enteric infections in HIV-infected patients is summarized in Table 43-2. Symptomatic therapy with tincture of opium, Lomotil, and Imodium is recommended. Octreotide has not proven to be beneficial in patients with chronic unexplained diarrhea.

IV. HEPATOBILIARY DISEASE IN AIDS. Abnormal results of liver chemistry tests occur in about 60% of patients with AIDS. Up to 80% of these patients have hepatomegaly, and nearly 85% have histologic changes in hepatic parenchyma.

The spectrum of hepatobiliary disease in patients with AIDS is summarized in Table 43-3. This spectrum includes viral hepatitis; granulomatous liver disease secondary to drugs; fungal, protozoan, bacterial, and mycobacterial infections; steatosis; nonspecific portal inflammation; sinusoidal abnormalities including peliosis hepatis; neoplasms such as KS and non-Hodgkin's lymphoma; and biliary diseases including acalculous cholecystitis, ampullary stenosis, and sclerosing cholangitis. These disorders may be superimposed on previous hepatobiliary disease resulting from alcoholism, intravenous (IV) drug abuse, and viral hepatitis.

A. Disorders

1. Viral infections (see also Chapter 50)

a. Hepatitis A virus (HAV) is transmitted through the fecal-oral route. It is prevalent in both IV drug users and homosexual men. Many anti-HIV–positive patients have anti-hepatitis A (IgG), which is the serologic evidence of past exposure to hepatitis A virus, with full recovery. There is no chronic form of HAV and no evidence that the clinical course of an acute HAV infection is altered in patients with AIDS. Treatment is supportive.

b. Hepatitis B virus (HBV) is transmitted parenterally by contaminated needles and sexually from infected people. IV drug users and homosexual men are at high risk of the development of HBV infection. In fact, approximately 90% of patients with AIDS have serologic evidence of HBV infection, and 10% to 20% are chronic carriers. Patients with AIDS and previous HBV infection have normal or slightly elevated serum transaminase levels. This is because HBV is not directly cytopathic to the infected hepatocytes and the degree of inflammatory response and liver damage is largely dependent on the host's immunologic status.

Patients with HIV-induced immune suppression are likely to have less inflammatory response and an improvement in the biochemical and histologic features of chronic HBV infection. However, it has been noted that there is increased replication of HBV in HIV-infected individuals, determined by an increase in the HBV deoxyribonucleic acid (DNA) polymerase activity and an increase in HBe antigen levels and HB core antigen–positive hepatocyte nuclei.

TABLE 43-3 Hepatobiliary Disorders in Patients with HIV Infection

Hepatitis	*Histoplasma capsulatum*
Hepatitis A	Microsporidia
Hepatitis B (acute and chronic)	Biliary tract disease
Hepatitis C (acute and chronic)	Ampullary stenosis
Hepatitis D (delta virus)	Sclerosing cholangitis
Cytomegalovirus	Cytomegalovirus
Epstein-Barr virus	*Cryptosporidium*
Herpes simplex virus	*Candida*
Drugs	Acalculous chloecystitis
Granulomatous liver disease	Neoplasms
Mycobacterium tuberculosis	Lymphoma
Mycobacterium avium-intracellulare	Kaposi's sarcoma
Cryptococcus neoformans	

Patients with AIDS who have acute hepatitis B have increased viremia and an increased risk of the development of chronic hepatitis B. Patients with hepatitis B who are also infected with HIV respond poorly to interferon therapy, even in the absence of AIDS. The presence of HIV antibodies is also associated with a suboptimal response to HBV vaccination in terms of both the level of anti-HBs and the percentage of patients responding to the vaccine. Higher doses of the vaccine may need to be used in this population. Measurement of HB surface antibody titers is recommended in HIV-positive people to determine whether the desirable titer of greater than 10 milli-International Units per liter (mIU/L) is present.

c. **Delta hepatitis.** Hepatitis delta virus (HDV) is a hepatotropic RNA virus dependent on HB surface antigen for its replication and expression. It is known to cause coinfection with HBV or superinfection in patients with chronic hepatitis B. Patients with HIV infection have slightly higher serum aminotransferase levels with HDV infection. Reactivation of HDV after HIV infection has been reported.

d. **Hepatitis C virus (HCV)** infection and positive serologic studies for HCV antibody are often seen in patients infected with HIV. Most patients have HCV, chronic active hepatitis, or cirrhosis. The response to antiviral therapy with ribovirin and pegylated interferon has been poorer in these patients, as compared to patients who are not co-infected with HIV. However, HCV co-infection should be treated in the apprapriate patient.

e. **Herpes simplex virus.** More than 95% of homosexual men with AIDS have serologic evidence of herpes simplex virus (HSV) infection. Patients with AIDS may have HSV encephalitis, esophagitis, or orolabial or genital HSV infections with pain, ulceration, and progressive tissue destruction. Hepatitis may occur with widely disseminated HSV infection. In most of these conditions, patients manifest orocutaneous or genital vesicles or both, ulcers, fever, hepatomegaly, and leukopenia. Fulminant hepatitis may develop with overwhelming infection, and patients may have coagulopathy, hepatic encephalopathy, and shock. Diagnosis may be established by histopathologic examination of a liver biopsy specimen. The virus may be cultured from the blood, urine, cutaneous lesions, or liver. Mortality is very high despite therapy with acyclovir sodium or vidarabine.

f. **Epstein-Barr virus infection.** The course of hepatitis in patients with AIDS who also have the Epstein-Barr virus has not been well characterized.

g. **CMV infection** usually produces subclinical disease in immunocompetent adults. Occasionally patients have fever, hepatomegaly, and slightly elevated aminotransferase levels. CMV infection may remain latent after primary infection and recur with immunocompromise.

Approximately 95% of homosexual men have serologic evidence of previous CMV infection. In HIV-infected patients, CMV may produce colitis, esophagitis, pneumonitis, and retinitis. It is usually disseminated when the liver is involved. In patients with CMV hepatitis, the serum alkaline phosphatase and aminotransferase levels are moderately increased. Hepatic involvement ranges from the asymptomatic carrier state to fulminant hepatic necrosis. The diagnosis is made by liver biopsy in affected patients. CMV commonly produces a parenchymal and portal mononuclear cell infiltrate and focal hepatic necrosis. Occasionally granulomas are present. Cytoplasmic inclusion bodies seen in the hepatocytes and in situ hybridization and immune fluorescence techniques can rapidly detect CMV. CMV can be cultured from urine, blood, and tissue from infected sites.

Treatment is with IV ganciclovir sodium, which may stabilize the clinical course of patients with CMV infection but may cause neutropenia. Foscarnet may be used as an alternative therapy without associated neutropenia.

2. **Bacterial and mycobacterial infections**

a. *Mycobacterium avium-intracellulare* **(MAI)** is the most common opportunistic pathogen causing hepatic infection in AIDS. It is usually found in patients with AIDS who have had previous opportunistic infections. The presentation is often with fever, malaise, anorexia, weight loss, diarrhea, hepatomegaly, and widely disseminated disease. The alkaline phosphatase level is usually highly elevated, with mildly elevated transaminases.

The diagnosis is confirmed by liver biopsy and the typical findings of acid-fast bacilli and poorly formed granulomas due to the suppressed activity of T lymphocytes. The organism may be obtained from cultures of liver, blood, lung, GI mucosa, bone marrow, and lymph nodes. The prognosis is poor due to severe immunosuppression in the patients. Therapeutic trials using a four-drug regimen consisting of rifampin, ethambutol, clofazimine, and ciprofloxacin hydrochloride have given promising results in bacteremia with MAI.

b. **Mycobacterium tuberculosis.** As their immunosuppression progresses, HIV-infected patients have an increased risk of the development of tuberculosis, usually from reactivation of a latent infection. In addition to the pulmonary infection, extrapulmonary tuberculosis involving peripheral lymph nodes, bone marrow, blood, and liver may occur. The liver involvement may be biliary, with disseminated infection or with formation of granulomas and frank abscesses. Hepatic failure may develop. Occasionally bile duct obstruction by tuberculosis or enlarged lymph nodes may present as cholestasis. Infections with drug-resistant strains of tuberculosis are being reported, especially in patients living in inner-city settings.

Symptoms and signs include fever, night sweats, weight loss, productive cough, pleuritic chest pain, abdominal pain, lymphadenopathy, hepatosplenomegaly, and jaundice. Chest x-rays may show only hilar or mediastinal lymphadenopathy. The purified protein derivative (PPD) is usually negative with concomitant cutaneous anergy. Serum alkaline phosphatase level is usually significantly elevated, but the transaminase and bilirubin levels are only mildly elevated in most patients.

The diagnosis is usually made by culture of sputum, urine, blood, lymph node, bone marrow, or liver tissue. Histologic stains for acid-fast bacilli are not as sensitive. Liver biopsy may show granulomas, Kupffer's cell hyperplasia, focal necrosis, parenchymal inflammation, sinusoidal dilatation, and occasionally peliosis hepatis.

Therapy includes isoniazid, rifampin, ethambutol, and pyrazinamide. Although most patients respond well to therapy, adverse drug reactions are common. The Centers for Disease Control and Prevention recommends that HIV-seropositive patients with a history of exposure to tuberculosis, or with a positive PPD even in the absence of active tuberculosis, receive prophylactic isoniazid therapy for at least 6 months.

c. **Other mycobacteria.** Infections with atypical mycobacteria such as **Mycobacterium xenopi** or **Mycobacterium kansasii** may rarely cause infection. Disseminated disease may occur in patients with hematologic malignancies, chronic renal failure, or advanced immunosuppression. Hepatic infection usually presents with hepatomegaly and greatly elevated serum alkaline phosphatase levels. Diagnosis requires positive cultures from infected tissues.

d. **Salmonella.** Patients with AIDS frequently have extraintestinal salmonellosis with bacteremia and frequently relapse despite antibiotic therapy. Patients usually have fever, headaches, diarrhea, nausea, abdominal pain, bloating, hepatomegaly, and abnormal results on liver chemistry tests. Diagnosis may be established by cultures of blood, stool, and liver tissue. Therapy includes ampicillin, chloramphenicol, trimethoprim/sulfamethoxazole, ciprofloxacin hydrochloride, or a third-generation cephalosporin.

3. **Fungal infections**

a. **Cryptococcus neoformans.** Patients with AIDS who are infected with *C. neoformans* usually have meningoencephalitis and pulmonary infections. With hematogenous dissemination, cryptococcal hepatitis may develop. The symptoms and signs are predominantly due to the neurologic, pulmonic, or disseminated infection. Chronic low-grade fever, headache, altered sensorium, meningismus, cough, dyspnea, and pleuritic chest pain may be present.

Diagnosis can be made by cultures and histochemical stains of involved tissue or by detection of cryptococcal antigen. Poorly formed granulomas may be seen in liver biopsy specimens. Therapy includes amphotericin B, flucytosine, and fluconazole. Patients with AIDS frequently relapse after initial therapy and may require chronic preventive therapy.

b. ***Histoplasma capsulatum.*** Hepatic histoplasmosis in patients with AIDS usually develops from widely disseminated disease of which the origin is often in the lungs. Most patients have either lived or traveled in endemic areas such as midwestern United States river valleys or Puerto Rico.

Symptoms include severe weight loss, malaise, chronic fever, and sometimes cough and dyspnea. Cutaneous lesions, lymphadenopathy, and hepatosplenomegaly may be present. Liver chemistry and serum alkaline phosphatase levels are moderately elevated. The diagnosis may be made by blood cultures or by biopsy of the bone marrow, liver, lymph node, or lung. Smears with Gomori's methenamine silver stain show the presence of budding yeast. Granulomas may also be present in the liver.

Treatment with amphotericin B often results in a dramatic response, but the disease may recur. Prophylactic therapy with ketoconazole or fluconazole may be necessary.

c. ***Candida albicans.*** Hepatic candidiasis in patients with AIDS should be suspected in the setting of dissemination from invasive esophagitis or another source or after chemotherapy for lymphoma or leukemia. Patients may have prolonged fever, right upper quadrant pain, tenderness, and hepatomegaly. The serum alkaline phosphatase level is usually greatly elevated, compared to a mild elevation in the transaminases. Microabscess may form in the liver and spleen. These lesions may be seen on CT as radiolucent areas and on ultrasonography as bull's-eye lesions with central hyperechoic foci within hypoechoic lesions.

Diagnosis may be established by cultures of blood or liver and histologic demonstration of granulomas and yeast forms or pseudohyphae with a silver stain. Treatment includes amphotericin B, 5-fluorocytosine, ketoconazole, or fluconazole.

d. **Other fungal infections.** Systemic **sporotrichosis** with hepatic infection has been reported in patients with AIDS, but it is rare. **Coccidioidomycosis** may become systemic in immunosuppressed patients including those with AIDS. In addition to pulmonary nodules seen on chest x-ray, the diagnosis is usually made by histologic examination with periodic acid–Schiff (PAS) stain of sputum, specimens obtained at bronchoscopy, bone marrow, and liver. The organism may be cultured from tissues, blood, and urine. The liver biopsy shows granulomas. Treatment of sporotrichosis and coccidioidomycosis is with long-term therapy with amphotericin B.

4. Protozoan infections

a. ***Pneumocystis carinii.*** Diffuse interstitial pneumonia is the most common serious opportunistic infection caused by *P. carinii* in patients infected with HIV. Immunodeficient patients may have concomitant hepatic infection with granuloma formation. These patients have elevated serum alkaline phosphatase and aminotransferase levels, usually associated with severe hypoalbuminemia. Therapy is with trimethoprim/sulfamethoxazole or pentamidine.

b. ***Microsporidia.*** Homosexual men have a high incidence of exposure to microsporidia, and immunosuppressed patients with AIDS are particularly susceptible to development of GI infection. Hepatic infection is rare but may occur. Histologic examination of the liver biopsy may show focal granulomas in the portal areas. The parasites or their spores may be seen with special stains within histiocytes and in extracellular locations.

c. ***Cryptosporidium.*** Infection of the liver with *Cryptosporidium* mainly involves the gallbladder and the biliary tract (see section II.A.7).

5. Drug-induced hepatitis. Approximately 90% of patients who have AIDS take at least one potentially hepatotoxic drug during the course of their illness. Drug-induced hepatotoxicity tends to present subclinically. It is often difficult to differentiate drug-induced hepatitis from that caused by infections or malignancies. Withdrawal of hepatotoxic drugs may result in normalization of the liver chemistry tests and clinical improvement. A liver biopsy or other appropriate workup may be necessary to determine the precise nature of the hepatobiliary abnormality in patients in whom the suspected drug is needed or in those in whom withdrawal of the drug does not result in improvement.

6. **Hepatic neoplasms**
   a. **KS** is the most common neoplasm found in patients with AIDS. It occurs primarily in homosexual men, in whom it behaves as an aggressive malignancy with visceral and cutaneous lesions. About one half of the patients have GI lesions, which appear as violaceous macules on endoscopy. The lesions are generally submucosal and may present with bleeding or obstruction.

   About one third of the patients have hepatic involvement. The liver chemistry tests may be normal, or there may be an elevation of the serum alkaline phosphatase levels. On CT scan, hepatic lesions have a nonspecific appearance. Unguided percutaneous liver biopsy is insensitive in the diagnosis of KS. Occasionally KS lesions can be seen on laparoscopy if the lesions are superficial and anteriorly located. In general, hepatic involvement is rarely documented antemortem.

   Macroscopically, the lesions are multifocal and may occur at subcapsular hilar and intrahepatic locations. Histologically, KS is seen as multifocal areas of vascular endothelial cell proliferation with pleomorphic spindle-shaped cells and extravasated red blood cells. Sinusoidal dilatation with vascular lakes may be present. The clinical spectrum may include peliosis hepatis and angiosarcomatous lesions.

   Treatment includes radiotherapy or chemotherapy with vinblastine, vincristine, or etoposide. Interferon therapy also may produce considerable tumor reduction.

   b. **Lymphoma.** In HIV-infected patients, the development of lymphoma is considered a criterion for AIDS. Patients with AIDS, like other immunosuppressed patients, have an increased risk of the development of non-Hodgkin's lymphoma, often of B-cell origin. Patients with AIDS in whom lymphoma develops are usually homosexuals.

   Lymphoma in patients with AIDS is often extranodal with involvement of unusual sites such as the central nervous system or rectum. Most patients have multiorgan involvement. Primary hepatic lymphoma also may occur.

   Patients initially may have lymphadenopathy, hepatomegaly, jaundice, right upper quadrant pain, and systemic symptoms such as fever, malaise, and night sweats.

   Hyperbilirubinemia and considerable elevations of serum alkaline phosphatase levels usually occur in advanced illness. CT and ultrasound are helpful imaging techniques in the diagnosis of hepatic lymphoma. The lesions are usually multifocal and may obstruct the biliary tract and result in ductal dilatation.

   Histologic examination of liver biopsy specimens obtained with CT or laparoscopic guidance confirms the diagnosis. The lymphomas are usually high grade and respond less well to chemotherapy than they do in immunocompetent patients.

   c. **Other malignancies.** Hepatic metastasis from cancers developing in other sites has been seen in patients with AIDS. These include malignant melanoma, adenocarcinoma, and small-cell cancers. The immunodeficiency may permit dissemination to distant sites, including the liver.

7. **Biliary tract disease.** In addition to diseases of the biliary tract seen in immunocompetent patients, opportunistic infections involving the gallbladder and the biliary tract occur in patients with AIDS and may present with atypical findings, sepsis, or acute abdomen.
   a. **Acalculous cholecystitis** is rarely seen in immunocompetent people. It is sometimes associated with total parenteral nutrition and biliary sludge. In patients with AIDS, it may have a subacute clinical course or may present with fever and right upper quadrant abdominal pain. Patients may also have

concurrent diarrhea. The disease is usually caused **by CMV, *Cryptosporidium,*** or ***Candida.***

Most patients do not have a leukocytosis. The levels of serum alkaline phosphatase and transaminase are moderately elevated. Ultrasound and CT typically show a dilated gallbladder with thickened wall and no gallstones. Therapy is surgical excision of the inflamed gallbladder. Pathologic examination reveals an inflamed, edematous gallbladder wall with mucosal ulceration. Often CMV inclusion bodies are seen near the mucosal ulcers. Coinfection with **bacteria, *Cryptosporidium,*** and ***C. albicans*** may be present.

b. Cholangitis secondary to papillary stenosis (stenosis of the ampulla of Vater) and sclerosing cholangitis-like findings are well-recognized complications in patients who have AIDS. Patients have fever, right upper quadrant pain, and elevated serum alkaline phosphatase levels. CT and ultrasonography are relatively insensitive in detecting these abnormalities. Retrograde endoscopic cholangiopancreatography (ERCP) usually defines the lesions, and endoscopic sphincterotomy, balloon dilation, and stent placement in the strictures may treat and remove the obstruction to bile flow.

The infectious organisms causing periampullary, choledochal, and cholangiolar narrowing and dilatation are CMV, ***Cryptosporidium,*** *Candida*, MAI, and HIV. Lymphoma and KS may involve the ampulla and the biliary tract, resulting in obstruction.

B. Diagnostic workup. When patients with AIDS have hepatobiliary disease, considerations include, in addition to the conditions discussed previously, hepatic disease secondary to alcoholism, malnutrition, sepsis, hypotension, drugs, and previous viral infections. Appropriate serologic studies should be obtained to document viral disease.

An ultrasound or CT examination of the liver may show ductal dilatation or mass-occupying lesions. Patients with ductal dilatation or suspected ductal disease should undergo ERCP. Mechanical decompression with sphincterotomy and stent placement may eliminate the obstruction.

Biopsies of the involved areas should be cultured and examined histologically. In patients with focal lesions, liver biopsy should be obtained under ultrasound or CT guidance. Percutaneous liver biopsy is recommended when CT or ultrasound is not helpful. In patients who have ascites, laparoscopic examination of the liver and guided biopsy decrease the risk of complications that occur with percutaneous biopsy techniques. Liver biopsy specimens should be cultured and histologically examined with special stains. In about 50% of these patients, the liver biopsy helps establish the diagnosis and provides a more rational basis for patient management.

Selected Readings

Abou Lafia DM. AIDs-related non-hodgkins lymphoma. *Infect Med.* 2007;24(11):470–481.

Bivi EJ, et al. Diagnostic yield and cost effectiveness of endoscopy in chronic human immuno-deficiency virus-related diarrhea. *Gastrointest Endosc.* 1998;48:354.

Blanshard C, et al. Investigation of chronic diarrhea in acquired immunodeficiency syndrome. A prospective study of 155 patients. *Gut.* 1996;38:824.

Carr A, et al. Treatment of HIV associated microsporidiosis and cryptosporidiosis with combination antiretroviral therapy. *Lancet.* 1996;38:824.

Dietrich DT, et al. Diagnosis and treatment of esophageal diseases associated with HIV infection. *Am J Gastroenterol.* 1996;91:2265.

Koziel MJ, et al. Viral hepatitis in HIV infection. *N Engl Med.* 2007;356:1445–1457.

Poles MA, et al. HIV-related diarrhea is multifactorial and fat malabsorption is commonly present, independent of HAART. *Am J Gastroenterol.* 2001;96:1831.

Re VI, et al. Prevalance, risk factors, and outcomes for occult hepatitis B infection among HIV-infected patients. *J Acquir Immune Defic Syndr.* 2007;44:315–320.

Smith JO, et al. Hepatitis C and HIV. *Curr Gastroenterol Rep.* 2007;9:83–90.

Soriano V, et al. Core of patients coinfected with HIV and hepatitis C virus. *Aids.* 2007;21(9):1073–1089.

Wilcox CM, et al. Fluconazole compared with endoscopy for human immunodeficiency virus infected patients with esophageal symptoms. *Gastroenterology.* 1996;110:1803.

Wilcox CM, et al. Review article: the therapy of gastrointestinal infections associated with acquired immunodeficiency syndrome. *Aliment Pharmacol Ther.* 1997;11:435.

Wilcox CM. Current concepts of gastrointestinal disease associated with human immune deficiency virus infection. *Clin Perspect Gastroenterol.* January/February 2001:9.

$\mathcal{T}$he management of patients with acute gastrointestinal (GI) bleeding is discussed in Chapter 14. Such patients typically have unequivocal evidence of bleeding, such as hematemesis, hematochezia, or melena. However, other patients bleed slowly or intermittently from lesions of the GI tract in a less dramatic manner or in amounts that are insufficient to be clinically evident but may be detected by testing of the stool for occult blood. If bleeding is intermittent, detection and subsequent diagnosis are sometimes difficult. Occult GI bleeding is usually more problematic in patients with occult bleeding disorders (i.e., von Willebrand's disease). Although the major worry of patients and physicians is that occult bleeding is due to a cancer of the GI tract, the range of causes for the bleeding is virtually the same as that for acute bleeding (see Table 14-1). Occult GI bleeding is often attributed to therapy with anticoagulants or aspirin. However, neither warfarin nor aspirin alone appears to cause positive fecal guaiac–based occult blood tests. A positive fecal blood test of patients on warfarin, heparin, or aspirin should lead to formal evaluation of the GI tract.

I. DETECTION OF OCCULT BLEEDING

A. Frequency of testing. The American Cancer Society recommends that people at average risk for colon cancer (i.e., people without a history of colon polyps or cancer, without a strong family history of colon cancer, and without inflammatory bowel disease) undergo yearly testing of the stool for occult blood beginning at age 40. People at higher than average risk should enter an appropriate surveillance program, which may include occult blood testing and periodic sigmoidoscopy or colonoscopy (see Chapters 37 and 39).

B. Method of obtaining stool for testing. If the stool obtained at digital rectal examination (DRE) is negative for occult blood, that is presumptive evidence that there is no clinically significant blood in the stool, provided the patient is not taking vitamin C (see section II.B.2.c). If the stool at DRE is positive for occult blood, however, one does not know whether it is truly positive or is falsely positive due to the trauma of the examination, dietary factors, or medications that may affect the test. Interestingly, it has been shown in several studies that testing stool for occult blood at the time of DRE does not increase the number of false-positive test results in asymptomatic patients and promotes more compliance to screening. However, the most reliable method of obtaining stool for occult blood testing is the following:

1. Give the patient three occult blood test cards. Each card has two windows for testing stool, so the patient can submit six smears.
2. Instruct the patient to:
   a. **Avoid red meat** and other foods with a high peroxidase content (e.g., broccoli, turnips, cauliflower, and uncooked cantaloupe, radish, and parsnips). Foods with high peroxidase contents may give a false-positive test result because the tests for occult blood depend on the pseudoperoxidase activity of heme in stool.
   b. **Consume a high-fiber diet.** A high-fiber diet is thought to promote larger stools and perhaps "irritate" the surface of any potentially bleeding lesions. This irritating function of fiber in the stool has not been proved.
   c. **Avoid vitamin C,** iron preparations, aspirin, and other nonsteroidal antiinflammatory drugs. Vitamin C has been shown to give a false-negative test

result for occult blood because ascorbic acid inhibits the pseudoperoxidase activity of heme. Aspirin and other nonsteroidal antiinflammatory drugs may injure the gastric mucosa and cause bleeding, thus making the occult blood test positive.

3. After 3 days of this regimen, the patient should smear stool on the two test windows of a diagnostic card each day for the next 3 days (or the next three stools, if stools are less frequent than daily) and return the cards to the physician. Rehydrating the cards before testing increases the diagnostic yield.

II. DIAGNOSIS

A. Clinical presentation. Patients with occult blood in the stool typically feel well. They may have symptoms related to the cause of the bleeding, for example, peptic complaints, or abdominal discomfort due to a GI tumor, but they usually do not have symptoms attributable to blood loss. They may be anemic (hemoglobin level of less than 12 g/dL for women and less than 13 g/dL for men and serum ferritin level of less than 45 mg/L) due to either the chronic loss of blood or, more likely, the underlying disorder, or they may have normal levels of hemoglobin and hematocrit. The presence of occult blood may be detected by routine screening examination or in response to the patient's symptoms.

B. Diagnostic studies

1. **Examination of the colon by colonoscopy** is the preferred diagnostic study in the evaluation of patients for occult GI bleeding. The use of flexible *sigmoidoscopy* and **air-contrast barium enema** has been used as an alternative to colonoscopy; however, the sensitivity and specificity is less. Virtual colonoscopy is in the process of development as an alternative to colonoscopy.

2. **Examination of the upper GI tract.** If the examination of the colon is nondiagnostic, examination of the upper GI tract is indicated. The clinician may elect to study the UGI tract first if the patient's history suggests UGI disease or lesion. **Endoscopy** is the preferred method of studying the UGI tract for mucosal lesions.

3. **Examination of the small intestine** may be accomplished by radiologic or endoscopic techniques. The most widely available technique is barium upper GI and small-bowel series. Unfortunately, the diagnostic yield of this technique is inferior to **small-bowel enema or enteroclysis,** which is more arduous and not widely available. Enteroclysis is performed by passing a tube by mouth into the proximal duodenum and instilling barium followed by air. This technique provides an excellent air–barium contrast and is effective in detecting mass lesions of the SI, but is ineffective in detecting mucosal lesions.

4. **Enteroscopy** is indicated for the evaluation of the SI for the detection of mucosal lesions. **Push enteroscopy** is the usual technique used and entails a perioral insertion of a push enteroscope or a pediatric colonoscope via the UGI tract into the distal duodenum, jejunum and possibly into the ileum. Biopsy and endoscopic therapy can be performed when a lesion is found. **Sonde enteroscopy** involves the passage of a long enteroscope into the SI via the upper GI tract and allowing peristalsis to carry it into the distal SI. The mucosa is visualized as the sonde endoscope is slowly removed. It is a very uncomfortable procedure and does not allow biopsy or endoscopic therapy of the lesion. **Double balloon enteroscopy** is available at specialized medical centers to visualize the SI and obtain biopsies or apply therapeutic interventions.

   Interoperative enteroscopy permits visualization of the SI by the use of enteroscope or pediatric colonoscope that is advanced through the SI during laparotomy. Push enteroscopy and interoperative enteroscopy have been reported to detect abnormalities in up to 70% of patients.

5. More recently, the mucosa of the SI has been visualized by Pill-cam or **capsule endoscopy.** The patient swallows the capsule that takes numerous pictures along its course down the SI. These pictures are then retrieved by downloading them via a computer.

6. **Special studies.** A small number of patients continue to bleed, usually intermittently, from a source that defies identification, even after repeated

evaluations. Unusual causes of bleeding must be considered in these patients, and occasionally, extraordinary measures are required to make the diagnosis.

   a. **A technetium 99m sulfur colloid** scan may show a Meckel's diverticulum that contains gastric mucosa. Although only about 20% of Meckel's diverticula contain gastric mucosa, these are the diverticula that ulcerate and bleed. Bleeding from a Meckel's diverticulum may be occult but typically is more vigorous and sometimes intermittent.

   b. **Selective arteriography** should be performed in patients with undiagnosed occult GI bleeding, not to identify active bleeding but to determine whether an abnormal vascular pattern suggests an angiodysplastic or neoplastic lesion.

III. The treatment of occult GI bleeding depends on the cause. See the appropriate chapter. Vascular ectasias of the SI are the most common source of bleeding in patients with **obscure GI bleeding.** Endoscopic and surgical therapy is most successful with large and discrete vascular ectasias. The treatment of diffuse and multiple vascular ectasias are difficult and less successful. Hormonal therapy with estrogen and progesterone has been tried and has been noted to be successful in some reported cases, but not in controlled studies.

Selected Readings

Amaro R, et al. Diagnostic and therapeutic options in obscure gastrointestinal blood loss. *Curr Gastroenterol Rep.* 2000;2:395.

de Leusse A, et al. Capsule endoscopy or push enteroscopy for first-line exploration of obscure gastrointestinal bleeding? *Gastroenterology.* 2007 Mar;132:855–862.

Goldstein JL, et al. Small bowel mucosal injury is reduced in healthy subjects treated with celecoxib compared with ibuprofen plus omeprazole, as assessed by video capsule endoscopy. *Aliment Parmacol Ther.* 2007 May 15;25:1211–1222.

Graham DY, et al. Visible small-intestinal mucosal injury in chronic NSAID users. *Clin Gastroenterol Hepatol.* 2005;3(1):55–60.

Manner H, et al. Push-and-pull enteroscopy using the double balloon technique (double-balloon enteroscopy) for the diagnosis of Meckel's diverticulum in adult patients with GI bleeding of obscure origin. *Am J Gastroenterol.* 2006;101:1152–1154.

Pennazio M, et al. Outcome of patients with obscure gastrointestinal bleeding after capsule endoscopy: Report of 100 consecutive cases. *Gastroenterology.* 2004;126:643–653.

Qureshi WA. Current and future applications of the capsule camera. *Nat Rev Drug Discov.* 2004;3:447–450.

Rockey DC. Occult gastrointestinal bleeding. *N Engl J Med.* 1999;341:39.

Tiester SL, et al. A meta-analysis of the yield of capsule endoscopy compared to other diagnostic modalities in patients with obscure gastrointestinal bleeding. *Am J Gastroenterol.* 2005; 100(11):2407–2418.

Yamamoto H, et al. Clinical outcomes of double-balloon endoscopy for the diagnosis and treatment of small-intestinal diseases. *Gastroenterol Hepatol.* 2004;2:1010–1016.

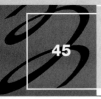

I. Acute pancreatitis is a discrete episode of inflammation resulting from intrapancreatic activation of digestive enzymes. It is a disease with a wide spectrum of severity, complications, and outcome.

   A. Acute edematous or interstitial pancreatitis. In this stage, the pancreatic inflammation and disease is mild and self-limited in most patients. The inflammation results in interstitial edema. The parenchymal damage is minimal, and the organ recovers its function after resolution of the inflammation.

   B. Hemorrhagic or necrotizing pancreatitis. In some patients, the inflammation may be extensive and progress to coagulation necrosis of the gland and the surrounding tissues, leading to hemorrhagic or necrotizing pancreatitis. The mass of inflamed pancreas containing necrotic tissue is referred to as a phlegmon.

II. COMPLICATIONS

   A. Spread of the inflammatory process. The retroperitoneal location of the pancreas and the absence of a well-developed pancreatic capsule allow the inflammatory process to spread freely. The activated pancreatic enzymes dissect through the tissue planes and affect any of the following organs: the common bile duct, duodenum, splenic artery and vein, spleen, pararenal spaces, mesocolon, colon, mesentery of the small bowel, celiac and superior mesenteric ganglia, lesser omental sac, posterior mediastinum, and diaphragm. The peritoneal surfaces may be involved with the inflammatory process, leading to exudation and fluid accumulation in the peritoneal cavity **(pancreatic ascites)** and the lesser omental sac. Involvement of the diaphragmatic lymphatics may lead to sterile pleural effusion and pneumonitis.

   Local effects of pancreatic enzymes and vasoactive materials include an intense chemical burn of tissue leading to leakage of protein-rich fluid from the systemic circulation into peritoneal and retroperitoneal spaces. This phenomenon may lead to hypovolemia. Systemic effects of these circulating materials include cardiovascular instability, respiratory failure, and renal failure.

   B. Hemorrhage within or around the gland may dissect along tissue planes and lead to a bluish discoloration in the periumbilical area **(Cullen's sign)** or in the costovertebral angle **(Turner's sign).**

   C. Pseudocysts. Necrotic tissue, blood, pancreatic juice, and fat from disrupted cells may accumulate within or adjacent to the pancreas, forming pseudocysts. Pseudocysts may resolve spontaneously as the inflammation subsides. If the pseudocyst is large or if there is a communication between the pseudocyst and a ruptured pancreatic duct with continued secretion of pancreatic juices into the enclosed space, the pseudocyst may not resolve.

   D. Pancreatic abscesses. The secondary infection of a pancreatic phlegmon or pseudocyst by enteric flora results in pancreatic abscess.

   E. Fat necrosis may occur in peritoneal, retroperitoneal, and distant locations such as in subcutaneous or intramedullary areas. **Calcium salts (soaps)** of free fatty acids liberated from fatty tissue may precipitate in these areas.

   F. Polyserositis and the adult respiratory distress syndrome. The entry of the activated pancreatic enzymes (e.g., trypsin, elastase, phospholipase A) into the circulation allows these potent digestive enzymes to attack distant sites.

Polyserositis involving pericardial, pleural, and synovial surfaces may occur. Left-sided **pleural effusion** is common. The pulmonary alveolar–capillary membrane may be disrupted, forming hyalin membranes lining the alveolar surface. A transudate fills the alveolar space and leads to a noncardiogenic pulmonary edema or adult respiratory distress syndrome.

G. Disseminated intravascular coagulation and microthrombi. The release of activated pancreatic enzymes into the circulation may result in disseminated intravascular coagulation with formation of intravascular microthrombi. These thrombi may affect the function of many organ systems. Pulmonary intravascular microthrombi result in intrapulmonary right-to-left shunting and hypoxia. Microthrombi in the glomerular capillaries, deposited in the mesangium and the glomerular basement membrane, results in renal dysfunction of varying severity.

H. Circulatory shock may occur in severe instances due to third-spacing of fluid and intravascular hypovolemia. If intravenous (IV) fluid replacement is inadequate, hypovolemia and hypotension may intensify the pancreatitis.

III. ETIOLOGY. There are many conditions implicated as causative factors in the pathogenesis of acute pancreatitis (Table 45-1).

A. Alcoholism and biliary tract disease. The two most common etiologic factors associated with pancreatitis are alcoholism and biliary tract disease **(gallstones).** These two factors account for 75% to 85% of all cases. In countries in which the incidence of alcoholism and excessive alcohol use is high, such as the United States, Australia, and South Africa, alcohol is the etiologic factor in more than 50% of patients. In contrast, in countries in which alcoholism is less prevalent, such as Britain and Israel, biliary tract disease is the most common cause of acute pancreatitis. The mortality of gallstone-associated pancreatitis is approximately 8% during the first attack and 1% during subsequent attacks. Chronic pancreatitis with pancreatic insufficiency rarely, if ever, occurs, even after multiple episodes of pancreatitis associated with gallstones.

TABLE 45-1	Causes of Acute Pancreatitis

Alcohol (ethanol, methanol) abuse (acute and chronic alcoholism)
Gallstones, biliary sludge (biliary tract disease)
Surgery (abdominal, cardiac, cardiopulmonary bypass, thoracic)
Trauma (blunt, penetrating)
Endoscopic retrograde cholangiopancreatography
Infections (viral: mumps, coxsackie, CMV, HSV, HIV; bacterial: *Mycoplasma*, *Legionella*, *Leptospira*; fungal: Aspergillosis; parasitic: *Salmonella*, *Mycobacterium*, *Toxoplasma*, *Cryptosporidium*)
Metabolic disorders (hypertriglyceridemia, pregnancy, hypercalcemia–hyperparathyroidism Vasculitis, ischemia
Drugs (see Table 45-2)
Anatomic abnormalities in the area of the ampulla of Vater with possible obstruction (Crohn's disease, duodenal diverticulum, annular pancreas, pancreas divisum, choledochal cyst, sphincter of Oddi dysfunction, ampullary neoplasm, pancreatic neoplasm, ampullary stenosis)
Penetrating gastroduodenal ulcer
Hereditary autoimmune factors
Miscellaneous (scorpion bite, parasites obstructing the pancreatic duct [Ascaris, fluke], severe systemic hypotension, cholesterol embolization, Reye's syndrome, fulminant hepatitis, refeeding in eating disorders)
Renal failure
Renal transplantation

TABLE 45-2	Drugs Associated with Pancreatitis

Definitely associated	Probably associated
Sulfonamides, sulfasalazine	Ethacrynic acid
Estrogens (oral contraceptives)	Chlorthalidone
Tetracyclines	Methyldopa
Azathioprine	L-Asparaginase
Mercaptopurine	Procainamide hydrochloride
Furosemide	Corticosteroids
Thiazides	Nonsteroidal antiinflammatory drugs
Valproic acid	Isoniazid
Ethanol	Nitrofurantoin
Methanol	Rifampin
Organophosphate insecticides	Metronidazole
Pentamidine	Erythromycin
ACE inhibitors	5-ASA
DDI	Salicylates

DDI, 2′,3′-dideoxyinosine; ACE, angiotensin converting enzyme.

There is a well-documented association between excessive alcohol consumption and pancreatitis. In most patients, the disease recurs many times, leading to chronic pancreatitis with irreversible functional and structural damage of the organ. Even though the mortality is considerably less than that of gallstone disease–associated pancreatitis, all the complications of acute pancreatitis may develop during the acute attacks.

B. Postoperative pancreatitis is infrequent but has a high mortality. It occurs after cardiopulmonary bypass, thoracic, and abdominal surgical procedures. Operations on and near the pancreas such as gastrectomy, biliary tract surgery, and splenectomy are involved in most of the cases.

C. Endoscopic retrograde pancreatography. Pancreatitis may occur in less than 1% of cases after endoscopic retrograde pancreatography (ERCP). However, hyperamylasemia is common after ERCP.

D. Blunt abdominal trauma is the most common cause of pancreatitis in children and young adults.

E. Some **metabolic disorders** are implicated as causes of pancreatitis.

1. **Hypertriglyceridemia** may precede and cause pancreatitis. Patients with some lipoprotein abnormalities, especially Frederickson type I, type IV, and type V hyperlipoproteinemia, are at increased risk of development of pancreatitis. An abrupt increase in serum triglycerides to greater than 2,000 mg/dL can precipitate a bout of acute pancreatitis. This can occur in patients with underlying hypertriglyceridemia who ingest either large amounts of lipid and moderate amounts of alcohol or large amounts of alcohol or who use birth control pills. Serum amylase may be normal in lipemic serum. Dilutions should be requested to ascertain the correct level of serum amylase.

2. **Hypercalcemia** from any cause can lead to acute pancreatitis. Causes of hypercalcemia include hyperparathyroidism, parathyroid adenoma or carcinoma, myeloma, excessive doses of vitamin D, familial hypocalciuric hypercalcemia, and hypercalcemia in patients receiving total parenteral nutrition (TPN) or using calcium carbonate–containing antacids. Acute pancreatic necrosis is frequent during hyperparathyroid crisis. Increased concentrations of calcium ions in pancreatic secretion and pancreatic tissue might promote activation of trypsinogen, initiating the proteolytic cascade.

F. Organ transplantation. Pancreatitis may complicate renal and liver transplantation.

G. Pregnancy. Women in whom acute fatty liver of pregnancy develops in the third trimester may also develop acute pancreatitis. However, 90% of instances of pancreatitis during pregnancy are associated with gallstones.

H. Infections. Viral agents, including mumps, hepatitis B, and Coxsackie virus group B, and some bacteria (e.g., *Mycoplasma pneumoniae*) have been implicated as causes for acute pancreatitis. Opportunistic protozoan, bacterial, and fungal pathogens, which may involve the pancreas, include *Cryptosporidium*, cytomegalovirus, *Legionella pneumophila*, and *Salmonella* species, *Mycobacterium avium*, and tuberculosis.

I. Connective tissue diseases. Pancreatitis may occur in patients with some connective tissue diseases, such as **systemic lupus erythematosus (SLE),** especially those complicated with vasculitis.

J. Vasculitis, present in other disorders such as Henoch-Schönlein purpura, thrombocytopenic purpura, and necrotizing angiitis, may also be implicated as a cause of acute pancreatitis.

K. Drugs have been associated with the development of pancreatitis in some patients. Table 45-2 lists the drugs in two groups: those for which there is a definite association and those for which the association is probable.

L. Anatomic abnormalities. Pancreatitis has been reported in patients with a number of anatomic abnormalities in the vicinity of the ampulla of Vater, possibly associated with its obstruction, such as duodenal Crohn's disease, duodenal diverticula, choledochocele, choledochal cysts, duodenal intussusception, and sphincter of Oddi dysfunction.

M. Pancreas divisum is a special condition that may lead to recurrent bouts of pancreatitis. Pancreas divisum results when the ducts of the embryologic ventral and dorsal parts of the pancreas fail to fuse. Wirsung's duct, which normally drains the entire pancreas, only drains the uncinate process in these patients. The rest of the pancreas is drained by the duct of Santorini through the minor papilla. In many of the patients with pancreas divisum and recurrent pancreatitis, the minor papilla has been found to be stenotic and may be implicated as the predisposing condition for the development of pancreatitis.

N. Duodenal ulcer. Penetration of a duodenal ulcer into the pancreas may result in local pancreatic inflammation. Even though there may be an elevation of serum amylase, extensive pancreatitis usually does not develop.

O. Hereditary pancreatitis in an autosomal dominant transmission pattern has been described in a number of families. Symptoms usually appear between the ages of 5 and 15 years and progress to chronic pancreatitis. There may be an increased incidence of pancreatic adenocarcinoma in these families.

P. Miscellaneous causes. There are numerous other reported causes of pancreatitis including **scorpion bite** by *Tityus trinitatis* found in the West Indies and pancreatic duct obstruction by **parasites** such as flukes (*Clonorchis sinensis*) and worms (*ascaris*). **Systemic hypotension, cholesterol embolization, Reye's syndrome,** and **fulminant hepatic failure** may also be associated with acute pancreatitis. **Refeeding pancreatitis** may occur in patients with eating disorders such as anorexia nervosa and bulimia.

IV. PATHOPHYSIOLOGY. The exact mechanism of the events that trigger the intrapancreatic activation of zymogens to active enzymes leading to autodigestion and inflammation remains unknown. However, there is evidence that more than one mechanism is involved. It is thought that **ischemia, anoxia, trauma, infections,** and **endo- and exotoxins** set the stage for activation of trypsinogen to trypsin with further activation of other zymogens to active enzymes, including phospholipase A, elastase, and lipase. The enzymes, along with the detergent effect of bile acids, then digest cell membranes and elastic fibers of blood vessels, leading to vascular damage with interstitial edema, hemorrhage, and parenchymal cell and fat necrosis of the pancreatic and peripancreatic tissues. Vasoactive substances such as bradykinin and histamine that are released lead to vasodilatation and increased permeability resulting in more edema and inflammation.

One popular theory to explain the initiation of the autodigestion cascade suggests obstruction to the outflow of pancreatic juice (i.e., with gallstone impaction at the ampulla resulting in intraductal hypertension) and inhibition of acinar cell zymogen secretion by exocytosis. In this setting, the zymogen-containing vacuoles in the acinar cells fuse with lysosomes, which contain proteases. This results in enzyme activation within the combined vacuoles. These vacuoles rupture into the acinar cell, resulting in acinar cell injury and death with consequent intra- and extraparenchymal injury. Reflux of duodenal contents into the pancreatic duct, presence of a common channel (communicating pancreatic and common bile duct) with or without impacted gallstone, and occlusion of pancreatic blood vessels are other popular theories. Other forms of ischemia may also lead to intracellular zymogen activation and result in parenchymal damage.

V. PROGNOSTIC FACTORS IN ACUTE PANCREATITIS. Acute pancreatitis is a disease of varying severity. In most individuals, the disease is mild or moderate with full recovery of the patient. However, in some individuals, the disease may be fulminant with very high morbidity and mortality. Thus, it is important to identify factors that increase the likelihood of a fatal outcome in patients with acute pancreatitis. Tables 45-3 and 45-4 summarize some of those factors. An increased mortality is observed when three or more risk factors are present. These include **hemoconcentration elevated hematocrit, hypotension,** need for massive fluid and colloid replacement from third spacing of fluids, **respiratory failure,** and **hypocalcemia.** Patients at high risk should be treated in an intensive care unit and may require surgical intervention.

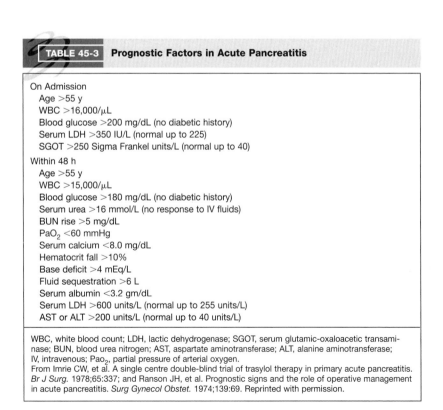

TABLE 45-3	Prognostic Factors in Acute Pancreatitis

On Admission
  Age >55 y
  WBC >16,000/μL
  Blood glucose >200 mg/dL (no diabetic history)
  Serum LDH >350 IU/L (normal up to 225)
  SGOT >250 Sigma Frankel units/L (normal up to 40)
Within 48 h
  Age >55 y
  WBC >15,000/μL
  Blood glucose >180 mg/dL (no diabetic history)
  Serum urea >16 mmol/L (no response to IV fluids)
  BUN rise >5 mg/dL
  PaO_2 <60 mmHg
  Serum calcium <8.0 mg/dL
  Hematocrit fall >10%
  Base deficit >4 mEq/L
  Fluid sequestration >6 L
  Serum albumin <3.2 gm/dL
  Serum LDH >600 units/L (normal up to 255 units/L)
  AST or ALT >200 units/L (normal up to 40 units/L)

WBC, white blood count; LDH, lactic dehydrogenase; SGOT, serum glutamic-oxaloacetic transaminase; BUN, blood urea nitrogen; AST, aspartate aminotransferase; ALT, alanine aminotransferase; IV, intravenous; Pao_2, partial pressure of arterial oxygen.
From Imrie CW, et al. A single centre double-blind trial of trasylol therapy in primary acute pancreatitis. *Br J Surg.* 1978;65:337; and Ranson JH, et al. Prognostic signs and the role of operative management in acute pancreatitis. *Surg Gynecol Obstet.* 1974;139:69. Reprinted with permission.

TABLE 45-4	Clinical Criteria for Severe Pancreatitis
Cardiac	BP <90 mmHg, tachycardia >130, arrhythmia and other ECG changes
Pulmonary	Dyspnea, rales PO_2 <60 mmHg, adult respiratory distress syndrome
Renal	Urine output <50 mL/h, rising BUN and creatinine
Metabolic	Calcium <8 mg/dL, albumin <3.2 g/dL
Hematologic	Falling hematocrit, diffuse intravascular coagulation
Neurologic	Irritability, confusion, CNS localizing signs
Abdominal	Tense distention, fluid wave, ileus

BP, blood pressure; ECG, electrocardiogram; PO_2, partial pressure of oxygen; BUN, blood urea nitrogen; CNS, central nervous system.

VI. DIAGNOSIS

A. Clinical presentation

1. **History.** Abdominal pain is the most common complaint in acute pancreatitis. It is usually located in the epigastrium, left upper quadrant, or periumbilical area, and often radiates to the back, chest, flanks, and lower abdomen.

   The pain is steady, dull, and boring in character. It is usually more intense when the patient is supine and may lessen in the sitting position with the trunk flexed forward and the knees drawn up. Patients also complain of nausea, vomiting, and abdominal distention secondary to ileus.

2. **Physical examination.** Patients with acute pancreatitis initially may present with fever, tachycardia, and hypotension. Shock is common in severe instances due to hypovolemia caused by third-space fluid sequestration (in retroperitoneal and other spaces) with increased vascular permeability and vasodilatation and other systemic effects of proteolytic and lipolytic enzymes released into the circulation. Jaundice may occur, due to obstructive cholelithiasis or, more commonly, the compression of the intrapancreatic portion of the common bile duct with edema of the head of the pancreas. Abdominal tenderness and rigidity may be present. Bowel sounds are diminished or absent. The presence of a bluish discoloration around the umbilicus **(Cullen's sign)** and at the flanks **(Turner's sign)** suggests hemoperitoneum and results from hemorrhagic necrotizing pancreatitis.

   Other findings such as pleural effusion (especially on the left side), pneumonitis and other pulmonary findings, such as ARDS, and subcutaneous fat necrosis resembling erythema nodosum may be present. Tetany due to hypocalcemia is a rare finding.

B. Diagnostic studies

1. **Laboratory studies**

   a. **Serum amylase.** Even though there is no definite correlation between the severity of pancreatitis and the degree of serum amylase elevation, serum amylase elevation is commonly equated to the presence of pancreatitis. However, hyperamylasemia may be present in many other conditions, as summarized in Table 45-5. Amylase is found in many organs, including salivary glands, liver, small intestine, kidney, and fallopian tubes, and in various tumors such as carcinoma of the esophagus, lung, and ovary. In 75% of the patients with acute pancreatitis, the serum amylase is elevated. Hyperamylasemia is noted within the first 24 hours and persists for 3 to 5 days. Amylase levels normalize unless there is extensive pancreatic necrosis, ductal obstruction, or pseudocyst

TABLE 45-5	Causes of Hyperamylasemia
Pancreatic trauma	Ruptured ectopic pregnancy
Pancreatitis	Ruptured or dissecting aortic aneurysm
Pancreatic pseudocyst	Splenic rupture
Pancreatic abscess	Renal insufficiency
Pancreatic cancer	Diabetic ketoacidosis
Biliary tract disease	Burns
Acute cholecystitis	Salivary gland disease
Common bile duct obstruction	Mumps
Perforated or penetrating peptic ulcer	Carcinoma
Intestinal obstruction	Lung
Intestinal ischemia or infarction	Esophagus
Peritonitis	Ovary
Acute appendicitis	Macroamylasemia

formation. Serum amylase levels may be spuriously normal in patients with hypertriglyceridemia and in patients with recurrent alcoholic pancreatitis.

  b. Serum lipase levels are elevated in approximately 70% of patients. When both serum amylase and serum lipase are determined, one enzyme is elevated in 80% to 85% of the patients with acute pancreatitis, thus increasing the diagnostic yield.

  c. Urine amylase is increased in acute pancreatitis and may remain elevated for 7 to 10 days after serum levels have returned to normal.

  d. Leukocytosis (10,000–20, 0000/μL) is frequent.

  e. Hemoconcentration due to third-space fluid sequestration may lead to hematocrit elevation to greater than 50%.

  f. Hyperglycemia is not uncommon and may result from decreased insulin and increased glucagon, catecholamine, and glucocorticoid release.

  g. Hypocalcemia occurs in about 25% of patients. Its pathogenesis is multifactorial and most likely results from sequestration of calcium in saponified fats as well as the presence of elevated levels of glucagon and calcitonin.

  h. Serum bilirubin, alkaline phosphatase, and **aminotransferase (alanine [ALT], aspartate [AST]) levels** may be transiently elevated and return to normal in 4 to 7 days unless there is persistent biliary obstruction from gallstones or other causes.

  i. Arterial hypoxemia may be present in 25% of patients. In some patients, adult respiratory distress syndrome (ARDS) may develop. Cardiovascular and electrocardiographic abnormalities may also occur, especially in severely ill patients.

2. Radiologic studies. Several radiologic studies are useful in the diagnosis and management of acute pancreatitis. These include flat film (kidneys, ureters, and bladder [KUB]) of the abdomen, chest x-rays, ultrasonography, computed tomography (CT), and ERCP.

  a. The **plain films** are useful in excluding other diagnoses, such as perforated viscus, mesenteric ischemia, or infarction. Findings suggestive of diffuse or localized ileus and presence of ascites are nonspecific.

  b. Ultrasound (US) and CT scans are helpful in determining the size and appearance of the pancreas, the peripancreatic spread of the inflammation and phlegmon, and the condition of the biliary tract. These noninvasive techniques should be used to confirm clinically suspected disease and its complications such as cholecystitis, choledocholithiasis, tumor, pseudocyst, and ascites.

When ileus is present, the US waves are scattered by the air in the intestinal lumen, and a clear picture of the pancreas cannot be obtained. However, US is the test of choice for documenting cholelithiasis and biliary ductal dilatation. CT scan of the abdomen gives a clearer picture of the pancreas and the surrounding areas than US does and should be obtained when there is a likelihood of severe pancreatitis (e.g., multiple positive Ranson's signs during the first 48 hours). If the CT scan is normal or shows mild pancreatic edema, the likelihood of a severe complication is remote even if many of Ranson's signs are positive. When a markedly swollen pancreas is seen with or without fluid collections, the presence of extensive necrotic areas within the pancreas **(necrotizing pancreatitis)** predisposes the patient to secondary infection and higher risk of mortality. The distinction between acute interstitial and necrotizing pancreatitis can be made if a CT scan is obtained following the administration of IV contrast medium **(dynamic CT scan).** In acute interstitial pancreatitis, the pancreas is well perfused and uniformly enhanced by the intravascular contrast agent. If necrosis is present, the areas of devitalized tissue are not perfused and are not enhanced.

The presence of air bubbles in the pancreatic and peripancreatic region is strong evidence of pancreatic infection. When fever, elevated white blood count, and clinical toxicity are associated with CT scan evidence of fluid collections or necrotizing pancreatitis, CT-guided percutaneous aspiration, staining, and culture of the obtained fluid may help to distinguish sterile pancreatitis from pancreatic infection. When infection is suspected or proved, surgical debridement may be lifesaving.

ERCP is generally contraindicated in patients with acute pancreatitis except when an impacted common bile duct stone may be the cause of the pancreatitis. Endoscopic sphincterotomy in these very ill patients may be immediately therapeutic. ERCP is also useful in establishing the diagnosis of pancreas divisum; annular pancreas; pancreatic cancer; periampullary, ampullary, and pancreatic ductal abnormalities; and the possible communication of the pancreatic duct with pseudocysts. These studies are usually performed after the patient has been clinically stabilized.

C. **Differential diagnosis.** Table 45-6 summarizes the differential diagnosis of acute pancreatitis. It may be difficult to distinguish between acute cholecystitis, ascending cholangitis, and pancreatitis, because they may present with similarly elevated serum amylase and abnormal liver tests. US and dimethylphenylcarbamylmethyliminodiacetic acid (HIDA) scans may be helpful in differentiating between these diseases. Gut ischemia, infarction, viscus perforation, aortic dissection, mechanical intestinal obstruction, myocardial infarction, and acute appendicitis need to be promptly diagnosed and surgically treated.

D. **Complications.** See Table 45-7.

VII. TREATMENT. In most patients (85%–90%) with acute pancreatitis, the disease is self-limited and resolves spontaneously. These patients are medically treated with

TABLE 45-6	Differential Diagnosis of Acute Pancreatitis
Acute cholecystitis	Mesenteric ischemia/infarction
Biliary colic due to choledocholithiasis	Vasculitis
Ascending cholangitis	Dissecting aortic aneurysm
Perforated viscus	Myocardial infarction
Penetrating peptic ulcer	Pneumonia
Alcoholic hepatitis	Renal colic
Viral hepatitis	Acute appendicitis
Acute intestinal obstruction	Diabetic ketoacidosis

| TABLE 45-7 | Complications of Acute Pancreatitis |

Pancreatic	Cardiovascular
Phlegmon	Cardiogenic shock
Abscess	Increased cardiac index
Pseudocyst	Decreased systemic vascular resistance
Nonpancreatic	Pulmonary
Inflammatory involvement of contiguous	Hypoxemia
organs	Pleural effusions
Obstructive jaundice	Pulmonary infiltrates, atelectasis
Pancreatic ascites	Adult respiratory distress syndrome
Intraperitoneal hemorrhage	Renal
Thrombosis of splenic vein	Decreased glomerular filtration rate and
Bowel infarction	renal plasma flow
Gastrointestinal bleeding	Acute tubular necrosis
Systemic	Acute renal failure
Metabolic	Hematologic
Hypocalcemia	Disseminated intravascular coagulation
Hyperlipidemia	Thromboses
Hyperglycemia	Increased factor VII or fibrinogen
Diabetes ketoacidosis	Skin and musculoskeletal
Nonketotic diabetic coma	Erythema nodosum–like lesions
Pancreatic encephalopathy	Angiopathic retinopathy
	Polyarthritis

supportive care with special attention given to analgesia, maintenance of normal intravascular volume, frequent monitoring of vital signs, and treatment of possible complications of the disease.

A. Meperidine (Demerol) in a dosage of 50 to 100 mg every 4 to 6 hours IV or intramuscular (IM) is better tolerated than morphine sulfate (MS), which may induce spasm of the sphincter of Oddi. In cases of severe pain, MS may be necessary.

B. The sequestration of fluid in the peripancreatic and retro- and intraperitoneal areas reduce the circulating plasma volume in most patients. **IV electrolyte and colloid solutions** should be given generously (i.e., 200–300 mL/L for the first 1–2 days) to replace the fluid deficit. Fluid volume status determination may require Swan-Ganz catheter placement.

C. It is believed that by **putting the pancreas "at rest"** by reducing pancreatic secretions, the pancreatic inflammation will be minimized. Patients usually are given nothing by mouth, and the upper gastrointestinal tract is decompressed by nasogastric suction. The rationale for nasogastric suction is to decrease gastric secretion and to prevent gastric contents from entering the duodenum. Nasogastric suction with a double-lumen sump tube is used in patients with nausea, vomiting, and ileus. It may not be necessary for the patient with mild disease.

D. No drugs have been shown to improve the course of acute pancreatitis. Clinical trials using inhibitors of gastric acid secretion such as histamine-2 blockers or proton pump inhibitors also are no more effective than nasogastric suction. Somatostatin or its analog octreotide may be beneficial by reducing pancreatic enzyme secretion.

E. Prophylactic antibiotics are not recommended in interstitial pancreatitis. Antibiotics should be reserved for patients with established infection. It is important to recognize and treat with the appropriate antimicrobial therapy possible secondary infection of the injured pancreatic tissue (phlegmon, pseudocyst, and abscess) or an obstructed biliary tract leading to ascending cholangitis.

In several studies, prophylactic antibiotics were found to be helpful in preventing either pancreatic infection or other infections among patients with necrotizing pancreatitis.

F. Nutritional support of the patient with acute pancreatitis should not be neglected. As the inflammation subsides, small feedings of a diet high in carbohydrate but low in protein and fat may be initiated. It is important to advance the diet slowly. The feedings should be stopped if symptoms return. Pancreatic secretion is stimulated equally in patients given elemental diets and those given regular diets intragastrically or intrajejunally. Parenteral administration of nutrition does not seem to increase pancreatic secretion. Thus, in patients who cannot receive feedings orally, parenteral nutritional support including intralipids should be instituted after the first few days. In some studies intragastric or intrajejunal feedings have shown decreased rate of infectious complications and should be preferred.

G. Patients with fulminant pancreatitis need intensive monitoring and therapy. These patients have very large fluid requirements. Most patients have respiratory insufficiency and acute respiratory distress syndrome and may require mechanical respiratory support. Hypocalcemia and hypomagnesemia should be promptly treated with IV replacement. Renal insufficiency and acute tubular necrosis are not uncommon, and patients may require dialysis.

H. Patients with severe disease should be closely followed by a surgical team. In patients with a deteriorating clinical condition, emergency laparotomy for drainage of the necrotic pancreas and peripancreatic spaces may be attempted. Some surgeons advocate subtotal pancreatectomy and a procedure to decompress the biliary tract. Alternatively, in clinically deteriorating patients with necrotizing pancreatitis demonstrated on CT scan, CT-guided percutaneous aspiration of the necrotic pancreas may be attempted. Gram's stain and culture should be performed on the aspirated material. Positive bacterial findings necessitate surgical debridement. In selected cases of infected necrosis, vigorous percutaneous drainage with multiple large tubes have been successful in either delaying surgery until the patient is a better surgical candidate or eliminating the need for surgery. Also, in selected incidences of infected necrosis, there may be a role for endoscopic drainage, particularly if the necrosis has organized.

Imipenem and/or other antibiotics covering gut pathogens should be given. In sterile necrosis, nonoperative medical management for the first 3 to 4 weeks is recommended.

VIII. Pancreatic pseudocysts are collections of necrotic tissue, fluid, and blood that develop in or near the pancreas over a period of 1 to 4 weeks after the onset of acute pancreatitis. They do not have a true capsule with an epithelial lining. A connection may be present to a disrupted pancreatic duct. Most pseudocysts (90%) are solitary lesions located in the body or tail of the pancreas. The main symptom is abdominal pain.

A. Pathogenesis. Most pseudocysts form during a severe episode of acute pancreatitis. Persistence of an elevated serum amylase level for more than a week after the onset of pancreatitis may signal the formation of a pseudocyst. Other causes of pancreatic pseudocyst include abdominal blunt trauma with disruption of a pancreatic duct, inadvertent surgical ductal trauma, and chronic pancreatitis. Neoplastic cysts, such as cystadenoma or cystadenoma-carcinoma, account for 10% of cystic pancreatic masses.

B. Diagnostic studies. Abdominal US and CT scans are the best imaging techniques used in the diagnosis of pancreatic pseudocysts. Serial scans help in following the size and course of the cysts. ERCP may be required to assess the possible connection of the pseudocyst with the pancreatic duct.

C. Complications and treatment. Most pseudocysts tend to resolve spontaneously. Symptomatic pseudocysts require decompression. This can be achieved by surgery or by percutaneous catheter drainage or by endoscopic techniques. Endoscopic and radiologic methods should be reserved for those institutions with extensive experience in these techniques. The serious complications of pancreatic pseudocysts are infection, perforation, and hemorrhage.

1. **Infection.** Patients with a pancreatic pseudocyst who have pain, fever, and leukocytosis need to be evaluated for infection. Percutaneous aspiration under US or CT guidance with Gram's stain and culture of the aspirate helps in confirming the diagnosis. Infected pseudocyst or abscess should be drained externally.
2. **Perforation.** Rupture or leak of a pseudocyst into the peritoneal cavity or retroperitoneum may result in shock and requires emergency surgery. The mortality from this complication is very high.
3. **Hemorrhage.** A pseudocyst may erode into a viscus (e.g., stomach, small or large bowel) or a blood vessel with subsequent hemorrhage. Angiography is often necessary prior to surgery for proper diagnosis of this complication.

Selected Readings

Amar S, et al. Sorofenibinducod pancreatitis. *Mayo Clin Proc.* 2007;82(4):516.

Badalov N, et al. Drug induced acute pancreatitis: An evidence-based review. *Clinical Gastroenterol Heptatol.* 2007;5(6):648–661.

Baron TH, et al. Acute necrotizing pancreatitis. *N Engl J Med.* 1999;340:1412.

Beger HG, et al. Surgical management of necrotizing pancreatitis. *Surg Clin North Am.* 1999;79:783.

Brown A, et al. Hemoconcentration is an early marker for organ failure and necrotizing pancreatitis. *Pancreas.* 2000;20:367.

DeWaele JJ, et al. Emergence of antibiotic resistance in infected pancreatic necrosis. *Arch Surg.* 2004;139(12):1371–1375.

Frakes JT. Biliary pancreatitis: A review emphasizing appropriate endoscopic intervention. *J Clin Gastroenterol.* 1999;28:97.

Freeman ML. Pancreatic stents for prevention of post ERCP pancreatitis. *Clin Gastroenterol Hepatol.* 2007;5(11):1354–1365.

Freeman ML, et al. Prevention of post-ERCP pancreatitis: A comprehensive review. *Gastrointest Endosc.* 2004;59:845–864.

German Antibiotics in Severe Acute Pancreatitis Study Group. Prophylactic antibiotic treatment inpatients with predicted severe acte pancreatitis. A placebo-controlled, double-blind trial. *Gastroenterology.* 2004;126(4):997–1000.

Jacobsen BC, et al. A prospective, randomized trial of clear liquids versus low fat solid diet as the initial meal in mild pancreatitis. *Clin Gastroenterol Hepatol.* 2007;5(8):946–951.

McClave SA, et al. Nutrition support in acute pancreatitis: A systematic review of the literature. *JPEN J Parenter Enteral Nutr.* 2006;30:143–156.

Meier R, et al. ESPEN guidelines on enteral nutrition: pancreas. *Clin Nutr.* 2006;25:275–284.

Shankar S, et al. Imaging and percutaneous management of acute complicated pancreatitis. *Cardiovasc Intervent Radiol.* 2004;27:567–580.

$\mathcal{C}$hronic pancreatitis results from progressive destruction and fibrosis of the pancreas with ongoing inflammatory lesions. The **exocrine** pancreatic tissue and function are lost in the earlier stages, followed by the loss of **endocrine** parenchyma and function. The disease frequently is complicated in the early stages of its evolution by attacks of acute pancreatitis, which are responsible for recurrent pain. After several years of ongoing inflammation and fibrosis, pancreatic insufficiency develops, with resulting malabsorption, steatorrhea, and diabetes mellitus. Acute attacks decrease and pain usually disappears.

I. CLASSIFICATION. Chronic pancreatitis may be classified into two forms that present with specific lesions and have different causes.

  A. Obstructive chronic pancreatitis is caused by the occlusion of pancreatic ducts, which precedes the onset of pancreatitis. The occlusion may be the result of tumors, scars of parenchymal inflammation, necrotic pseudocysts, or congenital anomalies **(e.g., annular pancreas, pancreas divisum).** The lesions are found in the part of the pancreas encompassing the occluded ducts. The ductal epithelium is relatively preserved, and intraductal protein plugs and stones are not present.

  Infiltrative and autoimmune diseases such as hemochromatosis and Sjögren's syndrome may also involve the pancreas, resulting in pancreatic insufficiency.

  B. Chronic calcifying pancreatitis (CCP) is the most frequent cause (95% of all instances) of chronic pancreatitis. It is significantly associated with chronic alcohol consumption and is exacerbated by cigarette smoking and by diets high in protein and high or low in fat.

  Less frequently, CCP occurs with hyperparathyroidism and hypercalcemia, and in some tropical countries (South India, Zaire, Nigeria, Brazil) it occurs in nonalcoholic young people (average age, 12–20 years) of both sexes living in areas where protein- and fat-poor diets are consumed. There is also a hereditary autosomal-dominant form of CCP with variable penetrance. Pancreatic insufficiency from **cystic fibrosis** may resemble CCP in morphology and presentation.

  1. Morphology. CCP is characterized by the lobular, patchy distribution of lesions of different intensity in neighboring lobules. **Protein plugs** are always found in the ductal and acinar lumina, and in the later stages these form **calcifications,** or **calculi (pancreatic calcification).** Atrophy of the epithelium and stenosis of the ducts are common. Recurrent attacks of acute pancreatitis, retention cysts, pseudocysts, and perineural inflammation are frequently associated.

  The first visible lesions are **protein precipitates** or plugs in the lumina of ducts and acini, which later calcify forming **pancreatic stones.** The ductal epithelium in contact with the protein plugs or stones loses its basement membrane, and the duct cells atrophy and disappear with the growth of periductal connective tissue and fibrosis leading to fibrotic strictures. Distal to the strictures, the exocrine tissue atrophies and disappears due to plugs, stones, and fibrosis. When a partially obstructed duct is distended by pancreatic juice under pressure of secretion, it may form an **intrapancreatic cyst.** These **retention cysts** may grow and extend into peripancreatic tissue, forming **retention pseudocysts.** Thus all lesions of chronic calcifying pancreatitis are thought to be secondary to the formation of protein plugs and stones in the pancreatic ducts and ductules, resulting in ductal obstruction, parenchymal inflammation, atrophy, and fibrosis.

2. **Pathophysiology.** The pathogenesis of **pancreatic lithogenesis** involves the precipitation of both a fibrillar protein—a form of **pancreatic stone protein (PSP)—and calcium carbonate.**

Normally the pancreatic juice is saturated with calcium. The precipitation of calcium in the pancreatic juice is prevented by the presence of a group of proteins, PSP-S_{2-5}, synthesized and secreted by the acinar cells. PSP-S_{2-5} acts as a calcium stabilizer of the pancreatic juice by blocking the growth sites of crystals. In the pancreatic juice, PSP-S_{2-5} may be hydrolyzed by active trypsin to give a shorter protein, PSP-S, which is insoluble at physiologic pH and does not prevent calcium carbonate crystallization. PSP extracted from pancreatic plugs and stones contain the same amino acid sequence as PSP-S_1. The relative concentration of PSP is significantly decreased in the pancreatic juice of patients who have CCP compared to normal controls; this is true even in the early stages of the disease, before the appearance of calcification on abdominal x-rays. This finding suggests that the formation of the calcified part of the stones is due to a decreased secretion of PSP, the stabilizer of calcium in pancreatic juice. PSP secretion is also decreased in hereditary chronic pancreatitis as well as in idiopathic and alcoholic forms; thus the condition may be either congenital or acquired.

The lesions of the ductal epithelium caused by the protein plugs and stones lead to transudation of protein- and calcium-rich interstitial fluid into ductal lumina, increasing the calcium concentration in the pancreatic juice and resulting in increased intraductal calcium crystallization. As the diseased ducts become obstructed by the precipitated protein and calcifications, the acini and the lobule, which the ducts drain, become atrophic and fibrotic, resulting in pancreatic parenchymal loss in a patchy distribution throughout the pancreas.

3. **Role of alcohol consumption and diet.** Acute recurrent pancreatitis is thought to be a complication of the initial stages of CCP. It occurs in chronic alcoholics who have recently increased their alcohol intake. Follow-up of these patients shows that in most of them, pancreatic calculi (calcifications) develop after a number of years.

Recurrent alcoholic pancreatitis progresses to overt pancreatic insufficiency at different rates in different people. However, there is a linear relation between the average daily consumption of alcohol and the logarithm of the risk. For a given amount of alcohol consumption, the risk increases with the increased duration of consumption. Even small quantities (1–20 g of alcohol per day) increase the risk. Rather than a statistical threshold of alcohol toxicity for the pancreas, there is a continuous spectrum of individual thresholds. The type of alcoholic beverage and the rhythm of alcohol consumption have no significant influence on the risk of development of CCP.

Chronic alcohol ingestion increases the total protein concentration of protein in pancreatic juice but decreases the concentrations of PSP, citrate, bicarbonate, trypsin inhibitory protein, and the pH. Decreased citrate concentration increases calcium availability. It is thought that the increased viscosity of the pancreatic juice, due to increased protein content and decreased concentrations of PSP and citrate, leads to formation of protein plugs and calcifications in these patients.

II. **DIAGNOSIS.** The insidious nature of chronic pancreatitis delays the early diagnosis of this disorder in many patients. Patients usually come to medical attention after considerable damage has occurred to the gland. In most cases, it is difficult to differentiate acute relapsing pancreatitis, in which the permanent pancreatic damage is mild to moderate, from chronic relapsing pancreatitis.

A. **Clinical presentations.** Chronic pancreatitis is an insidious process of parenchymal damage with necrosis and fibrosis of the gland. Approximately one half of the patients present with episodes of acute pancreatitis superimposed onto the damaged organ. One third of the patients may present with only abdominal pain. Other patients may have jaundice, weight loss, malabsorption, steatorrhea, diabetes mellitus, or upper gastrointestinal bleeding. Ten percent of the patients never experience pain. The average age of the patient at initial diagnosis is 35 to 50 years.

1. **Abdominal pain** accompanying chronic pancreatitis is described as a steady, boring, achy sensation usually associated with nausea with or without vomiting. It is commonly present in the mid-epigastrium, but it may also be perceived in the right or left upper quadrant or periumbilical area. It usually radiates to the back, increases in the supine position, and decreases on sitting up and leaning forward. Most patients require analgesics and may become addicted to narcotics.

   The course of the pain of chronic pancreatitis differs in different patient groups. In most patients, it is a constant experience in the first 5 years after its diagnosis. Thereafter, in about two thirds of the patients, it may resolve spontaneously or diminish in severity and frequency.

2. **Malabsorption.** Pancreatic exocrine function steadily diminishes with chronic pancreatitis.

   a. **Fat and protein malabsorption** becomes apparent after the loss of 90% of the pancreatic secretory capacity. Protein malabsorption may be compensated for with increased oral intake of protein without additional abdominal discomfort to the patient. However, increased fat intake results in more diarrhea and abdominal pain. The steatorrhea of chronic pancreatitis consists mainly of triglycerides (esterified fats) in contrast to steatorrhea of sprue, which contains free fatty acids: The esterified fats are hydrolyzed by pancreatic lipase to free fatty acids, but they are not absorbed by the diseased intestinal mucosa. Stool volume is also smaller in chronic pancreatitis, again due to the presence of esterified fats, because hydroxylated free fatty acids are the secretagogues of colonic chloride and water secretion.

   b. **Carbohydrate malabsorption** is rare in chronic pancreatitis, because loss of 97% of amylase secretion is necessary for maldigestion of starch.

   c. **Vitamin B_{12} malabsorption.** Decreased pancreatic exocrine function does not affect the absorption of bile salts, water- or fat-soluble vitamins, iron, or calcium. However vitamin B_{12} malabsorption may occur in some patients due to diminished secretion of trypsin. As vitamin B_{12} is ingested, a nonspecific protein (R protein) found in the upper gastrointestinal secretions binds with it and does not allow it to bind intrinsic factor (IF) from the stomach. Normally, trypsin in the second portion of the duodenum cleaves off the R protein and allows the association of vitamin B_{12} to intrinsic factor.

   The IF–vitamin B_{12} complex is necessary for the active absorption of the vitamin B_{12} at the terminal ileum. In chronic pancreatitis with diminished levels of pancreatic proteases, especially trypsin, in the duodenal lumen, the R protein is not cleaved off vitamin B_{12} and IF–vitamin B_{12} complex does not form, leading to vitamin B_{12} malabsorption.

3. **Diabetes mellitus.** Along with exocrine insufficiency, endocrine insufficiency with diminished insulin and glucagon release develops in these patients. Seventy percent of the patients with pancreatic calcifications develop diabetes mellitus. Microangiopathy and nephropathy do not seem to complicate diabetes mellitus resulting from chronic pancreatitis. However, due to concomitant diminished glucagon secretion, these patients are very sensitive to exogenous insulin and may develop hypoglycemia even with low doses.

4. **Physical examination.** There are no specific findings in chronic pancreatitis. Some patients have epigastric tenderness. A mass may be palpable if a palpable pseudocyst exists. Patients with malabsorption may have weight loss but do not present with signs of fat-soluble vitamin deficiency (vitamins A, D, E, and K) such as night blindness, hypocalcemia, osteomalacia, and bleeding tendency. Jaundice may exist in patients with common bile duct obstruction due to scarring in the pancreatic head. In these patients, it may be difficult to differentiate pancreatic cancer from chronic pancreatitis.

B. Diagnostic studies

1. **Serum chemistry profile.** There are no specific findings in the serum chemistry profile in patients with chronic pancreatitis. Even during acute attacks, the serum amylase or lipase level may not be elevated. The serum chemistry profile may reflect concomitant liver disease. With obstruction of the common bile duct, a cholestatic liver chemistry profile may emerge and should be confirmed by imaging techniques.

2. **Stool fat.** Steatorrhea is best confirmed by 72-hour stool collection for quantitative determination of fat. Most patients consuming 100 g of fat per day excrete more than 10 g of fat per day. In advanced pancreatic insufficiency, stool fat may reach 30 to 40 g per day.

3. **Radiologic studies**

   a. **Pancreatic calcifications** are present on plain abdominal radiographs in one third of patients with chronic pancreatitis.

   b. **Ultrasound** and, especially, **computed tomography (CT) scan** provide for more sensitive detection of pancreatic calcifications. The presence of pseudocysts, ductal dilatation, and tumors can also be delineated.

   c. **Angiography.** When a tumor is suspected, angiography may be helpful in identifying neovascularity of the tumor, deviation of normal vascularity due to tumor, or the lack of vascularity of the cystic lesions. When splenic vein thrombosis has occurred, angiography demonstrates the site of occlusion and the presence of gastric or esophageal varices.

   d. **Endoscopic retrograde cholangiopancreatography.** Pancreatic ductal anatomy is best delineated with endoscopic pancreatography: Dilatation, cystic changes, strictures, and calculi are demonstrated. Most patients with advanced chronic pancreatitis have a dilated common pancreatic duct with intermittent sites of narrowing, creating the "chain of lakes" appearance on the pancreatograms. The damage is also noted in the secondary ducts, with dilatation and blunting leading to loss of the fine "acinarization."

   Endoscopic retrograde cholangiopancreatography (ERCP) may also be helpful in the differentiation of pancreatic cancer from chronic pancreatitis. In pancreatic cancer, only that part of the duct involved with the tumor is abnormal, in contrast to generalized abnormal changes seen with chronic pancreatitis.

   e. **Endoscopic ultrasonography (EUS)** may be used in instances of CCP in which a tumor is suspected. The differentiation of sclerotic pancreatic cancer from atrophic and fibrotic pancreatic parenchyma may be difficult with this technique.

4. **Tests of pancreatic exocrine function.** Chronic pancreatitis or pancreatic insufficiency can be determined with certainty only by demonstrating diminished exocrine function during adequate stimulation of the pancreas. These tests may be necessary in situations in which no calcification is seen on radiographic studies and the ducts appear normal on ERCP.

   a. **Secretin stimulation test.** In this test, the duodenum is intubated under fluoroscopy and the duodenal contents are aspirated, collected, and analyzed after the patient receives intravenous secretin (1 U/kg of body weight) to stimulate pancreatic water and bicarbonate secretion. The total output of bicarbonate correlates well with the extent of pancreatic damage.

   The addition of cholecystokinin to secretin, to stimulate exocrine enzyme secretion (e.g., amylase or lipase), does not seem to increase the diagnostic accuracy. The secretin stimulation test is difficult to perform and requires technical expertise. It is reliably performed in specialized medical centers. The overall sensitivity is 74% to 90%.

   b. **The Lundh test meal** provides for endogenous stimulation of pancreatic exocrine secretion. After the patient is given a standard test meal, the proximal jejunal fluid is aspirated for 2 hours and analyzed for trypsin. This test is not as sensitive as the secretin stimulation test (sensitivity, 60%–90%).

c. **Bentiromide test.** Patients ingest 500 mg of N-benzoyl-L-tyrosyl-*p*-aminobenzoic acid (bentiromide), a synthetic peptide, which is specially cleaved by chymotrypsin to liberate PABA in the proximal small intestine. PABA is normally absorbed, conjugated in the liver, and excreted in the urine. Recovery of less than 60% of the liberated paraaminobenzoic acid (PABA) from a 6-hour urine collection is considered to be abnormal and suggests pancreatic insufficiency with decreased chymotrypsin output.

False-positive results may be obtained in patients with diffuse intestinal disease resulting in diminished absorption of PABA, with chronic liver disease resulting in decreased conjugation of PABA, and with renal insufficiency with reduced urinary output of PABA. The accuracy of the test may be increased with a concomitant d-xylose test or by giving a small amount of carbon 14–labeled PABA along with the test dose of the peptide. The ratio of urinary PABA to ^{14}C-PABA helps in differentiating false-positive results from pancreatic insufficiency.

Even though this test does not seem to be as sensitive as the secretin test in patients with mild pancreatic insufficiency, its ease of performance makes it a desirable alternative. Its overall sensitivity is 37% to 90%.

III. **LOCAL COMPLICATIONS.** Chronic pancreatitis in a minority of patients may be complicated by the development of pancreatic pseudocysts, abscess, ascites, common bile duct obstruction, duodenal obstruction, and portal and splenic vein thrombosis. The incidence of pancreatic cancer is not increased in patients with chronic pancreatitis.

IV. **The treatment of chronic pancreatitis** is mainly supportive and directed at the complications.
   A. **Management of pain**
      1. **In alcohol-related disease,** alcohol and tobacco consumption should be stopped. Patients should be advised to follow a diet with moderate fat and protein and high carbohydrate content.
      2. In some instances **pain relief** may be obtained by **small feedings and analgesics.** Many patients require narcotics.
      3. **Feedback control.** Oral treatment with large doses of pancreatic enzymes has been shown to decrease the abdominal pain experienced by patients with chronic pancreatitis by inhibiting pancreatic exocrine secretion and allowing the pancreas to rest. The presence of the proteases trypsin and chymotrypsin within the lumen of the proximal duodenum exerts a feedback control on pancreatic exocrine secretion. The patients in whom pain responds to pancreatic enzymes most readily are those with mild-to-moderate exocrine impairment. The use of pancreatic enzymes has also been shown to heal pancreatic fistulas and to decrease the frequency of attacks of acute, recurrent pancreatitis. The doses used are similar to those used for the treatment of malabsorption (see section IV.B).
      4. **Percutaneous injection of alcohol to destroy the celiac plexus** has been reported to relieve pain in some patients for as long as 6 months. Long-term effects of this treatment have not been determined.
      5. **Surgery** for relief of pancreatic pain is reserved for patients with intractable and disabling pain unresponsive to any other mode of therapy. The surgical procedures used depend on pancreatic and ductal anatomic abnormalities determined by preoperative CT scan and ERCP findings. In most patients, pain relief is achieved for the short term. The long-term effectiveness of these procedures in relieving pain is debated.

         Drainage procedures are used when there is generalized or localized pancreatic ductal dilatation, and **partial resection of the gland** is used when there is no ductal dilatation or the abnormality is confined to a segment of the pancreas.
         a. **Longitudinal pancreaticojejunostomy (the Puestow procedure).** In this procedure, the dilated pancreatic duct is filleted open longitudinally over the

length of the gland. A nonfunctioning segment of jejunum in a Roux-en-Y loop is also opened longitudinally and sewn over the open duct to allow for drainage of the pancreatic secretions.

b. **Caudal pancreaticojejunostomy (DuVal procedure).** When there is a ductal obstruction in the body of the pancreas with distal duct dilatation, the tail of the pancreas is resected and the remaining pancreas is placed in an end-to-end fashion into a nonfunctioning segment of jejunum.

c. **Sphincteroplasty of the sphincter of Oddi** or Santorini has been used in isolated strictures of these orifices (e.g., in pancreas divisum).

d. **Pancreatic resection.** In the absence of ductal dilatation and when abnormalities are confined to portions of the pancreas, 40% to 95% of the gland may be resected. When the disease is confined to the head of the pancreas, the Whipple's procedure (pancreaticoduodenectomy) may be used. Total pancreatectomy has been performed rarely when lesser procedures failed to relieve pain.

Although the short-term success of these procedures in relieving pain seems good, most patients experience pain recurrence. Also, pancreatic insufficiency and insulin-dependent diabetes mellitus become a problem after the resection of 50% of the gland in most patients. Surgical manipulation of the pancreas for relief of pancreatic pain should be reserved for truly refractory pain, and drainage procedures, when possible, are preferred to resection involving more than half of the gland.

B. **Malabsorption.** Steatorrhea is often an earlier and more severe problem than **azotorrhea** in chronic pancreatitis because secretion of lipase and colipase decreases earlier than that of the proteolytic enzymes. If steatorrhea is less than 10 g of fat per day, patients may do well with dietary restriction of fat. If the steatorrhea is greater than 10 g of fat per day, pancreatic enzyme supplementation is recommended in addition to dietary fat restriction.

1. **Pancreatic enzyme supplements.** Pancreatic extracts may be used for enzyme supplementation to reduce malabsorption. Table 46-1 lists some of the commercially available pancreatic enzyme preparations.

To eliminate malabsorption, the concentration of enzymes delivered to the duodenum need only be 5% to 10% of the concentration that is secreted into the duodenum after maximal stimulation of the pancreas. This means that approximately 30,000 IU of lipase must be present in the duodenum with each meal. Most commercial preparations contain only 3,000 to 4,000 units of active lipase per tablet. Therefore, if no lipase is inactivated in the stomach, six to ten tablets are required per meal to eliminate steatorrhea. Lesser amounts diminish but do not abolish steatorrhea.

The enzyme preparations are commonly given before each meal at the following doses: **Viokase,** eight tablets; **Cotazym,** six capsules; **Ilozyme,** four capsules; **Pancrease** MT16, three capsules; **Creon,** three capsules; **Entolase** H.P., three capsules; and **Zymase,** three capsules. If the patient has pancreatic pain, another one to two doses are given at bedtime. Although pancreatic enzyme preparations are free of serious side effects, patients ingesting large doses may complain of nausea, abdominal cramps, and perianal excoriation. The high content of nucleic acids contained in the enzyme preparations may result in hyperuricemia and kidney stones in some patients, especially in children. Allergy to pork protein may develop and cause adverse reactions.

Pancreatic lipase is irreversibly inactivated by a pH less than 4.0; therefore, it is important to maintain the gastric pH above 4.0 for at least 1 hour postprandially. Because different patients have different rates of gastric acid secretion, those who are achlorhydric or hypochlorhydric do well with the preceding dosages. However, in patients with normal gastric acid secretion, higher dosages of the enzymes or adjuvant acid-suppressant therapy or both may be necessary to keep the intragastric pH above 4.0 to deliver adequate active enzyme concentrations to the small bowel.

TABLE 46-1 Commercial Pancreatic Enzyme Preparations

Preparation	Type	Enzyme content (Units)		
		Lipase	Protease	Amylase
Pancrelipase				
Cotazym	C	8,000	30,000	30,000
Cotazym-S	ECMS	5,000	20,000	20,000
Festal II	ECT	6,000	20,000	30,000
Ku-Zyme HP	C	8,000	30,000	30,000
Pancrease	ECMS	4,000	25,000	25,000
Pancrease MT4	ECMT	4,000	12,000	12,000
Pancrease MT10	ECMT	10,000	30,000	30,000
Pancrease MT16	ECMT	16,000	48,000	48,000
Pancrease MT25	ECMT	25,000	75,000	75,000
Viokase	T	8,000	30,000	30,000
Zymase	ECS	12,000	24,000	24,000
Pancreatin				
Creon	ECMS	8,000	13,000	30,000
Creon 25	ECMS	25,000	62,500	74,700
Pancreatin 8×	T	22,500	180,000	180,000
Entozyme	T	600	7,500	7,500

C, capsule; T, tablet; ECT, enteric-coated tablet; ECS, enteric-coated sphere; ECMT, enteric-coated microtablet; ECMS, enteric-coated microsphere.

2. **Adjuvant acid-suppressant therapy** may be used to increase the gastric luminal pH and improve the survival of the exogenous enzymes during transit from the stomach.
   a. **Sodium bicarbonate** and **aluminum hydroxide** are the only antacids that are effective in reducing steatorrhea; they are administered before or at the beginning of the meal in a dosage that maintains intragastric pH above 4.0. This seems to be 16.6 g per 24 hours for sodium bicarbonate and 18.4 g per 24 hours for aluminum hydroxide gel. Other antacids, such as magnesium aluminum hydroxide or calcium carbonate, tend to increase steatorrhea.
      Sodium bicarbonate 650 mg before and after meals has been effective, especially with **Viokase.** If the patient is receiving a nighttime dose of the enzymes, the dose of sodium bicarbonate is increased to 1,300 mg at bedtime. Hypercalcemia and the milk–alkali syndrome have not occurred with this regimen. Enteric-coated enzyme preparations should not be used with sodium bicarbonate. They may release the contents of the microspheres in the stomach with the loss of enzyme activity if used concomitantly with sodium bicarbonate.
      Magnesium- and calcium-containing antacids effectively increase gastric pH but may aggravate steatorrhea by precipitating bile salts in the duodenum and forming calcium and magnesium soaps from the undigested free fatty acids, which increases intestinal secretion.
   b. **Gastric acid suppression with histamine-2 blockers or proton-pump inhibitors.** Adjuvant therapy with histamine-2 (H_2) blockers and proton pump inhibitors (PPIs) may be used. However, concurrent use of a pH-sensitive, delayed-release pancreatic enzyme preparation and an H_2 blocker or a PPI could result in premature release of the enzymes in the stomach.

c. **Enteric pH-coated pancreatic enzyme preparations** are effective if the intragastric pH remains at 4.0 to 5.0 and the duodenal pH above 6.0 to allow for dissolution of the coating and release of the active enzymes. These preparations have not been shown to be more advantageous than the other preparations. The newer preparations (e.g., Creon) with smaller microspheres may have better bioavailability in the duodenum.

Most patients with exocrine pancreatic insufficiency do quite well with adequate enzyme replacement. The dosage of the enzymes should be increased if symptoms are not alleviated.

C. **Nutritional support.** Patients with chronic pancreatitis tolerate small but frequent feedings that are high in protein better than large feedings. In debilitated patients, dietary supplements rich in protein should be used. If patients cannot tolerate enteral feedings, parenteral nutrition may be given.

Medium-chain triglycerides (MCTs) may be substituted for long-chain triglycerides to increase the total fat intake because MCTs are hydrolyzed much more rapidly by pancreatic lipase, and some are absorbed while still intact into the portal vein. MCT is sold as MCT oil for food preparation.

D. **Bacterial overgrowth.** As many as 25% of patients with chronic pancreatitis have concomitant bacterial overgrowth in the small intestine. These patients may need both pancreatic enzymes and antimicrobial therapy (e.g., tetracycline 500 mg p.o. three or four times daily; metronidazole 250–500 mg p.o. three times daily for 7–14 days; Xifaxan 400 mg p.o. daily for 10 days before diarrhea and steatorrhea can be effectively treated.

E. **Diabetes mellitus.** Patients who have diabetes mellitus with insulin deficiency as a result of chronic pancreatitis also have concomitant glucagon deficiency. Thus, these patients are very susceptible to hypoglycemia, and their insulin dosage needs to be closely monitored.

Selected Readings

Adler DG, et al. The role of endoscopy in patients with chronic pancreatitis. *Gastrointest Endosc.* 2006;63:933–937.

Cahen DL, et al. Endoscopic versus surgical drainage of the pancreatic duct in chronic pancreatitis. *N Engl J Med.* 2007;356:676–684.

Dragonuv P, et al. Idiopathic pancreatitis. *Gastroenterology.* 2005;128(3):756–763.

Dragonuv P, et al. A 54-year-old man with abdominal pain attributed to chronic pancreatitis. *Clin Gastroenterol Hepatol.* 2007;5(3):302–306.

Eleftheriadis N, et al. Long term outcome after pancreatic stenting in severe chronic pancreatitis. *Endoscopy.* 2005;37:223–230.

Elta GH. Is there a role for the endoscopic treatment of pain from chronic pancreatitis? *N Engl J Med.* 2007;356:727–729.

Etemad B, et al. Chronic pancreatitis: Diagnosis classification and new genetic developments. *Gastroenterology.* 2001;120:682–707.

Frey CF, et al. Comparison of local resection of the head of the pancreas combined with longitudinal pancreatic jejunostomy (Frey procedure) and duodenum-preserving resection of the pancreatic head (Berger procedure). *World J Surg.* 2003;27:1211–1230.

Gabrielli A, et al. Efficacy of main pancreatic duct endoscopic drainage in patients with chronic pancreatitis, continuos pain, and dilated duct. *Gastrointest Endosc.* 2005;61: 576–581.

Lankish MR, et al. The effect of small amounts of alcohol on the clinical course of chronic pancreatitis. *Mayo Clin Proc.* 2001;76:242–251.

Lowenfel AB, et al. Risk factors for cancer in hereditary pancreatitis study group. *Med Clin North Am.* 2000;84:565–593.

Morinville V, et al. Recurrent acute and chronic pancreatitis: Complex disorders with a genetic basis. *Gastroenterol Hepatol.* 2005;1(3):195–205.

Norton ID, et al. The role of transabdominal ultrasonography, helical computed tomography and magnetic resonance cholangiopancreatography in diagnosis and management of pancreatic disease. *Curr Gastroenterol Rep.* 2000;2:120.

Palanivelu C, et al. Laparoscopic lateral pancreatic jejunostomy: A new remedy for an old ailment. *Surg Endosc.* 2006;458–461.

Pickartz T, et al. Autoimmune pancreatitis. *Nat Clin Pract Gastroenterol Heptatol.* 2007;4(6):314–323.

Pitchumoni CS. Pathogenesis of alcohol-induced chronic pancreatitis: Facts, perceptions and misperceptions. *Surg Clin North Am.* 2001;81:379–389.

Ralmondo M. What is the role of EUS in screening for chronic pancreatitis? *Nat Clin Pract Gastroenterol Hepatol.* 2007;4(10)530–532.

Toskes PP. Alcohol consumption and chronic pancreatitis. *Mayo Clin Proc.* 2001;76:241.

Whitcom DC, et al. Mechanisms of disease: Advances in understanding the mechanisms leading to chronic pancreatitis. *Nat Clin Pract Gastroenterol Hepatol.* 2004;1(1):46–52.

PANCREATIC CANCER, AMPULLARY CANCER, CYSTIC TUMORS, AND NEUROENDOCRINE TUMORS OF THE PANCREAS

47

$\mathcal{E}$**xocrine pancreatic cancer** accounts for 95% of all the cancers that arise in the pancreas. Between 75% and 95% of exocrine pancreatic cancers arise from the ductular epithelium. Other cancers, such as acinar cell carcinoma, giant cell carcinoma, adenosquamous carcinoma, mucinous carcinoma, cystadenocarcinoma, papillary cystic tumor, mucinous ductal ectasia, intraductal papillary neoplasm, fibrosarcoma, leiomyosarcoma, and lymphoma are rare and account for less than 10% of the exocrine tumors.

Islet cell tumors of the pancreas make up approximately 5% of the carcinomas of the pancreas. These tumors often manifest themselves by the hormones they secrete. Tumors secreting gastrin, insulin, glucagon, vasoactive intestinal polypeptide (VIP), pancreatic polypeptide (PIP), neurotensin, and somatostatin may present as single tumors or as part of multiple neoplasm syndromes.

I. ADENOCARCINOMA OF THE PANCREAS

A. Epidemiology. The prevalence of adenocarcinoma of the pancreas is nine to ten per 100,000 persons in most Western countries. It is the fourth most common cause of death from carcinoma in males (after lung, colon, and prostate) and the fifth in females (after breast, colon, lung, and ovary). It can occur at any age but is most commonly seen in the sixth to eighth decades of life. It is more common in men than in women (1.3:1), in blacks than in whites (incidence 15.2/100,000 black men), and in Jews than in non-Jews.

There has been an increase in the incidence of pancreatic cancer in the last 30 years. Various substances have been implicated as possible etiologic factors. The risk of pancreatic cancer developing is increased 1.5 times in cigarette smokers. The risk increases as the number of cigarettes smoked increases, and the excess risk levels off 10 to 15 years after smoking cessation.

Diets rich in fat, red meat, or both have been implicated as risk factors. There seems to be a protective effect of diets rich in fruits and vegetables, carotenoids, and selenium. Other risk factors include history of peptic ulcer surgery (partial gastrectomy); cholecystectomy, possibly by increasing cholecystokinin (CCK) secretion; chronic pancreatitis (mostly hereditary and tropical types); hereditary nonpolyposis colorectal cancer; ataxia-telangiectasia; Peutz-Jeger syndrome; familial breast cancer; familial atypical multiple mole melanoma; and prolonged exposure to the gasoline derivatives 2-naphthylamine and benzidine and metal dusts. There is no conclusive evidence that drinking alcohol is related to the development of pancreatic cancer.

B. Pathophysiology. Adenocarcinoma of the pancreas forms a dense, fibrotic mass in the pancreas associated with a desmoplastic reaction. Seventy percent of the lesions are located in the head; the remainder is in the body and the tail of the gland or are multifocal or diffusely infiltrate the gland. By itself, the tumor may not cause symptoms. However, because the pancreas, which is a retroperitoneal organ without a mesentery, lies close to the porta hepatis, common bile duct, duodenum, stomach, and colon, the tumor mass may impinge on or penetrate into any of these structures and cause symptoms.

Pancreatic cancer metastasizes widely. It spreads locally by direct extension and to distant sites by lymphatic and vascular channels. It also invades nerves and nervous plexuses, especially in the celiac and mesenteric areas. The most common sites of extralymphatic metastasis are the liver, peritoneum, lungs, intestines, adrenals, kidneys, bones, and the diaphragm. Pancreatic tumors other than ductal adenocarcinomas (e.g., cystadenocarcinomas, islet cell tumors) often have a more indolent course. Tumors such as carcinomas of the breast, lung, thyroid, kidney, ovary, uterus, and prostate, and melanomas may metastasize to the pancreas and present as mass lesions in the organ.

C. Diagnosis

1. Clinical presentation

  a. History. The early symptoms of pancreatic cancer are vague and nonspecific. The most common symptoms are abdominal pain, back pain, weight loss, anorexia, nausea, jaundice, diarrhea, malabsorption, depression, and abdominal mass.

    i. An insidious weight loss with anorexia and nausea, accompanied by upper abdominal pain radiating to the back, is the most common presentation. Greater than 90% of the patients initially have jaundice. Common bile duct obstruction by a tumor in the head of the pancreas may result in jaundice while the mass is still small. Tumors located in the body and tail of the organ may result in jaundice in later stages either by extension or due to metastasis to the porta hepatis or the liver parenchyma.

    ii. Up to 70% of the patients may present with diabetes mellitus or **glucose intolerance**. The decreased or delayed insulin secretion is thought to arise from loss of B cells due to the desmoplastic reaction of the tumor.

    iii. Migratory thrombophlebitis (Trousseau's sign) may be a mode of presentation. However, this entity is not specific for pancreatic cancer. It may occur with other malignancies such as carcinomas of the stomach, colon, ovary, and lung.

    iv. A minority of the patients may also present with a picture of **acute pancreatitis, cholangitis, gastrointestinal bleeding, polyarthritis,** and **skin nodules** due to fat necrosis.

  b. The physical examination in most instances is not helpful. The major findings in a subpopulation of patients are jaundice, palpable gallbladder, epigastric mass, and nodular liver if metastases are present.

  c. Warning signs for early diagnosis. The initial symptoms of pancreatic cancer are usually ignored by the patient (patient delay) and the physician (physician delay). The mean duration of symptoms before diagnosis in most series is 3 to 4 months. Most of the tumors are unresectable and, therefore, the disease is fatal. The following warning signs may facilitate an early diagnosis of this malignancy:

    i. Recent upper abdominal or back pain consistent with retroperitoneal lesion.

    ii. Recent upper abdominal pain or discomfort with negative gastrointestinal investigations.

    iii. Jaundice with or without pruritus.

    iv. Weight loss greater than 5% of normal body weight.

    v. Unexplained acute pancreatitis.

    vi. Unexplained onset of diabetes mellitus.

  d. Differential diagnosis. A variety of malignant and benign disorders of other organs may present with features similar to pancreatic cancer. Also, it is important to remember that pancreatic cancer may coexist in a patient with a common benign disorder such as gallstones or peptic or diverticular disease, and normal contrast studies of the gastrointestinal tract, serum chemistries, and hemogram do not rule out the presence of pancreatic cancer, especially if the tumor is small.

2. Diagnostic studies

  a. Laboratory tests. There are no specific laboratory tests for the early detection of pancreatic cancer. If there is involvement of the liver or the biliary tract, this will be reflected in the serum chemistries. The serum amylase and lipase in most instances are normal. A subgroup of patients has elevated blood glucose levels.

b. Tumor markers. Various serologic tumor markers including tumor associated antigens, enzymes, and hormones have been investigated for early detection of pancreatic cancer. These are carcinoembryonic antigen (CEA), CA 19-9, alpha-fetoprotein, pancreatic oncofetal antigens, pancreatic ribonuclease, and galactosyl transferase isoenzyme II. The sensitivity and specificity of these assays have not been adequate for early diagnosis of this disease.

The most extensively studied serum marker is CA 19-9, which is used widely. It is not specific for pancreatic cancer, however, because it also can be elevated in other gastrointestinal tumors such as those in the bile ducts and colon. Because levels of CA 19-9 are frequently normal in the early stages of pancreatic cancer, the test is not reliable for use in screening. The presence of high levels may help differentiate between benign diseases of the pancreas and pancreatic cancer. When the pancreatic cancer is completely resected, the CA 19-9 levels fall, suggesting that it is a useful marker for follow-up surveillance.

The ratio of testosterone to dihydrotestosterone is below 5 (normal is 10) in more than 70% of men with pancreatic cancer, presumably because of increased conversion of testosterone by the pancreatic tumor. This ratio may be more sensitive than CA 19-9 in detecting smaller pancreatic cancers and more specific than the other markers.

c. Ultrasound and computed tomography. Ultrasonography usually is the first examination for suspected pancreatic cancer. Computed tomography (CT) with intravenous (IV) contrast is used when satisfactory imaging is not obtained with ultrasound (US). These two techniques are by far the most sensitive and specific for pancreatic disease. They both demonstrate enlargement of the gland, alteration in contour or consistency of the gland, the presence of masses, and biliary or pancreatic duct dilatation. CT scans may also delineate peripancreatic nodal enlargement as well as invasion of other organs and vessels. Metastasis to the liver and porta hepatis may be detected.

US and CT are complementary in imaging the pancreas. The lesions in the head of the pancreas are seen well by US, whereas those in the body and tail are detected better by CT scan. However, small lesions, especially in the body or tail, may be missed by both techniques. **Helical thin section CT scan with IV contrast and CT angiography (CTA)** increase the diagnostic yield.

d. Magnetic resonance imaging, contrast-enhanced magnetic resonance imaging (MRI) using IV gadolinium–DPTA is useful for detecting small pancreatic tumors. Ductal size is evaluated by **magnetic resonance cholangiopancreatography (MRCP). MR arteriography (MRA)** has obviated the need for angiography and improves the examination of the pancreas for tumor. Fat-saturation MRI is especially valuable in looking for suspected tumors in a pancreas that is not enlarged.

e. Endoscopic retrograde cholangiopancreatography (ERCP). The diagnosis of pancreatic cancer by ERCP depends on radiographic demonstration of pancreatic duct stenosis or obstruction caused by the tumor. An accompanying cholangiogram may further delineate abnormalities along the course of the common bile duct. It can also visualize and differentiate ampullary and duodenal carcinomas. In experienced hands, it has greater than 90% sensitivity and specificity in providing a definitive diagnosis of pancreatic cancer.

In addition, biopsies of periampullary tissue and cytologic examination of aspirated pancreatic juice may increase the diagnostic yield further. ERCP is usually performed if an abnormality is noted on the US or CT scan or if an abnormality is suspected but cannot be demonstrated by these methods.

In addition to diagnosis, ERCP may be used to place stents in the obstructed biliary and pancreatic ducts to relieve obstruction and palliate patients with unresectable tumors.

f. Endoscopic ultrasonography (EUS). The pancreas may be visualized clearly with this method from the lumina of the duodenum, antrum, and gastric fundus to localize pancreatic cancers that are too small to be seen by CT or transabdominal US. Associated lymph nodes and vascular involvement are accurately demonstrated. The sensitivity of EUS compares favorably with that of CT and angiography. Staging of pancreatic cancer with EUS may become routine before selection of therapy. EUS guided fine-needle aspiration allows cytologic evaluation.

g. Angiography. Celiac and superior mesenteric angiography with selective cannulation of the pancreatic vessels may provide a sensitive diagnostic tool. However, this invasive technique is best used to determine resectability of the tumor before surgery. Arterial encasement, venous occlusion, and tumor vascularity can be visualized, and angiography may save the patient an unnecessary abdominal exploration. If a tumor is resectable, the arterial blood supply and anatomic variations of the foregut vasculature can be delineated by angiography to help in the planning of surgery.

h. Cytologic diagnosis. Direct percutaneous fine-needle aspiration can be performed with US, CT, EUS, or angiographic guidance. The aspirated material is used for cytologic examination. This technique may provide the tissue diagnosis and allow differentiation of lymphoma or endocrine tumors from adenocarcinoma without surgery; it is especially useful in elderly patients in whom the morbidity and mortality of laparotomy are high.

The drawbacks of this procedure are that a negative result cannot exclude the presence of a malignant tumor, especially if the tumor is small, and that tumor seeding may occur along the needle tract with possible peritoneal spread of the tumor.

i. Percutaneous transhepatic cholangiogram. In patients with obstructive jaundice with dilated bile ducts, percutaneous transhepatic cholangiogram (PTC) may visualize the common bile duct and the site of its obstruction. A drainage catheter may then be introduced percutaneously for biliary decompression.

j. Laparoscopy. The most common sites of distant metastasis from pancreatic cancer are the liver, the peritoneum, and the omentum. These lesions, which may be too small to be detected by CT, may be directly visualized by laparoscopy. Because the presence of these metastases contraindicates surgery, laparoscopy may help increase the accuracy of staging.

D. Treatment. To decide on the appropriate mode of treatment for pancreatic cancer, a staging system has been devised.

Stage I: confined to pancreas alone.
Stage II: involving only neighboring structures.
Stage III: involving regional lymph nodes.
Stage IV: including liver and other distant spread.

Regardless of the mode of therapy chosen, all patients need to receive intensive supportive and nutritional therapy, either enteral or parenteral, as indicated. The importance of emotional support in this disease, both to the patients and their families, cannot be overstated. Optimal therapy requires a multidisciplinary approach by a team that includes a medical oncologist, an interventional radiologist, a gastroenterologist, a radiotherapist, an internist and a pain management specialist.

1. Surgery

a. Definitive surgery. In a large series of patients with pancreatic cancer, only 5% to 22% had a resectable tumor at the time of diagnosis. The standard operation for pancreatic cancer is **pancreaticoduodenectomy** (the Whipple's operation) or a modification of this procedure. The Whipple's operation consists of en bloc removal of the duodenum, a variable portion of the distal stomach, and the jejunum, gallbladder, common bile duct, and regional lymph nodes, followed by pancreaticojejunostomy and gastrojejunostomy. Vagotomy should be performed if more than 60% of the stomach is removed. **Total pancreatectomy** does not offer better results; however, it produces exocrine insufficiency and brittle diabetes, which is difficult to manage. In the United States, a less extensive operation that preserves the pylorus and avoids postgastrectomy symptoms is being used with no apparent compromise of long-term survival. In most of these patients, the cancer is at the head of the pancreas.

The 5-year survival of patients who undergo pancreatic resection is 17% to 24% in large centers. There may be a better prognosis for some subgroups of patients such as those with smaller tumors (<2 cm in diameter), patients without lymph node metastases or major vessel involvement, and those with no residual tumor. In such patients, the 5-year survival may be as high as 57%. The mortality of pancreaticoduodenectomy is less than 5% in many centers, and there are fewer complications than previously due to both technologic and procedural advances.

b. Palliative surgery

   i. Biliary obstruction. In patients with **unresectable tumors of the head of the pancreas with biliary obstruction,** a bypass procedure may be performed to decompress the biliary tract. The choice of operation depends on the location of the obstruction: A cholecystojejunostomy, choledochojejunostomy, or hepatojejunostomy may be done. Because approximately one third of the patients with ductal adenocarcinoma of the head of the pancreas eventually have duodenal obstruction, a gastrojejunostomy may be performed at the same time to spare the patient a second laparotomy.

   Mean postoperative mortality after biliary bypass is about 20% with an average survival of 5.4 months. In debilitated patients, a percutaneous or endoscopically placed biliary stent may decompress the biliary tract and reduce the morbidity and the length of hospitalization. The success rate of stents is more than 85% with less than 1% to 2% mortality. Patients treated with stents may have more frequent hospital admissions for stent occlusion, recurrent jaundice, and infection. However, the new, expandable metal stents seem to avoid these complications. Duodenal obstruction can be treated only by surgery.

   ii. Cancer of the body or tail of the pancreas is invariably diagnosed at a late stage. It is very important, however, to rule out endocrine cancer in these instances by tissue diagnosis because endocrine tumors are much more amenable to treatment and have a much better prognosis. See Section IV.

   iii. Abdominal and back pain. Most patients with pancreatic cancer complain of debilitating abdominal or back pain. The injection of phenol or absolute alcohol around the celiac plexus for the relief of pain is helpful in some patients. This procedure can be done operatively during laparotomy or percutaneously. Narcotics and radiotherapy may also be used.

2. Chemotherapy. Most patients with stages I and II and some with stage III disease who are reasonable surgical candidates should be treated surgically. However, some patients with stages III and IV disease have been treated with single- or multiple-agent chemotherapy with variable results. The drugs used are 5-fluorouracil (5-FU), mitomycin, carmustine (BCNU), lomustine (CCNU), methyl CCNU, streptozotocin, and Gematabine (Gemzar). Response rates have been 20% to 40% in small series. Combination chemotherapeutic regimens are also being tested. Additional controlled studies are needed in this area before chemotherapy can become an established treatment of this disease.

3. **Radiation therapy** alone has not been unequivocally successful in the treatment of nonresectable localized cancer of the pancreas. However, the combination of radiation therapy (4,000–6,000 rad) with chemotherapy (using 5-FU) has been found to result in enhanced radiation therapeutic efficiency. In one study, the survival was increased from 5.5 months to 11 months. Newer radiation techniques using iodine 125 directly implanted into the tumor tissue and neutron beam radiation show promise in the treatment of unresectable cancer of the pancreas.
4. **Intraoperative radiation therapy** offers the possibility of delivering higher doses of radiation to the pancreatic cancer with less risk of injury to the adjacent organs. In most centers, a single dose of 20 Gy is delivered to the surgically exposed cancer by an electron beam through a field-limiting cone. Median survivals of 13 to 16 months have been reported with excellent local control. Five percent of patients have lived 3 to 8 years. Relief of pain has been achieved in 50% to 90% of these patients. Unfortunately, in 30% of these patients unavoidable irradiation of the duodenum may result in bleeding, obstruction, and perforation. In most patients, therefore, protective gastrojejunostomy is performed at the same time as the intraoperative radiation.

II. **AMPULLARY CARCINOMA.** Ninety percent of ampullary or periampullary tumors are adenocarcinomas of pancreatic ductal origin and arise as a periampullary mass from the area of interface of the pancreaticobiliary ductal system, the ampulla of Vater, the pancreas, and the duodenum. They are considered separately from pancreatic cancer because of better resectability and prognosis.
   A. **Clinical presentation.** Most patients are elderly, in the sixth or seventh decade of life, and present with anorexia, weight loss, malaise, abdominal pain, and progressive jaundice (obstructive.) Iron deficiency anemia and cholangitis may be present. Recurrent acute pancreatitis of no identifiable etiology may be the presentation in some patients.
   B. **Diagnosis** of ampullary carcinoma is facilitated by UGI endoscopy and biopsy of tumor for histologic examination and EUS. For staging of tumor depth of invasion and presence of nodal spread, utilize IV contrast enhanced CT and MRI of the abdomen, MRCP, and ECRP.
   C. **Treatment.** Tumors confined to the ampulla that do not invade the muscularis propria on EUS may be resected endoscopically or preferably by surgical approach. Pancreaticoduodenectomy is the most effective and definitive treatment for periampullary carcinoma. Small tumors with metastases have a good prognosis.

III. **Cystic tumors of the pancreas** are a heterogeneous group of pancreatic neoplasms that include mucinous cystic neoplasms (50%), serous cystadenomas (30%), intraductal papillary mucinous neoplasms (12%), papillary cystic tumors (3%), and other tumors (5%).
   A. **Mucinous cystadenomas** are cystic lesions more commonly seen in the body and tail of the pancreas and occur more commonly in women. They are often asymptomatic and may be found during an abdominal US or CT examination. If there is a mass in the wall of the cystic lesion, CT or EUS guided fine-needle aspiration may be necessary for a diagnosis of **cystadenocarcinoma.** The aspirated fluid is usually viscous. Elevated levels of carcinoembryonic antigen (CEA) in the cyst fluid indicate malignancy. Surgical resection is indicated for malignant lesions.
   B. **Serous cystadenomas** may occur in any part of the pancreas. They are well-circumscribed, solitary, cystic lesions. On EUS or CT guided fine-needle aspiration the fluid has low viscosity and low levels of amylase and CEA. Elevated CEA indicates malignancy. In some cases, CT shows a cystic lesion, especially in the head and neck of the pancreas, that has a honeycomb appearance with an area of central fibrosis and calcification (stellate, or star shaped). Small serous cystadenomas may be monitored; larger ones and those which are malignant should be resected.

C. **Mucinous ductal ectasia** or **intraductal papillary mucinous neoplasm (IPMN)** or **ductal ectasia** or **ductal ectatic mucinous cystadenoma** is frequently seen in the head of the pancreas. It often causes dilatation and filling of the main pancreatic duct or its side branches with thick viscous mucus. When the tumor is localized to a branch of the duct, then it may resemble a cluster of grapes. On ERCP, the dramatic picture is of a patulous ampulla of Vater with extruding mucus. Some patients are asymptomatic, but others may complain of abdominal pain and others may have a long history of recurrent acute pancreatitis associated with steatorrhea and glucose intolerance. The appropriate treatment is surgical resection to relieve symptoms and to prevent invasive carcinoma.

D. **Papillary cystic neoplasm (solid and cystic tumor)** or **solid and papillary neoplasm of the pancreas** is a rare tumor mostly seen in young women. Palpable abdominal mass may be present. It may be asymptomatic or may cause abdominal pain. In symptomatic cases surgery may be indicated.

IV. **PANCREATIC ENDOCRINE TUMORS.** Pancreatic endocrine tumors are relatively rare. The incidence in the United States is less than 1 per 100,000 persons. These tumors may arise sporadically in persons with **multiple endocrine neoplasia type I (MEN I)**. MEN I is an autosomal dominant syndrome associated with mutations in the MEN I tumor suppressor gene. It is characterized by multiple neuroendocrine tumors involving the parathyroid, pituitary gland, and pancreas, especially with gastrinomas and insulinomas. In rare cases, pancreatic endocrine tumors may be associated with Von Hippel–Lindau disease.

A. **Clinical presentation.** The clinical presentation of pancreatic endocrine tumors is related to the symptoms of the specific hormonal hypersecretion. The best characterization of these syndromes are those associated with insulinoma, glucagonoma, gastrinoma, VIPoma, somatostatinoma and PPOma, the nonfunctioning pancreatic neuroendocrine tumors associated with high serum levels of pancreatic polypeptide.

1. **Insulinomas** have an incidence of 1 to 4 cases per 1 million persons per year. Ten percent of these patients also have MEN I. The predominant symptoms are due to hypoglycemia (blood sugar levels <50 mg/dL) with inappropriately high insulin levels. Patients may present with intermittent confusion, sweating, nausea, vomiting, weakness, and even loss of consciousness. In most cases, the tumors are diagnosed before they become >2.5 cm and before they metastasize.

   The diagnosis is confirmed by the detection of elevated fasting serum insulin, C-peptide levels, and the tolbutamide test. Endoscopic ultrasound (EUS) is the preferred imaging modality for the detection of the tumor. Intraoperative ultrasound is used to locate the tumor.

   The initial management is dietary modification and administration of diazoxide. For isolated tumors, the tumors are enucleated surgically. In patients with MEN I, a subtotal pancreatectomy may be undertaken due to the risk of multiple tumors and a higher rate of recurrence.

2. **Glucagonomas** are among the rarest of the pancreatic endocrine tumors. Eighty percent are sporadic and 20% are associated with MEN I. The age of occurrence is the seventh decade of life. Glucagonomas may be associated with diabetes mellitus. Most of the patients present with **necrolytic migratory erythema** characterized by raised erythematous patches beginning in the perineum and then involving the trunk and extremities. Plasma glucagon levels exceed 1,000 picograms per milliliter (pg/mL).

   Tumors are usually visible on CT scan and most patients present with metastases. Initial treatment involves use of somatostatin analogs. Those that are refractory may be treated with intravenous infusion of amino acids. Surgery may be curative with isolated tumors or palliative.

3. **Gastrinomas and Zollinger–Ellison syndrome (ZES)** is characterized by **elevated gastrin levels and gastric acid hypersecretion** resulting in peptic

ulcer disease (PUD), GERD, diarrhea, and abdominal pain. A positive secretin test (see Chapter 24) may be necessary to confirm the diagnosis. The majority of gastrinomas are found in the **"gastrinoma triangle"** which is an area bounded by the cystic and the common bile ducts, the duodenum, the surrounding lymph nodes, or in the pancreas. EUS and somatostatin scintigraphy may help in the localization of the tumor(s) preoperatively; however, intraoperative palpation and duodenectomy is usually necessary. Proton pump inhibitors are highly effective in controlling the symptoms of associated gastric acid hypersecretion.

4. **VIPomas** present with the Verner–Morrison syndrome or pancreatic cholera characterized by profound diarrhea, hypokalemia, and achlorhydria. The syndrome is due to the ectopic secretion of vasoactive intestinal peptide (VIP). VIP causes enterocyte intercellular elevation of cyclic AMP, resulting in intestinal smooth muscle relaxation, inhibition of electrolyte absorption, and profound secretory diarrhea.

   VIPomas often present in fifth decade of life. The diagnosis is based on the presence of elevated serum VIP levels. Most tumors are visualized with CT scan or MRI, EUS, or somatostatin scintigraphy. Surgical resection is used for localized disease to reduce tumor burden in patients with metastases. Somatostatin analogs are effective in suppressing VIP secretion and controlling the secretory diarrhea.

5. **Somatostatinomas and PPOmas** may be associated with diabetes mellitus, hypochloridemia, and diarrhea. **PPOmas** are associated with high serum levels of PP. Although high levels of PP do not cause symptoms, the tumors cause symptoms from tumor bulk. Most patients have metastatic disease at the time of diagnosis; however, surgical resection is curative in patients in the early stage of the disease.

Selected Readings

Alberts SR, et al. Treatment options for hepatobiliary and pancreatic cancer. Symposium of solid tumors. *Mayo Clin Proc.* 2007;82(5)628–637.

Arvanitakis M, et al. Predictive factors for pancreatic cancer in patients with chronic pancreatitis in association with K-RSA gene mutation. *Endoscopy.* 2004;36(6): 535–542.

Brugge WR, et al. Cystic neoplasms of the pancreas. *N Engl J Med.* 2004;351:1218–1226.

Brugge WR, et al. Diagnosis of pancreatic cystic neoplasms: A report of the cooperative pancreatic cyst study. *Gastroenterology.* 2004;126:1330–1336.

Dewitt J, et al. Comparison of endoscopic ultrasound and computed tomography for the preoperative evaluation of pancreatic cancer: a systematic review. *Clin Gastroenterol Hepatol.* 2006;4:717–725.

Farnell MB, et al. Pancreas cancer working group. A prospective randomized trial comparing standard pancreatoduoderectomy with extended lymph aderectomy in resectable pancreatic head adenocarcinoma. *Surgery.* 2005;138:618–628.

Giovannini M, et al. Endoscopic ultrasound-guided cystogastrostomy. *Endoscopy.* 2003;35:239–245.

Handrich SJ, et al. The natural history of the incidentally discovered small simple pancreatic cyst: Long-term follow-up and clinical implications. *Am J Roentgenol.* 2005;184:20–23.

Kalady MF, et al. Pancreatic duct strictures: Identifying risks of malignancy. *Ann Surg Oncol.* 2004;11(6):555–557.

Kim JE, Lee KT, et al. Clinical usefulness of carbohydrate antigen 19-9 as a screening test for pancreatic cancer in an asymptomatic population. *J Gastroenterol Hepatol.* 2004;19:182–186.

Li D, et al. Pancreatic cancer. *Lancet.* 2004;363:1049–1057.

Maire, F, et al. Differential diagnosis between chronic pancreatitis and pancreatic cancer: Value of the detection of KRAS II mutations in circulating DNA. *Br J Cancer.* 2002; 87(5):551–554.

Maire F, et al. Intraductal papillary mucinous tumors of the pancreas: The perioperative value of cytologic and histopathologic diagnosis. *Gastrointest Endosc.* 2003;58: 701–706.

Norton ID, et al. The role of transabdominal ultrasonography, helical computed tomography and magnetic resonance cholangiopancreatography in diagnosis and management of pancreatic disease. *Curr Gastroenterol Rep.* 2000;2:120.

Somagyi L, et al. Diagnosis and staging of islet tumors of the pancreas. *Curr Gastroenterol Rep.* 2001;2:159.

JAUNDICE AND INTERPRETATION OF LABORATORY LIVER TESTS

48

*L*aboratory tests have an important role in the recognition of liver disease and determination of the nature and extent of the liver dysfunction. There is no one specific test for assessment of liver disease. However, the combination of a number of tests that assess different parameters of liver physiology obtained serially over time and interpreted within the clinical context may serve in establishing the diagnosis and prognosis and help in following the course of the hepatic dysfunction. The most useful laboratory tests in liver disease may be grouped into **three categories.** These are tests that reflect **(a) liver cell injury and necrosis, (b) synthetic function of the liver, and (c) cholestasis** from intra- or extrahepatic biliary obstruction or infiltrative processes in the liver, or both.

I. SERUM ENZYMES AS MARKERS OF HEPATOCELLULAR INJURY AND NECROSIS

A. Serum transaminases. The transaminases, or aminotransferases, are a group of enzymes that catalyze the transfer of an amino group from amino acid to ketoacid. The two transaminases whose activities are measured most frequently in the assessment of liver disease are **serum glutamic-oxaloacetic transaminase (SGOT), or aspartate aminotransferase (AST), and serum glutamic-pyruvic transaminase (SGPT), or alanine aminotransferase (ALT).** Both ALT and AST require pyridoxal-5′-phosphate as cofactor. They are found in the liver, skeletal, and cardiac muscle, kidney, brain, pancreas, lung, leukocytes, and erythrocytes. High concentrations of ALT are found only in the liver.

Both of these enzymes are normally present in the serum. Normal values are less than 40 U/L. When tissues rich in transaminases are damaged or destroyed, the enzymes are released into the circulation. The increment in the serum activities reflects the relative rates at which the enzymes enter and leave the circulation.

Serum transaminases are sensitive indicators of liver cell damage. SGPT, or ALT, is a cytosolic enzyme, whereas SGOT, or AST, is both cytosolic and microsomal. The serum activity of these enzymes is increased in any form of liver cell injury, including viral-, drug-, or toxin-induced hepatitis; metastatic carcinoma; heart failure; and granulomatous and alcoholic liver disease. Rebounds of transaminase values or persistent elevations usually indicate recrudescences of hepatic inflammation and necrosis. Therefore, their serial determination reflects the clinical activity of the liver disease.

In the jaundiced patient, values greater than 300 to 400 U/L usually indicate acute hepatocellular disease. Extrahepatic obstruction usually does not cause as high a rise in serum transaminases. Values less than 300 U/L in a jaundiced patient are nondiagnostic and can occur with acute and chronic hepatocellular diseases as well as with obstructive jaundice. The largest elevation, in excess of 1,000 U/L, is observed in viral hepatitis, in acute toxic or drug-induced liver injury, in prolonged hypotension, and in acute common bile duct (CBD) obstruction.

The SGOT/SGPT ratio is most useful in detecting patients with alcohol-related liver disease. In these individuals, the SGOT/SGPT ratio is usually greater than 2, due to the decreased concentration of SGPT in the hepatocyte cytosol and serum of alcoholic patients. Patients with alcoholic liver disease are deficient in pyridoxal-5′-phosphate, a coenzyme necessary for the synthesis of aminotransferases in the liver, particularly ALT.

The degree of elevation of the serum transaminase activity has a low prognostic value. Rapid recovery may occur in cases of toxic hepatitis, in shock-related liver cell injury, or with relief of acute CBD obstruction, even with values greater than 3,000 U/L. In contrast, in most patients with cirrhosis and in those with terminal liver failure, values may be near normal.

Transaminase elevations are not specific for liver disease; they may also be elevated in patients with cardiac and skeletal muscle damage as well as after strenuous exercise such as jogging, running, and working out. The extent of enzyme elevation with muscle disease is usually less than 300 U/L except in acute rhabdomyolysis. However, with severe muscle injury, other enzymes such as aldolase and creatine phosphokinase (CPK) are also elevated.

Uremia may depress aminotransferase levels. This effect is reversible after dialysis, suggesting that a dialyzable inhibitor of the aminotransferase reaction is in the serum of uremic patients.

Lactic dehydrogenase (LDH) is a cytoplasmic enzyme found in most normal and malignant tissues. Of the five isoenzymes of LDH (1–5), the electrophoretically slowest one (LDH-5) corresponds to the liver. LDH is much less sensitive than the aminotransferases in measuring liver cell injury, even when isoenzyme analysis is used. It is most sensitive in revealing myocardial infarction and hemolysis.

II. TESTS OF BIOSYNTHETIC FUNCTION

A. Serum proteins. The liver is the major source of most of the serum proteins. Albumin, fibrinogens and other coagulation factors, plasminogen, transferrin, ceruloplasmin, haptoglobin, and β-globulins are all synthesized by the parenchymal cells of the liver. γ-globulins, on the other hand, are not synthesized in the liver but by lymphocytes and plasma cells.

Serum proteins are determined in the laboratory using several techniques. The most useful ones are the fractional salting-out techniques and paper electrophoresis. Salting-out methods, which are used in most chemistry profiles (e.g., SMA-12), separate and quantitate albumin and globulins, whereas electrophoretic techniques separate and give values for albumin, α_1-, α_2-, β-, and γ-globulins. Higher values for albumin are usually obtained by the salting-out method. Electrophoretic methods permit a more detailed fractionation of serum proteins by their migration due to their net charge in an electric field (Fig. 48-1).

In most forms of liver disease, there is a decrease in the concentration of serum albumin and other serum proteins synthesized in the liver and a rise in globulins. The magnitude of the serum protein alterations depends on the severity, extent, and duration of the liver disease. Albumin has a relatively long half-life (t1/2 = 17 + days). Thus its level may not change in acute disease. The rise in globulins, mainly

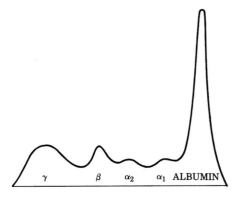

Figure 48-1. Electrophoretic pattern of normal serum.

γ-globulins, in liver disease is due to a decrease in the antigen-filtering function of the diseased liver. A serum albumin value of less than 3 g/dL (normal range, 3.5–5.0 g/dL) and serum globulins greater than 4 g/dL (normal range, 2.0–3.5 g/dL) usually suggest chronic or progressive liver disease. Hypoalbuminemia and hyperglobulinemia are characteristically noted in cirrhosis and tend to be more marked than in acute hepatic diseases. A normal albumin level with a polyclonal hypergammaglobulinemia may be seen in well-compensated cirrhosis.

Deficiency or absence of serum α_1-globulins may be seen in patients with a form of liver disease associated with the accumulation of α_1-antitrypsin in hepatocytes.

Information obtained from protein fractionation suggests the extent of hepatocellular damage and has prognostic significance. In a patient with cirrhosis, an increase in the albumin value of 2 to 3 g/dL toward normal with treatment implies an improvement in the hepatic function and a more favorable prognosis than if there were no rise despite therapy.

Protein determination has limited clinical value for several reasons. It is not a very sensitive indicator of liver disease; thus, it has limited value for differential diagnosis, and abnormal values may be seen in other, nonhepatic disorders.

B. Prothrombin time (PT). The liver synthesizes all the clotting factors except factor VIII. It is also involved in the clearance of the clotting factors and dissolution of the formed clot. The serum activities of several clotting factors are useful indicators of hepatic synthetic function.

The one-stage PT, which reflects the activities of prothrombin, fibrinogen, and factors V, VII, and X, is dependent on both hepatic synthesis of these factors and availability of vitamin K. Prolongation of PT (normal range, 11.5–12.5 seconds) by 2 seconds or more is considered abnormal.

A prolonged PT is not specific for liver disease. It may be present in congenital deficiencies of coagulation factors, in states of consumption of coagulation factors, and with ingestion of drugs that affect the coagulation cascade. PT is also prolonged in patients with hypovitaminosis K due to obstructive jaundice, steatorrhea, prolonged dietary deficiency, or intake of antibiotics that alter the bowel flora as well as due to poor utilization of vitamin K in parenchymal liver disease. Parenteral injection of vitamin K (10 mg subcutaneously) normalizes the PT in 24 hours in most patients, except those with parenchymal liver disease.

Although PT is not a very sensitive index of liver disease, it has a high prognostic value, especially in acute hepatocellular disease. Prolongation of PT more than 5 to 6 seconds heralds the onset of fulminant hepatic necrosis. In alcoholic liver disease as well as other chronic hepatocellular diseases, prolongation of PT by more than 4 to 5 seconds that does not respond to parenteral vitamin K therapy indicates poor long-term prognosis.

III. TESTS OF CHOLESTASIS

A. Enzymes

1. Serum alkaline phosphatase. Alkaline phosphatases are enzymes that catalyze hydrolysis of organic phosphate esters at an alkaline pH. These enzymes are found in many tissues. The serum enzyme is principally derived from three sources: (a) the hepatobiliary system: the bile canalicular surface of the hepatocytes and biliary epithelium; (b) bone: the osteoblasts; and (c) the intestinal tract: the brush border of the intestinal mucosal cells (10% of the total serum enzyme). The enzyme has a half-life of about 7 days in the body.

The alkaline phosphatase activity in individuals 18 to 60 years of age is higher in men than in women. After 60 years of age, the level increases in both genders and may be higher in women than men. It is much higher in children than in adults and corresponds to bone growth and osteoblastic activity. In pregnancy, placental phosphatase may cause doubling of serum alkaline phosphatase, especially in the third trimester.

In a patient with elevated alkaline phosphatase, the hepatobiliary system, bone, and occasionally the small intestine and kidney may be the source of the increased enzyme activity. To determine the source of the elevated enzyme, several approaches may be used. Polyacrylamide gel electrophoretic separation of isoenzymes is the most accurate. The heat susceptibility of the enzyme from different sources seems to be different. The heat stability at 56°C for 15 minutes decreases in the following order: the placenta, liver, and bone. Unfortunately, there is overlap, and results are difficult to interpret and not diagnostically useful.

The preferred approach to differentiate hepatobiliary enzyme from others is to measure the serum activity of another, similar enzyme elevated in liver dysfunction, such as 5'-nucleotidase, γ-glutamyltranspeptidase, or leucine aminopeptidase. However, lack of elevation of these enzymes in the setting of elevated alkaline phosphatase does not rule out liver disease because these enzymes do not necessarily rise in parallel with alkaline phosphatase.

Hepatobiliary alkaline phosphatase synthesis and leakage into the circulation seem to be mediated by bile acids. In intra- and extrahepatic biliary obstruction, alkaline phosphatase is elevated before jaundice develops. Values may be 3 to 10 times normal with a minimal rise in the transaminases. In hepatocellular diseases that primarily affect the liver parenchyma (cirrhosis, hepatitis), the alkaline phosphatase may not rise or may rise minimally with a concomitant large rise in transaminases.

Serum alkaline phosphatase elevation (2–10 times normal) is also helpful in the early diagnosis of infiltrative diseases of the liver, including granulomatous involvement with tuberculosis, sarcoidosis, fungal infection, tumors (primary or metastatic), and abscesses.

In summary, the major value of the serum alkaline phosphatase measurement is in differentiation of hepatocellular liver disease from obstructive liver diseases such as bile duct obstruction with stones, tumors, strictures, or granulomas within or outside the liver parenchyma (Table 48-1).

2. **5'-Nucleotidase.** This enzyme is another phosphatase found in many tissues but primarily located in the liver in the canaliculi and sinusoidal membranes. Serum values are elevated (normal range, 0.3–3.2 Bodansky units) in hepatobiliary diseases with a spectrum of abnormality similar to that found for alkaline phosphatase. It is specific for the liver and is not influenced by gender or race, but values increase with age, reaching a plateau after age 50. It does not rise in bone disease or in pregnancy. Serum 5'-nucleotidase may be particularly helpful in the diagnosis of liver disease in childhood and in pregnancy.

5'-Nucleotidase and alkaline phosphatase are both valuable in the diagnosis of biliary obstruction and hepatic infiltrative or space-occupying lesions. Even though the correlation between the two enzymes is high, the values may not rise

---

TABLE 48-1   Causes of an Isolated Alkaline Phosphatase Elevation

Primary or metastatic tumor of liver or bone
Granulomatous liver disease
Hodgkin's disease
Non-Hodgkin's lymphoma
Inflammatory bowel disease
Primary biliary cirrhosis
Hepatic abscess and intraabdominal infections
Congestive heart failure
Hyperthyroidism
Diabetes
Any bone disease with rapid turnover
Partial extrahepatic bile duct obstruction
Sclerosing cholangitis

proportionately in individual patients, and rarely 5′-nucleotidase may be normal in the presence of elevated hepatic alkaline phosphatase. Like alkaline phosphatase (AP), 5′-nucleotidase may be used to screen for liver metastases and to follow their evolution. In screening for liver metastases, it seems to have a higher predictive value and lower rate of false-positives than γ-glutamyl transpeptidase, alkaline phosphatase, or a combination of the three.

3. **Leucine aminopeptidase.** This protease has been demonstrated in all human tissues but especially in the liver in the biliary epithelium. It is not elevated in bone disease, and the values are similar in both adults and children. In pregnancy, however, the values rise progressively, reaching a peak at term.

   Serum leucine aminopeptidase is at least as sensitive as alkaline phosphatase and 5′-nucleotidase in the diagnosis of biliary obstructive, space-occupying, and infiltrative diseases of the liver. There is controversy regarding its specificity for these disorders versus hepatic parenchymal disease. However, values greater than 450 U/L are rarely seen in patients with hepatocellular disease such as cirrhosis or hepatitis.

4. **γ-Glutamyl transpeptidase (GGT).** This enzyme is particularly found in the liver, pancreas, and kidney. Values are comparable in both genders after age 4. Serum activity does not rise due to pregnancy or bone diseases.

   Elevated values are found in diseases of the liver, biliary tract, and pancreas. The degree of elevation of serum GGT is comparable in various liver diseases; thus, it has limited value in the differential diagnosis of jaundice. GGT values are elevated in individuals who have alcoholic liver disease or who ingest large quantities of alcohol and use barbiturates or phenytoin. A GGT/AP value greater than 2.5 is highly suggestive of alcohol abuse. Its serum values are diminished by female sex hormones, including those in birth control pills.

B. **Serum bilirubin reflects the capacity of the liver to transport organic anions and to metabolize drugs.** The **formation of bilirubin** from heme is essential for mammalian life because it provides the body with the main means of elimination of heme. Eighty percent of the circulating bilirubin is derived from heme of hemoglobin from senescent red blood cells destroyed in the reticuloendothelium of the bone marrow, spleen, and liver. Ten percent to 20% of the bilirubin comes from other sources such as myoglobin, cytochromes, and other heme-containing proteins processed in the liver. Initially, heme is oxidized at the alpha position to the green pigment biliverdin, which is then reduced at the gamma position to bilirubin.

   Bilirubin is virtually insoluble in aqueous solutions. In blood, it is reversibly but tightly bound to plasma albumin at a 1:1 ratio. Unbound bilirubin diffuses into tissues and can cross the blood–brain barrier; it may cause kernicterus and jaundice in infants. Sulfonamides, salicylates, free fatty acids, x-ray contrast media, diuretics, hypoxia, and acidosis have the ability to displace bilirubin from its binding site on albumin.

1. **Processing of serum bilirubin by the hepatocyte.** Newly formed bilirubin is removed from the circulation very rapidly by the liver. Normally, the plasma bilirubin concentration is less than 1 mg/dL. The processing of the serum bilirubin load by the hepatocyte occurs in **four steps.** These are **uptake, cytosolic binding, conjugation, and secretion.**

   a. **Uptake of bilirubin by the hepatocyte** occurs with the dissociation of the albumin–bilirubin complex facilitated by hepatocyte plasma membrane proteins with subsequent translocation of bilirubin into the hepatocyte through a saturable protein carrier, which also binds other organic anions but not bile salts.

      The hepatocellular uptake system operates well below saturation, and uptake does not limit bilirubin excretion. Approximately 40% of the bilirubin taken up by the hepatocyte after a single pass refluxes unchanged back to the plasma. This reflux may increase in hyperbilirubinemia.

   b. **Cytosolic binding.** Once in the hepatocyte, bilirubin binds to two cytosolic proteins: ligandin and Z protein. The binding limits the reflux of bilirubin back to the plasma and delivers it to the endoplasmic reticulum for conjugation.

c. **Conjugation of bilirubin** involves its esterification with glucuronic acid to form, first, a monoglucuronide, then a diglucuronide. The principal enzyme involved is uridine diphosphate (UDP)–glucuronyl transferase. Administration of microsomal enzyme inducers such as phenobarbital, glutethimide, and clofibrate causes increased activity of this enzyme. Conjugation renders bilirubin water-soluble and is essential for its elimination from the body in bile and urine. Most of the conjugated bilirubin excreted into bile in humans is diglucuronide with a lesser amount of monoglucuronide.

d. **Secretion of conjugated bilirubin from the hepatocyte to the bile canaliculi** involves a specific carrier and occurs against a concentration gradient. The carrier is shared by other anions, including anabolic steroids and cholecystographic agents, but not bile acids. In fact, bile acids facilitate bilirubin secretion. Secretion is the rate-limiting step in the transfer of bilirubin from plasma to bile.

Conjugated bilirubin is excreted in bile as a micellar complex with cholesterol, phospholipids, and bile salts. Bacteria in the colon deconjugate and convert it to a large number of urobilinogens. A minor portion of these pigments is absorbed into plasma through the enterohepatic circulation and is excreted in the urine; the rest is excreted in the stool.

2. **Urinary bilirubin.** Unconjugated bilirubin is not excreted by the kidney. Conjugated bilirubin may be excreted in the urine in considerable amounts when there is conjugated hyperbilirubinemia. Only the conjugated bilirubin not bound to albumin can be filtered through the glomerulus and appear in the urine. Compounds such as salicylates, sulfisoxazole, and bile salts that displace bilirubin from its binding site on serum albumin augment its renal excretion.

Detection of bilirubin in the urine implies the presence of hepatobiliary disease. Absence of bilirubin in the urine of a jaundiced patient suggests unconjugated hyperbilirubinemia.

3. **Serum bilirubin**

a. **Measurement.** Serum bilirubin is measured by van den Bergh's diazo reaction. Unconjugated bilirubin requires the presence of alcohol for the diazo reaction and gives an indirect van den Bergh's reaction. Conjugated bilirubin reacts directly without alcohol. **Total serum bilirubin** is measured with the diazo reaction carried out in alcohol, where both the conjugated and the unconjugated bilirubin react with the reagent. The conjugated bilirubin is then measured from the diazo reaction carried out without alcohol. The difference represents the concentration of the unconjugated bilirubin.

b. **The serum concentration of bilirubin** depends on a balance between the rate of production and hepatic removal of bilirubin.

i. **Increased bilirubin levels** may result from overproduction of bilirubin; impaired hepatic uptake, binding, conjugation, or secretion; and leakage of the bilirubin from damaged cells or bile ducts. Hyperbilirubinemia results in clinical jaundice at a serum bilirubin concentration greater than 2.0 to 2.5 mg/dL.

ii. **Unconjugated hyperbilirubinemia** results from overproduction or defective hepatic uptake or conjugation, whereas **conjugated hyperbilirubinemia** results from decreased hepatic secretion (excretion) or leakage of the conjugated bilirubin due to diffuse liver injury or impairment of biliary flow at the canalicular or bile duct level.

Unconjugated hyperbilirubinemia is present when the total serum bilirubin is greater than 1.2 mg/dL and the direct fraction is less than 20% of the total serum bilirubin. Causes of hyperbilirubinemia are summarized in Table 48-2.

IV. UNCONJUGATED HYPERBILIRUBINEMIA

A. **Hemolysis** causes increased production of bilirubin. When the excretory capacity of the liver is exceeded, serum levels of unconjugated bilirubin rise. Reduction of

TABLE 48-2	Causes of Hyperbilirubinemia

Unconjugated	Conjugated
Increased bilirubin production	Hereditary disorders
Hemolytic anemia	Dubin-Johnson syndrome
Hemoglobinopathies	Rotor syndrome
Enzyme deficiencies	Hepatocellular disease
Autoimmune	Viral hepatitis
Disseminated intravascular	A; B; non-A, non-B; D; Epstein-Barr virus;
coagulation	cytomegalovirus
Ineffective erythropoiesis	Chronic hepatitis
Pernicious anemia	Cirrhosis
Blood transfusions	Drug-induced liver injury
Hematoma	Alcohol-induced liver injury, fatty liver,
Hereditary disorders	hepatitis, cirrhosis
Gilbert syndrome	Infiltrative diseases
Crigler-Najjar syndromes type I, II	Tumors (primary, metastatic), infections
Drugs	(tuberculosis, parasites, abscess)
	Drug-induced cholestasis
	Recurrent jaundice of pregnancy
	Extrahepatic cholestasis, cholecystitis,
	choledocholithiasis, cysts, tumors,
	pancreatic disease (cysts, carcinoma,
	chronic pancreatitis)
	Postoperative jaundice
	Sepsis
	Parenteral nutrition
	Primary biliary cirrhosis
	Sclerosing cholangitis

red cell survival to one-half normal does not cause elevation of serum bilirubin. A sixfold increase in red cell destruction results in serum bilirubin elevation to less than 5 mg/dL.

In hemolytic hyperbilirubinemia, there may be a concomitant increase in conjugated bilirubin levels. However, if conjugated bilirubin is in excess of 15% of the total bilirubin level, hepatic dysfunction must also be present.

B. Ineffective erythropoiesis. Patients with hematologic disorders characterized by abnormalities of heme biosynthesis have increased bilirubin turnover without increased extramedullary red cell destruction. These disorders include iron-deficiency anemia, pernicious anemia, thalassemia, sideroblastic anemia, lead poisoning, and erythropoietic porphyria.

V. HEREDITARY UNCONJUGATED HYPERBILIRUBINEMIA. There is no definite evidence that abnormalities of hepatic uptake or cytosolic binding of bilirubin result in hyperbilirubinemia. However, deficiency of hepatic bilirubin UDP–glucuronyl transferase is known to result in unconjugated hyperbilirubinemia. The degree of enzyme deficiency allows this disorder to be divided into three types: Gilbert syndrome and Crigler–Najjar types I and II.

A. Gilbert syndrome. Gilbert syndrome may be the most common cause of mild unconjugated hyperbilirubinemia. It is present in up to 5% to 7% of white adults in the United States and Western Europe. These patients have a partial deficiency in bilirubin glucuronyl transferase. Some patients also have decreased uptake of bilirubin and organic anions and a mild compensated hemolytic state.

The syndrome is inherited as an autosomal dominant trait with incomplete penetrance and is characterized by mild, persistent unconjugated hyperbilirubinemia. The disorder usually does not become obvious until the second decade and often is diagnosed incidentally during a physical or laboratory examination. The serum bilirubin range is 1.3 to 3.0 mg/dL, rarely exceeding 5 mg/dL. The hyperbilirubinemia fluctuates and increases with fasting, surgery, fever, infection, excessive alcohol ingestion, and intravenous (IV) administration of glucose solutions. The other liver enzymes and the histologic studies of the liver are normal. Bilirubin monoglucuronide is the dominant pigment in the bile.

The diagnosis of Gilbert syndrome is made in patients with no systemic symptoms, no overt hemolysis, and normal liver serum tests and histologic studies. Patients with this disorder when placed on a 300-kcal diet without lipids for 24 to 48 hours have an elevation of their serum bilirubin by 100% or by 1.5 mg/dL. Also, administration of phenobarbital (180 mg/day in divided doses for 2 weeks) decreases the serum bilirubin levels by enhancing the activity of the glucuronyl transferase.

B. Crigler-Najjar type I syndrome is an extremely rare disorder with an autosomal recessive inheritance. It appears early in life with hyperbilirubinemia ranging from 24 to 45 mg/dL. In most infants, it is associated with kernicterus and cerebral damage. These patients lack the hepatic bilirubin glucuronyl transferase, and administration of microsomal enzyme inducers such as phenobarbital does not influence bilirubin levels. The patients have normal liver histologic studies and a normal liver enzyme profile but colorless bile. Phototherapy may transiently reduce the bilirubin level, but most affected individuals die within the first year of life with kernicterus. A few patients survive to the second decade, when encephalopathy develops.

C. Crigler-Najjar type II syndrome. Patients with this disorder have a partial deficiency of the glucuronyl transferase. This disorder is inherited as an autosomal dominant trait with incomplete penetrance. Serum unconjugated bilirubin levels are in the range of 6 to 25 mg/dL. The bile is rich in monoconjugates. Jaundice may not be apparent until adolescence, and neurologic complications are rare.

As in Gilbert syndrome, hyperbilirubinemia increases with fasting or removal of lipid from the diet. Liver histology and serum liver enzymes are normal. These patients also respond to treatment with phenobarbital, with the reduction of their bilirubin to less than 5 mg/dL.

D. Acquired deficiency of glucuronyl transferase. Neonatal jaundice may be aggravated or prolonged in infants treated with drugs such as chloramphenicol or vitamin K, or exposed to pregnane 3-β-20α-diol in breast milk due to inhibition of transferase activity. Hypothyroidism delays normal maturation of this enzyme and prolongs neonatal jaundice in these infants.

VI. CONJUGATED HYPERBILIRUBINEMIA. In jaundice from liver or biliary tract disease, both conjugated and unconjugated bilirubin levels are elevated, and the urine contains bilirubin. With bile duct obstruction, the level plateaus between 10 and 30 mg/dL. Levels greater than 30 mg/dL are more likely in patients with hepatocellular disease. Urinary excretion is the main means of obtaining bilirubin homeostasis in obstructive jaundice. Intra- or extrahepatic causes of jaundice cannot be differentiated on the basis of total serum bilirubin or the proportion of conjugated bilirubin. Fractionation of plasma bilirubin helps to distinguish predominantly unconjugated from conjugated hyperbilirubinemia. The most common causes of cholestasis are listed in Table 48-3.

A. Familial conjugated hyperbilirubinemia

1. Dubin-Johnson syndrome. This chronic intermittent form of jaundice is an autosomal recessive disorder with elevation of both the conjugated and the unconjugated serum bilirubin. Most patients are mildly jaundiced, but levels may be as high as 30 mg/dL. Patients exhibit normal liver enzyme profiles; however, histologically a yellow-black pigment is seen in the hepatocytes. This melaninlike substance is found in the lysosomes. The liver may be slightly enlarged and may be tender.

The principal defect in these patients is reduced ability to transport organic anions except for bile salts from the liver cell into the bile. Pregnancy and oral

TABLE 48-3	Causes of Cholestasis

Extrahepatic	Intrahepatic
Biliary	Drugs
Gallstone	Hormones
Stricture	Pregnancy
Cyst	Viral hepatitis
Diverticula	Alcohol hepatitis
Carcinoma	Hodgkin's disease, lymphoma
Bile duct	Sarcoidosis
Ampulla of Vater	Primary biliary cirrhosis
Lymph node involvement	Sclerosing cholangitis
Pancreas	Sepsis
Carcinoma	Parenteral nutrition
Pseudocyst	Postoperative
Chronic pancreatitis	Dubin-Johnson syndrome
	Rotor syndrome

contraceptives, which reduce hepatic excretory function, may unmask Dubin-Johnson syndrome by producing overt jaundice. These patients also have an abnormality in coproporphyrin excretion. The urine shows greater coproporphyrin I than III levels, which is a reversal of the normal pattern.

   2. Rotor's syndrome. This benign disorder is inherited as an autosomal recessive trait with defects in hepatic uptake and storage of conjugated bilirubin. There may be an additional excretory defect or a decrease in the intrahepatic binding of bilirubin, allowing conjugated bilirubin to reflux into the plasma. The hyperbilirubinemia is usually less than 10 mg/dL. Other liver enzyme tests and liver histology are normal. There is no pigment in the hepatocytes. The urinary coproporphyrin levels are higher than normal, and coproporphyrin I may be greater than III but not as great as in Dubin-Johnson syndrome. The pattern of coproporphyrin excretion is similar to that seen in other hepatobiliary disorders.

B. Recurrent jaundice of pregnancy. In a minority of pregnant women, usually after the seventh week of gestation but most commonly in the third trimester, an intrahepatic cholestasis occurs with jaundice and pruritus. The serum bilirubin level remains less than 8 mg/dL but is accompanied by considerably elevated alkaline phosphatase and cholesterol levels and mildly abnormal transaminases. Histologically, there are varying amounts of intrahepatic cholestasis but minor parenchymal cell changes.

   These patients have an increased sensitivity to the cholestatic (antiexcretory) effects of estrogenic and progestational hormones. The condition is benign and needs to be differentiated from fatty liver of pregnancy, which can be fatal. Pruritus responds to treatment with cholestyramine. The condition usually recurs with subsequent pregnancies, but all of the abnormalities revert back to normal promptly after delivery.

C. Drug-induced cholestasis

   1. The use of oral contraceptives in some women may result in intrahepatic cholestasis and jaundice due to the inhibitory effect of these drugs on hepatocellular biliary excretion. The liver function abnormalities resolve after the drug is discontinued, and chronic liver dysfunction does not occur.

   2. Male sex hormone analogs such as methyltestosterone may produce cholestatic jaundice and may result in chronic liver disease and biliary cirrhosis.

3. Many drugs produce cholestasis and liver cell injury, which may be accompanied by allergic manifestations such as fever, rash, arthralgia, and eosinophilia.

D. Postoperative jaundice. The cause of postoperative jaundice is multifactorial. Most patients have bilirubin pigment overload from blood transfusion with decreased red cell survival and resorption of blood from hematomas and large ecchymoses. Concurrent use of drugs may cause hepatic dysfunction, injury, or cholestasis. Hypotension, hypoxemia, sepsis, and shock contribute to impaired hepatic function. Renal insufficiency may decrease urinary excretion of conjugated bilirubin and enhance the degree of jaundice.

The hyperbilirubinemia may reach 30 to 40 mg/dL, with most of the bilirubin being conjugated. Serum alkaline phosphatase level may be elevated up to 10-fold, but the transaminases are usually only moderately elevated. Liver biopsy in most instances shows intrahepatic cholestasis. The course of the jaundice depends on the general condition of the patient. As the entire organ systems recover, the jaundice subsides and liver function returns to normal.

E. Sepsis from any source in the body may result in conjugated hyperbilirubinemia and mild-to-moderate elevation of the transaminases and alkaline phosphatases.

F. Hepatocellular disease. The most common disorders associated with jaundice are hepatitis and cirrhosis. With injury to the hepatocytes, all the steps in bilirubin metabolism are affected. Because secretion is the rate-limiting step, most of the bilirubin is conjugated. The hyperbilirubinemia in hepatocellular disease usually does not plateau and may exceed 60 mg/dL.

1. The major causes of intrahepatic cholestasis are
   a. Alcohol-related liver disease.
   b. Drugs (phenothiazines, sulfonylureas, allopurinol, azathioprine, thiazides, acetaminophen, and aspirin).
   c. Viral hepatitis (acute and chronic A, B, non-A, non-B, delta, Epstein-Barr virus, cytomegalovirus, and others).
   d. Toxic hepatitis.
   e. Sepsis.
   f. Infiltrative disorders (sarcoid, lymphoma, tuberculosis, primary or metastatic malignancy, sickle cell disease).

2. Laboratory studies
   a. In intrahepatic cholestasis, the laboratory tests reflect abnormal liver function (Table 48-4).
   b. In viral hepatitis, the transaminases may be elevated to 10 to 50 times normal (see Chapter 49).
   c. In alcoholic liver disease, the alkaline phosphatase usually rises up to about five times normal, SGOT (AST) is elevated less than 10 times normal, and the SGPT (ALT) is lower than the SGOT (AST). The SGOT/SGPT ratio is usually 2:1 to 3:1 (see Chapter 51).
   d. In drug-induced cholestasis, bilirubin may not be high, but there is usually a dramatic rise in alkaline phosphatase with a slight rise in transaminases (see Chapter 53).

3. The course of the jaundice depends on the general condition of the patient. As the entire organ systems recover, the jaundice subsides and liver function returns to normal.

G. Extrahepatic cholestasis
   1. Causes
      a. Extrahepatic biliary obstruction due to stones, strictures, lymphadenopathy, or tumors can occur anywhere along the route of the bile ducts from the hilum of the liver to the duodenal papilla. Gallstone disease accounts for most of the benign extrahepatic obstruction. Most of these patients have an abrupt onset of jaundice. The disease ranges from biliary colic to acute cholecystitis and ascending cholangitis, especially with CBD stones.
      b. Cancer. Pancreatic cancer, cholangiocarcinoma, adenocarcinoma of the duodenum and ampulla of Vater, metastatic or primary liver tumors, and

| TABLE 48-4 | Patterns of Laboratory Studies in Cholestatic Disease States |

Disease	Bilirubin (mg/dL)	Alkaline phosphatase	SGOT (AST)	SGPT (ALT)	Albumin
Alcoholic liver disease	0–20	5 × nl	10 × nl	2 × nl	nl or sl ∅
Acute viral hepatitis	0–20	nl–3 × nl	10–50 × nl	10–50 × nl	nl
Drug-induced intrahepatic cholestasis	5–10	2–10 × nl	nl–5 × nl	10–50 × nl	nl
Common bile duct obstruction	0–10	nl–10 × nl	nl–10 × nl	nl–10 × nl	nl
Malignant common bile duct obstruction	5–20	2–10 × nl	nl	nl	nl

SGOT, serum glutamic-oxaloacetic transaminase; AST, aspartate aminotransferase; SGPT, serum glutamic-pyruvic transaminase; ALT, alanine aminotransferase; nl, normal; sl ∅, slightly depressed.

enlarged nodes at the porta hepatis are common causes of extrahepatic biliary obstruction and jaundice.

2. **Laboratory studies**

   a. In general, **patients with gallstone disease** have less hyperbilirubinemia than those with intrahepatic cholestasis or extrahepatic malignant obstruction. The serum bilirubin is usually less than 20 mg/dL. The alkaline phosphatase may be elevated up to 10 times normal. The transaminases may abruptly rise about 10 times normal and decrease rapidly once the obstruction is relieved.

   b. In **pancreatic cancer and other obstructive cancers,** the serum bilirubin may rise to 35 to 40 mg/dL, the alkaline phosphatase may rise up to 10 times normal, but the transaminases may remain normal. See Table 48.4 for additional patterns of laboratory studies.

VII. DIAGNOSTIC STUDIES. The history, physical examination, and laboratory tests are usually not sufficient to make the diagnosis of the underlying disorder causing the jaundice. Additional diagnostic procedures are needed to arrive at a definitive diagnosis.

A. **Noninvasive techniques**

   1. **An abdominal flat plate** (kidneys, ureters, bladder [KUB]) obtained in the radiology department is the first test to be done on a patient with jaundice. Aside from providing information on other organs in the abdomen, it may show calcified gallstones, a "porcelain" gallbladder, air in the biliary tract, or air in the gallbladder wall.

   2. **Ultrasonography.** In most patients, the ultrasound should be the first procedure performed. It identifies with 95% accuracy the presence of extrahepatic bile duct obstruction, because the ducts proximal to the obstruction are usually dilated. It is a sensitive test for revealing stones in the gallbladder, but it fails to show small stones or strictures in the bile ducts. CBD stones are visualized reliably by ultrasound only in about one third of such patients. Ultrasound may also demonstrate tumors, cysts, or abscesses in the pancreas, liver, and other structures near the biliary tract. Ultrasound is limited in patients who are obese, who have had a recent barium study, or who have a

large amount of bowel gas. Absence of ductal dilatation on ultrasound does not exclude extrahepatic obstruction. Nondilated ducts caused by early, intermittent, or incomplete biliary obstruction; tumor encasement; sclerosing cholangitis; or the presence of cirrhosis of the liver may result in negative ultrasound results. Duct diameters measured by ultrasound are normal in 25% to 40% of patients with documented CBD stones. The significance of CBD dilatation in postcholecystectomy patients is controversial. If an abnormality of the bile ducts is suspected in such patients, direct visualization techniques (e.g., endoscopic retrograde cholangiopancreatography or percutaneous transhepatic cholangiography) should be used to allow both strictured and dilated areas to be evaluated.

3. **Computed tomography (CT) of the abdomen** provides excellent visualization of the liver, gallbladder, pancreas, kidneys, and retroperitoneum. It can differentiate between intra- and extrahepatic obstruction with 95% accuracy. However, CT may not define incomplete obstruction caused by small gallstones, tumors, or strictures. CBD stones are seen in only 30% of patients.

4. **Cholescintigraphy (dimethylphenylcarbamylmethyliminodiacetic acid [HIDA] scan).** When there is a suspicion of acute cholecystitis with cystic duct obstruction and ascending cholangitis with CBD obstruction even in the presence of a very elevated serum bilirubin level, the scintiscan may help provide the diagnosis. The nuclear scan is done following a single IV injection of a technetium 99m derivative of iminodiacetic acid (IDA). If the scintiscan demonstrates a patent CBD by the presence of the radionuclide within the small bowel but no filling of the gallbladder or the cystic duct within 2 hours after the injection of the tracer, acute cholecystitis or cystic duct obstruction is diagnosed. However, if the radionuclide fills the biliary tract and does not appear in the duodenum within 2 hours of injection, CBD obstruction is inferred.

5. **Radionuclide scanning.** The visualization of the liver by the ^{99m}Tc-sulfur colloid scan is dependent on the uptake of ^{99m}Tc-sulfur colloid by the Kupffer's cells of the liver. Space-occupying lesions, such as liver abscesses, cysts, and primary and metastatic tumors, appear as filling defects, whereas chronic hepatocellular disease (e.g., cirrhosis) with portal hypertension is associated with patchy uptake of the radionuclide with increased uptake by the spleen and bone marrow. This test is limited by its ineffectiveness in demonstrating small space-occupying lesions (i.e., <2–3 cm). It is most helpful in estimating liver size and in implicating the presence of cirrhosis in patients with normal or abnormal liver chemistries.

6. **The oral cholecystogram** is an old test that may be useful in patients with low-grade jaundice to demonstrate the presence of radiopaque or radiolucent stones in the gallbladder as well as to help assess gallbladder function. However, nonvisualization of the gallbladder may be due to a bilirubin level of 3 mg/dL, chronic liver disease, chronic gallbladder disease, the absence of a gallbladder, or failure of the patient to ingest the contrast material, to absorb it, or to remain in the fasting state.

7. **The IV cholangiogram** has been associated with a high frequency of allergic reactions and failure to visualize the biliary tract if the bilirubin is 2 mg/dL. Its use is not recommended.

8. **Magnetic resonance cholangiopancreatography (MRCP)** is a newer noninvasive technique for visualization of the biliary and pancreatic ductal system. It is especially useful in patients who have contraindications for endoscopic retrograde cholangiopancreatography (ERCP). Excellent visualization of biliary anatomy is possible without the invasiveness of ERCP.

B. **Invasive techniques**

1. **Liver biopsy.** Percutaneous liver biopsy is a safe, bedside procedure of low cost. It is helpful in evaluating the following: hepatocellular injury of unknown cause; hepatomegaly; fever of unknown origin; hepatic defects demonstrated by ultrasound, CT, or radionuclide scanning; and chronic hepatitis. It is also used

for staging of malignant lymphoma and confirming the diagnosis and assessing the severity of suspected alcoholic liver disease. A 2-cm piece of liver tissue is needed to ensure accurate diagnosis; however, a sampling error can be expected 10% of the time despite an adequate amount of tissue. Liver biopsy may be very helpful in evaluating the patient with cholestatic jaundice but only after extrahepatic bile duct obstruction has been ruled out. Contraindications include an uncooperative patient, hydatid cyst disease, suspected vascular lesion of the liver, right-sided pleural effusion, infection of the biopsy site, and clinically significant coagulopathy (i.e., PT 4 seconds prolonged and platelet count <75,000).

2. **Laparoscopy (peritoneoscopy)** can be performed with local anesthesia and allows direct visualization of the liver. It may be helpful in the diagnosis of portal hypertension, cirrhosis, and liver tumors in difficult cases and also allows for visually directed liver biopsies.

3. **Percutaneous transhepatic cholangiography (PTC)** is performed in the radiology department. Contrast material is injected directly under fluoroscopy into the intrahepatic biliary tract through a 22- to 23-gauge, 15-cm-long Chiba or skinny needle passed percutaneously from a right lateral intracostal approach. It allows the visualization of the intrahepatic bile ducts. An adequate study should be obtained in up to 75% of the patients with nondilated ducts and in more than 90% of patients with dilated ducts as diagnosed by a previous ultrasound or CT scan. The complication rate ranges from 1% to 10%.

The patients must be cooperative and have good bleeding parameters with a PT within 3 seconds of control and a platelet count greater than 50,000. Prophylactic antibiotics should be used in patients with suspected obstruction and infection. After the procedure, patients must be monitored for possible bleeding or leakage of bile into the peritoneum.

This procedure may be used therapeutically to decompress the biliary tract nonsurgically with the placement of a stent through an area of obstruction from malignancy or benign stricture of the bile duct. The drainage may be external or internal into the small bowel. The success rate is variable, and the procedure should be considered palliative for poor-risk patients or those with nonresectable masses.

4. **Endoscopic retrograde cholangiopancreatography (ERCP)** is the procedure of choice when obstruction of the pancreatic or distal CBD is suspected by ultrasound or CT scan. The duodenal lumen and papilla are visualized, and contrast material is injected into the pancreatic and bile ducts under fluoroscopic guidance. The technique is successful greater than 90% of the time whether the ducts are dilated or not. Visualization of the pancreatic duct may reveal chronic pancreatitis, pseudocyst, or tumor causing the obstruction; stones, strictures, and tumors causing obstruction of the bile ducts also may be delineated.

ERCP allows for biopsies of the periampullary duodenum and the papilla for tissue diagnosis. It may also be used as a therapeutic procedure in patients with recurrent or retained CBD stones. A sphincterotomy can be performed by cautery with incision of the papilla, relieving the obstruction and allowing the gallstones to pass into the duodenum. Retrieval of gallstones may also be accomplished with intraductal balloon or baskets or after intraductal crushing using special catheters. Nasobiliary stents may be placed in the CBD to allow drainage, and permanent biliary stents may be placed in the obstructed ducts as palliation in instances of inoperable carcinomatous obstruction.

5. **Angiography.** Visualization of the hepatic arterial and venous circulation is helpful in evaluating portal hypertension and determining the vascular supply, vascularity, and surgical resectability of a mass lesion in the liver.

VIII. SUMMARY. The algorithm shown in Figure 48-2 summarizes the diagnostic workup for the evaluation of jaundice.

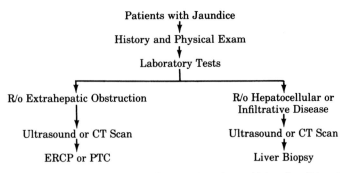

Figure 48-2. Interpretation of laboratory liver tests in patients with jaundice. (R/o, rule out or exclude.)

Selected Readings

Balisteri WF, et al. Intrahepatic cholestosis: summary of an American Association for the study of liver diseases single topic conference. *Hepatol.* 2005;42:222–235.

Heathcote EJ. Diagnosis and management of cholestatic liver disease. *Clin Gastroenterol Hepatol.* 2007;5(7):776–782.

Mendes FD, et al. Abnormal hepatic biochemistries in patients with inflammatory bowel disease. *Am J Gastroenterol.* 2007;102(2):344–350.

Pratt DS, et al. Evaluation of abnormal liver enzyme results in asymptomatic patients. *N Engl J Med.* 2000;342:1266.

Sorbi D, et al. An assessment of the role of liver biopsies in asymptomatic patients with chronic liver test abnormalities. *Hepatology.* 1999;30(suppl):487A.

Vuppalanchi R, et al. Etiology of new-onset jaundice: How often is it caused by idiosyncratic drug-induced liver injury in the United States? *Am J Gastroenterol.* 2007 Mar;102:558–562.

Wong K, et al. The diversity of liver diseases associated with an elevated serum ferritin. *Can J Gastro.* 2007;20:467–470.

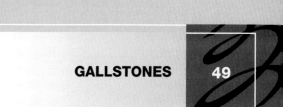
I. ANATOMY AND PHYSIOLOGY

A. The **biliary tract** starts at the hepatocyte canaliculi, which empty into biliary ductules. Larger ducts join the right and left hepatic ducts, which drain into the common hepatic duct (CHD) at the porta hepatis. When the cystic duct from the gallbladder joins the CHD, the common bile duct (CBD) is formed. The CBD is usually 8 cm long and 0.5 to 0.9 cm in diameter. It passes behind the first portion of the duodenum, through a groove in the head of the pancreas, and empties into the second portion of the duodenum at the ampulla of Vater. Distally the pancreatic duct may join the CBD before it also empties into the ampulla.

B. The **gallbladder,** a pear-shaped distensible organ, 4×8 cm in size with a normal capacity of 30 to 50 mL, lies in a fossa on the visceral surface of the liver on a line separating the right and left hepatic lobes. When distended with acute inflammation, the fundus comes in close contact with the anterior abdominal wall in the right upper quadrant near the ninth and tenth costal cartilages, giving rise to the Murphy's sign. Posteriorly, it abuts the first and second portion of the duodenum and the hepatic flexure of the colon. Thus, extension of the inflammation of the gallbladder may lead to spontaneous fistulas into these hollow organs.

C. Bile flow. Bile, formed by the hepatocytes (600 mL per day), consists of water, electrolytes, bile salts, cholesterol, phospholipids, bilirubin, and other organic solutes. The gallbladder stores and concentrates bile during fasting. Approximately 90% of the water and the electrolytes are resorbed by the gallbladder epithelium, resulting in bile rich in organic constituents. The stratification of this bile into a density gradient is thought to play a role in gallstone formation.

II. Gallstone disease

is a major health problem in the United States. It affects approximately 20% of adult Americans. Gallstones are formed by the precipitation of insoluble bile constituents: cholesterol, polymerized bilirubin, bile pigments, calcium salts, and proteins. Gallstones are classified into cholesterol, black pigment, and brown pigment stones. Cholesterol stones are most frequent in industrialized societies. Black pigment stones occur in patients with chronic hemolytic disorders, and brown pigment stones are associated with impaction in the biliary tract. These stones are more prevalent than cholesterol stones in the Far East. Cholesterol stones may be pure, large (>2.5 cm), solitary or mixed (>70% cholesterol), multiple, smooth, and faceted. Black and brown stones contain less than 25% cholesterol and are multiple and irregular. They contain polymerized bilirubin and calcium salts (bilirubinate, phosphate, and fatty acids). All types of gallstones may become calcified. The calcification is usually central in pigment stones and peripheral in cholesterol stones.

A. Pigment stones (black and brown)

1. Epidemiology. Clinically, black pigment stones are more prevalent in three major settings: hemolytic states, cirrhosis, and the elderly. In the United States, approximately 30% of gallstones are pigment (mostly black) stones. The incidence is age-dependent: Pigment stones are more common in the sixth and seventh decades. In Asia, biliary tract parasitism with *Clonorchis sinensis* and *Ascaris lumbricoides*, biliary ductal stasis, and chronic or repeated spasm at the sphincter of Oddi as a result of widespread use of opium may contribute to the increased prevalence (approximately 70%) of brown pigment cholelithiasis.

2. The **pathogenesis** of black pigment stone formation is not clear; however, there seems to be an increased concentration of the insoluble, unconjugated bilirubin and poorly soluble bilirubin monoglucuronide in the bile of these patients. Abnormal motor function of the gallbladder and reduced bile salt concentration may also contribute to the pathogenesis. Infections with organisms such as *Escherichia coli* reduce biliary pH and deconjugate bilirubin glucuronide, which may create a nidus for gallstone formation.

B. **Cholesterol gallstones**
   1. **Risk factors**
      a. **Heredity.** The prevalence of cholesterol gallstones varies in different populations. There is a strong correlation between the percentage of cholesterol saturation of gallbladder bile and gallstone formation, as in Pima Indian women in whom the prevalence reaches 80%. Thus hereditary mechanisms are important.
      b. **Age.** Gallstones may be found at all ages, but the incidence increases with age.
      c. **Gender.** Women, starting at puberty, have a two to three times greater risk of developing gallstones compared to men.
      d. **Pregnancy.** Supersaturation of bile with impaired gallbladder emptying during pregnancy due to an increase of estriol, progesterone, and other sex hormone levels increases the incidence of cholelithiasis.
      e. **Use of exogenous estrogens.** There is increased cholelithiasis among users of exogenous estrogens and progesterone, as in birth control pills and in postmenopausal estrogen replacement. The condition could be secondary to gallbladder stasis induced by these hormones and to reduced bile flow and altered lipid composition of bile.
      f. **Diabetes.** The increased prevalence of cholelithiasis in diabetes is largely due to obesity and increased biliary cholesterol secretion.
      g. **Obesity.** The bile of obese people is more lithogenic due to excessive cholesterol secretion caused by increased cholesterol synthesis.
      h. **Rapid weight loss.** Regardless of the method of weight loss, up to 25% of patients who lose weight rapidly will develop symptomatic gallstones. With weight loss, cholesterol is mobilized from peripheral adipose tissue and secretes into bile leading to cholesterol supersaturation. Also, the stimulus for gallbladder contraction from dietary fat is diminished leading to gallbladder stasis. Weight fluctuation is also a risk factor for gallstones.
      i. **Hyperlipidemia.** Patients with type I and IV hyperlipidemia have a high risk of cholesterol gallstone formation.
      j. **Cystic fibrosis and pancreatic insufficiency.** Malabsorption of bile salts decreases the bile salt pool and increases the lithogenicity of bile, leading to cholelithiasis.
      k. **Ileal disease, bypass, or resection.** Extensive disease of the distal small intestine as in Crohn's disease, or surgical resection of the distal ileum impairs bile salt resorption and predisposes to gallstone formation due to decreased bile acid pool.
      l. **Drugs.** Clofibrate used in the treatment of hyperlipidemia decreases serum cholesterol by inhibiting cholesterol synthesis. This stimulates tissue mobilization and increases cholesterol secretion into bile. Bile becomes more lithogenic, leading to cholelithiasis. The somatostatin analog octreotide predisposes to gallstone formation by inducing gallbladder stasis.
      m. **Diet.** A high-calorie diet, refined carbohydrates, and diets high in polyunsaturated fatty acids predispose to cholelithiasis. Increased dietary fiber seems to decrease the risk of cholelithiasis. Weight-reduction diets with severe caloric restriction leading to rapid weight loss also may result in cholelithiasis.
      n. **Genetic factors.** The prevalence of gallstones is highest in the American Indian tribes, especially the Pima Indians of Arizona. By the age of 30, 80% of Pima women have gallstones. There is also a high prevalence of gallstones

in Chile. In addition to genetic factors, it is thought that this high prevalence in Chile is due partly to the high intake of beans, which adversely affects biliary cholesterol saturation. Gallstones are more common in first-degree relatives of patients with gallstones than in the general population.

  o. Spinal injury, especially high spinal section, is associated with a high incidence of gallstones, probably secondary to gallbladder stasis.

  p. Total parenteral nutrition promotes gallbladder stasis and the formation of sludge and gallstones with prolonged use.

  q. Truncal vagotomy may be a risk factor for cholelithiasis secondary to decreased gallbladder motility.

2. Cholesterol gallstone formation. The first step in the formation of gallstones is the secretion by the liver of bile supersaturated with cholesterol. Cholesterol in dilute hepatic bile is transported in spherical vesicles of phospholipid and cholesterol into the biliary tract and the gallbladder. Hepatic bile is concentrated in the gallbladder.

The second step in gallstone formation is crystallization. The precipitation of cholesterol crystals initiates the formation of gallstones. When the gallbladder bile becomes abnormally supersaturated with cholesterol, nucleation, flocculation, and precipitation of cholesterol crystals occur, leading to the initiation of gallstone formation. The excessive presence of promoters of crystallization and relative deficiency of inhibitors of crystallization are also thought to be important in the initiation of nucleation and crystal formation. The promoters and inhibitors are most likely proteins such as mucous glycoprotein. The growth of the crystals to macroscopic stones is further facilitated by the gallbladder mucus.

Patients who have cholesterol gallstones may have defects leading to the production of abnormally supersaturated bile due to an absolute increase in the secretory rate of biliary cholesterol or an absolute decrease in the secretory rate of biliary bile salts, lecithin, and phospholipids. Changes in the concentration of one of the key promoters of crystallization, mucous glycoprotein, are mediated by mucosal prostaglandins (PGs). Aspirin and nonsteroidal antiinflammatory drugs (NSAIDs), by decreasing PG synthesis, also prevent microcrystal and gallstone formation, especially in obese people undergoing weight reduction through dieting.

Gallbladder motor dysfunction and stasis also contribute to gallstone formation and may be a primary phenomenon.

3. Clinical presentation. Long-term studies have shown that at least one half of the individuals with gallstones remain asymptomatic, one third experience severe symptoms, and one fifth experience serious complications.

  a. The complications of cholelithiasis include the following:

    i. Cystic duct obstruction, leading to

      a) Colic.

      b) Acute cholecystitis.

      c) Cholangitis, sepsis.

      d) Perforation, peritonitis.

      e) Fistulization, gallstone ileus.

    ii. Choledocholithiasis, which may cause

      a) Obstructive jaundice.

      b) Cholangitis, sepsis.

      c) Acute pancreatitis.

      d) Stricture formation.

    iii. There is some evidence to suggest that gallstones and chronic cholecystitis also may predispose to carcinoma of the gallbladder.

  b. Biliary colic. Dyspeptic symptoms such as heartburn, fat intolerance, and increased "gas" (bloating, flatulence, and belching) are not symptoms specific to gallbladder disease. Biliary colic is pain arising from a distended gallbladder due to obstruction of the cystic duct with a gallstone. Commonly, the "attacks" follow heavy meals. The pain is felt mostly in the right upper quadrant and may radiate to the epigastrium, back, or shoulder. It may be mild or severe, lasts 1 to 6 hours, and usually is accompanied by nausea and vomiting. At times, when the cystic duct obstruction is transient, biliary colic is relieved spontaneously. However, prolonged cystic duct obstruction with a gallstone usually results in acute cholecystitis, cholangitis, and their complications.

   c. **Prognosis.** Both complications and mortality from gallstones increase with age and with passage of time. The first attack may be severe, especially in the elderly and patients with other serious illness. Because the mortality for these patients from complications of gallstones may be as high as 15% to 20%, elective surgery should be considered when asymptomatic gallstones are found. Surgery is also recommended for patients with symptoms or complications of cholelithiasis.

4. **Differential diagnosis.** Other causes of severe upper abdominal pain need to be considered in the differential diagnosis of biliary colic. These causes include acute myocardial infarction, ruptured aortic aneurysm, perforated peptic ulcer, pneumonia, pneumothorax, pleurisy, intestinal obstruction, intestinal ischemia, pancreatitis, and renal colic.

5. **Diagnostic studies.** The demonstration of gallstones by ultrasound is currently the best diagnostic test, having the highest sensitivity (90%–95%) and specificity (98%). An oral cholecystogram may also demonstrate gallstones as well as gallbladder contractile function after ingestion of fat; however, this test is not as sensitive as ultrasound. Computed tomography (CT) scan of the gallbladder is much more sensitive than conventional radiography in detecting gallstone calcium. However, ultrasound is more sensitive than CT in detecting gallbladder sludge and stones.

   Endoscopic retrograde cholangiopancreatography (ERCP) is useful in identifying CBD stones. It is not specific for the diagnosis of gallbladder stones.

   Magnetic resonance cholangiopancreatography (MRCP) is a noninvasive method to screen for CBD stones as well as for strictures and cystic anomalies of the CBD and bile duct dilatation. The reported sensitivity is 70% to 100% and specificity is 80% to 100%.

6. **Management** of symptomatic but uncomplicated gallstone disease
   a. **Pain relief.** The immediate treatment of biliary colic is symptomatic. Pain relief is usually achieved with narcotic analgesics, excluding morphine, and antiemetics.
   b. **Laparoscopic cholecystectomy** is the recommended treatment for long-term management. If choledocholithiasis is suspected, preoperative ERCP with sphincterotomy or intraoperative cholangiography may be necessary. Open cholecystectomy is reserved for patients who have contraindications to the laparoscopic procedure. In the average patient, the mortality of elective cholecystectomy is less than 1%. The risk increases in patients with diabetes, renal insufficiency, cardiovascular disease, respiratory disease, and cirrhosis of the liver.
   c. **Extracorporeal shock-wave lithotripsy (ESWL)** is not currently used in the United States for uncomplicated gallbladder stones. In centers where ESWL is available, it may be used for problematic CBD stones not cleared by ERCP. ESWL in combination with oral bile acid therapy has been used for patients who are not surgical candidates and who have single or small cholesterol gallstones and a functioning gallbladder. Gallstones are localized by three-dimensional ultrasound, then extracorporeal shock waves are focused and fired on the gallstones and fragmentation is achieved. Up to three sessions may be needed to achieve fragmentation of the gallstones into pieces smaller than 3 mm. It is expected that these fragments pass spontaneously into the duodenum or dissolve by oral bile acids. Oral bile acid therapy may need to be continued for several months. Approximately 20% of patients develop biliary colic and 25% subsequently undergo cholecystectomy. Other side effects include pancreatitis (1%), local pain, petechia and bruising, and microscopic hematuria.

d. Gallstone dissolution with oral bile acid therapy is based on the theory that cholesterol stones should dissolve in bile rendered unsaturated with respect to cholesterol by increasing the concentration of bile salts. Gallstone clearance may not depend completely on stone dissolution. Cholesterol-rich stones can disintegrate as they dissolve, and the resultant fragments might pass out of the gallbladder in the bile via the cystic duct and into the CBD and duodenum.

The first bile acid used orally was chenodeoxycholic acid (CDCA). CDCA decreases the cholesterol saturation of bile by lowering cholesterol secretion, thus bringing about a gradual dissolution of cholesterol stones. In a controlled trial using 12 to 15 mg/kg per day (approximately 1 g daily), the stones dissolved in 40% to 60% of the selected patients during 2 years of continuous therapy.

i. Contraindications. Dissolution therapy is contraindicated in the presence of any of the following:

a) Pigment stones

b) Calcified stones

c) Stones larger than 1.5 to 2.0 cm

d) Multiple stones

e) Nonopacifying gallbladder on oral cholecystogram

f) Obesity

g) Pregnancy or women who may become pregnant

h) Concomitant liver disease

i) Severe symptoms

j) Nonresponders by oral cystography after 9 months of therapy

k) Poor patient compliance

7. Side effects. The most common side effect is secretory diarrhea induced by the bile acid in the colon. Occasionally, gallstones become small enough during therapy to pass into and obstruct the cystic or CBD, resulting in inflammation. Minor liver enzyme elevations may occur in 7% of the patients without any significant structural changes in liver histology. There may be a modest rise in plasma and low-density lipoprotein (LDL) cholesterol.

8. Maintenance of therapy. CDCA therapy needs to be maintained indefinitely in all patients because the bile reverts to its previous supersaturated state in 1 to 3 weeks after cessation of the therapy, and stones recur within 6 to 48 months.

9. Ursodeoxycholic acid (UDCA) is more potent than CDCA in lowering biliary cholesterol secretion and saturation. It also has fewer side effects. It does not affect the serum LDL levels or liver chemistry tests. A UDCA dosage of 10 mg/kg per day is optimal and equivalent to a CDCA dosage of 15 mg/kg per day. In some patients, stone rim calcifications may occur and limit dissolution.

10. The **combination of UDCA and CDCA** is at least as effective and free of side effects as monotherapy with UDCA and is less expensive. The dosage of CDCA is reduced to 7.5 mg/kg per day, and UDCA is used at a dosage of 5 mg/kg per day.

III. CHOLECYSTITIS

A. Acute calculous cholecystitis. Inflammation of the gallbladder is associated with gallstones in more than 90% of cases. It is a common problem, presenting as an acute abdomen, especially in middle-aged women. Acute calculous cholecystitis is caused by obstruction of the cystic duct either by an impacted stone or by the edema and inflammation caused by the passage of a stone to the CBD and duodenum. The obstructed gallbladder becomes distended, and the walls become edematous, ischemic, and inflamed. Secondary infection with enteric organisms complicates the inflammation and may lead to cholangitis and sepsis.

1. Diagnosis

a. Clinical presentation. The pain of acute cholecystitis usually starts in the right upper quadrant or epigastrium as a colicky pain followed by local signs and symptoms of inflammation. It may radiate to the flanks, intrascapular regions, and right shoulder. Nausea and vomiting are also common. Physical examination reveals a tender right upper quadrant, especially at the tip of the ninth costal cartilage during inspiration (Murphy's sign). The gallbladder may be palpable. Abdominal rigidity represents peritoneal inflammation. Fever, tachycardia, and tachypnea are common. Jaundice suggests obstruction of the CBD and may be present in one third of the patients.

b. **The differential diagnosis** includes acute appendicitis, pancreatitis, hepatitis, pneumonia, pyelonephritis, perforated peptic ulcer, and myocardial infarction.

c. **Diagnostic studies**

i. **Laboratory studies.** Leukocytosis of 10,000 to 15,000/μL with a shift to the left usually accompanies acute cholecystitis. Elevation of the serum amylase is not uncommon without the presence of concomitant pancreatitis. Elevation of alkaline phosphatase and bilirubin levels usually suggests obstruction of the CBD due to either an impacted stone or edema and inflammation as a result of the passage of a stone. Alanine aminotransferase (ALT) and aspartate aminotransferase (AST) elevations suggest concomitant parenchymal cholangitis.

ii. **Ultrasonography** is the test of choice in demonstrating gallstones, thickening of the gallbladder wall, and pericystic fluid. If the CBD is obstructed, dilatation of the biliary tract may be present.

iii. **Biliary scintigraphy (i.e., dimethylphenylcarbamylmethyliminodiacetic acid [HIDA] or PIPIDA scan)** uses technetium 99m–labeled derivatives of iminodiacetic acid excreted in the bile. In healthy individuals, scans obtained 15 to 30 minutes after intravenous (IV) injection demonstrate the filling of the bile ducts and the gallbladder and passage of the radionuclide to the CBD and small intestine. In acute cholecystitis due to an obstructed cystic duct, the gallbladder does not fill. Parenchymal liver disease and high bile duct obstruction may lead to failure of imaging of the extrahepatic biliary tract. False-positive scans may occur in chronic cholecystitis, and false-negative scans have been reported in acalculous cholecystitis. In general, the sensitivity of this test is very high.

2. **Treatment**

a. The patient should be admitted to the hospital. Oral intake should be stopped and, in those with severe nausea and vomiting, a nasogastric sump tube should be inserted to aspirate gastric contents with low suction. IV fluid and electrolytes should be provided. Antibiotic therapy to cover enteric organism may be used if secondary infection is suspected after appropriate cultures are obtained.

b. **Cholecystectomy** is the definitive treatment for acute cholecystitis. Most patients can be treated with laparoscopic cholecystectomy. Extensive previous laparotomy with scarring may render laparoscopy impossible in some cases. Controversy as to the timing of the surgery still exists for uncomplicated cases; however, most surgeons prefer early intervention, within 5 days of onset of symptoms, rather than waiting 6 to 8 weeks. In elderly patients with other systemic diseases, such as congestive heart failure, the operation may need to be delayed. Preoperative ERCP may be performed in selected patients if CBD stones are suspected. Sphincterotomy and stone extraction eliminate the need for operative CBD exploration. Cholecystectomy should be performed acutely in cases of emphysematous cholecystitis in which the gallbladder walls and bile ducts contain gas. The infective organisms are the gas-forming bacteria, such as *Clostridium, E. coli,* and other anaerobes.

c. **Cholecystostomy.** In severe illness, when laparotomy is contraindicated, a cholecystostomy may be performed. Cholecystostomy involves evacuation of the gallbladder of the stones and infected bile and placement of a Foley catheter into the gallbladder for drainage to outside the body. When the patient is stable, a tube cholangiogram should be performed to assess the patency of the biliary system and the presence of possible residual stones. If these abnormalities are detected, cholecystectomy should be performed when possible.

3. Complications

   a. Perforation is the most serious complication of acute cholecystitis. It may be localized or may extend into the peritoneal cavity with subsequent peritonitis or into an adjacent hollow organ, such as the stomach, duodenum, or colon with formation of a cholecystenteric fistula. Surgical intervention is necessary in all cases.

   b. Gallstone ileus is a form of mechanical intestinal obstruction caused by the impaction of a large gallstone that has entered into the intestine from a cholecystenteric fistula. The obstruction may be intermittent as the stone moves along the intestine until permanent obstruction occurs. Most obstructions occur in the ileum. Colonic obstruction is rare except at sites of previous narrowing due to another disease process, such as diverticular or inflammatory bowel disease. Gallstone ileus requires prompt diagnosis and laparotomy.

   c. Mirizzi syndrome. Rarely, a gallstone impacted in the cystic duct or the neck of the gallbladder may cause a localized obstruction of the common hepatic duct from direct pressure or inflammatory changes around the duct. The obstruction can cause right upper quadrant pain, jaundice, recurrent cholangitis, and possibly a fistula between the two ducts.

   Ultrasound examination may show dilated ducts above the point of obstruction as well as the stone. ERCP or percutaneous transhepatic cholangiography (PTC) confirms the site of obstruction. CT scan may be helpful in defining the stone and differentiating it from tumor or mass. Surgery is required in most instances.

B. Acute acalculous cholecystitis is a particularly severe form of inflammation of the gallbladder that occurs in the absence of cholelithiasis. There is a high incidence of necrosis, gangrene, and perforation of the gallbladder in this group of patients. The mortality may be as high as 50% if diagnosis is delayed and prompt therapy not instituted.

Most of the patients are elderly or debilitated as a result of coexisting disease or trauma. The condition is also seen in patients of all ages in the intensive care unit, after surgery, or on total parenteral nutrition. Absence of oral intake associated with gallbladder stasis, sludge formation, and increased biliary pressure due to narcotic drugs that increase the tone at the sphincter of Oddi may contribute to its pathogenesis.

1. Diagnosis

   a. Clinical presentation. Bile is usually infected with enteric bacteria, which may lead to sepsis. The clinical presentation may be nonspecific, and the diagnosis requires a high index of suspicion. Most patients complain of abdominal pain, nausea, and vomiting. Fever and chills may be present. Serum bilirubin, alkaline phosphatase, ALT, and AST may be elevated. There is usually a moderate leukocytosis (10,000–20,000 cells/μL) with a left shift. Serum amylase may be elevated.

   b. Diagnostic studies. The diagnostic test of choice in acute acalculous cholecystitis is ultrasound of the gallbladder, which identifies a distended gallbladder with thickened walls and biliary sludge. Nuclear scans with HIDA or PIPIDA may give equivocal results in these debilitated patients and are not reliable.

2. Treatment. Successful management of acute acalculous cholecystitis requires prompt diagnosis and early surgical intervention. Patients should be treated with antibiotics to cover enteric organisms and enterococci. Cholecystectomy is the surgical procedure of choice. Cholecystostomy is not recommended because, in most cases, the gallbladder is necrotic or gangrenous and its total removal is necessary to prevent perforation and other complications.

IV. CHOLEDOCHOLITHIASIS

A. Pathogenesis. Stones in the bile ducts may be primary (develop in the duct) or secondary (originate in the gallbladder). If they are discovered after cholecystectomy, they may have been overlooked (retained) or may have formed after the surgery (recurrent).

1. **Primary bile duct stones** are rare in Western countries. They are more common in the Orient and are often associated with biliary infections and parasitic infestations. They are usually pigment stones.

2. **Secondary bile duct stones.** Because 10% to 15% of patients with cholesterol gallstones also have stones in the CBD, it is thought that most CBD stones in the Western countries originate from the gallbladder. In fact, 95% of patients with ductal stones also have stones in the gallbladder.

3. **Stones found in the bile ducts** after cholecystectomy may be retained or may have formed de novo. Bile stasis associated with partial obstruction or marked dilatation of the duct may promote choledocholithiasis. Recurrent stones are often formed from bile pigments.

B. Diagnosis

1. **Clinical presentation**

   a. **Choledocholithiasis** may present in the following ways:

      i. Biliary colic–abdominal pain

      ii. Obstructive jaundice

      iii. Cholangitis

      iv. Pancreatitis

      v. Hemobilia

   b. **The biliary obstruction** caused by cholelithiasis and the ensuing increased biliary pressure and diminished bile flow result in the morbidity associated with duct stones. The rate of progression of the obstruction, its degree, and concomitant bacterial contamination of the biliary tract determine the severity of the syndrome. Thus acute obstruction usually causes colic with or without concomitant pancreatitis; gradual obstruction may present as jaundice. Cholangitis and abscess formation may follow if obstruction is not relieved. Chronic biliary obstruction, if not relieved, may give rise to secondary biliary cirrhosis resulting in hepatic failure and portal hypertension.

   c. **Signs and symptoms.** The most common complaint is right upper abdominal or epigastric pain, which is usually associated with nausea and vomiting. Jaundice, which may be fluctuating or progressive, is also common. If obstruction is severe, dark urine and pale stools may develop. Fever and chills, if present, will signal cholangitis or abscess formation.

2. **Diagnostic studies**

   a. **Laboratory studies.** Elevation of alkaline phosphatase and bilirubin levels is the hallmark of ductal obstruction. Serum amylase may be elevated without concurrent pancreatitis. Elevation of transaminases (ALT, AST) may be seen transiently with passage of a stone. If it persists, along with leukocytosis, cholangitis is suspected.

   b. **Ultrasonography** is the initial diagnostic test of choice in the workup of gallstone disease. Aside from the presence of stones in the gallbladder, dilatation of the biliary tract secondary to obstruction of the bile ducts is clearly seen on ultrasound. If the obstruction occurs acutely, dilatation may not be present.

   In patients who have undergone cholecystectomy, slight dilatation of the CBD (up to 0.8 cm) may be acceptable without the presence of distal obstruction.

   c. **Biliary scintigraphy** using ^{99m}Tc-labeled HIDA or PIPIDA may show obstruction of the CBD in 85% to 90% of cases. In a positive scan, if the cystic duct is patent, the passage of the radionuclide into the gallbladder and the major ducts but not into the small bowel is noted within 1 to 4 hours.

   d. **CT scan is** an excellent method to demonstrate CBD stones, especially those with calcium.

e. MRCP has excellent sensitivity and specificity in visualizing the CBD for stones as well as detecting other structural abnormalities such as ductal dilation, sclerosing cholangitis and cystic abnormalities.

f. ERCP demonstrates the location of the stone or stones in the bile ducts and is preferred in patients with suspected CBD obstruction without intrahepatic ductal dilatation. Endoscopic examination of the upper gastrointestinal tract and the duodenal ampullary orifice helps rule out pathology in these areas. Endoscopic sphincterotomy has replaced operative sphincteroplasty in patients with retained or recurrent CBD stones discovered after cholecystectomy. In most cases, CBD stones smaller than 1.5 cm spontaneously pass into the duodenum after endoscopic sphincterotomy. Stones larger than 1.5 cm can be fragmented and removed with special ERCP catheters, baskets, and balloons. This technique can also be used therapeutically in debilitated patients with CBD stones and intact gallbladders when cholecystectomy and bile duct exploration are medically contraindicated. If an impacted CBD stone is the cause of the pancreatitis, endoscopic removal by sphincterotomy is the preferred immediate mode of therapy. In all cases in which an obstructed CBD is manipulated, broad-spectrum IV antibiotic coverage must be provided to the patient to prevent sepsis.

g. PTC may be used diagnostically and occasionally therapeutically in some patients. If obstruction of the CBD and dilatation of the intrahepatic biliary tract has been demonstrated by ultrasound, the location and the nature of the obstruction can be delineated by PTC. Furthermore, it is possible to relieve the obstruction, even if temporarily, by the insertion of a stent, especially in debilitated patients in whom surgery is contraindicated. Dissolution of CBD cholesterol stones by infusion of solvents such as monooctanoin with a catheter percutaneously placed above the stone or attempts at dislodging and mobilizing the stone and facilitating its passage into the duodenum or withdrawing it percutaneously may be considered for therapy for such patients. Patients should be treated with IV broad-spectrum antibiotics before such attempts.

C. Treatment. In symptomatic patients presenting with stones in the gallbladder and the CBD, the treatment of choice is laparoscopic cholecystectomy and endoscopic stone extraction via ERCP pre- or postoperatively. Cholecystectomy and CBD exploration are reserved for patients with contraindications to the laparoscopic procedure or who require abdominal exploration. If stones are found in the CBD during CBD exploration, they should be removed, and a drainage procedure such as a sphincteroplasty or choledochoenterostomy may be performed to allow the passage of any residual stones into the gut. In these instances, a T tube is placed in the CBD to decompress the biliary duct and to allow the performance of postoperative cholangiograms.

In approximately 2% of the patients, a residual CBD stone is demonstrated on postoperative cholangiograms. These residual stones may be extracted either percutaneously through the T tube or endoscopically by means of ERCP. In situ dissolution of cholesterol stones with monooctanoin or MBTE infusion has also been successful in selected patients. If these methods fail, endoscopic sphincterotomy and stone removal or reoperation may be necessary.

V. Obstructive cholangitis is an inflammation of the bile ducts associated with enteric bacterial infection in the setting of biliary obstruction. Obstruction may be secondary to CBD stones, biliary strictures, choledochal cysts, biliary fistulas, stenosis of biliary–enteric anastomoses, and occasionally malignancy. Mechanical manipulation of the biliary ducts (i.e., during PTC, ERCP, or T-tube studies) may also result in cholangitis.

The **most common organisms** found in the bile in cholangitis are *E. coli, Klebsiella, Proteus, Enterobacter, Pseudomonas, Streptococcus fecalis,* and *Clostridium.* The spillage of the bacteria into the bloodstream often gives rise to bacteremia and sepsis. When infection is severe, invasion of the liver parenchyma may occur, resulting in abscess formation. Recurrent infection and inflammation of the bile ducts may result in strictures, areas of dilatation, and intraductular calcium bilirubinate stone formation. Secondary biliary cirrhosis and portal hypertension may be late sequelae.

A. Diagnosis

    1. Clinical presentation. Patients usually present with intermittent abdominal pain, fever, chills, and jaundice. Dark urine and pale stools suggest the presence of biliary obstruction.

    2. Diagnostic studies. Leukocytosis with a shift to the left and elevation of serum alkaline phosphatase and bilirubin levels are common. Serum ALT, AST, and amylase levels are usually elevated.

B. Treatment. When cholangitis is suspected, prompt diagnosis and relief of the obstruction is essential. Patients should be given IV antibiotics for enteric organisms to prevent sepsis.

    Ultrasonography, ERCP, PTC, and abdominal CT scan may be necessary to diagnose the extent, nature, and location of the obstruction. The choice of definitive treatment for relief of the obstruction depends on the findings. Surgery or other less invasive techniques such as PTC or ERCP may be required.

Selected Readings

Agrawal S, et al. Gallstones, from gallbladder to gut: Management options for diverse complications. *Postgrad Med.* 2000;108:143.

Chuang CZ, et al. Physical activity, biliary lipids and gallstones in obese subjects. *Am J Gastroenterol.* 2001;96:1860.

deLedinghen V, et al. Diagnosis of choledocholithiasis: EUS or magnetic resonance cholangiography? A prospective controlled study. *Gastrointest Endosc.* 1999;49:26.

Donovan JM, et al. Physical and metabolic factors in gallstone pathogenesis. *Gastroenterol Clin N Am.* 1999;28:75–97.

Germanos S, et al. Clinical update: surgery for acute cholecytitis. *Lancet.* 2007;369:1774–1776.

Ko C, et al. Gallbladder disease. *Clin Perspect Gastroenterol.* March/April 2000:87.

Kolla SB, et al. Early vs delayed laparoscopic cholecystectomy for acute cholecystitis: a prospective, randomized trail. *Surg Endos.* 2004;18:1323–1327.

Mendez SN, et al. Intestinal motility and bacterial overgrowth in patients with gallstones. *Gastroenterology.* 2001;120:1310.

Mulholland MW. Progress in understanding acalculus gallbladder disease. *Gastroenterology.* 2001;120:570.

Peng WK, et al. Role of laparoscopic cholecystectomy in the early management of acute gallbladder disease. *Br J Surg.* 2005;92:586–591.

Schirmer BD. Cholelithiasis and cholecystitis. *J Long Term Eff Med Implants.* 2005;15:329–338.

Shaffer EA. Gallbladder sludge: What is its clinical significance? *Curr Gastroenterol Rep.* 2001;3:166.

Throwridge RL, et al. Does this patient have acute cholecystitis? *JAMA.* 2003;299:80–86.

Tsai CJ, et al. Long-term intake of dietary fiber and decreased risk of cholecystectomy. *Am J Gastroenterol.* 2004;99:1364–1370.

Tsai CJ, et al. Dietary protein and risk of cholecystectomy in a cohort of US women: The Nurses Health Study. *Am J Epidemiol.* 2004;160:11–18.

Tsai CJ, et al. Glycemic load, glycemic index, and carbohydrate intake in relation to risk of cholecystitis in women. *Gastroenterology.* 2005;129:105–112.

Verma D, et al. EUS vs MRCP for detection of choledocholithiasis. *Gastrointest Endosc.* 2006;64:248–254.

*H*epatitis can be defined as the constellation of symptoms and signs resulting from hepatic inflammation and hepatic cell necrosis. If the insult is acute and occurs in a previously asymptomatic individual, the term **acute hepatitis** can be applied. The most common causes of acute hepatitis are **viruses, toxins, and alcohol.** Occasionally other disease entities such as Wilson's disease, leukemias, and lymphomas with acute infiltration of the liver may give rise to a clinical picture of acute hepatitis. Viruses, however, are the major etiologic agents of acute liver injury.

Systemic infection with several viruses results in hepatic inflammation and cell death. Viruses that cause hepatitis have been classified as hepatitis **A (HAV), B (HBV), C (HCV), delta (HDV), and E (HEV).** However, in some individuals, infection with the **Epstein-Barr virus (EBV) or cytomegalovirus (CMV)** also results in acute hepatitis.

In most patients, acute viral hepatitis presents as an acute illness characterized by the abrupt onset of malaise, fever, anorexia, nausea, headache, abdominal discomfort, and pain. Jaundice, itching, dark-colored urine, and light-colored stools often cause the patient to seek medical attention. At this stage, the disease caused by different viruses is usually indistinguishable; serologic studies and viral DNA or RNA determination by polymerase chain reaction (PCL) may provide the only means of identification. Pertinent factors regarding the five forms of acute and chronic viral hepatitis are summarized in Tables 50-1 and 50-2.

I. HEPATITIS ASSOCIATED WITH EPSTEIN-BARR VIRUS

   A. Pathogenesis. EBV is a herpes virus and is the causative agent of infectious mononucleosis (IM). Although clinical jaundice occurs in approximately 5% of the cases of IM, hepatitis caused by this virus may be as common as that from HAV and HBV. However, the hepatitis in IM is usually mild and is accompanied by other clinical features of IM.

   1. In most individuals, the **natural primary infection** with EBV occurs asymptomatically in childhood, conferring lifelong immunity to IM in the form of IgG antibodies to EBV. In the industrialized countries, 50% to 60% of the children by age 5 and more than 80% of the individuals by age 20 acquire seropositivity to EBV. Infection tends to occur earlier in lower socioeconomic groups, but symptomatic disease is frequent in college students who were not exposed to EBV in childhood. In adults, symptomatic disease develops in one half of the cases and may be severe in older individuals.

   2. Transmission of the virus occurs through contact with infected saliva. The virus is found in saliva droplets and in the epithelial cells. Blood transfusions have been implicated in a few cases.

   3. In most cases, **the virus initially infects oropharyngeal epithelial cells** with secondary infection of the B lymphocytes with further dissemination of the virus. The incubation period is usually 4 to 7 weeks. The virus can be isolated from oral secretions in 80% of patients with acute IM. The EBV genome is incorporated into some infected B lymphocytes, which incite a cytotoxic T-cell proliferation and response, seen in the peripheral blood smear as the atypical mononuclear cells of IM. Although the cellular and hormonal response brings the infection under control, infection persists in a subpopulation of B lymphocytes. In fact, EBV can be isolated from the saliva of 15% to 20% of asymptomatic adults. Persistent and reactivated infections are rare but do occur.

TABLE 50-1   Five Forms of Viral Hepatitis

	Hepatitis				
	A	**B**	**C**	**D**	**E**
Virus	HAV	HBV	HCV	HDV	HEV
Family	Picornavirus	Hepadnavirus	Flavivirus	Satellite	Calicivirus
Size	27 nm	42 nm	30–60 nm	40 nm	32 nm
Genome	ssRNA	dsDNA	ssRNA	ssRNA	ssRNA
Length	7.8 kb	3.2 kb	10.5 kb	1.7 kb	8.2 kb
Acute mortality	0.2%	0.2%–1.0%	0.2%	2%–20%	0.2%
Chronicity	None	2%–7%	50%–70%	2%–70%	None
Spread	Fecal-oral	Parenteral Sexual Perinatal	Parenteral ? Sexual	Parenteral ? Sexual	Fecal-oral
Antigens	HAV Ag	HBsAg HBcAg HBeAg	HCV Ag	HDV Ag	HEV Ag
Antibodies	Anti-HAV	Anti-HBs Anti-HBc Anti-HBe	Anti-HCV	Anti-HDV	Anti-HEV
Viral markers	HAV-RNA	HBV-DNA DNA polymerase	HCV-RNA	HDV-RNA	Viruslike particles

HAV, hepatitis A virus; HBV, hepatitis B virus; HCV, hepatitis C virus; HDV, hepatitis D virus; HEV, hepatitis E virus; ssRNA, single-stranded RNA; dsDNA, double-stranded DNA; kb, kilobase; Ag, antigen. From Hoofnagle JH, DiBisceglie AM. Serologic diagnosis of acute and chronic viral hepatitis. *Semin Liver Dis.* 1991;11:74. Reprinted with permission.

TABLE 50-2   Serologic Diagnosis of Acute Viral Hepatitis*

Disease	Serologic results	Comments
Hepatitis A	IgM anti-HAV	Reasonably specific
Hepatitis B	HBsAg	Can be negative (early loss)
	IgM anti-HBc	Indicates acute hepatitis
Hepatitis C	Anti-HCV	Can appear late in disease
Hepatitis D	HBsAg and anti-HDV	Anti-HDV can appear late in disease
	IgM anti-HBc present	Coinfection
	IgM anti-HBc absent	Superinfection
Hepatitis E	All negative	History of exposure

HAV, hepatitis A virus; HBsAg, hepatitis B surface antigen; HBc, hepatitis B core; HCV, hepatitis C virus; HDV, hepatitis D virus.
*Initially four tests should be obtained: IgM anti-HAV, IgM anti-HBc, HBsAg, and anti-HCV. In some situations, further testing for anti-HDV and anti-HCV are needed (see text).
From Hoofnagle JH, DiBisceglie AM. Serologic diagnosis of acute and chronic viral hepatitis. *Semin Liver Dis.* 1991;11:11. Reprinted with permission.

B. Clinical presentation. In patients 15 to 30 years old, IM classically presents with fatigue, malaise, fever, anorexia, distaste for food and cigarettes, nausea, vomiting, and headache. Periorbital edema and a rash may be present. Sore throat is common and may be caused by a secondary infection with β-hemolytic *Streptococcus*. Lymphadenopathy and splenomegaly are present in about half of the cases. Ten percent to 15% of the patients have hepatomegaly, and 5% develop jaundice. Hemolytic anemia may be present.

Occasionally in IM, the hepatitis may be the predominant presentation, especially in older patients, and may last 1 to 2 months. In some cases, the clinical presentation of fever, right upper quadrant pain, jaundice, and elevated alkaline phosphatase may mimic extrahepatic obstruction.

1. Diagnostic studies. Mild elevation of transaminases (more than twice normal) and alkaline phosphatase is common. Serum bilirubin is 1 to 8 mg/dL. The hepatitis is usually milder than seen with other viruses. Severe jaundice, liver failure, coagulopathy, and encephalopathy are rare.

In the acute disease, 60% of the patients have an absolute lymphocytosis, and 50% have the "atypical mononuclear cells." The monospot test has a specificity of 99% and a sensitivity of 80%. It may be negative initially in one sixth of the patients and should be repeated. The heterophil antibody is more sensitive and is positive in 90% of the patients. EBV-specific serology (IgM antibody [Ab]) allows for definitive diagnosis but may be negative in early mild IM. A single high virus-specific antibody (IgG) does not reliably distinguish current from previous infection.

C. Treatment. Currently there is no specific treatment for IM hepatitis. Corticosteroids may be of value in severe acute pharyngitis for the edema but do not provide any benefit for other manifestations of IM including hepatitis. Acyclovir sodium has been used in a few cases of persistent severe IM with some clinical improvement.

II. CYTOMEGALOVIRUS INFECTIONS OF THE LIVER

A. Pathogenesis. CMV is a common infectious agent resulting in asymptomatic infection in most individuals. Occasionally, an IM-like illness or hepatitis may occur. In immunosuppressed patients, a severe disseminated infection can result with multisystem disease and a high mortality. CMV infection in acquired immunodeficiency syndrome (AIDS) is discussed in Chapter 43. Transmission is through close contact with infected saliva, urine, and occasionally blood.

Once an infection occurs, the virus persists and cannot be eradicated from the host. The viral genome is incorporated into the host cells and remains latent most of the time. Occasionally, CMV reactivates and is shed in the patient's saliva and urine. In a normal host, these reactivations are controlled by the immune response, but they may present as opportunistic infections in immunocompromised and allograft patients. Viremia in these patients may result in hepatitis as well as infections of other organs. Reinfection is also possible with a different strain of CMV; thus, individuals may bear more than one type of CMV in their cells, which may reactivate at different times.

B. Diagnosis

1. Virus identification. CMV can be cultured from the urine, saliva, blood, and other tissues of infected individuals. The proper laboratory should be consulted ahead of time to expedite the proper method of sampling and delivery of the specimens for best results.

2. Immune response. Primary infection is usually diagnosed by seroconversion. CMV-specific IgG antibody is absent in the acute serum and positive later in the disease course. If an acute sample is not collected, high-titer IgG will not be diagnostic of an acute infection. However, CMV-specific IgM antibodies will be diagnostic for the presence of acute infection. In recurrent infections, virus isolation may be required for diagnosis. None of the normal hosts and only one third of the allograft patients has a rise in IgM titers during CMV recurrences.

3. Liver disease
   a. Primary CMV infections. In patients with primary CMV infections, sub-clinical liver involvement may be common with a mild rise in liver enzyme levels. In others, a mild, self-limited hepatitis with a mild or moderate rise in liver enzymes is present. There may be accompanying hemolysis and atypical mononuclear cells in the peripheral blood smear.
   b. CMV from blood transfusions. In these instances, the virus is thought to be present in blood leukocytes including neutrophils. The onset of disease is 3 to 6 weeks after transfusions. Hepatitis in most patients is accompanied by a mononucleosislike disease.
   c. Transplant patients. In most patients who have undergone transplantation, CMV is found to be a common cause of acute hepatitis. CMV may enter the patient through the transplanted organ or transfusions, or it may be reactivated during immunosuppression. In these patients, chronic infection of the liver may also exist without producing disease.
   d. Liver biopsy specimens may be cultured for CMV. Histologically, liver parenchyma contains the owl-eye inclusions in the hepatocytes and may contain noncaseating granulomas or granulomatous changes.
   e. It is debatable whether CMV can cause massive hepatic necrosis. There is no evidence that CMV causes chronic liver disease in normal hosts. However, in immunocompromised patients (e.g., in patients with AIDS), the hepatobiliary infection may be extensive and chronic. Concomitant liver infections with CMV and HBV have been described.
C. Treatment. In proven cases, intravenous (IV) therapy with ganciclovir sodium may be helpful. Doses used vary from 2.5 mg/kg q8h for 20 days to 5 mg/kg q12h for 14 days. Treatment may need to be continued indefinitely (see Chapter 43) in patients with AIDS.

III. HEPATITIS A. Infections with HAV account for approximately 25% of the clinical hepatitis cases diagnosed in industrialized nations. It occurs both sporadically and in epidemics. In general, it causes less morbidity and mortality than hepatitis virus types B, C, and delta.
A. Pathogenesis. HAV is endemic in underdeveloped countries, where infections usually occur in children and are clinically inapparent. The outcome of the infection seems to depend on the age of the patient and the infecting dose of the virus. The disease is of shorter duration and milder in children. Adults may present with clinically significant disease; fulminant hepatitis occurs with a frequency of 1 to 8 per 1,000 cases. HAV is a 27-nm, nonenveloped RNA enterovirus and belongs to the group picornavirus. All strains of the virus identified to date belong to one serotype. The infection is acquired by the fecal-oral route and can be isolated from the liver, bile, stools, and blood during the late incubation period and acute pre-icteric phase of the disease. Fecal viral shedding and viremia diminish once jaundice occurs.
B. Diagnosis
   1. Clinical presentation. The typical course of a case of acute hepatitis A is shown in Figure 50-1. Hepatitis A has an incubation period of from 2 to 7 weeks with a mean of 4 weeks. In clinically apparent cases, there is an abrupt onset of symptoms. Malaise, fever, anorexia with aversion to food and cigarettes, nausea, and abdominal pain are frequent. Within a few days after the onset of symptoms, there is a marked rise in serum alanine aminotransferase (ALT), aspartate aminotransferase (AST), and bilirubin levels, resulting in jaundice. In approximately 25% of the cases, hepatosplenomegaly is noted.
   2. The duration of the illness is usually less than 1 month, but elevated serum transaminases have been recorded for as long as 6 months.
   3. Complications from hepatitis A are rare. A cholestatic phase may occur in some patients and may mimic obstructive jaundice. Relapses have been seen within 4 to 15 weeks of recovery from the disease and may be precipitated by exertion or alcohol intake. The disease may last 16 to 40 weeks. There may be

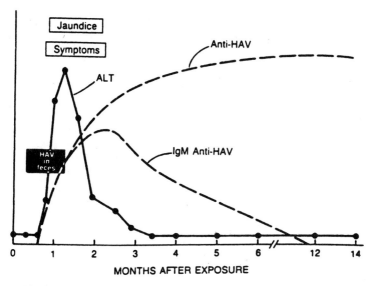

Figure 50-1. Typical course of acute hepatitis A. ALT, alanine aminotransferase; HAV, hepatitis A virus; anti-HAV, antibody to HAV. (From Hoofnagle JH, DiBisceglie AM. Serologic diagnosis of acute and chronic viral hepatitis. *Semin Liver Dis.* 1991;11:74. Reprinted with permission.)

complications from immune complex formation and deposition. There is no evidence that HAV causes a chronic carrier state or chronic liver disease; however, chronic carriers of HBV can be infected with HAV.

    4. Serology. The development of serologic assays for hepatitis A antigen (HAAg) and antibody (Haab) has allowed for accurate diagnosis of HAV infection. HAAg can only be detected in the stool and possibly the blood of viremic patients shedding the virus in the preclinical stages of the disease.

    High titers of HAV-specific IgM antibody develop in all patients by the time of clinical presentation. Thus, the presence of anti-HAV IgM in a jaundiced patient confirms the diagnosis of hepatitis A. The titers of IgM antibody decline over the next few months. IgG antibodies are slower to appear but can be detected in all patients after 3 weeks of disease. The presence of HAV IgG antibody in a patient in the absence of HAV IgM antibody denotes previous infection with HAV with full recovery.

C. The treatment of hepatitis A is supportive. Most patients do not require hospitalization. Patients should receive good nutrition and abstain from alcohol and other hepatotoxic agents. Enteric precautions are recommended to prevent fecaloral transport. In patients with severe cholestatic hepatitis A, steroid therapy may be beneficial. Prednisone 40 mg daily may be given for several weeks and gradually tapered.

D. Prophylaxis. Administration of normal serum immunoglobulin has been shown to provide protection if given before exposure to the virus or during the incubation period of the disease.

    1. Postexposure prophylaxis of 0.02 mg/kg is recommended for household and sexual contacts of patients with hepatitis A within 2 weeks of exposure. Similar prophylaxis is recommended for staff and members of daycare centers and institutions providing custodial care. It is not recommended for contacts in schools, offices, factories, and hospitals unless there is a problem with hygiene.

2. **Travelers** to endemic areas should receive prophylaxis, with the dose of the immunoglobulin dependent on the intended period of stay. For travel of less than 2 months' duration, 0.02 mL/kg should be given, and 0.06 mL/kg for longer periods.

3. **Vaccine.** Over the last several decades, the incidence of HAV infection has been decreasing in industrialized countries. Because infection in early childhood is becoming less common, a population of susceptible adolescents and adults, in whom hepatitis A can be more severe, is emerging. Passive immunization with serum immune globulin (IG) has a limited duration of protection of approximately 3 months. For a longer duration of protection, active immunization with a vaccine is required. Clinical trials with a killed whole virus vaccine have been successful, and the vaccine is now available. The vaccine is administered in three doses intramuscularly into the deltoid muscle at 0, 1, and 6 months. A recombinant complementary DNA vaccine for this RNA virus is also available.

A combination vaccine (Twinrit-Galaxo Smith Kline) containing 20 μg of HBsAg protein (Energix –B) and >720 ELISA units of inactivated Hep A virus (HAV VIX) provides dual protection with three injections at 0, 1, and 6 months.

IV. HEPATITIS B (HB). There are about 2.5 billion people worldwide infected with HB virus (HBV), of these about 350 million persons are chronic carriers and 4 million new HBV infections occur yearly. The highest prevalences of HBV (about 15%) are in the Far East and Southeast Asia, Middle East, Africa, and among Alaskan natives and Pacific Islanders. HBV causes acute and chronic liver disease and liver cancer.

HBV is spread **parenterally (horizontal transmission)** or by intimate contact since HBV is found not only in blood, but also in semen, saliva, and other body secretions. It is believed that transmission in Asia is **perinatal (vertical transmission)** from mother to infant.

The risk factors for transmission include high-risk sexual activity (multiple sexual partners, homosexual activity as in men having sex with men), injection drug use, hemodialysis, living or being born in an endemic area, and working in the health care profession.

There are eight **genotypes** (A–H) of HBV. Genotype A is found in Europe and North America, genotype B and C in the Far East and Southeast Asia, and genotype D mainly in southern Europe, Africa, and India. The clinical significance of genotypes are enfolding (i.e., genotype A and B are more sensitive to treatment with interferon than genotypes C and D).

A. **HBV is a DNA virus** belonging to a class of animal viruses called **hepadna viruses.** These viruses are hepatotropic, tend to cause persistent infections, and have been associated with the development of hepatocellular carcinoma. HBV is unique among human viruses in its genomic and antigenic structure and its replicative cycle.

The structure of HBV is shown in Figure 50-2. It consists of an outer shell made up of a protein (HBsAg) and a complex inner core. The complex inner core or the nucleocapsid core is a 27-nanometer (nm) icosahedral structure that consists of 180 copies of viral core protein (HBcAg) surrounding the viral DNA (genome) and virally encoded DNA polymerase. HBcAg protects the viral genome from

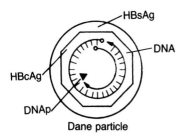

Figure 50-2. Structure of hepatitis B virus. (From Hoofnagle JH, Schafer DF. Serologic markers of hepatitis B virus infection. *Semin Liver Dis.* 1986;6:1. Reprinted with permission.)

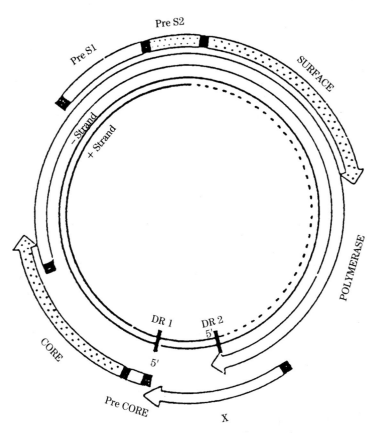

Figure 50-3. Structure of the HBV genome. The thick lines are the DNA strands, and the open reading frames that code for proteins are indicated outside the DNA. Black boxes indicate the start sites of the open reading frames. (From Foster GR, Carman WF, Thomas HC. Replication of hepatitis B and delta viruses: Appearance of viral mutants. *Semin Liver Dis.* 1991;11:122. Reprinted with permission.)

degradation by exogenous nucleases. Figure 50-3 depicts the structure of the HBV genome.

The HBV genome is composed of circular DNA of approximately 3,200 base pairs with a complete negative strand and an incomplete complementary positive strand. The negative strand contains overlapping genes that encode structural proteins (surface proteins and their derivatives and core) and two replicative proteins (polymerase and X). HBV is unique among DNA viruses in that it replicates in a way similar to that of the RNA retroviruses such as the human immunodeficiency virus (HIV) via an RNA intermediate.

Once HBV is blood borne in the host, the replication cycle begins with the attachment of HBV to the hepatocyte cell membrane and entry into the hepatocyte cytoplasm. The virus is then uncoated and the nucleocapsid and the viral DNA are transported into nucleus. Once in the nucleus, the viral genome is repaired by filing in the gap in the positive-strand DNA and forming the covalently closed circular DNA (cc cDNA.) Thus, complexly double-stranded HCV DNA is formed. Synthesis of cc cDNA is catalyzed by the viral DNA polymerase.

The cc cDNA is the template for synthesis of genomic and subgenomic transcripts, catalyzed by host RNA polymerase. Genomic or pregenomic RNA thus formed then acts as the template for future DNA minus-strand synthesis.

Viral RNA transcripts are then transported into the cytoplasm and their translation into proteins yields the viral envelope, core, precore protein, and viral DNA polymerase. Viral Packaging encapsidation occurs in the cytoplasm. Encapsidation involves the assembly of the viral core consisting of 180 molecules of core proteins and the synthesis of the viral DNA by reverse transcription. The template for the minus strand is pregenomic mRNA and the template for the plus strand is minus-strand DNA. The two DNA strands of HBV are made sequentially rather than simultaneously as occurs in conventional DNA replication. Once the DNA synthesis is completed, the template RNA is degraded by specific RNAase which resides in the viral polymerase.

After replication is complete, the viral core is either transported into the nucleus or passes through the endoplasmic reticulum and Golgi apparatus where the core acquires the envelope proteins before exportation from the cell by exocytosis.

Early in HBV infection, some of the nucleocapsid cores are transported back to the nucleus where synthesis of the plus strand is completed and stable cc cDNA molecules are formed. The cc cDNA molecules form a reservoir of transcriptional templates so that after cell division of the infected hepatocytes, infection will be propagated to daughter hepatocytes. When the HBV infection is well established, nucleocapsid cores are preferentially exported from the hepatocytes facilitating the horizontal spread of infection throughout the liver.

Integration of HBV-DNA either intact or more frequently in fragments into the host genome does occur in chronic HBV infection and is implicated in hepatic carcinogenesis.

B. Pathogenesis. At the entry of HBV and its invasion of hepatocytes, viral proteins are expressed on the hepatocyte membrane. These proteins are recognized by the host immune systems, both the humoral and the cellular arms. If the host immune response to the infected hepatocytes is strong enough to destroy all the involved cells, "hepatitis" results in clearance of the virus.

However, if the immune response is inadequate to completely obliterate the infected hepatocytes, an ongoing viral infection ensues with varying degrees of hepatic inflammatory response.

If the HBV infection occurs perinatally (i.e., by vertical transmission, before the immune system of the infant is fully developed), an inadequate immune response is mounted and viral persistence results (immune tolerance).

C. Serology. Infection with HBV results in an overproduction of HBsAg outnumbering the intact virus by 10 million to 1. Assays to detect various HBV-related antigens and antibodies in the serum of infected individuals are summarized in Figure 50-4.

Hepatitis B e antigen (HBeAg) is an internal antigen of HBcAg particles that can be detected in the serum of patients with high levels of circulating HBV. HBeAg is found only in HBsAg-positive serum and signals active ongoing infection and infectivity. HBcAg is found only within the infected hepatocytes and not in the serum. The hepatitis B antibodies (Ab) are described in the following sections.

D. HBV infection. Infection with HBV may present in one of six clinical states: **acute hepatitis, immune tolerant state, chronic hepatitis, inactive asymptomatic carrier state, and cirrhosis and hepatocellular carcinoma.** Infection with HBV in older children and adults can lead to several outcomes.

Approximately two thirds of the individuals infected with HBV have a transient subclinical infection, followed by rapid clearance of the virus with a strong immune response, production of high titers of HBsAb, and permanent immunity. HBcAb is also produced in these individuals but does not confer or suggest immunity.

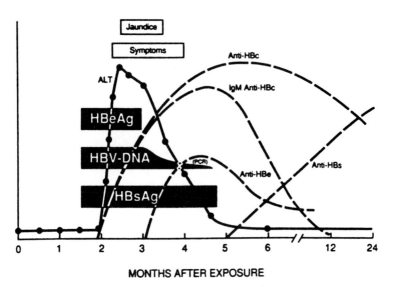

Figure 50-4. Typical course of acute hepatitis B. Initially, HBV-DNA can be detected by blot hybridization, but as the disease resolves, only low levels can be detected using polymerase chain reaction. ALT, alanine aminotransferase; HBsAg, hepatitis B surface antigen; HBeAg, hepatitis B e antigen; HBV-DNA, hepatitis B virus DNA; anti-HBc, antibody to hepatitis B core antigen; anti-HBe, antibody to HBeAg; anti-HBS, antibody to HBsAg; PCR, polymerase chain reaction. (From Hoofnagle JH, DiBisceglie AM. Serologic diagnosis of acute and chronic viral hepatitis. *Semin Liver Dis.* 1991;11:75. Reprinted with permission.)

E. Acute hepatitis. The outcomes of HBV infection are outlined in Figure 50-5. About one fourth of individuals with HBV infection develop clinically apparent acute hepatitis. The incubation period, or time between exposure and onset of symptoms, is 1 to 6 months. During this time, there is active viral replication, and the patient's serum becomes positive for HBsAg, DNA, and HBcAb IgM.

1. Clinical presentation. Before jaundice and typical clinical findings of hepatitis become apparent, these patients may present with rash, neuralgia, arthralgia, arthritis, glomerulonephritis, and polyarteritis nodosa, vasculitis, mixed cryoglobulinemia, pericarditis, pancreatitis, and aplastic anemia. These disease states are believed to result from circulating antigen-antibody complexes.

2. Laboratory tests

a. As the patient becomes symptomatic, there is a concomitant rise in serum ALT and AST (5–20 times normal) and a moderate elevation of the serum alkalie phosphatase (2–10 times normal). These enzymes represent hepatocellular damage. Serum bilirubin may reach very high levels (>30 mg/dL).

Prothrombin time (PT) and partial thromboplastin time (PTT) levels may also become abnormal depending on the severity of the liver disease.

b. Serum HBV-DNA becomes undetectable in these patients within 1 to 8 weeks after the onset of symptoms. HBcAg also disappears soon after the peak of serum transaminase. HBsAg usually remains detectable in the serum throughout the illness and may persist even into convalescence. This is because the initial HBsAg titers are very high, and because HBsAg has a long half-life of 8 days, it may take months to clear it to undetectable levels.

c. HBcAb is present in high titers in the serum of infected patients with HBV when jaundice appears. The initial antibody is of IgM type; with recovery, the IgM type disappears, and the IgG HBcAb titers reach high levels and persist for life.

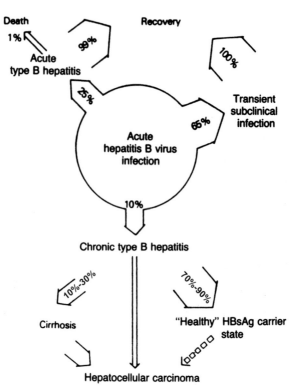

Figure 50-5. Outcomes of acute hepatitis B virus infection in adults. (From Hoofnagle JH, Schafer DF. Serologic markers of hepatitis B virus infection. *Semin Liver Dis.* 1986;11:1. Reprinted with permission.)

    d. HBeAb appears when HBeAg becomes negative and often disappears within a few months or years.

    e. HBsAb arises during recovery after HBsAg has cleared. There is usually a "window" period between the disappearance of HBsAg and the appearance of HBsAb. The only way to make the diagnosis of acute hepatitis in these individuals is to show the presence of HBcAb (IgM type). A minority of the patients (5%–15%) who clear HBV and recover normally never develop HBsAb. However, most of these individuals have positive IgM HBcAb.

    f. In some patients (10%), HBV clearance is very rapid, and HBsAg levels may be absent at the onset of symptoms. These acutely ill patients have positive IgM HBcAb titers and may have detectable HBeAg levels. These variations are more common in both mild and fulminant disease.

    g. HBV-DNA can be detected and measured quantitatively with specific assays. The hybridization assay measures replicating HBV-DNA whereas the amplication assay performed using the polymerase chain reaction (PCR) measures HBV-DNA nonspecifically.

3. Prognosis. In patients who can mount a vigorous immune response, the virus is cleared, and recovery is within a few months (1–6 months). A minority of the patients with acute hepatitis (1%–5%) develop fulminant hepatic failure (FHF) due to massive hepatic necrosis. The prognosis in these patients is poor and depends on hepatic regeneration.

The risk of HBV infection becoming chronic varies with the age of the patient at the initial infection. In an immunocompetent adult, the risk is <5%, in an immune compromised adult >50%, in early childhood 50%, and in the newborn 90%.

F. Chronic HBsAg carrier state and chronic hepatitis

   1. Clinical course and serology. About one tenth of adult patients infected with HBV do not clear the virus and remain HBsAg positive. Some of these patients develop chronic progressive hepatitis, and others may remain in a clinically quiescent "carrier" state. Figure 50-6 summarizes the serologic course of chronic type B hepatitis in immune competent adults.

      a. In patients who develop chronic type B hepatitis, the initial pattern of HBV markers is similar to that in patients with acute, self-limited hepatitis. However, in patients with ongoing active disease, HBeAg and HBV-DNA persist and accompany elevated serum transaminases even after 6 months of symptomatic disease.

      b. In most patients, the initial disease is mild, and some patients may be anicteric and symptomatic. These patients may present with only nonspecific symptoms of anorexia and fatigue and mild-to-moderate elevation of liver tests.

      c. IgM HBcAb levels remain elevated in chronic active type B hepatitis. As the disease wanes, the titers diminish with an increase in IgG HBcAb.

      d. Patients who remain HBsAg positive do not produce specific HBsAb. However, in 20% to 40% of HBsAg carriers, there may be low levels of HBsAb directed toward HBsAg subdeterminants not present in the serum.

      e. The course of chronic HBV infection varies. The activity of the liver disease and the serologic markers change over time. In approximately one half of these patients, HBeAg disappears and is replaced by HBeAb. Concomitantly, there is a flare of the hepatitis with elevated ALT and AST levels and loss of

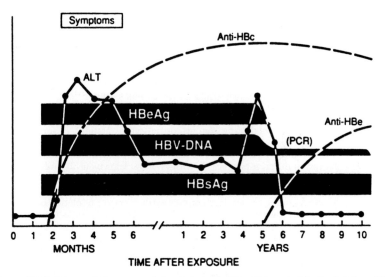

Figure 50-6. Representative course of chronic hepatitis B in which acute infection is followed by chronic infection. Ultimately, there is a remission in disease when seroconversion from HBeAg to anti-HBe occurs. ALT, alanine aminotransferase; HBeAg, hepatitis B e antigen; HBV-DNA, hepatitis B virus DNA; HBsAg, hepatitis B surface antigen; PCR, polymerase chain; anti-HBc, antibody to hepatitis B core antigen; anti-HBe, antibody to HBeAg. (Hoofnagle JH, DiBisceglie AM. Serologic diagnosis of acute and chronic viral hepatitis. *Semin Liver Dis.* 1991;11:75. Reprinted with permission.)

DNA from serum. This is followed by marked improvement of liver histology and a decrease in serum transaminases. The transition from the viral replicative phase, suggested by the presence of HBeAg, to the nonreplicative phase, suggested by the presence of HBeAb, is marked by an increased immune response of the patient to clear viral replication.

f. HBsAg persists in the serum of most of these patients even though there may be no evidence of viral replication. These individuals are referred to as the "healthy HBsAg carriers" or they are in the immune tolerant state.

g. If the HBV infection has occurred in adulthood, approximately 1% of the patients also clears the HBsAg and becomes HBsAb positive. Because previous liver damage has occurred in these patients, they are usually left with some degree of cirrhosis. These individuals account for some of the patients with "cryptogenic" cirrhosis.

h. In some patients, chronic HBV infection remains in the viral replicative stage. This may be continuous, with positive HBeAg titers; or intermittent or low grade, with undetectable HBeAg. The latter pattern is more common in the Far East and with HBV infection early in life.

Integration of HBV-DNA into the hepatocyte DNA occurs during chronic HBV infection and persistent viral replication. This may be a necessary step in the development of hepatocellular carcinoma in patients with previous HBV infection.

i. In 10% to 30% of the patients with chronic HBV hepatitis, cirrhosis develops accompanied by its complications of portal hypertension, esophageal varices, ascites, and encephalopathy. The level of IgM HBcAb correlates with the activity of the chronic hepatitis. High titers are found in severe exacerbations, moderate titers in moderately active disease, and low titers in mild cases. Patients who are healthy HBsAg carriers with no evidence of active liver disease have no detectable IgM HBcAb titers.

2. **The determining factors for development of chronic hepatitis after HBV infection** are (a) the age of the individual when initially infected, (b) the immune status of the host, (c) gender, and (d) the severity of the acute infection.

Ninety percent to 95% of infected neonates and about 30% to 50% of children but only 1% to 10% of adults develop chronic disease. Women are less affected than men, and the disease becomes chronic much more frequently in patients undergoing hemodialysis, in other intrinsically or iatrogenically immunocompromised patients, and in those with HIV coinfection. The severity of the initial disease appears to have little predictive value when the age of onset and the host immune status are taken into account.

3. **Reactivation of quiescent chronic HBV infection** occurs spontaneously or, more frequently, in individuals following the withdrawal of immunosuppressive drugs (e.g., chemotherapy, steroids, organ transplantation). In some patients, reactivation may precipitate fulminant hepatic necrosis. Most individuals with reactivation have positive HBsAg titers without positive HBeAg titers. In some patients, if the prior presence of HBsAg was not known due to subclinical acute disease, reactivation may be regarded as the initial acute infection. In these individuals, HBeAg, DNA and IgM HBcAb all may become positive. The initial loss of HBeAg in the carrier does not necessarily represent resolution of the infection, which suggests that HBV infection may become latent as the herpesvirus infections do. Recent data suggest that HBV may infect and reside quietly in the lymphocytes in the spleen of previously infected individuals.

4. **HBV mutants.** HBV polymerase is an RNA/DNA transcriptase that lacks a proofreading function. During viral replication, it frequently transcribes its template incorrectly, creating mutant viruses. Many of these mutants are incapable of forming infectious virions. However, several infectious HBV mutants have been identified by PCR. One of these mutants contains a point mutation in the gene coding the "surface" protein in the highly antigenic "a" determinant of HBsAg. This mutation alters the antigenic properties of the HBV, allowing it to escape the protective effects of the HBV vaccine.

Another mutant of HBV has been identified in patients who have active hepatitis B but lack HBeAg. These hepatitis B virions have a point mutation in the precore gene. This mutation prevents the synthesis of the precore-core protein and abolishes the formation of HBeAg, which modulates viral infection. Lack of HBeAg expression on the infected hepatocytes prevents immunologic recognition and destruction of these infected cells, resulting in chronic active hepatitis.

5. **Superinfection.** HBV carriers may develop hepatic superinfections with other hepatotropic viruses. Sudden increases in the serum transaminases may represent superinfection with HAV, HCV, or HDV.

   a. **HAV infection** may be a superinfection or simultaneous coinfection and is usually associated with more severe and fulminant hepatitis.

   b. **HCV superinfections** may be difficult to document accurately due to the delay of detectability of HBcAb in acute HCV infections. However, the diagnosis can be made in the face of increased serum transaminases with reduction of HBsAg titers due to viral interference, and negative tests for IgM HBcAb, IgM HAV, and anti-HDV. HCV DNA titers should be measured in ongoing hepatitis.

   c. **HDV** superinfection is discussed in section V.

   d. **Nonviral causes.** It should always be kept in mind that sudden increases in the serum transaminases may result from nonviral causes, such as drug and alcohol hepatotoxicity, shock, congestive heart failure, right ventricular failure, and extrahepatic biliary obstruction.

6. **The differential diagnosis of HBsAg-positive acute viral hepatitis** is summarized in Table 50-3.

7. **Primary hepatocellular carcinoma (HCC).** In the parts of the world where HBV infection is endemic (e.g., Far East, sub-Saharan Africa), PHC is the leading cause of death from cancer. It appears that persistent HBV infection is the leading cause of PHC. This suggests that HBV is an oncogenic virus. The presence of cirrhosis is not necessary for transformation into HCC.

   a. **Predisposing factors.** Some of the predisposing factors for development of HCC are race (e.g., Asians, Inuits), age at infection (especially infancy and early childhood), chronic-persistent infection, and the presence of environmental cocarcinogenic factors, such as ingestion of ethanol, cigarette smoking, and possibly exposure to aflatoxin.

 TABLE 50-3   **Differential Diagnosis of HBsAg-Positive Acute Viral Hepatitis**

Diagnosis	Suggestive features
Acute hepatitis B	IgM anti-HBc
Acute delta hepatitis (coinfection)	IgM anti-HBc and anti-HDV
Chronic hepatitis B with	
Acute hepatitis A	IgM anti-HAV
Delta hepatitis (superinfection)	Anti-HDV
Acute hepatitis C	Anti-HCV
Reactivation	Change in HBV markers
Other acute liver injury	Drug or alcohol history
	Evidence of other liver disease

HBc, hepatitis B core; HDV, hepatitis delta virus; HAV, hepatitis A virus; HCV, hepatitis C virus; HBV, hepatitis B virus.
Adapted from Hoofnagle JH, Schafer DF. Serologic markers of hepatitis B virus infection. *Semin Liver Dis.* 1986;6:1. Reprinted with permission.

b. **Pathogenesis.** It is thought that the integration of HBV-DNA into the DNA of the hepatocyte leads to alterations in cellular gene expression and cellular transformation. The resulting clones of transformed cells may become autonomous and form HCC.

c. **Diagnosis.** Early clinical detection of HCC is difficult. However, determination of elevation of serum alpha-fetoprotein (AFP) levels and demonstration of a mass in the liver by ultrasonography (US) or computed tomography (CT) scanning, or magnetic resonance imaging (MRI) are used currently on a yearly basis with reasonable success. Tissue diagnosis can be made by needle biopsy of the liver under US or CT guidance.

G. **Treatment**

1. **Acute HBV infection.** The treatment of acute HBV infection is supportive. Most patients recover promptly. Those in whom FHF develops require intensive care with appropriate treatment of the accompanying complications.

2. **Chronic HBV infection.** Advances have been made in the last decade in diagnosis and the treatment of chronic HBV infection. Chronic HBV infection is diagnosed by confirming the presence of HBsAg at least on two occasions 6 or more months apart. Serum transaminase levels, serologic tests, quantitative HBV-DNA level, and the liver histology can be used to categorize patients as belonging to one of the **three phases of chronic hepatitis B infection** (Table 50-4). These phases are **immune tolerant, immune reactive,** and **inactive carrier.**

It is important to note that patients do not remain in one of these groups indefinitely. Thus, the liver enzymes, HBV-DNA levels, and HBeAg and HBsAg status should be repeated every 6 to 12 months to detect changes in the status of the patient.

Patients in the **immune tolerant phase** are characterized by having normal or minimally elevated transaminases, minimal to no necroinflammatory activity on liver biopsy, positive HBeAg and negative HBeAb, and high HBV-DNA levels (10^5 copies/mL) Patients in this phase rarely respond to antiviral therapy and usually do not progress to severe liver disease. Antiviral therapy is not currently recommended for patients in the immune tolerant phase. However, many individuals in the immune tolerant phase will eventually enter a more active phase called the **immune reactive phase.** This is heralded by a rise in the transaminase levels and decreased HBV-DNA levels. Antiviral therapy is recommended at this phase of the disease.

| TABLE 50-4 | Clinical Characteristics of Three Phases of Chronic HBV Infection |

| | | | Immune reactive | |
Clinical profile	Inactive carrier	Immune tolerant	HBeAg+	HBeAg Mutant
HBeAg	−	+	+	−
HBeAb	+	−	−	+
HBV-DNA by PCR (copies/mL)	$<10^4$	$>10^5$	$>10^5$	$>10^4$
ALT	Normal	Normal	Elevated	Elevated
Liver biopsy	Inactive	Inactive	Active	Active
Treatment	Not recommended	Not recommended	Recommended	Recommended

If the patient appears to be in the immune tolerant phase and has normal transaminases, HBV-DNA >100,000 copies/mL, but has evidence of necroinflammation or fibrosis on liver biopsy, antiviral therapy is recommended.

There are data suggesting that high HBV-DNA levels may be associated with increased risk of hepatocellular carcinoma (HCC) even in patients with no active inflammation in the liver. This may be a reason to treat patients with HBV-DNA greater than 10,000 copies/mL. However, this is still controversial since there is no evidence currently that lowering HCV-DNA levels decreases the risk of HCC in patients with normal transaminases. A family history of HCC should lower the threshold for initiation of therapy in these patients.

In the **immune reactive phase** patients have variable degrees of elevation of the transaminases, evidence of necroinflammatory changes on liver biopsy, and often high HBV-DNA levels ($>10^5$ copies/mL). Patients in this phase are the ones most likely to benefit from antiviral therapy since, if left untreated, the ongoing necroinflammatory activity will more likely progress to cirrhosis and HCC.

In the immune reactive phase, most patients are HBeAg positive and HBeAb negative. However, there is a subgroup of patients who are HBeAg negative and HBeAb positive despite high levels of HBV-DNA. This type of infection is referred to **HBeAg mutant infection**. The mutation in these viruses occurs in the precore or core promoter region of the HBV genome giving rise to a strain of HBeAg that is incapable of producing HBeAg despite ongoing viral replication. Evolution of this strain usually follows a period of active disease. Approximately 30% to 50% of these patients intermittently have normal transaminases and low HBV-DNA levels. Patients infected with the HBeAg mutant virus are less likely to transition to an inactive state and appear to be at a greater risk of chronic liver disease complications even with lower HBV-DNA levels ($>10^4$ copies/mL). Antiviral therapy in these patients often results in lowering HBV-DNA and transaminase levels and results in histologic improvement. However, disease activity returns if antiviral therapy is stopped. Thus, most of these patients require lifelong therapy.

It is important to differentiate between patients infected with HBeAg mutant virus from inactive carriers who are also HBeAg negative and HBeAb positive. Inactive carriers have persistently low HBV levels ($<10^4$ copies/mL) and normal transaminases.

Inactive carrier state is characterized by normal transaminases, positive HBeAb, negative HBeAg, no evidence of inflammatory activity on liver biopsy, and very low nondetectable levels ($<10^4$ copies/mL) of HBV-DNA.

In this phase progression of liver damage does not occur and reactivation is uncommon. These patients do not require antiviral therapy. However, these patients should be followed clinically every 6–12 months.

Reactivation of viral replication and active HBV hepatitis may occur if the patients are treated with chemotherapy, corticosteroids, or other agents that may cause immunosuppression. Antiviral treatment of HBV should be instituted promptly with active disease.

The goal of therapy for chronic HBV infection ideally is to "cure" the patient by completely eradicating the HB virus. This is seldom possible. However, in a minority of patients, conversion from HBsAg to HBsAb may occur spontaneously or during other antiviral therapies.

Achievable qualitative goals include symptomatic improvement, prevention of long-term complications of chronic liver disease such as cirrhosis and HCC, reduction of morbidity and mortality, and prevention of spread of infection of HBV to others. Quantitatively, the goals of therapy include the suppression or loss of HBV-DNA, seroconversion from HBeAg positivity to HBeAb positivity, normalization of transaminases, and histologic improvement on liver biopsy.

a. **Interferons (IFN)** are endogenous glycoproteins with antiviral, antiproliferative, and immunoregulatory properties. Interferon-α, derived from leukocytes, and interferon-β, derived from fibroblasts, are similar and occupy the same receptor on the target cells. Interferon-γ, derived from T cells, is different and occupies a different receptor. Interferon has properties that have an impact on both viral replication and host HLA class I expression. These effects enhance the recognition of the infected hepatocytes by cytolytic T lymphocytes. Thus, both the antiviral and the immunoregulatory effects of interferons are necessary for effective antiviral therapy of chronic hepatitis B.

b. Recombinant interferon-α has been used with some success in the treatment of chronic HBV. In several studies, when 5 million units of IFN-α were given subcutaneously (SC) every day or 10 million units three fimes weekly for 4 to 6 months, approximately 28% to 35% of patients experienced a sustained loss of HBV-DNA, compared with none of the untreated, control patients. The loss of HBV-DNA is noted to occur after 6 to 12 weeks of interferon therapy and is accompanied by an acute hepatitislike elevation of aminotransferase activity, which suggests enhanced cytolytic T-cell (CTL) activity against virus-infected hepatocytes.

Outside of the above studies, treatment of patients with chronic HBV with recombinant IFN-α has not been very successful. The drug and treatment are poorly tolerated by patients and the above results have not been duplicated.

c. In more recent studies, treatment with Pegasys or PEG-IFN2b **(polyethylene glycol interferon-2b)** at a dose of 180 μg/week administered subcutaneously for 12 months gave more promising results (32% HBeAg seroconversion to HBeAb and 3% HBsAg conversion to HBsAb). Patients with HBV genotypes A and B seem to have greater success with PEG-IFN therapy than with the other HBV genotypes. Also, combination therapy or the addition of a nucleoside (i.e., Lamivudine, to PEG-IFN therapy) did not increase the therapeutic yield.

d. Side effects of interferon therapy. The side effects of interferon therapy are systemic flulike symptoms, bone marrow suppression, autoimmune phenomena (e.g., autoimmune thyroiditis, asymptomatic appearance of autoantibodies), and infections related to granulocytopenia, and psychiatric disturbances, especially depression.

e. Nucleoside and nucleotides. Lamivudine is the first oral nucleoside analog approved by the FDA to treat HBV infection. It works by inhibiting HBV-DNA replication when HBeAg-positive patients are treated with lamivudine at a dose of 100 mg/d over 1 year. HBeAb seroconversion is observed in approximately 15% to 18% of patients. Longer duration of therapy has been associated with higher HBeAb conversion rates. However, the treatment with lamivudine has limited efficacy due to the development of HBV-YMDD mutants that are resistant to the drug. The rate of resistance is 20% at the end of the first year of treatment and goes up to 70% in 3 or 4 years. Relapses of active hepatitis are common with the development of YMDD mutants and/or after discontinuation of therapy. In addition, the development of lamivudine resistance also negatively impacts the ability of the virus to respond to newer, more potent antiviral drugs.

Adefovir dipivoxil is an oral nucleotide that inhibits HBV-DNA replication by suppressing HBV-DNA polymerase. One-year therapy of HBeAg-positive patients with adefovir 10 mg daily results in 12% seroconversion to HBeAb, and the seroconversion increases up to 40% after 4 years of therapy. Determination of early response to therapy (by 6 months) is recommended since 50% of patients may not respond as indicated by a decrease of HBV-DNA viral load to <4/log copies/mL.

Resistance to adefovir is less than that toward lamivudine (1.5%–2% per year); however, it rises to 20% to 25% after 5 years of treatment. Fortunately, adefovir-resistant mutants are sensitive to lamivudine and adefovir is active against lamivudine-resistant strains of HBV. Resistant patients are treated with combination therapy. Adefovir as well as lamivudine may be used effectively in the treatment of HBeAg-negative patients. Monitoring of renal function is recommended during therapy.

Entecavir is a newer nucleoside analog approved by the FDA for use in the treatment of both HBeAg-positive and -negative patients. It has more potent antiviral activity against HBV than lamivudine and adefovir at doses of 0.5 mg or 1 mg daily taken orally. Approximately 20% of HBeAg-positive patients achieve HBe antibody seroconversion by the end of 1 year of treatment. The response increases up to 54% by the end of the second year of therapy with no emergence of resistance. Histologic improvement has also been demonstrated in these patients. In patients infected with lamivudine-resistant HBV mutants, 1-mg daily dose is effective. Unfortunately, up to 7% of patients infected with HBV resistant to lamivudine may also be cross-resistant to entecavir as well. Entecavir has no antiviral activity against HIV.

Tenofovir is a nucleotide analog which has been used in HIV treatment. It has been shown to be effective for the treatment of HBV and lamivudine-resistant HBV. It has a more potent treatment potential than adefovir with no side effects. It is ideal for treatment of patients coinfected with both HBV and HIV. However, resistant HBV develops similarly to Lamivudine after 2 years of therapy.

Newer agents include **telbivudine** 600 mg daily, an oral nucleoside analog that has been shown to have superior therapeutic benefit compared to lamivudine 100 mg daily in HBeAg-positive and -negative patients. So for no resistance has been seen after 2 years of therapy.

Clevudine and pradefovir are also close to being approved by FDA for the treatment of chronic HBV infection.

In summary, there is currently no standard therapy for patients with chronic HBV infection who are in immune reactive phase. In selected patients, especially those who were infected after early childhood and with no contraindication for interferon therapy, a one-year course of therapy with pegylated interferon alfa-2-a may provide a good chance of HBeAg seroconversion with a finite duration of treatment. This treatment has been shown to be more effective in patients infected with HBV genotype A.

In others, the most potent oral antiviral agent available with no or low resistance profile should be selected. In patients who clear HBV-DNA and achieve seroconversion of HBeAg to HBeAb, 6 to 12 months of further therapy is recommended. For patients with HBeAg-negative chronic infection, oral therapy with a nucleotide that has the least resistance profile should be selected since the treatment is expected to be indefinite.

Patients who have developed lamivudine resistance should be treated with combination therapy of adefovir or tenofovir or switched to entecavir at 1 mg daily. It is expected that combination therapy will be used in most patients in the future.

H. Hepatitis B vaccine and prophylaxis

1. Hepatitis B vaccine. HBV infection as acute or chronic disease is a major public health problem throughout the world. In Asia and Africa, HBV infection occurs primarily perinatally or in childhood, resulting in a 10% to 15% rate of chronic infection in the adult population. In the developed countries where the infection occurs mostly in adults, the chronic infection rate is lower (1%–10%) but still results in sizable morbidity and mortality.

Hepatitis B vaccine is indicated for immunization against infection caused by all known subtypes of HBV. Because hepatitis D (caused by the delta virus) does not occur in the absence of HBV infection, it can be expected that hepatitis D will also be prevented by hepatitis B vaccination. Immunization is recommended for people of all ages, especially those who are or will be at increased risk of exposure to HBV (Table 50-4).

a. The first-generation hepatitis B vaccines are derived from the plasma of chronic HBsAg carriers who are HBeAg negative. The vaccines are composed of purified HBsAg and induce protective HBsAb but no antibodies to the other HBV antigens. They have been available since 1980 and have been considered both effective and safe. Due to new concerns about the safety of this human plasma-derived vaccine, however, it is no longer in use in the United States.

b. The second-generation hepatitis B vaccines are manufactured using other methods (i.e., using HBsAg produced by other cell lines or organisms through recombinant DNA technology). The recombinant hepatitis B vaccine produced from yeast has been studied for safety and efficacy in humans and is as good as the plasma-derived hepatitis B vaccine. It has replaced the plasma-derived vaccine in the United States and is administered to children as part of the complete vaccination schedule.

There are two recombinant hepatitis B vaccines currently in use in the United States. Engerix-B contains 20 mg/mL, and Recombivax HB, 10 mg/mL of HBsAg protein. The dose for Engerix-B for neonates and children up to 10 years is 0.5 mL (10 mg), and for older children and adults, 1.0 mL (20 mg) is administered to the deltoid muscle at 0, 1, and 6 months. The vaccine is administered SC if the patient has a bleeding diathesis (e.g., hemophilia or a coagulopathy). An alternative dosing schedule with injections at 0, 1, and 2 months may be used for some populations (e.g., neonates born of HBV-infected mothers, others who have or might have been exposed to HBV, and travelers to high-risk areas). On this alternative schedule, an additional dose at 12 months is recommended for infants born of infected mothers and for others for whom prolonged maintenance of protective titers is desired. For hemodialysis patients, the dose is increased to 40 mg (2 mL) because the vaccine-induced protection is less complete and may persist only as long as antibody levels remain above 10 mIU/mL.

Recombivax HB is given in a similar dosing schedule to Engerix-B (0, 1, and 6 months) using different volumes (Table 50-5).

Protection against HBV infection by hepatitis B vaccines correlates well with HBsAb response produced in the host. Protection may not be complete before the antibody develops in the first few months after the first dose of the vaccine. The efficacy is increased if the intramuscular injection is given in the deltoid muscle rather than in the buttock. After immunization, 95% of healthy individuals develop the HBsAb. The antibody response depends on the individual's age and immune competence; younger persons respond better than older persons. Children and neonates respond quite well; however, immunodeficient patients such as those on hemodialysis or chemotherapy do not respond as well as healthy individuals. Most persons have substantial HBsAb levels even 5 years after their initial vaccination. The duration of the persistence correlates with the level of antibody response after the immunization. Thus, the timing of the booster doses remains controversial. However, levels of antibody below 10 mIU/mL sample-to-negative-control (S/N) counts per minute by radioimmunoassay may not be protective. This level may be used as a guide in individuals susceptible to the HBV infection for booster administration.

Interestingly, in healthy individuals even vaccines with minimal or undetectable HBsAb long after vaccination appear to be protective against clinically apparent HBV and chronic HBV infection. Based on the apparent long-term protection provided by vaccination and the absence of data demonstrating that booster immunization has an advantage over natural exposure, the U.S. Public Health Service has issued no recommendations for booster vaccination for healthy people. Hemodialysis patients and patients with immunosuppression may need booster injections when serum levels of HBsAb fall below 10 mIU/mL.

The recommended booster dose of Engerix-B is 10 mg for neonates and children up to 11 years of age, 20 mg for older children and adults, and 40 mg for hemodialysis patients. The dose of Recombivax-B for booster injection for hemodialysis patients is 40 mg; for other age groups, the dose is the same as in the initial injections.

A **combination vaccine** (Twinrix-Glaxo Smith Kline) containing 20 μg of HBsAg protein (Energix-B) and >720 ELISA units of inactivated hepatitis A virus (Havrix) provides dual protection against infection with HVA and SBV with three injections spaced 0, 1, and 6 months apart. It is indicated for all individuals with risk of both HAV and HBV infection.

It is recommended that all children receive HAV and HBV vaccination routinely.

TABLE 50-5 Recommended Dose and Schedule of Hepatitis B Vaccines

Recombivax HB

Group	Formulation	0 mo	1 mo	6 mo
Birth through 10 years of age	10 µg/mL	0.25 mL (2.5 µg)	0.25 mL (2.5 µg)	0.25 mL (2.5 µg)
11–19 years of age	10 µg/mL	0.5 mL (5 µg)	0.5 mL (5 µg)	0.5 mL (5 µg)
≥20 years of age	10 µg/ml	1.0 mL (10 µg)	1.0 mL (10 µg)	1.0 mL (10 µg)
Hemodialysis patients	40 µg/mL	1.0 mL (40 µg)	1.0 mL (40 µg)	1.0 mL (40 µg)
Infants born to HBsAg-positive mothers	10 µg/mL	0.5 mL (5 µg) + 0.5 mL HBIG	0.5 mL (5 µg)	0.5 mL (5 µg)

Engerix-B

Group	Formulation	0 mo	1 mo	2 mo/6 mo[a]	12 mo[b]
Birth through 10 years of age	20 µg/mL	0.5 mL (10 µg)	0.5 mL (10 µg)		0.5 mL (10 µg)
≥11 years of age	20 µg/mL	1.0 mL (20 µg)	1.0 mL (20 µg)		1.0 mL (20 µg)
Hemodialysis patients	20 µg/mL	2.0 mL (40 µg)	2.0 mL (40 µg)	2.0 mL (40 µg)	
Infants born to HBsAg-positive mothers	20 µg/mL	0.5 mL (10 µg) + 0.5 mL HBIG	0.5 mL (10 µg)	0.5 mL (10 µg)	
HBIG prophylaxis-postexposure		0.06 mL/kg			

[a]See Section VI for choice of 2 mo versus 6 mo for third dose.
[b]See Section VI for indication.
HB, hepatitis B; HBsAg, hepatitis B surface antigen; HBIG, hepatitis B immune globulin.

2. **Immune prophylaxis.** Hepatitis B vaccine alone is recommended for preexposure prophylaxis of susceptible individuals. When there is both an immediate and a long-term risk, hepatitis B immune globulin (HBIG) and hepatitis B vaccine (passive–active immunization) should be given in separate injection sites. This is recommended for people who have been exposed to HBV (a) through percutaneous (needle stick), ocular, or mucous membrane exposure to blood known or presumed to contain HBsAg; (b) from human bites by known or presumed HBsAg carriers that penetrate the skin; or (c) following intimate sexual contact with known or presumed HBsAg carriers. The HBIG (0.06 mL/kg) should be given intramuscularly as soon as possible after exposure—within 24 hours if possible. Hepatitis B vaccine (Engerix-B, Recombivax HB) should be given intramuscularly at a separate site within 7 days of exposure, and second and third doses should be given 1 and 6 months, respectively, after the first dose. An alternative schedule for Engerix-B is 0, 1, and 2 months.

V. HEPATITIS D (THE DELTA AGENT). The hepatitis D virus (HDV) was discovered in Italy by Mario Rizzetto in 1977 during an investigation of the distribution of the HBV antigens in liver biopsy specimens of patients chronically infected with HBV. He described a new antigen in the nuclei of infected hepatocytes that was obligatorily associated with HBsAg. This new antigen was named delta. Subsequently, large amounts of this antigen were extracted from the liver of a patient with chronic HBV infection and the delta agent. Using this antigen, a specific and sensitive radioimmunoassay was developed for the detection of both the delta antigen in liver biopsy specimens and the antibody directed at the delta antigen in the serum of infected individuals.

A. Epidemiology. HDV has a global distribution. It has been found to be endemic in the Mediterranean basin, southern Italy, eastern Europe, the Middle East, Asia, western Africa, Australia, New Zealand, islands in the South Pacific, and the Amazon basin. Epidemics of HDV have been reported in North and South America, Colombia, and Venezuela. In endemic regions, transmission occurs from close person-to-person contact with transmucosal exchange of body fluids. Perinatal transmission is rare. In nonendemic areas such as northern Europe and North America, transmission is by direct inoculation from infected blood products. Any population that has a high frequency of HBV infection is vulnerable to HDV infection, especially IV drug abusers, hemophiliacs, hemodialysis patients, homosexual men, and prisoners.

B. Pathogenesis. HDV is a defective hepatotropic RNA virus that requires the presence of HBV as a "helper virus" for its pathogenicity. It replicates only in hosts who have a concomitant HBV infection. HDV is a 36-nm spherical particle containing the D antigen and a single-stranded RNA molecule in the interior, which is coated by HBsAg on the exterior. The structure of HDV is shown in Figure 50-7.

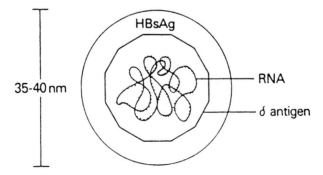

Figure 50-7. The delta agent. HBsAg, hepatitis B surface antigen; RNA, ribonucleic acid. (From Hoofnagle JH. Delta hepatitis and the delta agent in the American Association for the Study of Liver Diseases: Hepatobiliary disease–current concepts and controversies [postgraduate course] 1983.)

HDV seems to have a direct cytopathic effect on hepatocytes rather than causing immune-mediated hepatocyte damage, as results from HBV infection.

Individuals who are immune to HBV are protected from HDV infection. However, persons who are susceptible to both HBV and HDV infection (negative for all markers of HBV and HDV) and who are carriers of HBsAg may get hepatitis D.

C. Acute coinfection. In patients simultaneously exposed to HBV and HDV, coinfection occurs. The disease is usually self-limited, and the clinical course resembles that of classic acute hepatitis from HBV. Occasionally, coinfection results in extensive liver damage and FHF. This occurs more commonly in IV drug abusers. The diagnosis of coinfection with HBV and HDV is best made by the detection of positive titers for IgM HDV antibody, HBsAg, and IgM HBcAb, HBV-DNA and HDV-RNA (available only in research labs) in the patient's serum.

The coinfection may manifest itself as a single bout of elevated transaminases or more frequently as a biphasic illness with two separate transaminase peaks separated by weeks or even months. Expression of the disease due to HDV must wait for hepatocytes to be infected first by HBV. If the inoculations with the two viruses are close in time, HDV overwhelms the synthesis of HBV gene products in the HBV- and HDV-infected cells and causes the first bout of hepatitis. The second bout of hepatitis is caused by HBV expression. If the two peaks are very close in time, massive hepatic necrosis may occur and may be fatal to the patient. If the two bouts are separated by months, the first bout is usually from HDV. In either event, both viruses usually are cleared, and the patient completely recovers and develops both an HDVAb and HBsAb. Figure 50-8 summarizes the course of a case of acute HDV coinfection.

D. Superinfection. In chronic carriers of HBsAg, HDV superinfection usually causes severe liver disease, even FHF. In fact, 60% of FHF cases thought to be from HBV are actually due to HDV superinfection. Because most of the hepatocytes are already infected by HBV and contain HBsAg, HDV disseminates extensively and

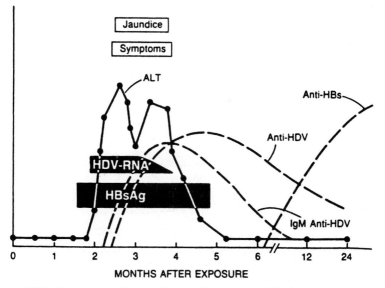

Figure 50-8. Typical course of acute delta hepatitis coinfection. ALT, alanine aminotransferase; HBsAg, hepatitis B surface antigen; HDV-RNA, hepatitis delta virus ribonucleic acid; anti-HDV, antibody to HDV; anti-HBs, antibody to HBsAg. (From Hoofnagle JH, DiBisceglie AM. Serologic diagnosis of acute and chronic viral hepatitis. *Semin Liver Dis.* 1991;11:79. Reprinted with permission.)

causes massive hepatic necrosis. Clinically, the disease may resemble fulminant type B hepatitis but can be recognized to be D hepatitis superinfection with the serologic presence of a strong IgM and IgG HDAb response and negative IgM HBcAb.

Anti-HDV arises late during acute HDV and is usually not detectable in serum at the onset of symptoms. In some cases of self-limited hepatitis D, anti-HDV is not detectable. For these reasons the serologic diagnosis of acute hepatitis D is often unsatisfactory and requires testing of both acute- and convalescent-phase serum samples. HDV antigen is present in both the serum and the liver of infected patients. Immune blotting for serum HDV antigen is available only in the research setting. However, the HDV antigen is detectable in the nuclei of hepatocytes and weakly in the cytoplasm in almost all patients with chronic hepatitis D. It has been detected in many pathology laboratories by a variety of immunostaining techniques, which can be applied to formalin-fixed, paraffin-embedded sections.

The hepatitis in these individuals tends to become chronic in almost all cases. In fact, very few patients clear both HBV and HDV after the superinfection. In HDV superinfection of HBsAg carriers, patients with negative HBcAg serology are probably the only ones in whom chronic HDV infection develops.

E. Chronic hepatitis D is characterized by a history of acute hepatitis. If the patient was a "silent carrier" of HBsAg, this acute illness may be the first episode of hepatitis for the patient. If the patient had chronic hepatitis from HBV, the disease may be thought of as an exacerbation or a superimposed hepatitis. Figure 50-9 summarizes the typical course of acute delta hepatitis superinfection.

Unfortunately, chronic HDV infection accelerates the progression of liver disease both in patients with ongoing chronic liver disease from HBV and in silent carriers of HBsAg. Most patients develop chronic active hepatitis, which often progresses to cirrhosis over a short span of time. The detection of high titers of anti-HDV is strongly suggestive of chronic HDV.

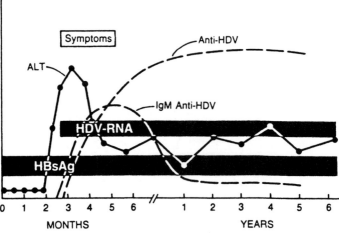

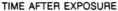

Figure 50-9. Typical course of acute delta hepatitis superinfection. ALT, alanine aminotransferase; HDV-RNA, hepatitis delta virus ribonucleic acid; HBsAg, hepatitis B surface antigen; anti-HDV, antibody to HDV. (From Hoofnagle JH, DiBisceglie AM. Serologic diagnosis of acute and chronic viral hepatitis. *Semin Liver Dis.* 1991;11:79. Reprinted with permission.)

F. Treatment. Currently there is no specific therapy for delta hepatitis, and the treatment for all forms of the disease is supportive. Steroids and other immunosuppressive drugs have not been effective. Interferon-α 9 MU three times weekly results in initial response in 50% of patients, but biochemical and virologic responses are rarely sustained. Monitoring of interferon-α therapy in chronic HDV is best accomplished by sequential testing for HDV-RNA in serum or in the liver.

Currently, the control of delta infection depends on its prevention. Because HDV infection requires the helper function of HBV, prevention of HBV infection and the HBsAg carrier state will also prevent HDV infection. Thus, the hepatitis B vaccine helps prevent new HBV and HDV infections. However, the large number of people carrying the HBsAg remains at risk for development of delta hepatitis. A vaccine against HDV is not yet available.

VI. HEPATITIS C
A. Epidemiology. Hepatitis C virus (HCV), identified in 1988 is a single-stranded enveloped RNA virus that belongs to the Flaviviridae family. It appears to be responsible for most instances of parenterally transmitted non-A, non-B hepatitis. The virus seems to mutate frequently and appear in many subtypes. Table 50-6 summarizes the differential diagnosis of elevated liver tests suggesting non-A, non-B hepatitis other than hepatitis C.

HCV is associated with transfusions of contaminated blood and blood products such as plasma, factor VIII, factor IX, fibrinogen, cryoprecipitate, and immune globulin prior to 1990. HCV is also transmitted by IV drug abuse, hemodialysis, and organ transplantation. It appears to be transmitted rarely by familial, sexual, or maternal–infant exposure. Heterosexual transmission seems to be much less frequent than homosexual transmission of the virus.

Health care workers exposed to a patient or the blood of a patient infected with HCV may acquire hepatitis C either from an accidental needle stick or without such an incident; however, the risk in such cases seems to be less than 10%. This occurrence has been documented in dialysis and oncology units and in plasmapheresis centers. Sporadic instances of hepatitis C occur and may account for 6% to 36% of the sporadic cases of hepatitis seen in urban areas. There may be unnoted percutaneous exposure among such patients (i.e., with use of intranasal cocaine, tattooing, body piercing, and exposure to blood through sharing toothbrushes, razors, or other personal items).

TABLE 50-6	Differential Diagnosis of Elevated Liver Tests Suggesting Non-A, Non-B Hepatitis
Disease	**Diagnostic features**
Mononucleosis	Lymphocytosis, IgM anti-VCA, Monospot
Cytomegalovirus	Lymphocytosis, anti-cytomegalovirus
Syphilis	VDRL test
Cholangitis	History and clinical course
Drug injury	History of drug intake
Autoimmune chronic active hepatitis	Antinuclear antibody, immunoglobulins
Ischemic liver injury	History, lactic dehydrogenase levels
Budd-Chiari syndrome	History
Wilson's disease	History, ceruloplasmin, copper

Anti-VCA = antibody to the viral capsid antigen of Epstein-Barr virus.
From Hoofnagle JH, Schafer DF. Serologic markers of hepatitis B virus infection. *Semin Liver Dis.* 1986;6:1. Reprinted with permission.

Vertical transmission of HCV from mother to child is uncommon (5% except for persons coinfected with HIV [50%]). Maternal HCV Ab crosses the placenta and HCV Ab may be detected in the child up to 1 year after birth. To detect active infection in the child, the presence of HCV-RNA by PCR needs to be determined. Cesarean section decreases the transmission of HCV from the mother to the child.

The disease is found worldwide and appears to be almost as common in economically developed countries as it is in underdeveloped countries.

HCV preferentially replicates in hepatocytes; however, replication extrahepatic sties also have been demonstrated. HCV inherently has a high mutation rate that results in considerable heterogeneity throughout its genome. It is classified into 6 **genotypes** that are genetically distinct groups of viral isolates that have arisen during the evolution of the virus. There are also 40 subtypes (i.e., a, b).

In the United States, **genotype 1** is most prevalent (approximately 70% of HCV infections) and is associated with lower response rates to interferon therapy than the other genotypes. **Genotype 2** accounts for 15% and **genotype 3** for 10% of the HCV-infected patients in the United States. **Genotype 4** is the most common genotype in Egypt and the Middle East. **Genotype 5** is found in South Africa, and **genotype 6** in Southeast Asia. Regardless of ethnicity, those infected with type 1 HCV are found to have higher circulating levels of HCV and a greater likelihood of developing cirrhosis and HCC.

B. Clinical presentation

1. Acute hepatitis

    a. The mean incubation period for transfusion-associated hepatitis C is 7 to 8 weeks with a range of 2 to 26 weeks. Shorter incubation periods of 1 to 2 weeks have also been recorded.

    b. The acute illness associated with hepatitis C usually cannot be distinguished from hepatitis caused by other heterotropic viruses. However, it tends to be less severe. Usually patients complain of flulike symptoms, easy fatigability, malaise, and anorexia with occasional nausea and vomiting; fever, arthralgia, and skin rash are rare.

    c. Approximately 25% of patients with hepatitis C are icteric. Jaundice usually lasts less than a month. The serum transaminase (ALT, AST) levels are only moderately elevated (<800 IU/L).

    d. Transient agranulocytosis and aplastic anemia have been observed in patients with hepatitis C.

    e. A clinical feature characteristic of hepatitis C is its episodic, fluctuating pattern of serum transaminase (ALT, AST) activity. Periods of elevation of these enzyme levels are interrupted by months of normal or near-normal levels of liver enzyme activity (Fig. 50-10).

2. Chronic disease

    a. Long-term follow-up studies in patients with hepatitis C have revealed that at least 90% of patients infected with HCV have chronic disease. The disease may continue to appear to resolve both biochemically and histologically, followed by intermittent or constant elevation of serum transaminases. Persistent viremia can prevail in the presence or absence of elevated ALT activity. In fact, spontaneous total resolution of the disease may occur in only a small proportion of infected individuals.

    b. The progression to chronic hepatitis cannot be predicted from the clinical or biochemical severity of the acute illness. Anicteric as well as icteric disease may become chronic.

    c. In most studies, the frequency of development of chronic liver disease from transfusion-associated hepatitis C is 85% to 90%. When biopsied, approximately 70% to 80% of these patients have chronic active hepatitis, and 10% to 20% have cirrhosis. The chronic active hepatitis in these patients is progressive and progresses to cirrhosis in most cases over 10 to 30 years.

    d. Cofactors such as concomitant alcoholism, hemochromatosis, and chronic hepatitis B coinfection with HIV are important contributors to progressive liver disease and cirrhosis in patients with chronic hepatitis C.

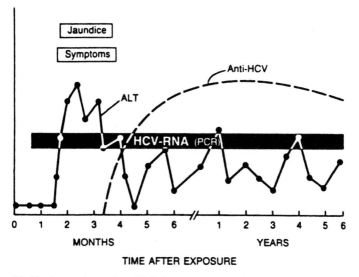

Figure 50-10. A case of acute hepatitis C that progressed to chronic infection and disease. ALT, alanine aminotransferase; HCV-RNA, hepatitis C virus ribonucleic acid; anti-HCV, antibody to hepatitis C virus; PCR, polymerase chain reaction. (From Hoofnagle JH, DiBisceglie AM. Serologic diagnosis of acute and chronic renal hepatitis. *Semin Liver Dis.* 1991;11:78. Reprinted with permission.)

    e. Several studies have linked essential mixed cryoglobulinemia (EMC) (an immune complex vasculitis associated with joint, skin, and sometimes kidney involvement), porphyria cutanea tarda (PCT), and lymph-proliferative diseases such as lymphoma and lymphocytic leukemia with HCV infection.

  3. Hepatitis C and hepatocellular carcinoma. There is convincing evidence that HCV infection is associated with the development of hepatocellular carcinoma. Several patients have been reported to develop hepatocellular carcinoma 9 to 18 years after the onset of transfusion-associated hepatitis C.

C. Diagnosis

  1. Serologic tests. Serologic assays are used for screening for HCV infection and for first-line diagnosis. There are two types of anti-HCV (HCVAb) assays, the enzyme immunoassay (EIA) and the recombinant immunoblot assay (RIBA). Both detect antibodies to different HCV antigens. Three successive generations of EIAs have resulted in increased sensitivity in detecting HCVAb and thus, with the third-generation EIA confirmatory, RIBA testing is rarely needed.

  2. Virologic tests. Currently there is no method available for culturing HCV from serum samples. Viral detection is accomplished by amplification methods for HCV-RNA such as with the polymerase chain reaction (PCR). **Qualitative PCR testing** for HCV-RNA is very sensitive and can detect as few as 100 viral copies/mL within one week of infection with HCV. The **quantitative** PCR testing allows the measurement of serum HCV-RRN levels (viral load) and are used in assessing the effectiveness of antiviral therapy.

  3. Histopathologic examination of liver biopsy specimens from HCV-infected patients has been standardized to differentiate and quantitate inflammation and fibrosis. These are expressed in fractions of 0-4/4, with the high numerator used for increasing severity.

D. Treatment of chronic HCV. There is no vaccine against HCV and there is no reliable postexposure prophylaxis. So prevention of spread of HCV depends on diagnosing and treating persons who are likely to be infected. Infected patients should be vaccinated against HAV and HBV because of the high risk of severe liver disease if superinfection occurs with these viruses.

1. **Monotherapy.** Treatment of chronic HCV infection is based on parenteral interferon (IFN) therapy. Initially, the treatment consisted of IFN monotherapy using 3 million units given subcutaneously three times per week for 6 months and yielded about 10% end of treatment response (ETR). However, with this therapy, there is a >90 % relapse rate 6 months after cessation of therapy, giving a sustained viral response (SVR) of about 3%. When this treatment was extended to 12 months, the SVR increased to about 10%.

2. **Combination therapy**

   a. **Combination therapy** using IFN-α with ribavirin, an oral guanosine nucleoside analog, has been shown to greatly improve sustained response rates in naive and relapsing patients. In treatment of naive patients with IFN-α at a dose of 3 million units given sc three times a week, in combination with oral ribavirin 800 to 1,200 mg per day for 12 months, achieves sustained virologic response rates of approximately 30%. These rates are higher (up to 40%–50%) for patients with low viral loads and with HCV genotypes II and III. In patients with HCV genotypes II and III, combination therapy for 24 weeks achieves the same efficacy as combination therapy administered for 48 weeks. The impact of combination therapy on interferon monotherapy nonresponders is less impressive.

   b. **The current standard of therapy** for a patient with chronic HVC is a combination of pegylated interferon and ribavirin.

      The addition of polyethylene glycol (PEG) to interferon increases the half-life of the drug in the patient, thereby allowing once-weekly administration. When pegylated IFN therapy is combined with oral ribavirin, the rate of SVR is greatly increased especially in patients with HCV genotype 1. The optimal dose of PEG interferon-α-2b (PEG-IFN) is 1.5 μg/kg per week sc and for PEG interferon-α-2a (Pegasys) is 180 μg per week sc. The preferred ribavirin dose is weight-based (>10.6 mg/kg) for PEG-IFN and with Pegasys it is 1,000 to 1,200 mg per day.

      For naive patients with HCV genotype 1 infection, treatment is recommended for 48 weeks. Early viral response is assessed by quantitative determination of HCV-RNA by PCR (viral load) at the end of the first month. In patients who have undetectable viral load after one month of therapy, the SVR is >90%.

      For patients with undetectable viral load at 3 months of therapy or those with a 2 log drop in the viral load, the SVR is in the range of 48%.

      Patients with HCV genotypes 2 and 3 with the same treatment plan have SVR >80% after treatment.

      Patients who fail to respond to above therapy or those who relapse after treatment may be offered therapies involving longer duration of therapy, higher ribavirin and interferon doses, and/or treatment with **consensus interferon (Infergen)** which is a synthetic interferon at a dose of 15 μg sc daily and ribovirim for 48 weeks. These treatments are still under study and are evolving.

   c. There are numerous **side effects** of interferon and ribavirin therapy. Aside from the flulike symptoms, fatigue, and depression, interferon causes cytopenia and autoimmune thyroiditis. Ribavirin causes hemolytic anemia and psychiatric and mood disorders and insomnia. It is paramount that these side effects are treated promptly and effectively for patients' comfort and to ensure patient compliance. Growth factors, especially erythropoietin is being used in many patients to alleviate anemia. Patients with mood disorders or changes need to be treated with appropriate drugs and should be followed by mental health professionals as needed.

      Patients with HIV and HCV coinfection should be treated for HCV as well as HIV.

      Since ribavirin is teratogenic, patients who are taking ribavirin and are sexually active need to use barrier contraception during the treatment and 6 months posttherapy.

Newer oral agents are being developed to enhance the eradication of HCV in infected patients. Polymerase and protease inhibitors and other antiviral drugs show promise. However, these agents, when used alone, have not been shown to be effective in achieving SVR due to the rapid development of viral resistance. When added to the current regimen of interferon and ribavirin-based therapies, though, they seem to enhance SVR and also possibly shorten the treatment duration.

VII. The hepatitis E virus (HEV) is a small (27–30 nm) RNA virus that causes acute epidemics of enterically transmitted hepatitis in underdeveloped areas of the world. HEV is transmitted by the fecal-oral route and is associated with contamination of food or water sources.

   A. Diagnosis. HEV antigen can be detected in the liver, bile, and stool during the incubation period and symptomatic phase of hepatitis E. Anti-HEV can be detected by immune electron microscopy in serum during acute illness. Titers of anti-HEV rise during convalescence; however, immunity to reinfection may not be absolute. HEV-RNA has been cloned. Recombinant immunoassays are being developed for both anti-HEV and HEV antigen. Diagnosis of acute HEV can be made in patients presenting with acute hepatitis with a recent history of living in or travel to endemic areas of the world (Central and South America, Mexico, Asia, Africa, and the Middle East) and absence of serologic markers of acute hepatitis A, B, and C.

   B. Clinical course. HEV causes an acute hepatitis in adults with varying severity. In pregnant women, especially in the third trimester, it is associated with high mortality—approximately 10% to 35% of instances. HEV infection does not lead to chronic hepatitis or to the carrier state.

Selected Readings

Berg T, et al. Extended treatment duration for hepatitis C virus type 1: comparing 48 versus 72 weeks of peginterferon-alpha-2a plus riboviron. *Gastroenterology*. 2006;130:1086–1097.

Chen CJ, et al. Risk of hepatocellular carcinoma across a biological gradient of serum hepatitis B DNA level. *JAMA*. 2006;295(1):65–73.

Derenci P. Predictors of response to therapy for chronic hepatitis C. *Semin Liver Dis*. 2004;24(suppl 2):25–31.

Fartoux L, et al. Effect of prolonged interferon therapy on the outcome of hepatitis C virus-related cirrhosis: A randomized trial. *Clin Gastroenterol Hepatol*. 2007;Apr;5:502–507.

Hoofnagle JH, et al. Management of hepatitis B: summary of a clinical research workshop. *Hepatology*. 2007;45:1056–1075.

Krawczynski K, et al. Hepatitis E virus: Epidemiology, clinical and pathological features, diagnosis and experimental animal models. In: Thomas HC, Lemon S, Zuckerman AJ, eds. *Viral Hepatitis*. 3rd ed. Malden, Mass.: Blackwell; 2005:624–634.

Lok ASF. Navigating hepatitis B treatments. *Gastroenterol*. 2007;132:1586–1594.

Lok ASF and McMahon BJ. AASLD practice guidelines: Chronic hepatitis B. *Hepatology*. 2007; 45:507–539.

McLean OR, et al. Acute Hepatitis C: Diagnosis and management. *Pract Gastroenterol*. 2007;(Sept)66–77.

Niro GA, et al. Peglyated interferon alpha-2b as monotherapy or in combination with riboviron in chronic hepatitis delta. *Hepatology*. 2006;44:713–720.

Oldfield EC, et al. The A's and B's of vaccine—Preventable hepatitis: Improving prevention in high risk adults. *Rev Gastroenterol Disord*. 2007;7(1):1–21.

Pungpapong S, et al. Natural history of hepatitis B virus infection: an update for clinicians. *Mayo Clin Proc*. 2007;82(8):967–975.

Re VL, et al. Prevalence, risk factors, and outcomes for occult hepatitis B virus infection among HIV-infected patients. *J Acquir Immune Defic Syndr*. 2007;44:315–320.

Sarazin C, et al. A normal hepatitis C virus protense inhibitor, plus pegylated interferon alpha-2b for genotype 1 nonresponders. *Gastroenterology*. 2007;132:1270–1278.

Shiffman ML, et al. Peginterferon Alpha-2a and Riborvirin for 16 or 24 weeks in HCV genotype 2 or 3. *N Eng J Med*. 2007;357:124–134.

Shresthas MR, et al. Safety and efficacy of a recombinant hepatitis E vaccine. *N Engl J Med*. 2007;356:895–903.

Sorjano V, et al. Core of patients with HIV and Hepatitis C virus. *AIDs*. 2007;21(9):1073–1089.

Zeuzem S, et al. Efficacy of 24 week treatment with peginterferon alpha—2b plus ribovirin in patients with chronic hepatitis C infected with genotype 1 and low pretreatment viremia. *J Hepatol*. 2006;44:97–103.

51 ALCOHOLIC LIVER DISEASE (ALD)

I. EPIDEMIOLOGY. The association of alcohol abuse and liver damage has been known since the time of the ancient Greeks. The availability of alcoholic beverages, licensing laws, and economic, cultural, and environmental conditions all influence both per capita alcohol consumption and mortality from alcohol-related liver disease. Alcoholism is, in part, inherited, and aberrant alcohol-drinking behavior is genetically influenced. The risk factors that may affect the susceptibility to development of alcoholic liver disease include genetic factors, malnutrition, female gender, and viral agents (hepatitis virus B, C, and D).

Ninety percent to 95% of people with chronic alcohol consumption develop **fatty liver.** In almost all instances, this lesion is thought to be reversible on cessation of alcohol intake. Ten percent to 30% of individuals go on to perivenular sclerosis (collagen deposition in and around central veins). Ten percent to 35% of chronic alcoholics, however, have acute liver injury that may become recurrent or chronic. Some of these patients recover, but 8% to 20% go on to sinusoidal, perivenular, and pericentral fibrosis and cirrhosis. Even during the inflammatory stage without the presence of cirrhosis, patients may have portal hypertension, ascites, and esophageal varices.

II. RELATION OF CIRRHOSIS TO ALCOHOL CONSUMPTION. The alcohol content of various beverages is shown in Table 51-1. The development of alcoholic cirrhosis correlates with the quantity and duration of alcohol consumption. For men, the relative risk of cirrhosis has been estimated to be 6 times greater when consumption is 40 to 60 g of alcohol per day than when it is up to 20 g per day, and 14 times greater at 60 to 80 g per day. The average "cirrhogenic" dose has been calculated to be 40 to 80 g of ethanol per day consumed for approximately 10 to 12 years.

In a case-controlled study in men, the relative risk for cirrhosis was 1.83 for men consuming 40 to 60 g of absolute alcohol per day compared to men consuming fewer than 40 g per day. The relative risk rose to 100 for men consuming more than 80 g per day. The average cirrhogenic and threshold doses are lower in women than in men. Binge drinking compared to drinking with meals and beer and spirits compared to wine drinking increases the risk for ALD.

III. ETHANOL METABOLISM
  A. Absorption, distribution, and elimination. In a healthy man, about 100 mg of ethanol per kilogram of body weight is eliminated in an hour. Heavy alcohol consumption for years may increase the rate of ethanol elimination up to 100%.

Ethanol is absorbed from the gastrointestinal tract, especially the duodenum and jejunum (70%–80%), by simple diffusion because of its small molecular size and low solubility in lipids. The rate of absorption is decreased by delayed gastric emptying and by the presence of intestinal contents. Food delays gastric absorption, producing a slower rise and lower peak value of blood alcohol in fed than in fasting patients.

The systemic distribution of alcohol is very rapid. In organs with a rich blood supply, such as the brain, lungs, and liver, alcohol rapidly equilibrates with the blood. Alcohol is poorly lipid-soluble. At room temperature, tissue lipids take up only 4% of the quantity of alcohol dissolved in a corresponding volume of water.

| | TABLE 51-1 | Alcohol Content of Various Beverages |

Beverage	Alcohol concentration* (g/100 mL)	Alcohol in standard measures
Beer	3.9	13.3 g; 12-oz bottle/can
Red wine	9.5	11.0 g/glass; 71 g/bottle
Rosé	8.7	10.0 g/glass; 65 g/bottle
White wine, dry	9.1	10.0 g/glass; 64 g/bottle
White wine, medium	8.8	10.0 g/glass; 62 g/bottle
White wine, sweet	10.2	11.0 g/glass; 71 g/bottle
White wine, sparkling	9.9	11.0 g/glass; 74 g/bottle
Port	15.9	124 g/bottle
Sherry, dry	15.7	123 g/bottle
Sherry, medium	14.8	115 g/bottle
Sherry, sweet	15.6	122 g/bottle
Vermouth, dry	13.9	122 g/bottle
Vermouth, sweet	13.0	100 g/bottle
Cherry brandy	19.0	148 g/bottle
Hard liquor 70% (brandy, gin, whiskey)	31.7	240 g/bottle; 7.5 g/single-shot

*Percentage alcohol $\times$ 0.078 = g alcohol/100 mL.
Key: 1 fl oz = 30 mL; 1 pint = 470 mL; 1 wine bottle = 757 mL.

In an obese person, therefore, the same amount of alcohol per unit of weight gives a higher blood alcohol concentration than in a thin person. The mean volume of distribution of ethanol is less in women than in men, resulting in higher peak blood concentrations and greater mean areas under the ethanol concentration–time curves.

In humans, less than 1% is excreted in the urine, 1% to 3% via the lungs, and 90% to 95% as carbon dioxide after it is oxidized in the liver.

B. Chemical metabolism

1. Alcohol dehydrogenase. Although most of the ingested ethanol is metabolized by the liver, other tissues such as the stomach, intestines, kidney, and bone marrow cells oxidize ethanol to a small extent. There is an alcohol dehydrogenase (ADH) present in the mucosa of the stomach, jejunum, and ileum, which results in a considerable first-pass metabolism of alcohol. The gastric ADH activity is less in women than in men and decreases with chronic alcoholism.

In the liver, the main pathway for ethanol metabolism is by its oxidation to acetaldehyde by ADH. Alternative pathways of oxidation in other subcellular compartments are also present. Multiple molecular forms of ADH exist, and at least three different classes have been described on the basis of structure and function. Various ADH forms appear in different frequencies in different racial populations. This polymorphism may explain, in part, individual variation in the rate of acetaldehyde production and first-pass elimination.

The hepatic metabolism of ethanol proceeds in three basic steps. First, ethanol is oxidized within the hepatocyte cytosol to acetaldehyde. Second, acetaldehyde is oxidized to acetate via catalysis mainly by aldehyde dehydrogenase (ALDH) in the mitochondria. Third, acetate ALDH is released into blood and is oxidized by peripheral tissues to carbon dioxide and water.

When ethanol is oxidized to acetaldehyde via ADH, nicotinamide-adenine dinucleotide (NAD) is required as a cofactor and is reduced to NADH during the reaction, resulting in an increase in the liver of the NADH/NAD ratio. This increase in the redox state of the liver has serious metabolic effects such as inhibition of hepatic gluconeogenesis, impairment of fatty acid oxidation, decrease in citric acid cycle activity, and increase in conversion of pyruvate to lactic acid resulting in lactic acidosis.

2. **The microsomal ethanol oxidizing system (MEOS)** is located in the endoplasmic reticulum (ER) of the hepatocyte. It is a cytochrome P-450-, NADPH- (reduced nicotinamide-adenine–dinucleotide phosphate), and oxygen-dependent enzyme system that oxidizes ethanol to acetaldehyde. Because chronic consumption of ethanol leads to the proliferation of the ER, the activity of the MEOS is also increased (induction). However, its quantitative contribution to the total ethanol metabolism is still controversial. The current nomenclature for MEOS is P45011E1. In addition to ethanol, this enzyme system oxidizes other alcohols, carbon tetrachloride (CCl_4), and acetaminophen (Tylenol).

3. **ALDH** rapidly metabolizes acetaldehyde to acetate. Multiple molecular forms of ALDH have been demonstrated. Two major hepatic ALDH isoenzymes (I and II) exist in humans. The mitochondrial isoenzyme (ALDH I) has been reported to be missing in about 50% of liver specimens in Japanese people. The deficiency of ALDH I in Asians has several metabolic and clinical consequences.

4. **Change in hepatic redox state.** When ethanol is oxidized to acetaldehyde in the hepatocyte cytosol via ADH, NAD is required as a cofactor. NAD is reduced to NADH. Also, ALDH-mediated conversion of acetaldehyde to acetate requires NAD conversion of NADH in the mitochondria. Thus, both the cytosolic and mitochondrial redox states are altered. This effect is manifested by respective increases of both liver and blood lactate to pyruvate and of β-hydroxybutyrate to acetoacetate ratios. This state leads to inhibition of hepatic gluconeogenesis, fatty acid oxidation, and citric acid cycle activity, which may clinically exhibit as fatty liver, hypoglycemia, and lactic acidosis (Fig. 51-1).

5. **Alterations in metabolism** of ethanol, acetaldehyde, and acetate during chronic alcohol consumption. Chronic ethanol consumption enhances ethanol clearance except in the presence of clinically significant liver damage or severe food restriction. This effect is attributed to increased ADH activity, MEOS activity, a hypermetabolic state in the liver, and possible increased mitochondrial reoxidation of NADH, which is the rate-limiting step in ethanol elimination and metabolism. The explanation for increased ethanol elimination by corticosteroids is the induced increase in NADH conversion to NAD as a result of steroid-induced gluconeogenesis.

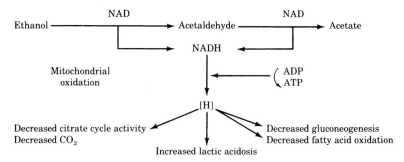

Figure 51-1. Metabolic consequences of change in hepatic redox state secondary to oxidation of ethanol.

In healthy people, almost all the acetaldehyde formed during ethanol oxidation is effectively oxidized in the liver. However, detectable concentrations of acetaldehyde have been found in the peripheral blood of chronic alcoholics and in Asians, who experience alcohol-related flushing. The unusually high blood acetaldehyde levels found in severely intoxicated, chronic alcoholics are thought to result from an increased rate of ethanol oxidation of ADH and a decrease in the liver ALDH activity associated with both liver injury and chronic ethanol consumption.

IV. PATHOGENESIS OF ALCOHOLIC LIVER INJURY

A. Hepatocyte injury. Alcoholic liver injury is multifactorial. Ethanol causes physical changes. It "fluidizes" all biologic membranes including hepatic mitochondria, endoplasmic reticula, and cell surface membranes by changing their lipid composition. There is an increase in the cholesterol ester content of plasma membranes and a decrease in the enzyme activity of such enzymes as succinic dehydrogenase and cytochromes *a* and *b*, and in the total respiratory capacity of the mitochondria. Chronic alcohol consumption also potentiates the release of alkaline phosphatase and γ-glutamyl peptidase from liver plasma membranes.

In addition to the metabolic effects resulting from the changed redox state and the inhibition of fatty acid oxidation during the oxidation of ethanol (Fig. 51-1), acute large doses of ethanol mobilize fat from adipose tissue to the liver. Administration of ethanol with a high-fat diet potentiates alcoholic fatty liver. This effect is attenuated with chronic alcohol consumption.

B. Acetaldehyde is thought to be the major initiating factor in the pathogenesis of alcoholic liver damage. It has been shown to form covalently bound adducts with hepatocyte proteins. Acetaldehyde-protein adducts could inhibit hepatic protein secretion, impair biologic functions of proteins, and combine with tissue macromolecules and thereby cause severe tissue injury. Acetaldehyde may also initiate lipid peroxidation via the generation of free radicals. Normally, free radicals are inactivated by glutathione. However, acetaldehyde may bind with glutathione or with cysteine and inhibit the synthesis of glutathione, which may contribute to the depression of liver glutathione seen in chronic alcoholics; this reaction may also increase lipid peroxidation.

Humoral immune response by production of antibodies to acetaldehyde adducts, microtubules, and other proteins may play a role in the liver injury. There is also some evidence that cytotoxic reactions mediated by mononuclear cells may take place to increase cellular damage.

Chronic alcohol consumption induces the MEOS, which also contributes to increased acetaldehyde production. However, MEOS induction also enhances oxygen consumption and potentiates hypoxia, especially in the centrolobular (perivenous) area because the P45011E1 is predominantly localized to this area in the lobule. The induction of P45011E1 also increases hepatotoxicity of other chemicals such as CCl_4 and acetaminophen, which may contribute to the liver injury, especially in zone 3 (perivenular zone).

In addition to the accumulation of fat in the hepatocytes with chronic alcohol consumption, there is also an accumulation of protein in and around hepatocytes such as microtubular protein (alcoholic hyalin) and exportable proteins secondary to impairment of their synthesis and transport out of hepatocytes. The result is an additional decrease in the sinusoidal area and perfusion of hepatocytes.

C. Hepatic fibrogenesis. Alcohol-induced hepatocyte necrosis and inflammation may trigger fibrogenesis and the development of cirrhosis. However, ethanol itself and its metabolites also have significant effects on collagen metabolism and fibrogenesis. Thus alcoholic hepatitis is not a necessary step in the development of cirrhosis.

Chronic alcohol consumption has been associated with the induction and proliferation of perisinusoidal and perivenular mesenchymal cells called Ito cells and of myofibroblasts, which produce increased amounts of types I, III, and IV collagen and laminin. Myofibroblasts are contractile cells and may contribute to scar contraction and portal hypertension in cirrhosis. Ito cells and myofibroblast processes extend into the space of Disse around the hepatocytes, and their concentrations correspond to the degree of collagen formation in the space of Disse. Fibronectin formation is also stimulated; the fibronectin may form a skeleton for collagen formation. The increased collagenization of the space of Disse results in reduction of the fenestration between sinusoids and the space of Disse and, therefore, may isolate the hepatocyte from its blood supply. These changes also increase the resistance to blood flow and contribute to increased portal pressure. Perivenular and perisinusoidal fibrosis has a predictive value for the development of alcoholic cirrhosis. The presence of alcoholic hepatitis and steatosis also correlates with the development of cirrhosis.

Various cytokines including tissue necrosis factor (TNF), interleukin-2 and interleukin-6, transforming growth factors (TGF-α and -β), and platelet-derived growth factor (PDGF) all seem to contribute to stimulation and transformation of Ito cells and reinforcement of liver cell injury.

  D. Nutritional factors in alcoholic liver disease. The role of nutritional factors in the development of alcoholic liver injury has been controversial. However, it is thought that protein-calorie malnutrition may contribute to liver injury. Because of the metabolic alterations caused by ethanol and because of the present liver injury, however, the malnutrition noted in people with chronic ethanol abuse may be, in part, secondary rather than primary. There is some evidence that a high-protein diet and phenyl phosphatidylcholine (extracted from soybeans) have a protective effect on the liver in alcohol-induced cirrhosis.

V. DIAGNOSIS

  A. Clinical presentation. Alcoholic hepatitis (AH) is an acute or chronic illness associated with severe chronic alcoholism, involving extensive hepatocellular necrosis, inflammation, and scarring. It is extremely variable in clinical presentation and may be superimposed on other forms of alcoholic liver disease such as fatty liver and Laënnec's cirrhosis.

    Alcoholic liver disease may occur without any symptoms. The most common complaints in symptomatic patients with alcoholic hepatitis are anorexia, nausea, vomiting, and abdominal pain, especially in the right upper quadrant. Most patients lose weight due to anorexia and nausea. One fourth of patients have fever. Fever may be due to severe liver damage in the absence of an infection; however, infections should be excluded in these immunocompromised patients. Jaundice, when present, is usually mild, but in 20% to 35% of the patients who present with a cholestatic picture, it is severe. Diarrhea and symptoms related to complications of portal hypertension such as ascites, peripheral edema, and esophageal varices are less common. Most patients with acute hepatitis have a tender and somewhat enlarged liver. Jaundice, splenomegaly, ascites, peripheral edema, spider angiomata, palmar erythema, parotid enlargement, gynecomastia, testicular atrophy, finger clubbing, and Dupuytren's contractures may also be present.

  B. Diagnostic studies

    1. Laboratory studies

      a. The most characteristic laboratory findings in acute alcoholic hepatitis are elevated serum transaminases and bilirubin. Serum glutamic-oxaloacetic transaminase (SGOT, or aspartate aminotransferase [AST]) levels are usually 2 to 10 times normal. Values greater than 500 U/L are rare. Serum glutamic-pyruvic transaminase (SGPT, or alanine aminotransferase [ALT]) levels are also elevated, but they are increased less than SGOT levels. The reduced SGPT levels may be related to mitochondrial injury in alcoholic hepatitis. The SGOT/SGPT ratio in alcoholic hepatitis is usually greater than 1.

      b. Serum alkaline phosphatase level is moderately elevated in at least one half of the patients. In patients presenting with a cholestatic picture, the elevation may be marked. **γ-Glutamyltranspeptidase (GGTP)** activity is also often elevated in alcoholic hepatitis. This enzyme is quite sensitive for alcoholic injury.

c. **Serum globulins** are often increased, and, interestingly, IgA levels are disproportionately elevated compared to the other immunoglobulins. Serum albumin levels may be normal initially in well-compensated and well-nourished patients but are usually decreased.

d. Because the liver is the main site of synthesis of the coagulation factors, in severely ill patients the **prolongation of prothrombin** time by greater than 7 to 10 seconds predicts a poor prognosis.

e. The **hematologic parameters** are usually abnormal in alcoholic hepatitis. Leukocytosis with a shift to the left is common. Anemia and thrombocytopenia are usually present. Platelet count of <100 usually indicates the presence of cirrhosis. Aside from the fact that alcohol is toxic to the bone marrow, patients may have hypersplenism, disseminated intravascular coagulation (DIC), and bone marrow suppression from their acute and chronic disease state.

f. Other causes of liver injury should be ruled out by appropriate serologic tests and a careful drug history. **Acetaminophen** even in therapeutic doses may be toxic in alcoholic patients. Aspirin and acetaminophen levels may be helpful in selected patients.

g. **Hepatitis C infection** increases the risk of developing cirrhosis in ALD. This is also true in reverse. Thus, patients with ALD should be tested for hepatitis C antibody and if the test is positive, treatment of hepatitis C should be recommended.

2. **Ultrasound.** Even though the diagnosis may be easily established in most patients from the history, physical examination, and blood work, it may be helpful in some patients, especially in those presenting with the picture of cholestasis, to obtain an abdominal ultrasound to rule out biliary tract disease, ascites, and the presence of hepatocellular carcinoma. Some patients may require computed tomography (CT) scan of the abdomen and endoscopic retrograde cholangiopancreatography (ERCP).

3. **Liver biopsy** should be performed early in the course of the disease in most patients to confirm the diagnosis and to stage the severity of the liver injury. With deterioration of liver function (excessive prolongation of the prothrombin time or the presence of ascites), liver biopsy may not be possible later in the disease process.

   Microscopic examination of the liver biopsy is essential for classification of the alcoholic injury with regard to steatosis, early fibrosis, alcoholic hepatitis, or Laënnec's cirrhosis. In patients with alcoholic hepatitis, pathologic features may include the following:

a. **The hepatocellular necrosis** is mainly centrilobular but may be panlobular. Hepatocytes in various stages of degeneration are usually present. Many hepatocytes are swollen, balloonlike, or vacuolated and often contain a fibrillar material or alcoholic hyalin called Mallory bodies. This cytoplasmic material, even though commonly seen in patients with alcoholic hepatitis, is not limited to this disease. It has also been reported in diseases such as hepatoma, Indian childhood cirrhosis, and liver disease in patients with intestinal bypass surgery, obesity, diabetes, and drug reaction. Occasionally it is seen in primary biliary cirrhosis, primary sclerosing cholangitis, and Wilson's disease.

b. **The inflammatory exudate** consists predominantly of polymorphonuclear (PMN) leukocytes in addition to some mononuclear cells. PMNs are seen in portal tracts and sinusoids and are usually concentrated in areas of hepatocellular necrosis with or without alcoholic hyalin. In 50% to 75% of the cases, rosettes of PMNs are seen around degenerating hepatocytes containing Mallory bodies. This finding constitutes the hallmark of the disease.

c. **Fibrosis** is usually extensive and seen early in the disease. It frequently surrounds the central veins and extends into the perisinusoidal areas. The stellate fibrosis often remains after inflammation resolves and leads to micronodular cirrhosis.

    d. Fatty infiltration is commonly seen in patients with alcoholic hepatitis. The extent of steatosis depends on recent alcohol intake, dietary fat, and the concomitant presence of obesity or diabetes.

    e. Severe cholestasis may be seen in one third of patients. In these patients, in addition to pericentral injury and scar formation, there is marked periportal necrosis, inflammation, and destruction of small bile ducts.

    f. Hemosiderosis may be seen in some of these patients.

VI. CLINICAL COURSE. In patients with steatosis only, abstinence from alcohol may lead to resolution of the liver injury. However, if perivenular and sinusoidal fibrosis is present, abstinence may halt further damage, but the scarring may remain.

    Alcoholic hepatitis is a disease of varying severity. The overall mortality is 10% to 15%. Healing is slow, and most patients require 2 to 8 months for recovery after stopping consumption of alcohol. The disease usually worsens after the first several days, regardless of the initial presentation. Patients may have encephalopathy and other complications during this stage, such as gastrointestinal bleeding from esophageal varices, gastritis or peptic ulcers, coagulopathy or DIC, infections especially of the urinary tract and lungs, spontaneous bacterial peritonitis, and hepatorenal syndrome. A combination of serious complications often leads to death of the patient.

    Many patients with a history of chronic alcoholism have episodes of acute alcoholic hepatitis superimposed on existing cirrhosis. It is thought that repeated bouts of alcoholic liver injury, necrosis, and fibrosis lead to extensive scarring and Laënnec's cirrhosis.

VII. TREATMENT. The most important component of therapy of alcoholic liver disease is **strict abstinence from alcohol.** Alcohol is the most common cause of liver disease in the Western world. In many countries, the incidence of alcoholic liver disease is increasing at a time when the incidences of other liver disorders are remaining steady or declining.

    A. Supportive therapy. The mainstay of therapy for alcoholic hepatitis is supportive. Most patients require bed rest. Seriously ill patients should be admitted to an intensive care unit. If complications of portal hypertension exist, they should be promptly treated. Infections and concomitant pancreatitis should be ruled out or appropriately treated.

    B. Diet. Alcohol intake should be strictly forbidden. Patients should be given thiamine, folic acid, and multivitamins. The electrolyte, calcium, magnesium, phosphate, and glucose levels should be strictly monitored and corrected.

    Protein-calorie malnutrition is present in most patients. The energy expenditure and protein degradation are increased. Insulin resistance is a ubiquitous finding. This causes fat to be preferred over carbohydrate as an energy source. Frequent feedings with a high-carbohydrate, high-fiber, and low-fat diet may decrease insulin resistance and improve nitrogen balance. In patients who cannot eat, enteral tube feedings may be given with standard formulas. Special formulations such as Hepatic-Aid may be reserved for the small minority of patients for whom encephalopathy remains a major problem after a fair trial of standard therapy. Patients should receive sufficient daily calories to provide basal energy expenditure (BEE) × 1.2 to 1.4 total kcal or 25 to 30 kcal/kg of ideal body weight. Thirty percent to 35% of total calories should be given as fat and the remainder as carbohydrate. Protein should not be restricted below 1 mg/kg unless encephalopathy necessitates further restriction.

    In patients in whom enteral therapy is not possible, parenteral nutrition should be given promptly following guidelines similar to those outlined for enteral nutrition. The use of solutions rich in branched-chain amino acids such as HepatAmine is controversial and is not necessary except in cases of hepatic encephalopathy and coma.

    C. Alcohol withdrawal. Initially, symptoms of alcohol withdrawal may be present. Alcoholic seizures and delirium tremens should be prevented by strict attention to the patient's metabolic status and by the careful administration of benzodiazepines. Because the metabolism of these drugs is altered in the presence of the "sick" liver and encephalopathy may easily be induced, reduced doses of diazepam or chlordiazepoxide should be used; oxazepam is preferable and may be used in regular doses.

D. Controversial therapies. Other therapies used in the treatment of alcoholic hepatitis are still controversial. They should be used only in carefully selected and controlled settings.

1. **Corticosteroids—prednisone or prednisolone**—given for 4 to 6 weeks at 40 mg have been shown in several studies to improve mortality in severely ill patients with alcoholic hepatitis and encephalopathy. No benefit has been reported for less seriously ill patients.

   An equation has been developed to assess the severity of alcoholic hepatitis:

$$\text{Discriminant function (DF)} = 4.6 \times \text{PT (sec)} - \text{control PT} + \text{serum bilirubin}$$

   where PT = prothrombin time

   DF greater than 32 has been equated with severe disease. Using DF, several multicenter trials have confirmed the usefulness of prednisone in severely ill patients. Hepatic encephalopathy was noted to be a predictor of early mortality. Based on these studies, corticosteroid therapy for 28 days may reduce early mortality in severely ill patients with alcoholic hepatitis.

2. **Anticytokine therapy.** Serum levels of tumor necrosis factor (TNF) as well as IL-1, IL-6, and Il-8 are elevated in AH and correlate with mortality.

   a. **Pentoxifylline** has been shown to reduce the production of TNF-2, IL-5, IL-10 and IL-12. In an animal model it has been shown to reduce portal pressure in cirrhosis. In a study with 101 patients with severe AH, pentoxifylline 400 mg t.i.d. was compared to placebo and the in-hospital mortality was lower in patients receiving pentoxifylline. The difference in mortality between the two groups suggests a number needed to treat of 4.7 which is identical to the number comparing the use of steroids to placebo in patients with severe AH.

   b. **Infliximab (IgG monoclonal antibody to TNF)** has been used in two small uncontrolled pilot studies and suggested a benefit. However, in a trial infliximab at 10 mg per kg in combination with prednisolone 40 mg per day resulted in a higher incidence of death due to increased risk of infections.

   c. **Etanercept,** a P75-soluble TNF receptor: FC fusion protein neutralizes soluble TNF. In a small study of 13 patients with severe AH, etanercept therapy for 2 weeks increased the 30-day survival rate to 92%; however, in 23% of patients etanercept therapy had to be prematurely discontinued due to infection, GI bleeding, or hepatic decompensation.

3. **Antioxidants**

   a. **Vitamin E** alone or in combination with other antioxidants may improve outcome of patients with AH.

   b. **Sadenosylmethionine (SAMe)** is a precursor of cysteine, one of the amino acids of the tripeptide glutathione, and is produced in the body from methionine and adenosine triphosphate by the enzyme SAMe synthetase. This enzyme's activity is decreased in patients with cirrhosis and results in a low level of glutathione. SAMe given to patients with Child's A or B cirrhosis decreased the 2-year mortality rate from 29% to 12%.

4. **Silymarin,** the active ingredient in **milk thistle,** is thought to exert hepatoprotective actions through free-radical scavenging and immunomodulatory effects. In patients with alcoholic liver disease, improvement in liver chemistry tests and liver histology is thought to be the result of decreased lipid peroxidation and lymphocyte proliferation.

5. **Anabolic steroids** might benefit patients with alcohol-related liver disease because of their effects on protein and nucleic acid synthesis. A number of trials have been undertaken to assess the effects of these drugs. Currently, there is

no consensus as to their value in any stage of alcoholic liver disease. Moreover, long-term use may promote peliosis hepatis and hepatocellular carcinoma.

6. **Propylthiouracil (PTU)** at doses of 300 mg per day for 45 days has been tried in patients with mild-to-moderate alcoholic hepatitis. Therapy with PTU may reverse the relative tissue anoxia in the centrilobular zone of the liver by decreasing the rate of oxygen consumption. Patients receiving PTU in several studies recovered more rapidly than controls. The effect of PTU on severely ill patients is not known.

7. **Colchicine** has been advocated for therapeutic use in alcoholic liver disease because of its antiinflammatory, antimicrotubular, and antifibrotic actions; however, its effectiveness has not been established.

8. **Potential new therapies.** Thalidomide, misoprostol, adiponectin, and probiotics have all been shown in preliminary studies to have anticytokine properties. Also, leukocytapheresis or other extracorporeal recirculating systems to remove cytokines are being studied; therapies inhibiting apoptosis may also be beneficial.

E. **Liver transplantation.** The suitability of patients with alcoholic liver disease as candidates for liver transplantation has been debated since the advent of transplantation programs. Clear guidelines are still lacking. Abstinence from alcohol is associated, in most patients, with improved liver function and prolonged survival. However, progressive liver failure develops in some patients despite abstinence. Because no effective therapy exists for decompensated alcoholic cirrhosis, patients with end-stage disease should be considered for liver transplantation. Unfortunately, the demand for donor livers exceeds the availability, and thus transplantation cannot, at present, supply each deserving patient. In patients referred for liver transplantation, it is important to rule out other alcohol-related medical problems, such as cardiomyopathy, pancreatitis, neuropathy, and malnutrition, which may worsen the overall prognosis. Posttransplant compliance with the medical regimen, continuation of strict abstinence from alcohol, and the availability of family or social support systems are important. When liver transplantation has been carried out, the outcomes have been good and do not differ substantially from those reported in patients with nonalcoholic liver disease.

Selected Readings

Bridle K, et al. Hepcidin is down regulated in alcoholic liver injury: implications for the pathogenesis of alcoholic liver disease. *Alcohol Clin Exp Res.* 2006;30:106–112.

Clouston AD, et al. Steatosis as cofactor in other liver diseases: Hepatitis C virus, alcohol, hemochromatosis, and others. *Clin Liver Dis.* 2007;11(1):173–189.

Foody W, et al. Nutritional therapy for alcoholic hepatitis: New life for an old idea. *Gastroenterology.* 2001;120:1053.

Kapadia C. Alcoholic steatosis: The Kupfer cell—A villain? *Gastroenterology.* 2001;120:581.

Purohit V, et al. Role of S-adenosylmethionine, folate, and betaine in the treatment of alcoholic liver disease: summary of a symposium. *Am J Clin Nutr.* 2007;86(1):14–24.

Tilg H, et al. Cytokines in alcoholic and nonalcoholic steatohepatitis. *N Engl J Med.* 2000;343:1467.

Yipw W, et al. Alcoholic liver disease. *Semin Diagn Pathol.* 2007;23:149–160.

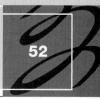

I. DEFINITION. Nonalcoholic fatty liver disease (NAFLD) is a spectrum of liver diseases with histologic features of alcohol-induced liver disease that occurs in individuals who do not consume significant quantities of alcohol. The spectrums of the liver diseases include **hepatic steatosis (fatty liver); nonalcoholic steatohepatitis (NASH)** with histologic evidence of hepatitis, hepatocellular injury, necrosis, and fibrosis; and **cirrhosis** with eventual portal hypertension and other complications including **hepatocellular carcinoma.**

NAFLD is believed to be one of the most common causes of abnormal liver chemistry tests in American adults. It is thought to be the major cause of cryptogenic cirrhosis. Ten percent to 20% of patients with NASH progress to cirrhosis or end-stage liver disease in a decade or more. The survival of patients with NAFLD is lower than in general population.

Clinically, NAFLD should be a diagnosis of exclusion. It should be suspected as a cause of chronic liver disease in patients who deny alcohol consumption and have negative serologic tests for active viral, congenital, and acquired causes of liver disease.

Hepatis C virus (HCV) or hepatitis G virus infections are not implicated as causes of NAFLD; however, NAFLD may increase the severity of HCV-related liver disease. Obesity-related steatosis seems to have deleterious effects similar to those of alcohol-induced steatosis on HCV-infected patients, exacerbating the liver damage.

In the United States the prevalence of NAFLD is estimated to be 20% and NASH 3%. The prevalence of NAFLD is 50% in people with diabetes, 74% in obese persons, and nearly 100% in morbidly obese individuals. NAFLD affects both adults and children: 2.6% of all children and 22.5% to 52.8% of obese children. Evidence for an association between arterial hypertension and atherosclerosis is accumulating. In fact, NAFLD is an independent risk factor for cardiovascular mortality.

II. ASSOCIATED CONDITIONS. Conditions associated with NAFLD include Type 2 diabetes mellitus, obesity, and dyslipidemia, all of which are related to **metabolic syndrome.**
   A. Obesity. Obesity is the condition most often reported to be associated with NAFLD. Obesity is described in 40% to 100% of patients with NASH. NASH has been documented in 9% to 36% of obese patients. The prevalence and severity of hepatic steatosis has been noted to be directly proportional to the grade of obesity, and the severity of NASH has been noted to be proportional to the degree of hepatic steatosis. The distribution of body fat seems to be important in the development of hepatic steatosis. In one study, a significant correlation was found between the degree of hepatic steatosis and waist-to-hip ratio, suggesting a relationship between visceral and intraabdominal fat and accumulation of fat in the liver.
   B. Hyperglycemia, insulin resistance, hyperinsulinemia, glucose intolerance, and Type 2 diabetes mellitus have been described in 25% to 75% of adult patients with NASH.
   C. Hyperlipidemias, including hypertriglyceridemia and hypercholesterolemia or both, have been found to be present in 20% to 80% of patients with NASH.
   D. Most patients with NASH seem to have multiple risk factors including obesity, Type 2 diabetes mellitus, and hyperlipidemia.
   E. Other risk factors include female gender, rapid weight loss, acute starvation, total parenteral nutrition, and small-bowel diverticulosis.

  F. Genetic conditions associated with NAFLD include Wilson's disease, homocystinuria, tyrosinemia, a-beta- and hypobetalipoproteinemia, and Weber–Christian disease.

  G. Surgical procedures associated with NAFLD, particularly NASH, include gastroplasty for morbid obesity, jejunoileal bypass, extensive small-bowel resection, and biliopancreatic diversion.

  H. Drugs. The use of a number of drugs has been implicated in the development of NAFLD. The list includes glucocorticoids, amiodarone, synthetic estrogens, tamoxifen citrate, 4,4′-diethylaminoethoxyhexesterol (DHEAH), isoniazid, methotrexate, perhexiline maleate, tetracycline, puromycin, bleomycin, dichloroethylene, ethionine, hydrazine, hypoglycin, l-asparaginase, azacytidine, azauridine, and azaserine. Chronic industrial exposure to petrochemicals has also been reported as a risk factor for NAFLD.

III. DIAGNOSIS

A. Clinical findings

  1. Symptoms. Most patients with NAFLD are asymptomatic; however, fatigue, malaise, or vague right upper quadrant pain or discomfort may cause patients to seek medical attention.

  2. Signs. Hepatomegaly may occur in up to 75% of patients. Splenomegaly may be present in 25% of patients. Stigmata of portal hypertension and cirrhosis occur rarely. In a subset of patients with NAFLD, especially in association with certain drugs and toxins (i.e., certain nucleoside analogs, antimitotic agents, or tetracycline) fulminant hepatic failure may develop rapidly. Cirrhosis may develop rapidly in patients with steatosis and inborn errors of metabolism (i.e., tyrosinemia).

  3. Laboratory findings. Laboratory features of NAFLD are nondiagnostic. Mild-to-moderate increases in serum aminotransferases (alanine [ALT] and aspartate [AST]) are the predominant laboratory abnormalities in patients with NASH. Typically, the liver test abnormalities are noted during routine testing or when patients seek medical attention for other complaints. However, liver enzymes are not always sensitive markers for NASH because some patients present with normal transaminases in the presence of severe liver disease. Also, there is no significant correlation between the degree of serum aminotransferase elevation and the histologic findings and severity of the hepatic inflammation or fibrosis. Serum ALT levels are often higher then AST levels, in contrast to the pattern seen in alcoholic hepatitis in which the AST/ALT ratio is higher and serum alkaline phosphatase levels may be mildly elevated; serum bilirubin and albumin levels are usually normal. Prolongation of prothrombin time (PT) is suggestive of hepatic decompensation. A small percentage of patients with NASH may have positive low-titer antinuclear antibody (ANA) levels. However, antimitochondrial antibody (AMA), antibody to hepatitis C virus, and hepatitis B surface antigen are negative, and serum ceruloplasmin and antitrypsin levels are normal. Elevated serum ferritin and transferrin saturation seem to occur commonly in patients with NASH. Men with NASH may have higher iron stores than women. One third of patients with NASH may have one or two copies of the Cys282Tyr mutation in the HFE gene (genetic marker for hemochromatosis). Trends toward more severe hepatic fibrosis in patients with NASH with this gene mutation have been reported.

  4. Imaging modalities. Several noninvasive imaging techniques including abdominal ultrasound (US), computerized tomography (CT), and magnetic resonance imaging (MRI) can reveal hepatic steatosis. None of the tests are significantly sensitive for the detection of hepatic inflammation or fibrosis. CT and MRI may be helpful only when extrahepatic manifestations of cirrhosis and portal hypertension (i.e., ascites, splenomegaly, varices) are present. Thus, none of these imaging modalities is sensitive or specific enough to definitively establish the diagnosis of NASH or reliably grade its severity.

  5. Liver biopsy is the only diagnostic test for confirming the clinical suspicion of NAFLD and NASH, staging the severity of the liver disease, and determining the extent of fibrosis. It is still uncertain as to whether liver biopsy is essential in the average patient, because biopsy results may not change clinical management. Liver biopsy should be considered for patients with metabolic syndrome and for patients with persistently elevated liver enzymes despite optimal treatment of associated metabolic conditions.

B. Histology. NAFLD is histologically indistinguishable from alcoholic liver disease. Histologic stages of NAFLD include steatosis, steatohepatitis, and cirrhosis. Steatosis involves macrovesicular fat accumulation in the hepatocytes. NASH histology includes macrovesicular steatosis, lobular inflammation, hepatocyte degeneration, hepatocyte ballooning, and hepatic fibrosis. Steatosis may be diffuse or located primarily in the central zones of hepatic lobules. Parenchymal inflammation of varying degrees is present in all cases and the cellular infiltrate may consist of neutrophils, mononuclear cells, and lymphocytes. Hepatocyte necrosis with ballooning and cellular dropout, Mallory's hyaline, and Councilman's bodies may be present.

Stainable iron may be present in 15% to 65% of patients. Pericellular, perisinusoidal, and periportal fibrosis have been described in 35% to 85% of patients with NASH. The extent of fibrosis may vary considerably from patient to patient, ranging from mild fibrosis around small veins or groups of cells (chicken-wire fibrosis) to extensive, severe fibrosis with bridging of portal tracts and central veins and distortion of the hepatic architecture. Cirrhosis is found at initial liver biopsy in 7% to 16% of patients with NASH and is indistinguishable from Laënnec's cirrhosis.

IV. The pathogenesis of NAFLD is complex, potentially involving multiple tissues including the liver, adipose tissue muscle, and other peripheral tissues. Adipose tissue and insulin resistance play a dominant role in the pathogenesis of NAFLD. It is known that visceral adipose tissue stores and mobilizes lipids. In the presence of caloric excess, adipose stores respond pathologically and affect the rates of both lipogenesis and lipolysis and results in an increased release of free fatty acids (FFA) from adipose tissue into the circulation. This then influences the accumulation of lipids in the liver and striated muscle. During this process cytokines are released and impair insulin signaling and reduce insulin-mediated glucose uptake into muscle. Also, an impaired insulin signal in the liver decreases glucose utilization and promotes glucose production, increasing hepatic glucose output. In addition, the availability of FFA in the liver stimulates de novo lipogenesis and FFA esterification. This is accompanied by impaired apolipoprotein (Apo) B100 and the formation of very low density lipoprotein (VLDL). All of these factors trigger lipid accumulation and oxidation in the liver, oxidative stress, the release of inflammatory cytokines, and hepatic stellate cell activation.

In summary, although the specific mechanisms involved in the pathogenesis of NASH are not completely clear, it is thought that NASH develops as a consequence of a two-hit process. The first hit is steatosis, and the second hit involves oxidative stress and proinflammatory cytokines which induce progressive liver disease. There is increasing evidence that the adipokines released from white adipose tissue seem to mediate the second hit involved in the pathogenesis of NAFLD and NASH.

Adiponectin is an adipokine with antiinflammatory properties. It also increases insulin sensitivity, regulates hepatic FFA metabolism, and reverses hepatic stellate cell activation. Low levels of adiponectin are strongly associated with visceral adiposity, hyperlipidemia, and insulin resistance. **Leptin,** another adipokine, is proinflammatory. It enhances hepatic fibrogenesis by increasing the expression of **transforming growth factor B (T6F-B)** and hepatic stellate cell activation. **Tumor necrosis factor (TNF)** and interleukin (IL)-6 are proinflammatory cytokines also produced by visceral adipose tissue. These cytokines play a central role in insulin resistance by impairing insulin signaling in hepatocytes and promoting inflammation. They also have a negative influence on the immune system. **Resistin** and **angiotensin** are two other factors that may contribute to the pathogenesis of NAFLD.

V. NATURAL HISTORY AND PROGNOSIS. The natural history of NAFLD is related to its histopathology. Simple steatosis does not appear to be a progressive disease; however, approximately 20% of patients with NAFLD–NASH progress to cirrhosis.

Although NASH is generally thought to be a clinically stable disease in most patients, it can progress to significant liver disease in a subgroup of patients. The risk factors for developing fibrosis and cirrhosis with NASH include older age, metabolic syndrome, obesity, diabetes mellitus, and AST/ALT higher than 1. Liver-related mortality has been found in 11% of patients with NAFLD with hepatic fibrosis who were followed up for 10 years. NAFLD may be as important as alcohol or HCV infection in causing cirrhosis in the United States. In fact, orthotopic liver transplantation is currently being performed for decompensated liver disease caused by NAFLD. Better understanding of the mechanisms involved in the pathogenesis of NAFLD is expected to help identify patients with hepatic steatosis who are at high risk of developing progressive liver disease, portal hypertension, and other complications of cirrhosis including hepatocellular carcinoma.

VI. TREATMENT. Currently, there is no effective therapy for NAFLD. Available treatment modalities attempt to eliminate the factors that are commonly associated with NAFLD. Weight loss, treatment of hyperglycemia, hyperlipidemia, and discontinuation of alcohol and potentially toxic drugs such as corticosteroids, estrogens, amiodarone, and perhexiline are recommended. Treatment for morbid obesity (i.e., bariatric surgery) should be considered. In small, short-term studies, the use of ursodeoxycholic acid, vitamin E, gemfibrozil, betaine (a metabolite of choline), N-acetylcysteine, and metformin resulted in improvement in liver chemistry tests and hepatic steatosis, but no significant change in histological grade of inflammation or fibrosis has been observed.

   Thiazolidinediones (TZDs) (i.e., **pioglitazone [Actos]** and **rosiglitazone [Avandia]**) is a class are drugs known as **"insulin sensitizers"** since they allow the adipose and muscle cells to become more sensitive to insulin and allow better uptake of serum glucose into these cells. In ongoing studies, TZDs show promise in reversing NASH, especially in the diabetic patients. (Avandia has been removed from the U.S. market for increasing cardiac risk factors.)

   Newer treatment modalities using anticytokine (e.g., TNFa antibodies, antioxidants, glutathione prodrugs, and insulin sensitizers) are being evaluated. Patients with NAFLD who develop hepatic decompensation should be evaluated for liver transplantation. In a number of patients, NASH has been observed to recur after successful liver transplantation.

Selected Readings

Day CP. From fat to inflammation. *Gastroenterology.* 2006;130:207–210.

Ekstedt M, et al. Long-term followup of patients with NAFLD and elevated liver enzymes. *Hepatology.* 2006;44:865–873.

Farrell GC, et al. Nonalcoholic fatty liver disease: from steatosis to cirrhosis. *Hepatol.* 2006;43(2 suppl I):S99–S112.

Gholam PM, et al. Nonalcoholic fatty liver disease in severely obese subjects. *Am J Gastroenteraol.* 2007 Feb;102:399–408.

Hubscher SG. Histological assessment of nonalcoholic fatty liver disease. *Histopathology.* 2006;49:450–465.

McClaine CJ, et al. Good fat/bad fat. *Hepatology.* 2007;45:1343–1346.

*M*ore than 1,100 drugs and herbal remedies have been reported to cause liver injury. Drug-induced liver injury can mimic almost all patterns of liver injury seen in humans. Among causes of acute liver failure, drug-induced liver injury accounts for more than 50% of them. The injury can be hepatocellular necrosis, cholestatic disease, deposition of microvesicular fat in hepatocytes, or mixed patterns. In most cases, the damage is caused by toxic metabolites of the drug or immune response to the drug or its metabolites. It may result in chronic hepatitis and cirrhosis. Antimicrobials, psychotropic drugs, lipid-lowering agents and nonsteroidal antiinflammatory drugs (NSAIDS), phenytoin, propylthiouracil antituberculosis drugs, sulfa compounds, and disulfirams are implicated most often. Table 53-1 is a partial list of drugs for which liver chemistry test monitoring is recommended. For the majority of drugs the risk of drug-induced liver injury is in the range of 1:104–105 in the United States. The risk is greater in women and the elderly, and the risk varies depending on the nutritional and other susceptibility characteristics of the patients and the drug class.

I. **HEPATOCELLULAR NECROSIS.** Drug-induced hepatocellular necrosis is clinically indistinguishable from cell injury from other causes such as viruses or ischemia. Thus it is important to obtain a drug history and note the presence of any hypersensitivity reactions such as rash or eosinophilia.

   A. **The diagnosis** is usually established by a history of drug ingestion and the elimination of other possible causes such as viruses or ischemia by appropriate serology and clinical data.

   1. **The severity** of the disease can range from minimal symptoms to fulminant hepatic failure. In fact, 20% to 50% of patients with fulminant hepatic failure have drugs, especially acetaminophen, as the cause of their liver failure.

   2. **Laboratory studies.** Serum glutamic-oxaloacetic transaminase (SGOT, or aspartate aminotransferase [AST]) and serum glutamic-pyruvic transaminase (SGPT, or alanine aminotransferase [ALT]) levels are elevated (2–30 times normal). These enzymes leak into the circulation from the cytoplasm of damaged or dying hepatocytes. The alkaline phosphatase and albumin levels are usually affected to a lesser extent. Serum bilirubin levels and the increase in prothrombin time (PT) correlate with the severity of the liver damage.

   3. A **percutaneous liver biopsy** performed early in the course of the disease can be helpful in identifying the type and extent of injury.

      a. Drugs such as carbon tetrachloride, acetaminophen, and halothane cause injury to the centrilobular or perivenular area.

 TABLE 53-1   **Drugs Recommended for Liver Chemistry Monitoring**

Piroxicam, diclofenac, sulindac, aspirin, pyrazine, fluconazole, itraconazole, dapsone, isoniazid, rifampin, labetalol hydrochloride, amiodarone hydrochloride, atorvastin calcium, lovastatin, nicotinic acid, valproic acid, carbamazepine, phenytoin, tolcapone, tacrine hydrochloride, rosiglitazone maleate, pioglitazone hydrochloride, methotrexate, propylthiouracil

    b. Drugs such as aspirin, nonsteroidal antiinflammatory drugs (NSAIDs), thiazide diuretics, nicotinic acid, clofibrate, gemfibrozil, oxacillin, sulfonamides, rifampin, ketoconazole, flucrocytosine, zidovudine, isoniazid, tacrine, trazodone, calcium channel blockers, beta blockers, and methyldopa cause diffuse parenchymal injury similar to viral hepatitis.

    c. Valproic acid, amiodarone, and intravenous tetracycline can cause extensive microvesicular fat infiltration of the hepatocytes and liver failure, as seen in Reye's syndrome or fatty liver of pregnancy.

  B. Treatment consists of prompt discontinuation of the offending drug and supportive measures. In most cases, patients recover over weeks to months. However, fatality in fulminant cases is still significant.

II. CHOLESTASIS. Drug-induced cholestasis is due to impairment of bile secretion by the hepatocytes. It may be caused by a change in the chemical and physical properties of the hepatocyte membranes as with estrogen and ^{17}C-alkyl-steroids. In addition, drugs, directly or by their toxic metabolites, may induce cholestasis by their effects on cytoskeletal elements, inhibition of membrane Na-K-ATPase, or immunologic damage to the hepatocytes or to the small bile ducts. Drugs most commonly involved in cholestatic liver injury are phenothiazines, tricyclic antidepressants, erythromycin, carbamazepine, cyproheptadine, tolbutamide, captopril, phenytoin, trimethoprim-sulfamethoxazole, sulfasalazine, and lipid-lowering drugs.

  A. Diagnosis. Patients with drug-induced cholestatic liver disease may present with clinical and laboratory findings very similar to those in intra- or extrahepatic bile duct obstruction, septic cholangitis, or acute cholecystitis.

    1. Clinical presentation and laboratory studies. Fever, pain, and tenderness in the upper abdomen (especially in the right upper quadrant), jaundice, and pruritus are commonly present. The serum alkaline phosphatase level is usually significantly elevated (2–10 times normal), with a mild increase in serum transaminases. Conjugated hyperbilirubinemia may be severe (2–30 mg/dL). There may be an accompanying rash or other signs of hypersensitivity.

    2. Diagnostic studies. Ultrasound should be performed in most patients to rule out possible bile duct obstruction. Endoscopic retrograde cholangiopancreatography (ERCP), percutaneous transhepatic cholangiography (PTC), or computed tomography (CT) may be necessary in difficult cases.

    3. Liver biopsy should be considered if the diagnosis cannot be made with the preceding clinical data. Histology usually shows cholestasis with or without inflammation. Microscopic cholangitis, infiltration of the portal tracts with inflammatory cells, and limited hepatocellular necrosis may be present.

  B. Treatment is supportive. Prompt withdrawal of the drug is essential.

III. MIXED-PATTERN LIVER INJURY. In most cases, drug-induced liver injury causes a combination of cholestasis and hepatocyte necrosis. Patients usually have moderate elevation of the serum transaminases, bilirubin, and alkaline phosphatase levels. Most of these reactions are the result of hypersensitivity to the drug and affect only a few susceptible individuals.

  A. Phenytoin (Dilantin) toxicity resembles viral mononucleosis. Patients present with fever, lymphadenopathy, and a tender liver. The liver biopsy shows portal lymphocytic infiltration and spotty necrosis of parenchymal cells.

  B. Drugs such as quinidine, allopurinol, nitrofurantoin, diltiazem, and many others cause a granulomatous reaction with some hepatocytic necrosis.

  C. For a detailed list of drugs and their liver toxicity see the article by Lewis in the Selected Readings.

IV. AMIODARONE HEPATOTOXICITY. Recently three cardioactive drugs—amiodarone, perhexiline maleate, and colalgia (4,4′-diethylaminoethoxyhexestrol)—have been found to cause liver injury resembling alcoholic hepatitis.

  A. Pathogenesis. Amiodarone has been reported to cause corneal and skin deposits, hypo- and hyperthyroidism, pulmonary infiltrates and interstitial fibrosis, peripheral neuropathy, and hepatomegaly with transaminase elevation in 20% to 40% of the patients receiving the drug. Liver histology in these patients resembles that of alcoholic hepatitis. There may be bile duct proliferation, fibrosis, and cirrhosis. Electron microscopy shows the presence of trapped phospholipids in secondary lysosomes. Amiodarone has been found to accumulate in acidic lysosomes and to competitively inhibit lysosomal phospholipases and phospholipid degradation leading to accumulation of phospholipids in lysosomes of liver cells. The relation of this phospholipidosis to the formation of a state resembling alcoholic liver injury and cirrhosis is not known.

Amiodarone has a long half-life and a large volume of distribution. The blood levels remain elevated, and the drug is present in the liver for months after the drug is stopped. The hepatotoxicity is usually clinically insidious. It usually develops after a year of therapy but can occur after 1 month.

B. Diagnosis. Liver disease is diagnosed by the findings of hepatomegaly, a moderate rise in serum transaminases, and occasionally elevated bilirubin. Liver biopsy with histologic and electron microscopic examination may be necessary.

C. Treatment and clinical course. Therapy is supportive after discontinuation of the drug. Even though hepatomegaly usually reverses in time, the liver disease may progress, leading to cirrhosis and its complications.

V. ASPIRIN HEPATOTOXICITY. Aspirin (ASA) and other salicylates have been noted to cause liver injury in patients with rheumatic and collagen vascular diseases such as juvenile and adult rheumatoid arthritis, rheumatic fever, and systemic lupus erythematosus. Normal subjects and patients with nonrheumatic diseases such as orthopedic problems may also be affected.

A. Pathogenesis. The blood level of the drug (>5 mg/dL) and the duration of intake (>6 days to weeks) seem to play an important role in the production of liver damage. The injury appears to be a cumulative phenomenon, appearing after many days of intake of large therapeutic doses. A single, toxic overdose of aspirin produces little or no hepatic injury.

Patients with rheumatic and collagen vascular disorders may be more susceptible to liver injury with aspirin than others. This may be due to the presence of hypoalbuminemia allowing higher serum levels of unbound aspirin, underlying liver damage, and possibly altered metabolism of the salicylates. The mechanism of hepatic injury seems to be intrinsic toxicity of the salicylate moiety rather than host idiosyncrasy to the drug. Salicylate choline and sodium salicylate also can induce hepatic injury. The liver disease is usually mild, acute, and reversible. Lowering the dose of ASA without totally discontinuing its use may be sufficient to reverse the injury. There is strong evidence to suggest that aspirin in the setting of a viral infection may provoke the development of Reye's syndrome in children.

1. Clinical presentation. Clinical manifestations of hepatic injury are not prominent. Most patients remain asymptomatic. Some patients complain of anorexia, nausea, and mild abdominal distress. Almost all patients are anicteric.

The liver disease is usually mild. However, encephalopathy, severe coagulopathy, and fatal liver failure have been reported. There is no established evidence that aspirin causes chronic liver injury.

2. Diagnostic studies. Serum transaminases are usually moderately elevated (2–10 times normal). In 10% of the individuals, SGOT levels are greater than 100 IU/mL. The SGOT (AST) levels are usually higher than the SGPT (ALT) levels. The alkaline phosphatase levels are usually normal or only modestly elevated. Serum bilirubin levels have been elevated only in about 3% of the reported cases.

3. Treatment is supportive. In most instances, it is not necessary to discontinue the drug for reversal of liver injury. Decreasing the dosage to attain blood levels less than 15 mg/dL seems to be sufficient.

VI. ACETAMINOPHEN HEPATOTOXICITY. Acetaminophen (Tylenol or Paracetamol) is an analgesic-antipyretic with few side effects when taken in therapeutic doses in most individuals. However, it is a potent hepatotoxin leading to hepatic necrosis when taken in large overdoses.

Most instances of acetaminophen-related liver injury result from a large, single overdose (>10 g or >30 regular-strength or >15–20 extra-strength tablets) taken in a suicide attempt. Multiple small doses taken with therapeutic intent can reach a total dose large enough to produce liver injury. Alcoholics have an enhanced susceptibility to liver injury from a single dose as low as 3 g or multiple therapeutic dosages (4–8 g per day for 2–7 days). Preexisting hepatic disease, malnutrition, and wasting diseases may also predispose patients to hepatic injury from acetaminophen with multiple therapeutic doses.

A. Pathogenesis. Following oral ingestion in therapeutic doses, acetaminophen is rapidly absorbed, and peak plasma concentrations are reached in 30 to 60 minutes. It is metabolized primarily in the liver by conjugation (70% to 80%) with glucuronide or sulfate, which are excreted in the urine. About 5% to 10% of the drug is oxidized to catechol metabolites and 3-hydroxy- and 3-methoxy-acetaminophen. Another 5% to 10% of the drug is processed by the cytochrome P-450 mixed-function oxidase (MFO) system and converted to a reactive metabolite N-acetyl-p-benzoquinone imine (NAPQI). Normally, this toxic intermediate reacts with the cysteine moiety of cytosolic glutathione and is excreted in the urine as thioethers. If the toxic metabolite is in excess of the cellular glutathione, it binds to vital hepatocyte proteins, leading to cell death. Figure 53-1 summarizes the metabolism of acetaminophen.

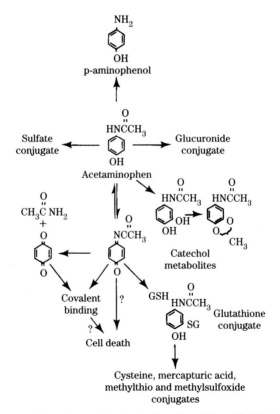

Figure 53-1. Major metabolic pathways of acetaminophen. (From Nelson SD. Molecular mechanisms of the hepatotoxicity caused by acetaminophen. *Semin Liver Dis.* 1990;10:268. Reprinted with permission.)

1. **Likelihood of hepatic injury.** The likelihood that a large dose of acetaminophen will lead to hepatic injury depends on the following:

   - Age of the patient
   - Total quantity ingested
   - Blood level achieved
   - Rate of disposition
   - Activity of the P-450 MFO system
   - Adequacy of glutathione stores

   a. **Age of the patient.** Acetaminophen overdose in young children is generally associated with a much lower incidence of hepatotoxicity than in adults.

   b. **Total quantity ingested.** The toxic total single dose in most instances is greater than 15 g. However, lower single doses of 3 to 6 g have been toxic in some situations.

   c. **Blood level achieved.** There is a correlation between blood levels at 4 and 10 hours after ingestion and the severity of the liver injury. If the blood levels exceed 300 mg/dL at 4 hours, the injury is often severe. Levels below 150 mg/dL are usually nontoxic. A nomogram that helps predict liver damage associated with particular blood levels of acetaminophen measured 4 to 12 hours after ingestion is shown in Figure 53-2.

   d. **Rate of disposition**

   e. **Activity of the P-450 MFO system.** The rate of production of the toxic metabolite clearly affects the toxicity of acetaminophen when large doses (>10 mg) are ingested. The capacity of the liver to sulfate and glucuronidase the drug is overwhelmed, and the absolute and relative amounts that are metabolized by the P-450 MFO system to the toxic metabolite are increased. Also, previous induction of the P-450 MFO system by chronic alcohol ingestion or by drugs known to stimulate the P-450 system such as barbiturates and phenytoin increases the biotransformation of the acetaminophen to the toxic metabolite.

   f. **Adequacy of glutathione stores.** Hepatic tissue levels of glutathione are critical to the toxic effects of acetaminophen. Toxicity and cell necrosis ensue when more than 70% of hepatic glutathione stores are used up by the toxic metabolite or when the tissue glutathione levels are depleted by previous fasting, malnutrition, or alcohol ingestion.

2. **Hepatotoxicity in alcoholics.** Serious hepatotoxicity has been reported with therapeutic doses of acetaminophen in alcoholics. This is because chronic alcohol ingestion enhances the formation of toxic metabolite by the previously induced P-450 MFO system, and malnutrition reduces the removal of the toxic metabolite due to reduced levels of hepatic glutathione.

3. The **location of hepatic injury** is centraxonial and corresponds to the location of the enzymes responsible for the metabolism of the drug. Sinusoids are often congested and dilated centrally. There is extensive hemorrhagic hepatocellular necrosis with minimal inflammatory infiltrate but without steatosis.

B. **Diagnosis**

1. **Clinical presentation.** A few hours after ingesting a large dose (>10 g) of acetaminophen, the patient usually has nausea and vomiting. If sedating drugs were also ingested, the patient may be obtunded. These symptoms usually disappear within 24 hours, and the patient appears fully recovered. Liver injury becomes apparent 48 to 72 hours after ingestion. The patient may complain of pain and tenderness in the right upper quadrant.

2. **Diagnostic studies.** SGOT (AST) and SGPT (ALT) levels are usually elevated into the thousands with lesser increases in serum alkaline phosphatase. In most cases, there is an early and severe coagulation abnormality with elevation of the prothrombin time. Values greater than twice normal forebode a grave prognosis. Usually bilirubin levels are mildly elevated.

3. **The severity of the liver injury** is variable. Progression to fulminant hepatic failure and death may occur 4 to 18 days after drug ingestion.

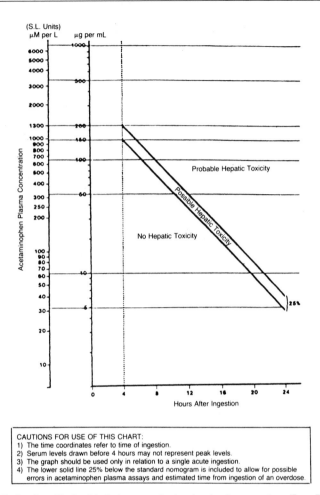

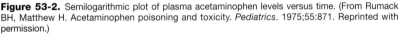

Figure 53-2. Semilogarithmic plot of plasma acetaminophen levels versus time. (From Rumack BH, Matthew H. Acetaminophen poisoning and toxicity. *Pediatrics*. 1975;55:871. Reprinted with permission.)

4. **Damage to other organs.** Other organs may be damaged by acetaminophen toxicity. Renal failure with acute tubular necrosis and myocardial damage evidenced by electrocardiographic changes may occur.

5. **Recovery.** If the patient recovers from the acute episode, there is a return of the hepatic architecture to normal within 3 months.

C. **Treatment**

1. Therapeutic approaches to acetaminophen overdose have included measures to reduce the absorption of the drug from the gastrointestinal tract by administration of activated charcoal or cholestyramine or to enhance its clearance from plasma by hemoperfusion or hemodialysis. None of these techniques has been found to be totally effective.

2. *N*-Acetylcysteine. Because glutathione is critical to detoxification of the toxic metabolite, replenishing hepatic stores of glutathione by providing its precursor cysteine in the form of N-acetylcysteine (NAC) (Mucomyst) has been shown to

be an effective antidote if administered within 10 hours of ingestion of the overdose of acetaminophen. Use of NAC within 24 hours of ingestion of acetaminophen overdose is recommended, but its usefulness beyond the first 10 hours is less dramatic. Oral NAC is well tolerated by most patients; it causes mild nausea and occasional vomiting. The intravenous route may be used if oral administration is not possible.

The protocol for treatment consists of identification of the patient and determination of the time and amount of acetaminophen ingested. If the ingestion has occurred within 24 hours of presentation, the patient should be intubated with a large-bore nasogastric tube, and gastric lavage should be performed. A loading dose of NAC, 140 mg/kg body weight, should be given orally and followed by 17 maintenance doses of 70 mg/kg each at 4-hour intervals for a total treatment period of 72 hours. While therapy is being administered, the blood level of acetaminophen should be determined and plotted on the nomogram shown in Figure 53-2. If the blood level of the drug falls in the range likely to lead to hepatotoxicity, the full course of therapy should be completed. The therapy can be discontinued if the level is below the toxicity range. If an oral dose of NAC is vomited within 1 hour of administration, that dose should be repeated. An antiemetic can be given to patients who are intolerant of oral NAC. In patients who persistently vomit the medication, NAC may be administered through a nasogastric or jejunal tube. NAC may be diluted 3:1 with cola, fruit juice, or water to produce a more palatable solution.

3. **Severely ill patients** should be given full supportive care as for severe viral hepatitis. Patients should be intensively monitored for maintenance of normal vital signs and urine output and for cardiac, renal, and hematologic status. Any abnormalities of fluid, electrolytes, or acid-base balance should be corrected immediately.

4. The Rocky Mountain Poison Center in Denver, Colorado, may be contacted day or night (telephone: 800-525-6115) to advise on any aspects of therapy.

VII. DRUG-INDUCED CHRONIC HEPATITIS. Drugs that have been documented to cause chronic hepatitis (CH) include oxyphenisatin, alpha-methyldopa, nitrofurantoin, dantrolene, isoniazid, propylthiouracil, sulfonamides, and halothane. The incidence of CH with any one drug is low, and the total number of cases is small. However, a drug history should be obtained from each patient suspected to have CH. In most cases, if drug-induced CH has not developed into cirrhosis, it improves or resolves with discontinuation of the drug.

A. **Methyldopa (Aldomet).** The incidence of hepatitis with methyldopa is very low; however, if the hepatitis is not noted in early stages, the disease may progress to chronic active hepatitis (CAH). Hepatitis occurs within weeks after starting the drug, suggesting a role for hypersensitivity. If the lesion is recognized early on, the injury and inflammation regress with discontinuation of the drug.

B. **Oxyphenisatin.** This laxative, although taken off the market in the United States, is still in popular use, especially among women in Europe and South America. Oxyphenisatin has been shown to cause acute and chronic hepatitis resembling "lupoid hepatitis." The disease may progress to cirrhosis if the drug is continued after the onset of liver injury. In most instances, however, after the withdrawal of the drug, the disease is halted and even reversed.

C. **Isoniazid (INH).** Isoniazid produces asymptomatic elevation of serum transaminases with mild liver injury in up to 20% of the patients within the first 2 to 3 months of therapy. However, approximately 1% of the individuals develop severe hepatic injury, even fulminant hepatic failure, associated with a high mortality. Chronic hepatitis generally does not develop if the drug is stopped within the first few weeks of recognition of the hepatitis. However, severe CAH accompanied by cirrhosis develops with persistent administration of INH.

1. **Pathogenesis.** INH-induced liver injury is thought to result from hepatotoxic reactive intermediates of INH metabolism. INH is first acetylated and then converted to acetylphenylhydrazine, which is a potent hepatotoxin. There are some

data to suggest that rapid acetylators (e.g., most East Asians) are more susceptible to INH-induced liver injury.

2. **Clinical presentation.** The clinical features of hepatitis induced by INH are nonspecific and resemble those of viral hepatitis. Fatigue, malaise, anorexia, nausea, vomiting, and abdominal discomfort are commonly noted. Jaundice is the presenting complaint in 10% of the patients. Signs and symptoms of hypersensitivity, rash, lymphadenopathy, arthralgia, and arthritis are rare.

   Older patients, especially older women, have a higher susceptibility to INH-induced hepatitis. Hepatitis is rare in patients younger than 20 years of age. The risk increases to 0.5% in patients 20 to 35, 1.5% for patients 35 to 50, and 3% for those over 50 years old. Alcohol and drugs that induce the hepatic P-450 enzyme system such as rifampin seem to increase susceptibility to INH injury. Continuation of INH after the onset of prodromal symptoms increases the severity of the hepatitis. Thus it is crucial to stop INH therapy in symptomatic patients immediately during the first 1 to 2 weeks.

3. **Treatment.** There is no specific therapy for INH hepatitis other than prompt withdrawal of the drug. Patients should be given supportive care. There is no role for corticosteroid therapy.

Selected Readings

Buckley NA, et al. Oral or intravenous N-acetylcysteine: Which is the treatment of choice for acetaminophen (paracetamol) poisoning? *Toxicol Clin Toxicol.* 1999;37:759.

Hanje AJ, et al. Thalidomide-induced severe hepatotoxicity. *Pharmacotherapy.* 2006;26: 1018–1022.

Kafrouni MI. Hepatotoxicity associated with dietary supplements containing anabolic steroids. *Clin Gastroeterol Hepatol.* 2007;5(7)809–812.

Lewis JH. Drug induced liver disease. *Med Clin North Am.* 2000;84:1275.

Lewis JH, et al. Drug and chemical induced cholestasis. *Clin Liver Dis.* 1999;3:433.

Marino G, et al. Management of drug induced liver disease. *Curr Gastroenterol Rep.* 2001;3:38.

Woo OF, et al. Shorter duration of oral N-acetylcysteine therapy for acute acetaminophen overdose. *Ann Emerg Med.* 2000;35:363.

I. Chronic hepatitis (CH) refers to a condition of hepatic inflammation, necrosis, and fibrosis that is present for at least 6 months. There are numerous causes of CH. The natural history and response to therapy depend on the etiology and the age and condition of the patient. However, the end stage of all forms of chronic hepatitis, cirrhosis, and its complications is the same for all causes.

A. Forms of CH. Histologically, CH has been subdivided into three forms:

1. **Chronic mild hepatitis** refers to mild disease in which the inflammation is confined to the portal tracts. Serum transaminases may be near normal or moderately elevated.

2. **Chronic active hepatitis (CAH)** refers to symptomatic CH in which the liver tests and histology are compatible with active inflammation, necrosis, and fibrosis, which may lead to cirrhosis. On histology, there is active inflammation spilling out of the portal tracts into the parenchyma with piecemeal necrosis and fibrosis.

3. **Chronic lobular hepatitis (CLH)** refers to lobular inflammation with spotty necrosis.

The histologic classification emphasizes the importance of liver biopsy in the diagnosis, management, and prognosis of the disease. Any of the causes described in section B can take any of these forms in histologic appearance; hence histology alone is not sufficient for diagnosis and proper management of these patients.

B. The causes of CH can be classified into several basic groups: viral, metabolic, autoimmune, and drug-induced CH. It is also important to exclude Wilson's disease, α_1-antitrypsin deficiency, and hemochromatosis in these patients. Table 54-1 summarizes the causes of CH.

1. **Autoimmune hepatitis (AH)** is a progressive inflammatory liver disease of unknown cause in which immune reactions against host antigens are believed to be the major pathogenic mechanism. Exclusion of other liver diseases that have similar features are very important before diagnosis of AH is made. These

---

TABLE 54-1   Causes of Chronic Hepatitis

Viruses	Metabolic causes
Hepatitis B virus	Primary biliary cirrhosis
Hepatitis C virus	Sclerosing cholangitis
Hepatitis D virus	Alpha$_1$-antitrypsin deficiency
Drugs	Wilson's disease
Alpha-methyldopa	Hemochromatosis
Oxyphenacetin	Autoimmune hepatitis
Isoniazid	Type I (antiactin)
Alcoholic liver disease	Type II (anti-KLM)
Nonalcoholic steatohepatitis	Type III (anti-SLA)
	Cryptogenic

include Wilson's disease, chronic viral hepatitis, alpha-1-antitrypsin deficiency, hemochromatosis, alcoholic and nonalcoholic steatohepatitis, drug-induced liver disease, primary biliary cirrhosis, and primary sclerosing cholangitis.

a. **Three types of AH have been recognized. These are Types I, II, and III.**

   i. **Type I (or Lupoid) AH** is the most common type in the United States and affects all ages. The majority (78%) of patients are women of northern European descent. Most patients also may have concurrent extrahepatic autoimmune diseases including autoimmune thyroiditis, Graves disease, ulcerative colitis, Crohn's disease, rheumatoid arthritis, pernicious anemia, progressive systemic sclerosis, systemic lupus erythematosus, Coombs positive hemolytic anemia, idiopathic thrombocytopenic purpura, leukoclastic vasculitis, nephritis, erythema nodosum, and fibrosing alveolitis. HLA-DR$_3$ and DR$_4$ are independence risk factors of susceptibility.

     Most patients (40%) present with an acute onset, and a subset of patients present with fulminant hepatitis. Others (25%) may present with cirrhosis indicating an indolent progressive subclinical disease.

    a) Prevalence in Europe and the United States is approximately 17 per 100,0000. AH accounts for 11% to 23% of chronic hepatitis in the United States.

    b) Diagnosis

       1) Clinical features. Most common symptoms are malaise and easy fatigability. Hepatomegaly and jaundice are usually present.

       2) Laboratory findings. Serum transaminases are usually elevated up to 10 times normal. Hyperbilirubinemia is usually below 3 times normal. Serum alkaline phosphatase level is frequently increased, but usually below 2 times normal. Patients also have hypergammaglobulinemia in the range of 50 to 100 g/L with a predominance of IgG fraction. Autoantibodies necessary for diagnosis included ANA, SMA, and anti-LKMI, but other antibodies may also be present. These include antiactin, SLA/LP, ASGPR, liver cytosol type I. Cryoglobulinemia may occur. The autoantibody and gamma globulin profiles are discussed in Table 54-2.

       3) On **pathologic examination** of the liver biopsies there is moderate to severe interface hepatitis and no biliary lesions, granulomas, or prominent changes suggestive of another liver disease. Plasma cells and rosettes may be seen.

TABLE 54-2 — **Clinical and Immunologic Comparison of the Three Types of Autoimmune Chronic Hepatitis**

Characteristic	Type I (lupoid) anti-SM (antiactin)	Type II anti-KLM-I	Type III anti-SLA
Age at presentation (y)	10–30 and 40–70	<17	30–40
Other autoimmune disorders	10%	15%–20%	
Autoantibodies (%)			
Anti-SM	100		35%
ANA	30–90	1–5	
AMA	10–20	1–5	
LE cells	10–50		
Gamma globulins (g/L)	30–100	20–30	
IgG	20–50	20–30	
IgA	3–5	1–3	
IgM	1–2	2–5	

SM, smooth muscle; KLM, kidney-liver-microsomal; SLA, soluble liver antigens; ANA, antinuclear antibody; AMA, antimitochondrial antibody; LEZ, lupus erythematosus.

ii. **Type II: anti-KLM (kidney-liver-microsomal) antibody–positive.** Type II is less prevalent than type I and has been described most often in Continental Europe. It tends to present predominantly in the pediatric age group (ages 2–14); however, it may also occur in adults and is more often associated with other autoimmune diseases, such as insulin-dependent diabetes mellitus, autoimmune thyroid disease, and vitiligo. The presentation is often acute, even fulminant, and has a propensity to progress rapidly to cirrhosis.

iii. **Type III: Anti-SLE-LP (soluble liver antigen).** These patients constitute a small group of AH patients who are, in general, negative for antinuclear antibody (ANA) and KLM antibodies. Type III AH may be a variant of Type I AH rather than a separate entity.

However, up to 30% of these patients may have smooth muscle antibody (SMA) and liver membrane antibody (LMA), rheumatoid factor, antithyroid antibodies, or antimitochondrial antibody (AMA). Nevertheless, there is no evidence that these patients differ in any significant respect from those with type I AH.

b. **Other findings.** Anti-liver specific protein (anti-LSP) and anti-asialoglycoprotein receptor (anti-ASGP-R) are found in virtually all AH patients with positive ANA or SMA and KLM-I. Anti-LSP is found in a number of chronic liver disorders, primarily those with an underlying immunopathology and in which periportal inflammation is a feature. Titers of anti-LSP and anti-ASGP-R correlate with histologically assessed disease severity and fluctuate in response to immunosuppressive therapy.

The distinction between AH and primary biliary cirrhosis is not always clearcut; histologic, clinical, and immunologic overlaps have been well described. In some young patients, AH may progress to sclerosing cholangitis.

Viral hepatitis (A, B, C, D, and E) should be excluded initially. The frequent finding of false-positive anti-HCV in patients with AH should be confirmed with HCV viral titer determination by the polymerase chain reaction (PCR).

AH runs a slow course in most patients. In some cases, however, a dramatic acute episode may develop, which may result in sudden death.

c. **Treatment.** In the past, patients with AH were diagnosed with histologic features showing advanced liver disease, and the disease was noted to be progressive and fatal within 4 to 5 years. In current practice, most patients come to medical attention in the earlier stages of the disease before the development of cirrhosis; thus, the life expectancy is improved. The mortality figures in the placebo groups of the major controlled trials all showed that more than half of the untreated patients died within 3 to 5 years. There is considerable evidence that immunosuppressive therapy that includes corticosteroids leads to a decrease in mortality. The goals of therapy are to diminish hepatic inflammation and fibrosis and prevent the progression of the chronic hepatitis to cirrhosis.

Following assessment of alternative causes of chronic hepatitis and of the extent of liver injury by liver biopsy, a therapeutic trial should be initiated. A response should occur within 3 months or will not occur at all. Soon after initiation of corticosteroid therapy, patients with AH feel better with abatement of fatigue, malaise, anorexia, and fever. Serum AST, ALT, and bilirubin levels fall, and there is a reduction in serum gamma globulin levels.

i. **Corticosteroids.** There is general agreement that the treatment of ACH should begin with a corticosteroid. **Prednisone** and **prednisolone** are equally effective. An acceptable regimen is prednisone or prednisolone 30 to 40 mg per day for 2 to 4 weeks. If the patient has a good response, the dose of the corticosteroid is reduced every 2 weeks according to serum ALT and AST levels. Once remission is obtained, some patients do remarkably well at low doses (2.5–7.5 mg per day) only to relapse if the drug is discontinued. In most (about 75%) of the patients, lifelong treatment is required. When a patient is in remission, a trial of drug withdrawal may be reasonable. If relapse occurs, however, treatment should be instituted promptly and continued indefinitely.

Patients who receive long-term corticosteroid therapy are at risk for progressive osteoporosis and vertebral compression fractures. Regular exercise, calcium 1.0 to 1.5 g daily and vitamin D 400 U daily and a bisphosphonate are indicated and recommended.

Corticosteroids have well-established, predictable dose-related side effects including hypertension, cataracts, diabetes mellitus, osteoporosis, and a predisposition to a variety of infections and weight gain. Most of these side effects are manageable if the dose is kept at less than 10 to 15 mg per day.

ii. **Azathioprine and 6-Mercaptopurine (6-MP).** The use of azathioprine has been of considerable value in permitting a lower dose of corticosteroids to be used to achieve remission.

It is recommended that azathioprine be started along with the corticosteroid at 2 mg/kg dose. Although azathioprine alone has not been effective in achieving remission, in some patients its use alone has been sufficient in maintaining remission. The dose is decreased to 75 to 50 mg when patients reach remission.

6-MP is an active metabolite of azathioprine, but the drugs are not equivalent in the treatment of AH. In small clinical trials, it was noted that 6-MP initially at 50 mg daily and increased to 1.5 mg/kg daily can salvage patients who have failed therapy with azathioprine.

Homozygous deficiency of thiopurine methyl transferase (TPMT) (an enzyme in the metabolic pathway of azathioprine and 6-MP) occurs in 0.3% of the population and heterozygous (intermediate deficiency) in 11% of the population. These deficiencies increase the potency of a given dose and enhance toxicity such as neutropenia, bone marrow suppression. Thus, TPMT enzyme genetics should be determined prior to onset of therapy with azathioprine and 6-MP.

Side effects of this therapy include nausea, vomiting, rash, pancreatitis, and cytopenia in less than 10% of patients. Side effects are reversible with dose reduction or termination of therapy. Risk of extrahepatic malignancy is about 1.4-fold in age- and sex-matched normal population.

iii. **Alternative therapeutic approaches.** Cyclosporine 5 to 6 mg/kg has been reported to be effective in treating patients with ACH in whom there has been no response to corticosteroids and in whom drug sensitivity prevents the use of azathioprine.

Other drugs including **tacrolimus** (4 mg twice daily), **mycophenolate** mofetil (1 g twice daily), **6-thioguanine** (0.3 mg daily), **sirolimus** (1–3 mg daily), and **budesonide** (9 mg daily) have been tried in small numbers patients with variable results.

iv. **Treatment results.** Remission is accomplished in 65% of patients within 18 months and 80% of patients within 3 years. Histologic resolution lags behind clinical resolution by 3 to 8 months.

Drug withdrawal may be tried in patients who satisfy remission criteria; however, it is achievable in about 21% of patients. Relapse after drug withdrawal occurs in 50% within 6 months and 70% to 86% within 3 years. Reinstitution of original therapy usually induces another remission, but relapse commonly occurs if therapy is stopped. Thus maintenance therapy either with low-dose prednisolone or azathioprine is recommended.

Treatment failure occurs in about 10% of patients. Higher doses of prednisone (60 mg daily) or prednisolone (30 mg daily) in conjunction with azathioprine (150 mg daily) results in improvement in 70% of these patients. Therapy needs to be continued indefinitely. Dose decrease of the drugs may be tried after remission is attained.

Ten-year life expectancy for treated patients is about 90%. Histologic cirrhosis does not alter treatment response and these patients should be treated similarly as those without cirrhosis.

Hepatocellular carcinoma (HCC) occurs in 0.5% of patients with AH, but only in patients with cirrhosis. Yearly abdominal ultrasound may be used for surveillance.

v. **Liver transplantation** may be offered to patients who have advanced liver disease and have failed medical therapy It is recommended that patients with AH be considered for liver transplantation at early stages of disease, before severe complications of cirrhosis develop. Survival ranges from 83% to 92% and 10-year survival is 75%. Recurrent disease may be seen mainly in recipients who are inadequately immunosuppressed. De Novo AH occurs in 3% to 5% of recipients transplanted for nonautoimmune disease, especially children receiving cyclosporin.

II. PRIMARY BILIARY CIRRHOSIS

A. Epidemiology. Primary biliary cirrhosis (PBC) is one of the more common forms of chronic liver disease. Its cause is unknown; however, genetic and immunologic factors appear to play a role. The lack of concordance of PBC in identical twins suggests that a triggering event is necessary to initiate PBC in a genetically susceptible person. It is characterized by chronic inflammation and destruction of small intrahepatic bile ducts, leading to chronic cholestasis, cirrhosis, and portal hypertension.

PBC primarily (>90%) is a disease of middle-aged women. The disease has not been seen in children. The age of onset ranges from 30 to 70 years. It affects all races and socioeconomic classes and seems to be associated with HLA-DR8 and DPQ1 gene.

PBC is associated with other autoimmune diseases including thyroiditis, hypothyroidism, Sjögren's syndrome, scleroderma, rheumatoid arthritis, and CREST syndrome (calcinosis, Raynaud's, esophageal dysmotility, sclerodactyly, and telangiectasia).

Patients with PBC also have abnormalities of cellular immunity, impaired T-cell regulation; negative delayed hypersensitivity skin tests, decreased numbers of circulating T lymphocytes, and sequestration of T lymphocytic with hepatic portal triads.

B. Histopathology of PBC includes gradual destruction of interlobular bile ducts with a lymphocytic and plasma cell rich inflammatory reaction, leading to progressive cholestasis, disappearance of bile ducts, portal fibrosis, and ultimately cirrhosis. The disease can be divided histologically into four stages of increasing severity. However, because the inflammation is patchy throughout the liver and the typical changes of all four stages sometimes can be found in a single liver biopsy specimen, it is often difficult to follow the course of the disease or the efficacy of a treatment program.

1. In **Stage I,** there is a florid destruction of small bile ducts with mononuclear cell (mostly lymphocytic) infiltrate. The infiltrate is confined to the portal tracts. Granulomas may be seen.
2. In **Stage II,** the lesion is more widespread with inflammation spilling into the periportal parenchyma. There is loss of bile ducts with few remaining irregular-appearing ones. Diffuse portal fibrosis may be present.
3. In **Stage III,** histology is similar to Stage II; however, fibrous septa extend between triads and form fibrous bridges.
4. **Stage IV** represents the end stage with frank cirrhosis and absence of bile ducts in portal tracts.

   Hepatic copper accumulation occurs due to chronic cholestasis, and levels of hepatic copper may be higher than those found in patients with Wilson's disease.

C. Diagnosis
1. **Clinical presentation.** In 50% to 60% of patients, the disease progresses insidiously and patients present with fatigue and pruritus. Usually, jaundice follows months or years later. In 25% of patients, jaundice may be the presenting

symptom. Darkening of the skin, hirsutism, anorexia, diarrhea, and weight loss may also be present. Less commonly, patients may present with a complication of portal hypertension, such as variceal bleeding or ascites, or have the disease identified during the workup of an accompanying connective tissue disease such as Sjögren's syndrome, scleroderma or CREST syndrome, systemic lupus erythematosus (SLE), or thyroiditis, or during routine blood screening. In fact, up to 50% of the patients are asymptomatic when initially diagnosed. Physical findings are variable and depend on the extent of the disease. Hepatomegaly, splenomegaly, spider angiomata, palmar erythema, hyperpigmentation, hirsutism, and xanthomata may be present. Complications of malabsorption, especially of fat-soluble vitamins and calcium, and those patients with Sjögren's also may have pancreatic insufficiency.

Renal tubular acidosis with defective urinary acidification after an acid load occurs frequently in PBC, but it is usually subclinical. Deposition of copper in the kidneys may cause the renal dysfunction. An increased susceptibility to urinary tract infection has been observed in women with PBC; the cause of this susceptibility is unknown. Also, there appears to be an increased prevalence of hepatocellular and breast cancer among patients with PBC.

2. **Laboratory studies**

   a. **Serum tests.** Serum alkaline phosphatase level is usually elevated markedly (2–20 times normal). The values for 5'-nucleotidase and γ-glutamyltranspeptidase (GGTP) parallel those for alkaline phosphatase. Serum **transaminase** levels are slightly elevated (1–5 times normal). The degree of elevation of these chemistry tests does not have prognostic significance. The serum **bilirubin** level usually rises with the progression of the disease and is a prognostic indicator of the disease. Serum **albumin** and the prothrombin time are normal early in the course of the disease. A low serum albumin level and **prolonged prothrombin** time that are not corrected by vitamin K therapy indicate advanced disease: Both findings are poor prognostic signs. Serum **lipid** levels may be strikingly elevated. Patients with early PBC tend to have slight elevations of low-density lipoproteins (LDL) and very-low-density lipoproteins (VLDL) and striking elevations of high-density lipoproteins (HDL). Patients with advanced disease have marked elevations of LDL and decreased HDL; lipoprotein X is present in patients with chronic cholestasis. Serum ceruloplasmin is normal or elevated in contrast to Wilson's disease. Elevated **thyroid stimulating hormone** (TSH) levels may be present.

   b. **Serology and immunologic abnormalities.** Serum IgM levels are markedly increased (4–5 times normal), whereas IgA and IgG levels are commonly within normal limits. The hallmark of the disease is the presence of **AMA,** which is present in more than 99% of the patients. It is usually present in high titer and is predominantly IgG. AMA has no known inhibitory effect on mitochondrial function and it does not affect the course of the disease. The finding of a significant AMA titer (>1:40) is strongly suggestive of PBC, even in the absence of symptoms and the presence of normal levels of serum alkaline phosphatase. The liver biopsy in these patients shows the characteristic lesions of PBC. Demonstration of AMA by indirect immunofluorescence lacks complete diagnostic specificity, however, because AMA may be found in other disorders using this technique. Newer techniques now available are more sensitive than immunofluorescence in detecting AMA. These include radioimmunoassays (RIA), enzyme-linked immunosorbent assays (ELISA), and immunoblotting technique. A PBC-specific mitochondrial antibody termed **M2** has been characterized. The M2 autoantibody reacts with four antigens on the inner mitochondrial membrane. These are the **E2** components and **protein X** of the pyruvate dehydrogenase complex (PDC). PDC is one of the three related multienzyme complexes (the 2-oxo-acid dehydrogenase complexes) of the Krebs cycle. These complexes are loosely associated with the inner face of the inner mitochondrial membrane. Two other antimitochondrial antibodies that are associated with PBC are anti-M4 and anti-M8, which react with antigens on the outer mitochondrial membrane. Anti-M8 is found only in patients who have anti-M2, and its presence may be associated with a more rapidly progressive course. The presence of anti-M4 with anti-M2 identifies the CAH–PBC overlap syndrome, and anti-M9 may identify cases with a benign clinical course. Other AMAs are found in syphilis (anti-M1), drug-induced disorders (anti-M3 and -M6), collagen vascular diseases (anti-M5), and some forms of myocarditis (anti-M7). Other autoantibodies such as ANA, rheumatoid factor, antithyroid antibodies, antiacetylcholine antibodies, antiplatelet antibodies, and antihistamine and anticentromere antibodies may also be present in some patients.

The complement system appears to be in a chronically activated state in patients with PBC due to activation of the classic complement pathway. There are decreased numbers of circulating T lymphocytes (both T4 and T8) and abnormalities of the regulation and function of these cells. Bile duct cells in patients with PBC express increased amounts of the class I histocompatibility-complex antigens HLA-A, HLA-B, and HLA-C and class II HLA-DR antigens on their cell membrane, in contrast to normal bile duct cells. These bile duct cells in patients with PBC are good targets for attack by activated cytotoxic T cells. Indeed, the bile duct lesion in PBC resembles that found in graft-versus-host disease and in instances of rejection of hepatic allografts—disorders that are known to be mediated by cytotoxic lymphocytes.

3. Diagnosis of PBC is not difficult in a middle-aged woman presenting with pruritus, an elevated alkaline phosphatase level, and the presence of AMA in the serum. Pathopneumonic findings in the liver biopsy confirm the diagnosis. However, if atypical features are present, such as absence of the mitochondrial antibody, male gender, or young age, other possibilities need to be excluded.

4. The differential diagnosis of PBC includes gallstones, tumor, cyst, postoperative or other causes of extrahepatic bile duct obstruction, primary sclerosing cholangitis, cholangiocarcinoma, sarcoidosis, drug-induced cholestatic liver disease, autoimmune hepatitis, alcoholic hepatitis, chronic active hepatitis, and cholestatic viral hepatitis.

The anatomy of the extra- and intrahepatic ducts may be satisfactorily demonstrated with endoscopic retrograde cholangiography or MRCP to rule out the first three of these possibilities.

D. The prognosis for asymptomatic patients with PBC is better than that for symptomatic patients. Patients who are asymptomatic at the time of diagnosis may have a normal life expectancy. Cases of prolonged survival with minimal progression of the disease and symptoms are well described. In symptomatic patients, advanced age, elevated serum bilirubin levels, decreased serum albumin levels, and cirrhosis each correlate with shortened survival.

E. The treatment of PBC can be divided into three areas: (a) management of symptoms, (b) specific drug treatments to halt the progression of the disease, and (c) hepatic transplantation.

1. Relief of symptoms

a. Pruritus is the most distressing symptom of PBC. The cause of pruritus is not known. It may be related to the retention of bile salts or other chemicals in the skin, or it may be immunologically mediated.

i. Cholestyramine. Oral cholestyramine is the treatment of choice. By binding and removing bile salts in the intestine, it interrupts the enterohepatic circulation and thus decreases the blood levels of bile salts. The usual dosage is 4 g before and 4 g after breakfast. Many patients require another 8 g with the evening meal. Cholestyramine reduces vitamin A, D, E, and K absorption and may contribute to worsening of osteoporosis, osteomalacia, and hypoprothrombinemia.

    ii. Colestipol hydrochloride (5 g orally t.i.w.) is as affective as cholestyramine with similar side effects; however, it may be more palatable.

    iii. Rifampin, at 150 mg p.o. b.i.d., a potent inducer of hepatic drug metabolizing enzymes, also relieves itching. Naloxone, naltrexone, cimetidine, phenobarbital, UVB light, and metronidazole have also been reported to be of benefit in some patients.

    iv. Plasmapheresis relieves itching in refractory cases.

  b. Hyperlipidemia. Skin xanthomas and xanthelasmas are likely to occur when the total serum lipids exceed 1800 mg/dL. Cholestyramine, 12 to 16 g per day, is the treatment of choice. Treatment with corticosteroids, phenobarbital, and plasmapheresis also has been reported to result in regression of the lipid deposits. Repeated plasmapheresis or plasma exchange may relieve symptoms of xanthomatous neuropathy. Clofibrate therapy of hypercholesterolemia is contraindicated in PBC.

  c. Gallstones. The incidence of gallstones is increased in PBC, occurring in about 40% of the patients. Gallstone disease may complicate the course of PBC and should be addressed appropriately by endoscopic sphincterotomy or surgery.

  d. Malabsorption and malnutrition. Steatorrhea is common and may reach levels as high as 40 g of fat per day in patients with PBC. In such patients, nocturnal diarrhea, weight loss, and muscle wasting may be prominent. **Malabsorption** in PBC is multifactorial. The progressive bile duct lesion in these patients reduces bile salt concentrations in the small intestine and markedly decreases micelle formation and fat absorption.

    The incidence of **celiac sprue** is increased in this patient population, which in itself causes further malabsorption.

    Pancreatic dysfunction may also be present. Since medium-chain triglycerides (MCT) do not require micelle formation for absorption, 60% of the dietary fat intake may be given as MCT to these patients.

    Patients should be screened for **fat-soluble vitamin deficiency.** Oral vitamin A (25,000–50,000 units per day) should be given to patients with advanced PBC to prevent night blindness, with monitoring of serum levels to prevent toxicity. Some patients may require oral zinc supplementation for improved dark adaptation. Vitamin E deficiency is also common in patients with PBC, but routine supplementation is not indicated. Vitamin K deficiency and hypoprothrombinemia may be monitored by following the prothrombin time. Oral vitamin K supplementation usually corrects this deficiency.

  e. Hepatic osteodystrophy is **osteoporosis and osteomalacia** with **secondary hyperparathyroidism.** In PBC, fat malabsorption and steatorrhea interfere with calcium absorption both by malabsorption of vitamin D and by loss of calcium with unabsorbed long-chain fatty acids. Vitamin D deficiency in PBC may be corrected with oral doses of vitamin D, between 400 and 4,000 IU daily. Since the hepatic and renal hydroxylation of vitamin D remains intact with PBC, the more expensive hydroxylated vitamin D preparations are not necessary. For the correction of osteoporosis, postmenopausal patients with PBC should be given calcium supplements together with vitamin D prophylaxis and bisphosphonates.

2. Specific drug treatment. Even though the etiology of PBC is unknown, it is well accepted that it is an autoimmune disease. Defects of both cellular and humoral immunity have been demonstrated. Also, with chronic cholestasis, there is intraparenchymal copper deposition and progressive hepatic fibrosis. Thus, drugs chosen to treat the hepatic lesion of PBC are those that stimulate or suppress the immune response, chelate copper, or decrease collagen formation. Corticosteroids, cyclosporin, azathioprine, chlorambucil, D-penicillamine, triethylene tetramine dihydrochloride, and zinc sulfate have been used in controlled trials in the treatment of PBC and have been found to be ineffective.

  a. Ursodeoxycholic acid at doses of 12 to 15 mg/kg of body weight per day is now used as the initial therapy of PBC. It improves the serum alkaline phosphatase, aminotransferase, IgM, and bilirubin levels. Histologic improvement is less impressive, but the rate of worsening may be slowed. Also, the need for cholestyramine is decreased in patients with pruritus. It appears that ursodeoxycholic acid is safe, effective, and well tolerated and its efficacy is usually maintained for up to 10 years.

   b. Colchicine, an antiinflammatory and anticollagen agent at doses of 0.6 mg daily or twice daily, has been shown in some studies to slow the progression PBC and to improve serum levels of bilirubin, albumin, alkaline phosphatase, aminotransferases, and cholesterol. After 2 to 4 years, however, there is no improvement in histology, symptoms, or physical findings. Except for diarrhea in a few patients, there is no toxicity. It seems likely that colchicine is of some benefit to patients with PBC.

   c. Methotrexate. Low-dose oral pulse methotrexate 0.25 mg/kg per week may induce striking improvement in biochemical tests, fatigue, and pruritus in some patients with PBC. Histologic improvement also has been seen. In one study 15% of patients with PBC treated with methotrexate developed interstitial pneumonitis. This high incidence has not been seen in other studies. At this time, methotrexate is best reserved for patients with PBC who do not respond to UDCA and/or colchicine and are noted to be clinically worsening.

   Most patients with PBC are initially treated with UDCA 12 to 15 mg/kg body weight per day. In patients whose liver chemistry tests do not normalize in 6 months and/or whose liver biopsies fail to improve or worsen after 1 year of treatment with UDCA, colchicine is added to the treatment regimen. Methotrexate is added if the liver biopsy does not improve or worsens after one year of treatment with UDCA and colchicine. It is reported that using this individualized approach of stepwise combination therapy more than 80% of patients with precirrhotic PBC has responded by improvement of their symptoms, normalization of the liver chemistry tests, and some improvement of the liver histology.

3. Liver transplantation is an effective treatment for PBC, with 1- and 5-year survival rates of 75% and 70% in most centers. Transplantation markedly improves chances for survival, and results are better with earlier transplantation. Patients developing cirrhosis should be referred to transplant centers and placed on waiting lists. Clinical variables have been determined at transplant centers to help in assessing the timing of transplantation. Recurrence of PBC in the grafted liver is rare.

III. PRIMARY SCLEROSING CHOLANGITIS

   A. Definition. Primary sclerosing cholangitis (PSC) is a chronic, fibrosing inflammation of the biliary ductal system leading to cholestasis, bile duct obliteration, and cirrhosis of the liver. Most patients are male (67%). PBC may present in two forms:

   1. Large-duct PSC. Involvement of the larger bile ducts can be identified by cholangiography. In the classic manifestation of the disease, large-duct PSC may be accompanied by small-duct PSC.

   2. Small-duct PSC (pericholangitis). Involvement of microscopically identifiable bile ducts may be the major manifestation of PSC. Changes in large bile ducts may accompany small-duct PSC.

   B. Pathogenesis

   1. The **etiology** of PSC remains unclear. Injury from infection of the bile ducts due to portal bacteremia, viremia, toxins, or ischemia from hepatic arterial damage has been proposed but not substantiated. There is a close relation between PSC and inflammatory bowel disease (IBD). In the United States approximately 75% of all patients with PSC have coexisting ulcerative colitis (UC) or Crohn's enterocolitis. PSC is the most common form of chronic liver disease accompanying UC; about 5% to 10% of all patients with UC eventually have PSC. Immunologic injury may be the most likely cause of the disease.

a. **Genetic factors.** A close association has been found between the HLA-B8 phenotype and PSC in 60% to 80% of patients with or without UC. Also, HLA-DR3 has been found in 70% of patients with PSC. It appears that a patient with UC who possesses HLA-B8, DR3 haplotype has a 10-fold increase in the relative risk of development of PSC. Of patients who do not possess HLA-B8, DR3, an association with HLA-DR2 has been found in 70%. HLA-B8, DR3 and HLA-DR2 are equally distributed in patients with PSC, with or without UC. It appears that HLA-DR3, HLA-DR2, and UC are separate, independent risk factors for the development of PSC.

b. **Humoral immune abnormalities.** As in primary biliary cirrhosis, adult patients with PSC usually have hypergammaglobulinemia and increased levels of IgM. High levels of IgG are found in all children with PSC, and 50% of these children also have elevated IgM levels. Smooth muscle antibody (SMA) and antinuclear antibody (ANA) may also be present in patients with PSC. However, there is no correlation between the presence of circulating autoantibodies and any clinical parameter of the disease.

Circulating anticolonic antibodies have been detected in 60% to 65% of patients with PSC and UC. Antineutrophil cytoplasmic antibody (ANCA) is present in 80% of patients.

Elevated levels of circulating immune complexes also have been found in both sera and bile of patients with PSC. Whether this finding is primary or an epiphenomenon is not clear. There is also activation of the complement system via the classic pathway, supporting the involvement of humoral immune mechanisms in PSC.

c. **Cellular immune abnormalities.** A significant reduction in the total number of circulating T cells, especially in the suppressor-cytotoxic (T8) cells, has been noted in PSC, leading to an increased ratio of helper suppressor (T4/T8) cells. There is also an increase in the number and percentage of B cells.

In the liver, the portal T4/T8 ratio has been found to be higher in the portal tract than around proliferating bile ductules. Cytotoxic (T8) cells tended to localize in areas of bile duct proliferation and infiltrate the ductal epithelium.

d. **Bile duct expression of HLA-DR.** Intra- and extrahepatic bile ducts in normal subjects do not express HLA class II (HLA-DR) antigens. It has been shown that most intrahepatic bile ducts in patients with PSC express HLA-DR antigens on the surface cell membrane of the bile duct epithelial cells. This aberrant expression may play a role in the pathogenesis of bile duct damage in PSC.

e. **Conclusion.** There is strong evidence that genetic and immunologic factors are important in the pathogenesis of PSC. The immunologic destruction of bile ducts seems to be triggered in genetically predisposed individuals, possibly by viruses, bacteria, or toxins. The association with IBD and UC may be explained by the passage of these microorganisms or toxins across the damaged colonic epithelial barrier into the portal circulation.

2. **The prevalence of PSC** in the United States is approximately 5 cases per 100,000 persons. It affects predominantly young males with an age range of 15 to 75+ years. At the time of diagnosis, most patients are younger than 45 years. PSC has been reported in children 4 to 14 years old.

3. **Associated disorders.** PSC may be associated with a variety of autoimmune disorders. These include Sjögren's syndrome, retroperitoneal and mediastinal fibrosis, thyroiditis, myasthenia gravis, Type 1 diabetes mellitus, celiac sprue, sarcoidosis, cystic fibrosis, Peyronie's disease, idiopathic chronic pancreatitis, lupus, rheumatoid arthritis, systemic sclerosis, immune thrombocytopenic purpura, and autoimmune hemolytic anemia.

4. **Cholangiocarcinoma.** Clinical experience and pathologic evidence strongly support an association between PSC and cholangiocarcinoma. Cholangiocarcinoma arises in 5% to 10% of patients with preexisting PSC and can present in a synchronous fashion with PSC. The most frequent location is the bifurcation of the

common right and left hepatic ducts (Klatskin tumor); however, it can be multifocal. It is usually heralded by rapid clinical deterioration with progressive jaundice, weight loss, and abdominal discomfort. Regardless of therapy, including transplantation, the prognosis for patients with cholangiocarcinoma complicating PSC has been poor. Active smoking and alcohol abuse may increase the risk of developing cholangiocarcinoma in patients with PSC. PSC may also be an independent risk for colorectal carcinoma.

C. Diagnosis. The diagnosis of PSC is based on clinical, biochemical, radiologic, and histologic criteria. The disease is suspected in patients with a cholestatic biochemical profile for longer than 3 to 6 months.

1. Clinical presentation

a. History. Most patients are initially asymptomatic but have a chronic indolent form of the disease, which may remain quiescent for many years. When fatigue, pruritus, and jaundice develop, patients typically have advanced disease. Weight loss, abdominal pain, and sometimes complications of cirrhosis or portal hypertension such as variceal bleeding, ascites, or encephalopathy may be the presenting findings.

Approximately 15% of patients with PSC present with an acute relapsing type of disease with fever, chills, night sweats, recurrent upper quadrant pain, and intermittent episodes of jaundice. This "cholangitic" group of patients may have self-limited, recurrent episodes of bacterial cholangitis caused by biliary sludge, which may intermittently obstruct strictured bile ducts.

The distinction between these two presentations of PSC may merge with progression of disease. In both types, intrahepatic bile duct obstruction may develop with sludge or pigment stones and recurrent symptoms of bacterial cholangitis.

b. Physical examination. Many patients, especially asymptomatic ones, have a normal physical examination. However, with advanced disease, patients may have jaundice and hepatosplenomegaly, xanthomas, signs of portal hypertension, and stigmata of chronic liver disease.

2. The **differential diagnosis** should include extrahepatic bile duct obstruction; drug-induced cholestasis; primary biliary cirrhosis; chronic active hepatitis, autoimmune hepatitis, and alcoholic hepatitis with a cholestatic profile; cholangiocarcinoma and secondary sclerosing cholangitis arising in patients with choledocholithiasis; and congenital or postsurgical abnormalities of the biliary tract such as Caroli's disease, choledochal cyst, or strictures. In immunodeficient patients, infections with HIV, cytomegalovirus, and *Cryptosporidium* should be considered. Vascular damage to the hepatic arterial tree by cytotoxic drugs, chemotherapy, and graft-versus-host disease after liver transplantation may mimic PSC.

3. Diagnostic studies

a. Laboratory tests. All patients with PSC have an elevated serum alkaline phosphatase level (>2 times normal). Serum transaminases are also usually elevated (2–5 times normal). Serum bilirubin level is variable. Serum albumin and prothrombin time are dependent on the severity of the liver dysfunction. CA-19-9 levels greater than 100 U/mL may raise the suspicion for the presence of cholangiocarcinoma.

Hepatic copper concentration is elevated in most of these patients due to cholestasis; however, serum ceruloplasmin levels are also elevated. Serum gamma globulin and IgM levels are elevated in half of the patients with PSC.

b. Radiologic visualization of the biliary tree is necessary for the diagnosis of PSC. Endoscopic retrograde cholangiopancreatography (ERCP) is the preferred technique over percutaneous endoscopic cholangiography (PTC) since the intrahepatic ducts are not dilated. Cholangiography typically shows the presence of multifocal stricturing and irregularity of intra- or extrahepatic biliary ducts, or both, giving a "beaded" appearance. There are bandlike short strictures and diverticulumlike outpouchings in the biliary tree in one fifth of patients. Up to 20% of patients have an abnormal pancreatic duct resembling that seen in chronic pancreatitis. The cystic duct and the gallbladder are usually spared but are involved in 5% of the patients. ERCP, in addition to defining the extent of ductal disease, allows for brushings to be obtained for cytologic examination to rule out malignancy. It also allows therapeutic dilatation and stenting of the abnormal bile ducts when indicated.

c. **Magnetic resonance cholangiography (MRC) and positron emission tomography (PET)** are noninvasive radiologic techniques that may be used in the diagnosis of PSC. However, not enough experience has accumulated with these techniques at the present time. Further experience and advances in MRC and PET may allow these modalities to be useful adjuncts in discriminating benign from malignant disease.

d. **Ultrasound.** In many patients, an initial ultrasound of the biliary tree may help rule out choledocholithiasis and ductal dilatation as well as pancreatic pathology.

e. **A liver biopsy** is recommended for diagnosis and staging of PSC. As in PBC, four arbitrary stages have been assigned to describe the severity of PSC. In the initial stages, the abnormal findings of fibrosis and obliterative cholangitis are confined to the portal tracts. Later, scar formation, ductal obliteration, and parenchymal liver involvement with fibrous piecemeal necrosis and septum formation are seen, leading eventually to cirrhosis.

4. **Complications**

a. **Progressive cholestasis** may eventually lead to fat malabsorption, steatorrhea, and fat-soluble vitamin (A, D, E, K) deficiencies. Hepatic osteodystrophy, visual abnormalities, and coagulation defects may occur but are uncommon in these patients.

b. When **cirrhosis** and **portal hypertension** develop, patients may present with ascites, hemorrhage from esophageal varices, or encephalopathy.

c. The prevalence of **cholelithiasis, choledocholithiasis, and cholangiocarcinoma** is increased in patients with PSC. Ascending cholangitis may complicate each of these disease entities. Cholangitis may also occur in patients with PSC without biliary stones. However, it is much more common and recurrent in patients with previous biliary surgery.

d. **Intra- or extrahepatic cholangiocarcinoma** in patients with preestablished PSC is usually multicentric and may be found as carcinoma in situ in areas of fibrous cholangitis. Thus PSC seems to be a premalignant lesion of the bile ducts.

D. **Treatment**

1. **Medical therapy.** The medical management of patients with PSC may be divided into two categories:

a. **Management** of complications of chronic cholestasis and bile duct obstruction, such as malabsorption, itching, and recurrent cholangitis.

i. **Malabsorption.** Fat-soluble vitamin deficiency should be established with measurement of serum levels of vitamin A and 25-OH vitamin D, and prothrombin time. Vitamin A replacement therapy consists of 15,000 units per day. Vitamin D replacement may be done using doses similar to those used in PBC (see section II.E.1.e). The value of calcium supplementation in PSC is unknown. Steatorrhea may be diminished with the use of medium-chain triglycerides instead of long-chain triglycerides, as recommended for PBC (see section II.E.1.d).

ii. **Pruritus.** Itching appears to present later in the course of PSC than in PBC. It is worse at night and may result in insomnia and excoriation. The mainstay of therapy is cholestyramine as long as there is adequate bile flow into the intestine. The dose is 4 to 8 g before breakfast and 4 to 8 g after breakfast. If stools are acholic, there is insufficient bile flow for cholestyramine to work. It usually takes 2 to 4 days for the itching to diminish. Once the itching has resolved, the dose may be adjusted downward. However, if itching does not diminish after 2 to 4 days, the dosage may be increased to 8 g three times daily. Additional increases in dosage have not been shown to be effective.

In patients who cannot tolerate cholestyramine, colestipol hydrochloride may be substituted. If constipation occurs with either drug, laxatives and fiber supplements may be added. Activated charcoal capsules also have been used for pruritus. Phenobarbital 60 to 90 mg at bedtime may increase bile flow and act as a sedative. Ultraviolet B light and large-volume plasmapheresis may be helpful in intractable cases. The use of ursodeoxycholic acid is discussed in the next section. Intractable pruritus suggests intensive bile duct scarring and obstruction and is an indication for liver transplantation. Also see the recommendation mentioned for PBC-related pruritus in section II.E.1.a.

iii. Recurrent cholangitis. Antibiotics may be used to treat episodes of ascending cholangitis. Prophylactic antibiotics such as daily doses of ciprofloxacin hydrochloride, amoxicillin, or double-strength trimethoprim/sulfamethoxazole may decrease the frequency and severity of such episodes.

b. Treatment of the underlying disease process. A variety of immunosuppressive, antifibrotic, and antiinflammatory drugs have been tried in the treatment of PSC. The slow progression of PSC and spontaneous fluctuation in bilirubin levels make it difficult to evaluate treatment. However, no drug has been shown to improve its natural history.

i. Cyclosporin, azathioprine, penicillamine, colchicine, and **prednisone** have been studied and found ineffective.

ii. Ursodeoxycholic acid (UDCA) at 20 mg/kg of body weight per day has given promising results in the long-term treatment of PSC in several studies. UDCA is postulated to decrease serum aminotransferase by stabilizing hepatocyte membranes rather than by decreasing levels of other bile acids. It also alkalinizes bile and increases the bile flow. Theoretically, the result should be a decrease in the formation of pigment stones in the biliary tract.

iii. Methotrexate. In a small number of patients with PSC, methotrexate 15 mg/kg of body weight per week has resulted in dramatic improvement in symptoms and biochemistry. In several patients, cholangiographic improvement also has been noted with no worsening of liver histologic findings. However, it is not certain that methotrexate is effective in most patients with PSC.

iv. Tacrolimus decreased the serum bilirubin by 75%, alkaline phosphatase by 70%, and aminotransferase by 83% after 1 year when given to 10 patients with PSC. The dose of tacrolimus was that which kept trough levels between 0.6 and 1.0 mg/mL. There are no data on liver biopsy or ERCP findings.

v. Combination therapy with **prednisolone,** 1 mg/kg of body weight per day, **azathioprine** 1.0 to 1.5 mg/kg of body weight per day, and **ursodiol** 500 to 750 mg per day in 15 patients has shown promising results with significant improvement in liver enzyme levels and liver histology. Studies using **tumor necrosis factor (TNF) inhibitors (etanercept** and **remicade)** are under way.

vi. Summary. Because damaged or destroyed bile ducts either lack the capacity to regenerate or do so slowly and ineffectively, diseases such as PBC and PSC should be treated at early stages before the loss of much of the biliary system and while there are still adequate numbers of functioning bile ducts.

2. Surgical therapy

a. Biliary drainage procedures, either percutaneously, endoscopically, or surgically performed, provide only temporary benefit and are riddled with complications such as infection, obstruction, perforation, leakage, and hemorrhage.

b. Balloon dilatation and stenting. In patients with one or two dominant strictures of the extrahepatic bile ducts or at their bifurcation, balloon dilatation, either by percutaneous or endoscopic approach and stenting, offers a less invasive alternative to surgery; however, a surgical backup is necessary in such cases.

c. Liver transplantation offers an important, successful therapeutic option, especially in young patients with advanced PSC in whom any of the following indications exist: (a) clinically significant gastroesophageal varices, (b) persistent bilirubin level greater than 10 mg/dL, (c) spontaneous bacterial peritonitis, (d) repeated bouts of cholangitis, (e) loss of synthetic liver function, and (f) refractory pruritus. Colectomy does not ameliorate PSC in patients who also have ulcerative colitis.

One-year survival rates after liver transplantation are in the range of approximately 85% to 90%. Previously undiagnosed cholangiocarcinoma has been noted in some of the patients who have undergone transplantation, with a very high incidence of recurrence in the transplanted livers. Increased risk of development of colonic malignancy with long-term immunosuppression in patients with chronic ulcerative colitis who have had a transplant is highly suspected and warrants periodic colonoscopic surveillance. In 20% of patients, PSC recurs in the new liver.

Selected Readings

Alvarez F, et al. International autoimmune hepatitis group report: Review of criteria for diagnosis of autoimmune hepatitis. *J Hepatol.* 1999;31:929.

Angulo P, et al. Primary biliary cirrhosis and primary sclerosing cholangitis. *Clin Liver Dis.* 1999;3:529.

Charatcharoenwitthaya, et al. Long-term survival and impact of ursodeoxycholic acid treatment for recurrent PBC after liver transplantation. *Liver Transpl.* 2007;131:1236–1245.

Corpechot, et al. Assessment of biliary fibrosis by transient elastography in patients with PBC and PSC. *Hepatology.* 2006;43:1118–1124.

Czaja AJ. Ursodeoxycholic acid in autoimmune hepatitis. *Hepatology.* 1999;30:138.

Czaja AJ. Autoantibodies in liver disease. *Gastroenterology.* 2001;120:239.

Donaldson PT, et al. HLA class II alleles, genotypes, haplotypes, and aminoacids in primary biliary cirrhosis: A large scale study. *Hepatology.* 2006;44:667–674.

Ghali P, Marotta PJ, et al. Liver transplantation for incidental cholangiocarcinoma: analysis of the Canadian experience. *Liver Transpl.* 2005;11:1412–1416.

Gong T, et al. Ursodeoxycholic acid for patients with primary biliary cirrhosis: an updated systematic review and meta analysis of randomized clinical trials using Bayesian approach as sensitivity analysis. *Am J Gastroenterol.* 2007;102:1799–1780.

Graziadei IW, et al. Long-term results of patients undergoing liver transplantation for primary sclerosing cholangitis. *Hepatology.* 1999;30:1121

Kaplan MM, et al. Primary biliary cirrhosis. *N Engl J Med.* 2005;353:1261–1273.

Kessler WR, et al. Fulminant hepatic failure as the initial presentation of acute autoimmune hepatitis. *Clin Gastroenterol Hepatol.* 2004;2:625–631.

Lee J, et al. Transplantation trends in primary biliary cirrhosis. *Clin Gastroenterol Hepatol.* 2007; 5(11): 1313–1315.

Lempinen M, et al. Enhanced detection of cholangiocarcinoma with serum trypsinogen-2 I patients with severe bile duct strictures. *Journal of Hepatology.* 2007;47(5):677–683.

Lindor KD. Ursodeoxycholic Acid for the treatment of primary biliary cirrhosis. *New Engl J Med.* 2007;357:1524–1529.

Manns MP, et al. Autoimmune hepatitis: Clinical challenges. *Gastroenterology.* 2001;120:1502.

Montano-Loza AJ, et al. Improving the end point of corticosteroid therapy in type 1 autoimmune hepatitis to reduce the frequency of relapse. *Am J Gastroenterol.* 2007;May;102:1005–1012.

Panjala C, et al. Risk of lymphoma in primary biliary cirrhosis. *Clin Gastroenterol Hepatol.* 2007;5(6):761–764.

Pompon RE, et al. Quality of life in patients with primary biliary cirrhosis. *Hepatology.* 2004;40:489–494.

Rudolph G, et al. The incidence of cholangiocarcinoma in primary sclerosing cholangitis after long-time treatment with ursodeoxycholic acid. *Eur J Gastro & Hep.* 2007;19(6):487–491.

Suzuki A, et al. Clinical predictors for hepatocellular carcinoma in patients with primary biliary cirrhosis. *Clin Gastroenterol Hepatol.* 2007;Feb;5:259–264.

Tischendorf JJ, et al. Transpapillary intraductal ultrasound in the evaluation of dominant bile duct stenoses in patients with primary sclerosing cholangitis. *Scand J Gastro.* 2007;42:1001–1017.

Ueno Y, et al. Primary biliary cirrhosis: what we know and what we want to know about human PBC and spontaneous PBC Mouse models. *J Gastroenterol.* 2007;42:189–195.

I. WILSON'S DISEASE

A. Pathogenesis. Wilson's disease is a treatable, genetic disorder. The metabolic defect leads to progressive accumulation of copper in the liver, brain (particularly in the basal ganglia), cornea, and kidneys, causing severe functional impairment leading to irreversible damage. If not treated, this disease is invariably fatal, but with early diagnosis and treatment, the clinical manifestations can be prevented and reversed.

Wilson's disease is an autosomal recessive disorder. The abnormal gene is distributed worldwide with a prevalence of heterozygotes of 1 in 200 and homozygotes of 1 in 30,000. The genetic defect is on chromosome 13 near the red-cell esterase locus. In 95% of patients, there is also an absence or deficiency of serum ceruloplasmin, the main copper-transporting protein in blood. This deficiency is caused by a decrease in transcription of the ceruloplasmin gene located on chromosome 3.

B. Copper metabolism

1. **Copper concentration in the liver.** The liver of a human newborn contains six to eight times the copper concentration of an adult liver. Within the first 6 months of life, this diminishes to a concentration of 30 mg/g of dry tissue. Thereafter, throughout life, the liver concentration of copper is maintained at this steady state by careful regulation of intestinal absorption and transport and of the liver stores through the synthesis of plasma and tissue copper proteins and excretion of copper from the body in the bile.

2. **Absorption and excretion.** Approximately 50% of the average dietary intake of 2 to 5 mg of copper is absorbed from the proximal small intestine and loosely binds to albumin. It is promptly cleared by the liver, where it is incorporated into specific copper proteins such as cytochrome oxidase and ceruloplasmin or is taken up by lysosomes before being excreted in bile. There are two main routes by which copper is mobilized from the liver.

   a. Synthesis of copper-containing ceruloplasmin and its release into the circulation.

   b. Biliary excretion amounting to 1.5 mg of copper per day. This is the principal route of elimination of copper from the body.

3. **Genetics.** The copper excess seen in Wilson's disease has been shown to be the result of decreased biliary excretion and not an increase in the absorption of copper. The defect is caused by mutations in the Wilson's gene (ATP7B) on chromosome 13 gene. The gene ATP7b encodes a cation-transporting P-type adenosine triphosphatase that is expressed in the liver, kidney, and placenta. Mutations in ATP7b result in disordered export of copper from the liver into bile with resultant accumulation of copper cation in hepatocytes. The ATP7b protein is present primarily in the trans-Golgi where it is critical for excretion of copper into bile, as well as providing appropriate copper for binding to ceruloplasmin. Lack of functional ATP76 limits the availability of copper for ultimate incorporation into ceruloplasmin. When copper is not available for binding, an apoprotein is secreted from the hepatocytes that is rapidly degraded in the plasma, resulting in the hallmark of Wilson's disease, diminished circulating ceruloplasmin levels.

4. Family screening. More than 200 mutations have been identified in the Wilson's gene. Once a proband has been identified as having Wilson's disease, it may be possible to screen siblings on the basis of genetic analysis. As an autosomal recessive disorder, 1 in 4 siblings may be expected to be homozygous for the gene defect. Genetic testing of siblings requires the sequencing of both alleles of the ATP7b gene in the proband and then subsequent comparison of those alleles to the ATP7b alleles in the siblings.

C. Copper toxicity

1. Acute toxicity. Ingestion of gram quantities of copper causes serious gastrointestinal and systemic injuries and occasionally hepatic necrosis. Generally, however, the vomiting and diarrhea that follow the ingestion of copper salts protect the patient from serious toxic effects.

2. Chronic toxicity. Hepatic copper overload may occur in disorders other than Wilson's disease. These include primary biliary cirrhosis, extrahepatic biliary artesian, Indian childhood cirrhosis, and other chronic cholestatic disorders. The excess hepatic copper may aggravate the underlying pathologic process by direct damage to the organelles or through promotion of fibrosis.

D. Diagnosis

1. Clinical presentation. Wilson's disease has many modes of presentation. It may simulate several different neurologic and psychiatric disorders. It may present as asymptomatic elevation of the transaminases, chronic active hepatitis, fulminant hepatitis, cirrhosis of the liver, acquired hemolytic anemia, renal disease, or eye abnormalities such as sunflower cataracts and Kayser-Fleischer (K-F) rings.

a. Liver disease is the most common presentation of Wilson's disease in childhood. About 40% of all patients with Wilson's disease come to medical attention with evidence of liver disease. Because an increase of 30 to 50 times the normal hepatic concentration of copper can occur without any clinical manifestations, symptoms of liver disease do not appear before 6 years of age. However, one half of the patients have symptoms by 15 years of age. Thus, overt Wilson's disease is encountered predominantly in older children, adolescents, young adults, and rarely in older adults.

i. Forms. The hepatic disease may take several different forms.

a) Commonly it begins insidiously and runs a chronic course characterized by weakness, malaise, anorexia, mild jaundice, splenomegaly, and abnormal liver chemistry tests. The disease may mimic acute viral hepatitis, mononucleosis, or chronic active hepatitis.

b) Fulminant hepatitis may occur suddenly, characterized by progressive jaundice, ascites, and hepatic failure. The outcome is usually fatal, particularly when the disorder is accompanied by hemolytic anemia.

c) Some patients present with the typical picture of postnecrotic cirrhosis with spider angiomata, splenomegaly, portal hypertension, ascites, bleeding esophageal varices, or thrombocytopenia mimicking idiopathic thrombocytopenic purpura (ITP). The liver enzymes may be normal. The diagnosis of Wilson's disease should always be considered in patients younger than 30 years with negative serology for viral hepatitis; with a history of chronic active hepatitis; or with juvenile, cryptogenic, or familial cirrhosis. Although fewer than 5% of such patients have Wilson's disease, it is one of the few forms of liver disease for which specific and effective therapy is available.

ii. Histology. There is no one specific histologic profile to identify Wilson's disease in liver biopsy specimens. In the early stages of copper accumulation, when copper is diffusely distributed in the cytoplasm, it is undetectable by rhodanine or rubeanic acid stains. At this stage, lipid droplets are seen in the hepatocytes with ballooned, vacuolated nuclei containing glycogen. This initial steatosis progresses to fibrosis, then ultimately to cirrhosis. With time and progression of the liver disease, the hepatocyte lysosomes seem to sequester the excess copper, which is detectable throughout some nodules by routine histochemical staining. Because of the variable stainability and the irregular distribution of copper among adjacent nodules, absence of a positive rhodanine or rubeanic acid stain on a histologic slide does not exclude the diagnosis of Wilson's disease. The parenchyma usually is infiltrated with mononuclear cells. There may be cholestasis, focal necrosis, and Mallory's hyalin. In other cases, the histology may resemble that of acute or chronic active hepatitis.

Once macronodular cirrhosis develops, the microscopic findings are nonspecific. Hepatocytes may contain some cytoplasmic lipid, vacuolated glycogen-containing nuclei, and cytoplasmic inclusions containing copper-rich lipofuscin granules.

b. Neurologic disease is the most common presentation of Wilson's disease. The usual age of onset is 12 to 32 years. The most common symptoms are as follows:

  i. Incoordination particularly involving fine movements such as handwriting, typing, and piano playing.

  ii. Tremor is usually at rest but intensifies with voluntary movement and emotion. It ranges from a fine tremor of one hand to generalized tremor of the arms, tongue, and head. It may be slow, coarse, or choreoathetoid. Dystonia, ataxic gait, spasticity, and rigidity are late neurologic manifestations.

  iii. Dysarthria begins with difficulty in enunciating words and progresses to slurring of speech, microphonia, and aphasia.

  iv. Excessive salivation occurs early in the course of the disease.

  v. Dysphagia is progressive and oropharyngeal; patients have difficulty initiating swallowing, leading to regurgitation and aspiration.

c. K-F rings are corneal copper deposits laid in the Descemet's membrane in layers appearing as granular brown pigment around the periphery of the iris. They may be absent in early stages but are present in all patients in the neurologic stage of Wilson's disease. Most K-F rings can be visualized by the naked eye, but some require slit-lamp examination.

d. Psychiatric disease. Almost all of the patients demonstrate some form of psychiatric disturbance, which may appear as teenage adjustment behavior, anxiety, hysteria, or a manic-depressive or schizoaffective disorder. Psychotropic drugs may accentuate the neurologic manifestations of Wilson's disease and increase the patient's problems.

e. Hematologic disease. In a few patients, Wilson's disease presents as a Coombs-negative hemolytic anemia with transient jaundice. It may be intermittent and benign, or it may occur with fulminant hepatitis. The hemolysis occurs during phases of hepatocellular necrosis with sudden release of copper from necrotic hepatocytes into the circulation. This effect is indicated by a marked rise in the concentration of nonceruloplasmin copper in the blood and in the amount of copper excreted through the urine.

With portal hypertension and splenomegaly, hypersplenism may result in thrombocytopenia and pancytopenia. Progressive liver disease also gives rise to clotting factor deficiencies and bleeding.

f. Kidney disease. Renal abnormalities result from accumulation of copper within the renal parenchyma. These abnormalities range from renal insufficiency with decreased glomerular filtration rate to proximal tubular defects resembling Fanconi's syndrome, renal tubular acidosis, proteinuria, and microscopic hematuria.

g. In disorders involving "inflammation" and metabolic syndrome iron overloading may occur due to reduced iron egress. Iron is essential for many bacterial and viral pathogens. Hepciden plays a key role in protecting the body's precious iron from these pathogens. In response to inflammatory cytokins, hepcidin degrades ferroprotin, thus preventing iron from entering the bloodstream where it could be used by the invading pathogens. This leads to iron accumulation in the macrophages. With chronic inflammation this may lead to iron restricted erythropolisis and anemia.

2. **Diagnostic studies**

   a. **Serum ceruloplasmin.** Ninety-five percent of patients with Wilson's disease have a serum ceruloplasmin concentration less than 20 mg/dL. Because approximately 20% of heterozygotes also have diminished levels, deficiency of ceruloplasmin is not sufficient for the diagnosis of Wilson's disease. Patients with fulminant hepatitis and 15% of patients with Wilson's disease presenting with only a hepatic disorder may have a ceruloplasmin concentration of 20 to 30 mg/dL due to a slight increase of this acute-phase reactant protein with inflammation. Hypoceruloplasminemia also may be found in patients with nephrotic syndrome, protein-losing enteropathy, or malabsorption; these conditions can be distinguished easily from Wilson's disease.

   b. **Serum copper.** Because ceruloplasmin is the main copper-transporting protein in the blood, **total serum copper levels** are often decreased in patients with Wilson's disease, but free copper is elevated and is therefore responsible for excess copper deposition in various tissues. The determination of the serum **free copper** concentration represents the most reliable finding for the initial diagnosis of Wilson's disease. This value is calculated as the difference between total serum copper concentration and the amount of copper bound to ceruloplasmin (0.047 mmol of copper per mg of ceruloplasmin).

   c. **Urinary copper excretion.** Serum free copper is readily filtered by the kidneys and accounts for the increased urinary copper excretion seen in Wilson's disease. Most patients have urinary copper excretion levels greater than 1.6 mmol per day. However, urinary copper levels often are elevated also in patients with cirrhosis, chronic active hepatitis, or cholestasis. This measurement does not distinguish these entities from Wilson's disease, therefore, despite the administration of D-penicillamine, an agent that increases urinary copper excretion.

   d. **Liver biopsy** should be obtained for histologic studies and quantitative hepatic copper concentration in excess of 250 μg/g. Edition of dry tissue is compatible with the diagnosis of Wilson's disease. To obtain a reliable result, it is essential that contamination of the specimen with traces of copper be avoided (a disposable biopsy needle minimizes this hazard) and that an adequate sample (ideally 1 cm in length) be submitted for analysis. A trasjugular biopsy is inadequate for quantitative purposes. Other disorders such as primary and secondary biliary cirrhosis and long-standing bile duct obstruction can also lead to a very elevated hepatic copper concentration by interfering with hepatic excretion of copper into bile. These patients, however, have elevated ceruloplasmin levels.

   e. In the rare patient with a normal serum ceruloplasmin concentration in whom a liver biopsy is contraindicated because of clotting abnormalities, a **radio copper loading test** can be performed using ^{64}Cu, with a half-life of 12.8 hours, given to patients by mouth (p.o.) (2 mg) or intravenous (IV) (500 mg); the serum concentration of radioactive copper is plotted with time in hours.

      In individuals who do not have Wilson's disease, radioactive copper appears and disappears from the serum within 4 to 6 hours. A secondary rise of radioactivity appears in the serum after the isotope is incorporated by the liver into freshly synthesized ceruloplasmin. In patients with Wilson's disease, this secondary rise in radioactivity is absent, since the rate of hepatic incorporation of radio copper into ceruloplasmin is diminished.

   f. **K-F rings** are present in all patients with Wilson's disease who have neurologic manifestations, but they may be absent in patients presenting only with hepatic disease. If they are not visible, they should be sought with slit-lamp examination.

   g. In **Wilson's disease** presenting as fulminant hepatitis, the combination of a disproportionately low serum alkaline phosphatase level and a comparatively modest aminotransferase Mia with jaundice and clinical and histologic evidence of hepatic necrosis suggests Wilson's disease. The ratio of the serum alkaline phosphatase to the total serum bilirubin also may be used.

   h. All siblings of known patients should be screened for the possibility of Wilson's disease by physical examination, slit-lamp examination of the corneas, and determinations of serum ceruloplasmin and aminotransferase concentrations.

E. Treatment. Untreated Wilson's disease causes progressive damage of the liver, brain, and kidneys. Until the late 1940s, patients usually died before reaching 30 years of age. The prognosis improved substantially after the introduction of the copper-chelating agent D-penicillamine in the 1950s. It is important to establish a firm diagnosis of Wilson's disease, because the patient will be on lifelong therapy.

   1. Diet. The dietary intake of copper should be less than 1.0 mg per day. Foods rich in copper such as organ meats, shellfish, dried beans, peas, whole wheat, and chocolate should be avoided.

   2. D-Penicillamine was the first oral drug used for the treatment of any stage of Wilson's disease. Penicillamine chelates heavy metals, especially copper, and facilitates their urinary excretion, thus shifting the equilibrium from tissues to plasma. It is also antiinflammatory and may interfere with collagen synthesis and fibrosis. Pyridoxine, 25 mg daily, is given to compensate for the weak antipyridoxine effects of penicillamine.

   The usual daily dose is 0.75 to 2.0 g p.o. The effectiveness of therapy can be monitored using the calculated free serum copper concentration, which should be less than 1.6 mmol/L. The earlier the therapy is instituted, the better the results. The histologic abnormalities and many of the symptoms are reversed; however, already established cirrhosis, portal hypertension, and some neurologic abnormalities such as dystonia, rigidity, dysarthria, and dementia may not be reversible.

   Up to 20% of patients have sensitivity reactions within weeks of the institution of penicillamine therapy. These reactions include fever, rash, lymphadenopathy, polyneuropathy, leukopenia, and thrombocytopenia. Dose reduction or short-term interruption of penicillamine therapy followed by restarting treatment at slowly increasing doses is usually successful in overcoming these side effects. For the 5% to 10% of patients who have serious penicillamine toxicity (lupus, nephrotic syndrome, pemphigus, and elastosis of skin, myasthenia gravis, thrombocytopenia, or severe arthralgias), another chelating agent, and **trientine dihydrochloride,** may be used.

   3. Trientine dihydrochloride is another chelating cupruretic agent used in the treatment of Wilson's disease. It has less of a cupruretic effect than penicillamine, but its clinical effectiveness is comparable. Typical dosage for initial therapy in adults is 750 to 1,500 mg per day in divided doses, and 750 to 1,000 mg per day for typical maintenance therapy. Trientine dihydrochloride has a better safety profile than penicillamine. No hypersensitivity reactions have been reported. Reversible sideroblastic anemia and bone marrow toxicity have been observed in patients who were overtreated with resultant copper deficiency. Due to its better safety profile, trientine dihydrochloride is now the drug of choice in the treatment of Wilson's disease. Both D-penicillamine and trientine dihydrochloride should be continued without interruption during pregnancy. Noncompliance with or interruption of the penicillamine or trientine dihydrochloride regimen is often followed by recurrence of symptoms or fulminant hepatitis.

   4. Oral zinc. Orally administered zinc sulfate (200–300 mg t.i.d.) has been found to be effective in the treatment of Wilson's disease, especially in patients who cannot tolerate cupruretic treatment. Orally administered zinc induces the synthesis of intestinal metallothionein, thus increasing the capacity for copper binding by the epithelial cells and trapping the metal in the intestinal mucosa, thereby preventing its systemic absorption. In addition, zinc may exert a protective effect by inducing metallothionein in the hepatocytes, thus decreasing the toxic effects of copper. In some patients, large doses of zinc are associated with headaches, abdominal cramps, gastric irritation, and loss of appetite. Zinc also interferes with absorption of iron, alters immune responses, and affects the serum lipoprotein profile.

Oral zinc therapy may serve as an adjunct to standard chelation therapy with D-penicillamine or trientine; however, there are reports that have raised concerns regarding the formation of zinc-penicillamine complexes that may diminish or abolish the therapeutic effectiveness of both drugs when used in combination.

Zinc is not recommended as the sole agent for initial therapy of symptomatic patients, but it is recommended as maintenance therapy at 150 mg per day in three divided doses to keep patients at negative copper balance. Zinc acetate is better tolerated than zinc chloride or sulfate.

5. **Tetrathiomolybdate,** an agent that appears to block the absorption of copper by holding the metal in a tight, metabolically inert bond, has been used in some patients intolerant to penicillamine. It is not commercially available for use in North America. Although the drug is generally well tolerated, at least two cases of bone marrow suppression have been documented. Further clinical trials are needed before it may be used as a primary therapy for Wilson's disease.

6. **Monitoring.** Periodic physical examinations, slit-lamp examinations of the cornea for documentation of the disappearance of K-F rings, and measurements of 24-hour urinary copper excretion and serum free copper should be performed to assess the effectiveness of therapy.

7. **Significant clinical improvement** may occur only after 6 to 12 months of uninterrupted treatment.

8. **Fulminant hepatic failure** may develop in a number of patients with Wilson's disease, either as an initial manifestation of the disease or as a consequence of noncompliance with medical therapy. A smaller subset of patients will have cirrhosis and hepatic decompression unresponsive to medical interventions outlined above.

9. **Orthotopic liver transplantation (OLT)** is a lifesaving procedure for patients with fulminant hepatitis or irreversible hepatic insufficiency due to Wilson's disease. The metabolic abnormality is reversed and the disease is cured. One-year survival following liver transplantation is now approximately 80%. The replacement of the affected liver expressing the mutant A7P7b gene protein product with a donor organ that expresses the normal gene protein product is expected to correct the defect in hepatic copper metabolism. Thus, the allograft is not susceptible to copper accumulation.

However, the resolution of the extra hepatic manifestations of Wilson's disease after OLT has been less than universal. Thus, OLT in the absence of decompensated liver disease and solely for the management of extrahepatic disease such as neurologic defects is not routinely recommended. Liver cell transplantation is currently under study as an alternative to liver transplantation.

II. **HEMOCHROMATOSIS.** Hemochromatosis refers to a group of disorders in which excessive iron absorption, either alone or in combination with parenteral iron loading, leads to a progressive increase in total body iron stores. Iron is deposited in the parenchymal cells of the liver, heart, pancreas, synovium, and skin, and the pituitary, thyroid, and adrenal glands. Parenchymal deposition of iron results in cellular damage and functional insufficiency of the involved organs.

A. **Classification of hemochromatosis**
   1. **Genetic.**
      a. Heredity hemochromatosis (HH) associated with HFE, TPR2, HJV, and HAMP.
      b. Ferroportin disease
      c. Aceruloplasminemia
      d. Hyporovatransferrinemia
      e. Frederick's ataxia
   2. **Acquired**
      a. Refractory anemias (e.g., thalassemia, spherocytosis, aplastic, sideroblastic anemia).
      b. Chronic liver injury (e.g., alcoholic cirrhosis, chronic viral hepatitis B and C, post–portacaval shunt).

    c. Dietary iron overload (e.g., Bantu, medicinal).

    d. Porphyria cutanea tarda.

    e. In thalassemia; sideroblastic, hypoproliferative, anemias with increased bone marrow turnovers; and repeated transfusions combined with increased intestinal iron absorption can lead to iron overload.

        Each unit of transfused blood contains 200 mg of iron; thus a patient receiving 4 units of blood per month over a period of 2 years will receive about 20 g of iron, an amount that overwhelms the limited capacity of the reticuloendothelial system to excrete the element.

  3. Parenteral iron overload

    a. Multiple blood transfusions.

    b. Excessive parenteral iron. Hemodialysis (rare since the introduction of recombinant erythropoietin).

B. Iron metabolism

  1. The total body iron in healthy, iron-replete individuals is approximately 4 to 5 g. Hemoglobin iron constitutes about 60%, and myoglobin, cytochromes, catalase, and peroxidase about 10% of the total body iron. Less than 1% is present as circulating iron bound to transferrin. About 35% is in the storage form as ferritin and hemosiderin, located mainly in the macrophages of the liver, spleen, and bone marrow as well as the parenchymal cells of the liver, muscle, and other organs. Approximately one third of the storage iron is found in the liver, primarily as ferritin. This provides an internal reserve that can be mobilized when needed.

  2. Absorption. A normal adult on the average ingests about 10 to 15 mg of iron per day. Only about 10% of this is absorbed into the circulation through the mucosal cells of the duodenum and proximal jejunum. Heme iron (meats) is absorbed four times more effectively than inorganic iron (vegetables and grains). There is no physiologic mechanism for excretion of iron out of the body in any appreciable quantity. Therefore, the intestinal absorption of iron is finely regulated in the normal individual. This permits the entry of only the amount necessary to replace the iron lost from exfoliated epithelial cells of the gastrointestinal tract and skin, and menstrual blood loss in women, which amounts to 1.0 mg per day in men and 1.5 mg per day in women.

C. Iron transport and storage proteins

  1. Transferrin is a beta globulin found in the plasma that transports inorganic ferric irons from the gastrointestinal tract to the reticulocyte and tissue stores as well as from the tissue stores to the bone marrow. The rate of synthesis of transferrin by the liver is regulated by the total body iron stores rather than the hemoglobin level. Thus the decreased transferrin levels in hemochromatosis are due to increased total body iron stores. Low transferrin levels are also seen in conditions such as inflammation, ineffective erythropoiesis, and liver diseases. Normally transferrin is about 30% saturated with iron; thus the total iron binding capacity (TIBC) of the serum is about 250 to 400 mg/dL.

  2. Ferritin is an intracellular protein made up of 24 subunits that sequesters inorganic iron within its core. When fully saturated, iron composes 23% of molecule. It is found in the macrophages, reticulocytes, intestinal mucosa, testis, kidney, heart, pancreas, skeletal muscle, and placenta. Serum and tissue ferritin are regulated by total body iron stores, with each 1 mg/mL of ferritin in the serum corresponding to 8 to 10 mg of stored tissue iron. The serum level of ferritin is a good estimation of total body iron stores.

  3. Hemosiderin. Multiple aggregates of ferritin make up this more stable form of iron storage. Iron stored in ferritin, as well as hemosiderin, can be mobilized by venisection.

D. Pathogenesis of HH.

  1. Iron excess in the bloodstream due either to increased intestinal iron absorption or parenteral iron administration will lead to the progressive accumulation of iron in the parenchymal cells of key organs creating the risk of toxicity and disease.

2. The circulating forms of iron that lead to tissue iron overload are not tightly associated with plasma transferring and are referred to as **non-transferrin bound iron (NTBI)**. NTBI increases whenever the capacity of transferring to incorporate incoming iron from the gut or reticulo endothelian cells becomes a limiting factor. A fraction of NTBI, called Labile plasma iron (LPI), is translocated across cell membranes in a non-regulated manner and leads to excessive iron accumulation in various organs. The extent of organ damage depends on the rate and magnitude of plasma iron overload. In transfusion dependant iron overload and juvenile forms of hemochromatosis early damage of the heart and endocrine glands predominate. In milder forms of iron overload late onset liver disease is more common.

3. The **control center** that keeps blood levels of iron within the narrow physiological range is in the hepatocyte. "Special sensors" respond to the iron and stimulate the synthesis and release of the **iron-hormone hepcidin**, which is encoded by HAMP gene. Hepcidin circulates through the body and interacts with the **iron-exporter ferroprotin** expressed in the surfaces of iron rich macrophages and intestinal cells. As a result of this interaction, ferroportin is internalized and degraded. The unneeded iron remain in the cells where it is saved for future use in the form of ferritin. The diminished release of iron restores blood levels to the non-toxic range, thus reinsuring the stimulus for further hepcidin synthesis and ferroportin gradually resumes its iron-exporting activity.

4. The mechanisms underlying hepatocyte iron sensing are still being investigated. However, as a result of their involvement in transferring and non-transferrin mediated iron uptake, HFE (the hemochromatosis gene) and transferrin receptor 2 might play a role in conveying iron signals to the hepatocyte control center. The details of this process are still unclear. However, both are important for hepcidin expression. Their functional loss causes hepcidin insufficiency and iron overload.

5. Hepcidin production can be impaired by genetic as well as acquired factors. Hepcidin deficiency has been associated with loss of HAMP, HJV, HFE, or TFR2. Even though there is genetic heterogeneity of HH, all forms identified so far originate from the presence of unneeded iron in the circulatory pool caused by insufficient hepcidin.

   Nongenetic factors which affect hepcidin output and lead to iron overload include **ethanol abuse**, toxic and viral insults, e.g., hepatitis C virus, diminished functional hepatic virus, e.g., in acute hepatic failure, end-stage liver disease or immune mediated liver disease.

6. "Hepcidin resistance or insensitivity" may also result from genetic or acquired factors that impair hepcidin-ferroprotein interaction. Mutations in ferroprotin gene have been noted to cause disease similar to HFE-hemochromatosis.

7. All forms of iron overload above the same basic features. Iron overload initially involves the plasma compartment signified biochemically by increased saturation of the iron transporter, parenchymal cells of key organs is reflected by increasing serum ferritin levels.

8. Expansion of the pool of non-transferrin-bound iron and its preferential uptake by parenchymal cells as the iron level and transferrin saturation increase in plasma. The result is total body iron overload with predominant deposition in parenchymal liver cells, leading to hepatic fibrosis and cirrhosis. A growing body of experimental evidence suggests that iron induces membrane lipid peroxidation, possibly as a consequence of free radical formation. This process damages lysosomal, microsomal, and other cellular membranes, resulting in cell death. Because iron is a cofactor for proline and lysine hydroxylase, two critical enzymes involved in the synthesis of collagen, some investigators have postulated that elevated tissue iron levels may promote an increased deposition of collagen and hepatic fibrosis. In addition, iron overload may activate and enhance the expression of some target genes in the liver, such as genes for ferritin and procollagen.

   Parenchymal cell deposition of iron also occurs in other tissues and may result in cardiac failure, diabetes mellitus, gonadal insufficiency, and arthritis.

E. Incidence. It has been estimated that the prevalence of homozygous and heterozygous HFE associated HH in populations of Northern European descent is about one in 250 and 1 in 8 to 10, respectively. The HFE associated HH disease is rarely identified in Africans or Asians. It is more common in men. The male-female ratio is 5 to 10:1. Nearly 70% of the patients have their first symptoms between the ages of 40 and 60 years. It is rarely clinically evident below the age of 20.

F. **Genetics.** In 1966 the HFE gene was identified in the short arm of chromosome 6. HFE-linked HH is responsible for 85% to 90% of cases of HH. HFE-linked HH is inherited as an autosomal recessive disorder. Its phenotypic expression is dependent on diet, gender, and other factors. An affected individual is often the offspring of two heterozygotes.

At least 30 missense mutations have been identified in HFE. One results in a change of cysteine to tyrosine at amino acid (AA) position 282**(C282Y);** a second mutation results in a change in histidine to aspartate at AA position 63**(H63D);** and a third mutation results in a change of serine to cysteine at AA 65**(S65C).** Homozygosity for the C282Y mutation has been identified in approximately 90% of individuals who have typical phenotypic HH. The clinical impact of H63D and S65C mutations is small. Approximately 83% of patients with HH are homozygous for C282Y mutation; an additional 4% are compound heterozygotes (C282Y/H63D).

Heterozygosity for C2824 is approximately 1 in 10 in the United States. Approximately one third of the males and one sixth of the females sharing one haplotype (heterozygotes) exhibit partial biochemical expression; however, these individuals rarely develop clinical manifestations of the disease.

Phenotypic expression of the inherited abnormality is modified by a variety of factors, including dietary iron intake, iron supplementation, chronic hemodialysis, alcohol consumption, menstrual blood loss, multiple pregnancies, and accelerated erythropoiesis.

Ten percent to 15% of patients have a clinical syndrome similar to HH, but do not have C282Y mutation.

The other inherited forms of iron overload, which do not involve mutations of the HFE, include iron overload resulting from mutations in transferrin receptor-2. Juvenile HH, which is caused by either mutation in **hemojuvelin** (HJV) or in the **hepcidin** gene, or **HAMP**. **Neonatal iron overload** is a rare disorder that is thought to be caused by an intrauterine hepatic viral infection resulting in an excessive uptake of iron into the fetal liver.

Decreased cell iron efflux may also cause HH. Iron egress from mammalian cells depends on the activity of a specialized membrane associated iron exporter, **ferroportin** and a circulating protein, **ceruloplasmin**, which oxidizes $Fe2+$ to $Fe3+$ and helps loading iron onto circulating transferring. Genetic or acquired factors that impair the function of these proteins lead to iron overload due to impaired iron egress. In such disorders, the reduced ability to deliver iron into circulating transferring causes low saturation of transferring with iron. Inefficient iron exit out of the cells causes tissue iron overload and organ injury.

Ferroportin disease is associated with the A77D mutation of ferroportin as an autosomal dominant disorder which causes progressive iron retention predominantly in reticuloendothelial cells of the spleen and liver. It is characterized by steadily increasing serum ferritin, marginal anemia and mild organ disease. The disorder appears to be spread worldwide in the different ethnic groups. So far 32 pedigrees of ferroportin mutations have been reported. Mutations of ferroportin cause impairment of iron recycling, particularly by reticuloendothelial macrophages which normally process and release a large quantity of iron derived from the lysis of senescent erythrocytes.

In **hypo or aceruloplasminemia**, an autosomal recessive neurodegenerative disease characterized by iron accumulation with brain as well as visceral organs such as the liver and pancreas is caused by mutations in the ceruloplasmin gene. Cerulopasmin plays a role in brain iron traffic. Patients due to diminished exit of iron from cells often present with iron deficiency anemia, neurologic disorder, retinal degeneration and diabetes velitus.

G. **Pathophysiology of HFE.** Since the discovery of HFE as the gene responsible for HH, its role in the dysregulated iron absorption seen in HH has been elucidated. In addition to leading to diminished hepcidin expression, HFE protein is also found in the crypt cells of the duodenum, associated with B_2-microglobulin and transferrin receptor. It is thought that HFE protein may facilitate transferrin receptor-dependent iron uptake into crypt cells and that mutant HFE protein may lose this ability, leading to a "relative" iron deficiency in the duodenal crypt cells. In turn, this may result in an increase in the expression of an iron transport protein called divalent metal ion transporter 1 (DMI-1) that is responsible for dietary iron absorption in the villous cells of the duodenum.

H. Diagnosis

1. **Clinical presentation.** Early in the course of IHC, patients may have the following signs or symptoms: lethargy, weight loss, and change in skin color, congestive heart failure, loss of libido, abdominal pain, joint pain, or symptoms related to diabetes mellitus. Hepatomegaly, skin pigmentation, testicular atrophy, loss of body hair, and arthropathy are the most prominent physical signs.

   Patients with hemochromatosis secondary to transfusion therapy for chronic anemia present with clinical symptoms at a young age. The typical patient with thalassemia, having received more than 100 blood transfusions, experiences failure of normal growth and sexual development in adolescence and hepatic fibrosis. Many patients die of cardiac disease by early adulthood.

   a. **Liver disease.** The liver is the first organ affected in IHC, and hepatomegaly is present in 95% of the symptomatic patients. Hepatomegaly may exist in the absence of symptoms and abnormal liver tests. In fact, serum aminotransferases are frequently normal or only slightly elevated in patients with IHC, even in the presence of cirrhosis. This finding reflects the relative preservation of the hepatocyte integrity, which usually persists throughout the course of the disease.

   Palmar erythema, spider angiomata, loss of body hair, and gynecomastia are often seen. Manifestations of portal hypertension may occur but are less common than in alcohol-related cirrhosis. Hepatocellular carcinoma (HCC) develops in approximately 30% of the patients with cirrhosis. This increased incidence of HCC may be due to chronic iron-overload-induced damage to hepatic DNA.

   b. **Skin pigmentation**, which may be absent early in the course of the disease, is present in a large percentage of symptomatic patients. The dark metallic hue is largely due to melanin deposition in the dermis. There is also some iron deposition in the skin, especially around the sweat glands. Pigmentation is deeper on the face, neck, exterior surfaces of the lower arms, dorsa of hands, lower legs, and genital regions, and in scars. Ten percent to 15% of the patients have pigmentation of the oral mucosa. Skin is usually atrophic and dry.

   c. **Endocrine disorders**
      i. **Diabetes mellitus** develops in 30% to 60% of the patients with advanced disease. The presence of a family history of diabetes mellitus and the presence of liver disease and direct damage to the beta cells of the pancreas by deposition of iron all probably contribute to the development of diabetes mellitus in IHC. Complications of diabetes mellitus such as retinopathy, nephropathy, and neuropathy may occur. IHC spares the exocrine pancreas.
      ii. **Loss of libido and testicular atrophy.** Hypogonadism is common with symptomatic IHC and is most likely due to hypothalamic or pituitary failure with impairment of gonadotropin secretion. Liver damage, alcohol intake, and other factors may contribute to sexual hypofunction.
      iii. **Other endocrine disorders.** Addison's disease, hypothyroidism, and hypoparathyroidism are less common in IHC.

   d. **Arthropathy** is present in about one fifth of the patients with IHC. It is more common in patients over 40 years of age and occasionally may be the presenting symptom.
      i. **Osteoarthritis** involving the metacarpophalangeal and proximal interphalangeal joints of the hands, and later of the knees, hips, wrists, and shoulders, is most commonly seen.

    ii. Pseudogout (chondrocalcinosis) occurs in approximately 50% of the patients with arthropathy. Knees are most commonly affected, but wrists and metacarpophalangeal joints are also usually involved.

    iii. The pathogenesis of arthritis is not known. However, iron deposition in the synovial cells may predispose to calcium pyrophosphate deposition.

  e. Cardiac involvement. Approximately 15% to 20% of the patients present with cardiac disease, most commonly cardiomyopathy, leading to heart failure. The heart is diffusely enlarged. Because iron is also deposited in the conduction system, a great variety of arrhythmias, such as tachyarrhythmias, conduction blocks, and low-voltage patterns, may also be present.

  f. Infection. Patients with hemochromatosis seem to have an increased risk of development of severe bacterial infections, particularly with *Yersinia enterocolitica, Yersinia pseudotuberculosis, Vibrio vulnificus, Neisseria species,* enteric gram-negative bacteria, *Staphylococcus aureus,* and *Listeria monocytogenes.* Sepsis, meningitis, enterocolitis, peritonitis, and intraabdominal abscesses have been reported. The ingestion of raw seafood appears to contribute to the risk of these infections and should be avoided. It is hypothesized that the increased availability of iron heightens susceptibility to infection because most bacteria utilize iron in growth.

2. Diagnostic studies. Diagnostic criteria are based on demonstration of excessive parenchymal iron stores in the absence of other causes of iron overload such as refractory anemia, thalassemia, and alcoholic cirrhosis.

  a. Serum iron and TIBC. The normal range for serum iron is 50 to 150 mg/dL. If the level is greater than 180 mg/dL, the patient should be questioned with regard to intake of iron-containing medicines. The serum iron should be rechecked 1 month after these medicines are discontinued. The serum iron and percentage of saturation of transferrin (TS) or TIBC are elevated (>45%), especially early in the course of the disease.

  b. Serum ferritin reflects both hepatic and total body iron stores. The levels are lower in women than in men. It is the most specific screening test for increased iron stores. However, normal levels may be found occasionally in patients with latent or precirrhotic HH. Ascorbic acid deficiency in patients with iron overload results in inappropriately low serum ferritin concentration. Elevated serum ferritin levels in the absence of iron overload may be attributable to infection, acute or chronic liver disease especially when associated with hepatocellular necrosis (e.g., viral, drug-related, or steatohepatitis), lymphoma, lymphocytic leukemia and other malignancies, rheumatoid arthritis, hyperthyroidism, and uremia.

  c. Genetic testing is recommended in patients with an elevated fasting TS or ferritin level. If individuals are C282Y-homozygotes or compound heterozygotes (C282Y/H630) younger than 40 years with normal liver enzyme (alanine aminotransferase [ALT] and aspartate aminotransferase [AST]) levels, no further workup is necessary. In patients with abnormal liver tests or who are older than 40 years, a liver biopsy is recommended to define the liver disease and extent of fibrosis.

  d. Liver biopsy. For patients older than 40 years with elevated liver chemistry tests, liver biopsy should be performed. Liver biopsy permits the following:

    i. Estimation of tissue iron by histochemical staining. The amount of stainable parenchymal iron is graded from 0 to 4, but the relation between histochemical grading and hepatic iron concentration is not linear. Grades 1 and 2 (slight-to-moderate siderosis) are quite common in the normal liver. Grade 4 siderosis indicates heavy iron excess. Grade 3 (submaximal siderosis) is difficult to interpret in quantitative terms.

      Early in HH, stainable iron is almost exclusively present in the hepatocytes, whereas in early secondary iron overload, the iron is predominantly in the Kupffer's cells. With progressive iron accumulation, the histologic features and pattern of stainable iron in various etiologic types of iron overload become indistinguishable, and iron is seen throughout the lobule, biliary duct epithelium, Kupffer's cells, and connective tissue.

    ii. Measurement of hepatic iron concentration by dry weight by chemical analysis is the most objective means of assessing total body iron stores. The normal range is 7 to 100 µg/100 mg of dry weight of liver tissue. In IHC, values are greater than 1,000 µg/100 mg of dry weight.

    Patients with alcoholic cirrhosis and increased stainable iron usually have a hepatic iron concentration less than twice normal. There is evidence that alcoholic patients with gross iron overload carry the IHC gene.

    The **hepatic iron index,** which is the hepatic iron concentration in mol/g of dry weight per age, seems to discriminate homozygous from heterozygous HH before the development of frank iron overload in homozygotes.

    iii. Histologic assessment of liver damage. In the early stages, the histologic appearance of the liver may be normal despite increased iron in the hepatocytes. Necrosis and inflammation are usually absent. Before cirrhosis is fully established, there is fibrosis radiating from expanded portal tracts. The hepatic iron concentration and the duration of exposure are critical determinants of the extent of liver injury. In the absence of coexistent alcoholic liver disease, fibrosis or cirrhosis usually does not occur in HH until the hepatic iron concentration reaches 4,000 to 5,000 mm/g liver (wet weight), or 2.2% dry weight. In patients with thalassemia major, the apparent threshold concentration for the development of hepatic fibrosis is about twice this level. Whether this difference is due to the initial location of iron in the reticuloendothelial cells or a shorter duration of exposure of the hepatocytes to high iron concentration is uncertain. As cirrhosis develops, the histology may resemble cirrhosis from chronic biliary obstruction. Some patients may have histology similar to that of alcoholic cirrhosis.

I. The treatment of IHC involves the removal of excess iron and therapy of functional insufficiency of the organs involved, such as congestive heart failure, liver failure, and diabetes mellitus.

    1. Phlebotomy. Iron is best removed from the body by phlebotomy. There are 250 mg of iron in 500 mL of blood. Because the body burden of iron in IHC may be in excess of 20 g, 2 to 3 years of weekly phlebotomy of 500 mL of blood may be necessary to achieve hemoglobin of 11% and serum ferritin level of 10 to 20 mg/L. Thereafter, the frequency of phlebotomy may be decreased to 1 unit of blood every 3 months for the rest of the patient's life.

    2. Chelating agents such as deferoxamine remove only 10 to 20 mg of iron per day. In patients with anemia, hypoproteinemia, or severe cardiac disease precluding phlebotomy, this technique may be used. However, it is difficult to achieve a negative iron balance by this means. In patients with refractory anemia, if it is initiated early in the course of iron loading, this approach can lower the risk of cardiac disease, promote sexual maturation, and generally improve the prognosis.

    Nightly subcutaneous infusion of deferoxamine induces excretion of chelatable iron into urine and, probably via the bile, into stool. The recommended dosage is approximately 40 to 80 mg/kg per day. At daily dosages of more than 50 mg/kg, the potential increases for hypersensitivity and ocular and otologic complications, including night blindness, visual field changes, irreversible retinal pigmentation, optic neuropathy, deafness, and other adverse reactions. In addition, the iron chelator deferoxamine can promote infections, including gram-negative sepsis and abscesses, by functioning as a siderophore, delivering iron to bacteria that use it in growth. Chelating compounds that can be taken orally, most notably including **β-hydroxypyridine,** are being developed.

    Despite the potential of vitamin C deficiency to exacerbate iron overload, vitamin C supplementation is contraindicated in patients with hemochromatosis. Sudden cardiac deaths have occurred in patients receiving chelation therapy and vitamin C supplements. The cause of these events may involve sudden shifts of iron from reticuloendothelial to parenchymal cells of the myocardium or increased cellular injury from increased lipid peroxidation.

3. **Prognosis.** In patients treated with phlebotomy, there is a decrease in the size of the liver and spleen, skin pigmentation, cardiac failure, serum aminotransferases, and glucose intolerance. Removal of iron has no effect on hypogonadism, arthropathy, or portal hypertension. Hepatic fibrosis may decrease, but cirrhosis is irreversible. Hepatocellular carcinoma occurs in one third of the patients with IHC and cirrhosis, despite iron removal. This complication does not seem to develop if the disease is treated in the precirrhotic stage. Hepatomas in IHC are usually multicentric and not amenable to surgical resection. Only 30% to 40% of the patients have elevated serum alpha-fetoprotein levels.

4. **Liver transplantation** is an option for patients in whom HH is diagnosed late in the course of their disease (i.e., with decompensated cirrhosis). Patients should be carefully evaluated for cardiac disease, arrhythmias, and left ventricular function and hepatocellular carcinoma.

   HH patients seem to have diminished posttransplant survival rates in comparison to patients with other forms of liver disease. This is most likely related to unrecognized cardiac disease and increased propensity for infections. Patients who are successfully "de-ironed" prior to transplant have more successful outcomes. Recurrent HH disease does not appear to develop in the allograft.

J. **Early diagnosis of IHC in family members.** To prevent the development of permanent organ damage, cirrhosis, and hepatocellular carcinoma, it is very important to diagnose and treat the disease in relatives at an early stage. The following are guidelines for screening relatives of patients with HH:

   Once a proband with HH is identified, genetic family screening is recommended for all first-degree relatives. In young proband with children, it is useful to perform HFE mutation analysis in the spouse to accurately predict the genotype in the children. If the spouse has either mutation, then the children will also need to undergo HFE mutation analysis. If C282Y homozygosity or compound heterozygosity (C282Y/H63D) is found in adult relatives of the proband, serum iron studies should be obtained. If ferritin or TS levels are increased, therapeutic phlebotomy should be considered. If ALT and AST levels are normal and ferritin is <1,000 µg/L, liver biopsy is probably not necessary.

III. α_1-ANTITRYPSIN DEFICIENCY

A. **α_1-antitrypsin (AAT)** is an acute-phase reacting α-1 globulin found in serum, various body fluids, and tissues. It is a potent protease inhibitor (PI) synthesized by hepatocytes, monocytes, and bronchoalveolar macrophages for protection against tissue injury resulting from proteases such as trypsin, chymotrypsin, elastase, and collagenase as well as from proteases released from polymorphonuclear leukocytes and macrophages. AAT is responsible for 90% of the serum protease-inhibiting capacity and approximately 90% of the alpha-1 band on serum protein electrophoresis.

1. AAT is a glycoprotein consisting of a single polypeptide chain with four carbohydrate side chains. Due to genetic mutations, at least 60 variants of AAT have been identified by their mobility on acid starch gel electrophoresis followed by crossed immunoelectrophoresis on agarose gel. Isoelectric focusing in polyacrylamide (PIEF) has replaced the starch gel techniques and offers increased resolution of PI variants. These variant proteins (phenotypes) have been designated by different letters of the alphabet. The faster moving proteins have been assigned earlier letters of the alphabet: PIM is the most common protein with medium mobility, PI S is slow, and PI Z is the slowest.

2. The inheritance of AAT is autosomal codominant. Each allele acts independently of the other and contributes its own active protein. The PI locus is on chromosome 14. Phenotypes are usually expressed as two alleles. Common PI variants associated with decreased plasma concentration of AAT are PI S at 60% and the classic deficiency phenotype PI Z at 10% to 15% of normal levels. The rare alleles PI I, PI P, PI M malton, and PI M Duarte also have low plasma levels. PI null (PI φ or PI–) phenotypes result in no detectable circulating AAT. PI S is relatively common in Spain, whereas PI Z is most common in Scandinavia.

3. The PI MM phenotype is associated with an average serum level of 220 mg of AAT/dL. Serum levels of AAT may be increased by acute and chronic inflammation

as a response to tissue injury, estrogen or oral contraceptive ingestion, pregnancy, carcinoma, and typhoid inoculation in normal individuals. In severely deficient individuals, the level rises only slightly with such stimuli.

4. When the livers of severely deficient subjects are examined histologically, accumulation of an amorphous material within most hepatocytes has been demonstrated. This material, like glycogen, takes the periodic acid–Schiff (PAS) stain but, unlike glycogen, is resistant to digestion with diastase. This PAS-positive material is a variant of AAT that has been excreted out of the hepatocytes. The greatest accumulation of this material is in the smooth endoplasmic reticulum (SER). The basic difference in the structure of this protein (PI Z) from that of the normal (PI M) is the replacement of a glutamic acid by a lysine. This limits its transport out of SER to the Golgi and thus its excretion from the hepatocytes, resulting in low serum levels of AAT. Other, less severe types of AAT deficiency have other amino acid substitutions. PI M Duarte and M malton have nearly normal electrophoretic mobilities but are associated with low plasma levels, intracellular aggregates, and lung and liver disease. PI S has decreased stability and does not accumulate in the liver cells. The non-PI M alleles are rare in African Americans. PI Z has its greatest frequency in northern Europe. In the United States, approximately 1 in 676 whites have severe AAT deficiency.

5. It is clear that subjects of phenotype PI ZZ and probably PI SZ and possible PI MZ are much more susceptible to the development of emphysema or chronic bronchitis or both than the general population. This tendency is potentiated by smoking. The emphysema is usually of the panlobular type and affects the lower lobes first.

6. Whereas emphysema is inversely related to plasma AAT levels, liver disease correlates with intracellular accumulation of AAT. Liver injury occurs in AAT phenotypes associated with intracellular protein accumulation (PI Z, PI M malton, PI M Duarte, PI ZZ, and possibly PI MZ). In contrast, no liver disease is seen in deficiency phenotypes due to intracellular protein degradation (PI S, PI null). The pathogenesis of the liver injury is not clear.

B. Liver disease. The first genetic association of AAT deficiency with liver disease and cirrhosis was made in children. Subsequently, its association with cirrhosis in adults has been confirmed. There is also an increased incidence of hepatic cancer in patients with cirrhosis.

1. In clinical studies involving PI ZZ infants, it has been found that 12% present with cholestasis and another 7% present with other evidence of liver disease during early infancy. By 6 months of age, these infants appear to recover clinically from their liver disease but continue to have elevated liver enzymes. At 3 months of age, 47% of "normal" PI ZZ infants have elevated liver enzymes. Only 34% of PI ZZ infants have no clinical or laboratory evidence of liver injury. At 4 years of age, approximately one half of the PI ZZ children continue to have elevated serum hepatic enzyme concentrations.

2. Roughly 75% of children with AAT deficiency and clinically apparent liver disease present with jaundice and cholestasis during infancy. The remainder present with evidence of portal hypertension in later childhood. Only 25% of the cholestatic infants recover without evidence of chronic liver disease.

3. The severe degree of cholestasis in some infants with AAT deficiency may simulate extrahepatic biliary obstruction with respect to both clinical evaluation and liver pathology. Surgical exploration in these instances has revealed "physiologic hypoplasia" of the extrahepatic biliary tract, secondary to decreased bile flow. Atresia of the ducts has not been demonstrated.

4. Approximately 25% of the children with AAT deficiency who present with cholestasis persist in having grossly abnormal liver function tests. These patients develop cirrhosis and portal hypertension with ascites and esophageal varices, and die from hepatic complications in the first 10 years of life. Another 25% have evidence of persistently abnormal liver function tests but are slower in developing clinical signs of cirrhosis and die of complications of their liver disease between 10 and 20 years of age. Another 25% have minimal liver dysfunction, minimal organomegaly, and less severe liver fibrosis

and live to adulthood. The remaining 25% appear to recover from their initial insult and return to normal liver function with minimal evidence of residual liver fibrosis.

5. In adults, as in children, men are twice as likely to have liver disease as women. In studies done with patients with PI ZZ phenotype from Sweden or of Northern European ancestry, the relative risk for cirrhosis was noted to be 37% to 47%, and of hepatoma, 15% to 29%. In studies done in heterozygotes of PI MZ or PI SZ phenotypes, the relative risk for cirrhosis was noted to be 1.8 and for hepatoma 5.7, compared with other patients investigated for liver disease.

6. **Diagnosis**

   a. Diagnosis of AAT deficiency should be considered in any chronic liver disease of uncertain cause in children and adults of white and particularly Northern European populations. The probability of AAT deficiency as a cause of the disease increases in patients with a family history of liver or obstructive lung disease and in patients in whom alcohol or viral hepatitis may be excluded. Children with neonatal hepatitis, giant cell hepatitis, juvenile cirrhosis, or chronically elevated liver chemistry tests should be investigated for AAT phenotype. Adults with chronic active hepatitis lacking serologic markers, or with cryptogenic cirrhosis, with or without hepatoma, also should be evaluated.

   b. The initial discovery of AAT deficiency is usually made by the absence of the alpha-1 peak on serum protein electrophoresis. This method is not very sensitive, and quantitative determination of serum AAT level and PI typing is usually necessary for accurate diagnosis. Liver biopsy further supports the diagnosis and helps to stage the extent of liver damage.

   c. **Biochemical studies.** Plasma AAT levels may be determined in most clinical laboratories by electroimmunoassay. Plasma levels should be related to the normal reference range for each laboratory. Functional analysis may also be performed by determination of total trypsin inhibitory capacity, 90% of which is due to AAT activity. Discrepancies may occur between immunologic and functional analyses due to the presence of dysfunctional or inactive species. Subnormal levels suggest a genetic AAT variant and are only rarely secondary to a disease process. Low levels have been described, however, in the infant respiratory distress syndrome, in protein-losing states, and in terminal liver failure. Levels below 20% of normal suggest the homozygous deficiencies PI Z, PI M malton, PI M Duarte, and PI null or heterozygous combinations of these alleles. Levels in the range 40% to 70% are compatible with heterozygous deficiency (PI MO, SZ, MZ, etc.). Heterozygotes with liver disease or active inflammation may well exhibit normal levels.

   d. **Phenotype determination.** Isoelectric focusing is the method of choice for phenotyping. A monoclonal antibody specific for PI Z AAT has been developed and is useful in detecting the presence of the PI Z allele. It has been used for mass population screening in an enzyme-linked immunosorbent assay (ELISA). Such antibodies also may be used for specific staining of histologic material.

   Specific diagnosis of most phenotypes also may be performed at the DNA level. Some genetic mutations may be identified by Southern blotting due to their fortuitous localization at a restriction endonuclease site (restriction fragment length polymorphism). This method may be performed on DNA purified from very few cells and therefore is ideally suited to prenatal diagnosis.

   e. **Liver biopsy and histopathology.** α_1-antitrypsin globular inclusions are localized predominantly in periportal hepatocytes, are weakly acidophilic, and may be overlooked easily on routine hematoxylin-eosin sections. After diastase treatment to remove glycogen, the remaining immature glycoprotein is strongly PAS-positive, reflecting high mannose content. In general, the number and size of globules increase with age and disease activity. Globules may be missed entirely in liver biopsies from heterozygotes due to sampling error.

   Immunofluorescence and immunoperoxidase staining with nonspecific antisera against AAT are more sensitive than PAS-D staining for the detection of intrahepatocellular aggregates. These techniques can be applied to both frozen and formalin-fixed tissue. Electron microscopy can reveal AAT, in the endoplasmic reticulum (ER), with dilatation in other periportal hepatocytes in which biosynthesis generally predominates, in both hereto- and homozygotes. Adult liver disease in AAT deficiency is usually characterized by relatively low-grade inflammation radiating from portal tracts. Inflammatory cells (primarily lymphocytes) are distributed in close proximity to areas of abundant PAS-D globules. There may be piecemeal necrosis. As the disease progresses, the liver becomes more fibrotic with the development of macronodular cirrhosis. Hepatoma of a hepatocellular or cholangiocellular type may accompany the cirrhosis.

C. Treatment

1. **Prevention.** As in all genetic disease, the diagnosis of α_1-antitrypsin deficiency in a patient, regardless of the mode of clinical presentation (lung, liver, or other symptoms), should lead to investigations of the family. It is desirable to identify homozygotes in an asymptomatic stage. Patients should be advised against smoking. Genetic counseling should be provided to families with one or more children affected by liver disease.

2. **Medical therapy.** No medical therapy is beneficial in patients with liver disease.

3. **Liver transplantation.** Liver transplantation provides a new source of plasma AAT. In these patients, the PI typing converts to that of the donor. The 1-year survival is 90% and the 5-year survival of juvenile patients in most transplant centers is 80% to 85%. The experience of liver transplantation for cirrhosis in PI Z adults is limited. In the absence of serious pulmonary manifestations, indications for liver transplantation are essentially those for decompensation due to chronic liver disease of any cause. Preoperative evaluation of pulmonary function and the exclusion of hepatoma are essential.

IV. CYSTIC FIBROSIS

A. Epidemiology. Cystic fibrosis (CF) is one of the most common, serious inherited diseases in Caucasians. It predominantly affects the lungs and the pancreas and causes early mortality in most patients. The overall prevalence of overt liver disease in patients with CF is 5% to 10%. However, as the general care of patients with CF has continued to improve, the proportion of patients living to adulthood has increased, thus the relative importance of liver disease has also increased.

The incidence of liver disease rises steadily with age and peaks in the adolescence years. It is rare for liver disease to have its onset after 20 years of age. It is more common in males compared to females with a ratio of 3:1.

B. Pathogenesis of the liver disease in CF is not fully understood. It is thought that there is altered bile ductular secretion resulting in concentrated viscous bile causing plugging and inflammation.

Several forms of hepatobiliary disease are seen in patients with CF. Neonatal cholestasis occurs in 2% to 20% of affected infants and may persist for several months. Hepatic steatosis is commonly seen. Micronodular cirrhosis occurs in 2% to 5% of patients.

Patient with CF have a high incidence of biliary tract disease including hyperplastic gallbladders, gallstones, common bile duct (CBD) strictures and CBD obstruction form severe pancreatic fibrosis, and a cholangiopathy indistinguishable from primary sclerosing cholangitis.

C. Treatment. Ursodeoxycholic acid has been shown to be helpful in the management of patients with hepatobiliary disease in the setting of CF. Special attention should be given to pulmonary function, infection, dosage of medications in the setting of malabsorption and blood sugar control due to high incidence of diabetes mellitus in patients with CF.

Liver transplantation has been used in children and adults with end-stage liver disease associated with CF. Survival rates were approximately 75%. For CF patients with severe pulmonary and liver disease, combined lung/liver or heart/lung/liver transplantation may be offered.

Selected Readings

Wilson's Disease

Brewer GI, et al. Treatment of Wilson's disease with zinc, XVII: Treatment during pregnancy. *Hepatology*. 2000;31:304.

Eghtesad B, et al. Liver transplantation for Wilson's disease: A single center experience. *Liver Transplant Surg*. 1999;5:467.

Ferenci P, et al. Late onset Wilson's disease. *Gastroenterol*. 2007;132:1294–1298.

Mufti AR, et al. Is a copperbinding protein deregulated in Wilson's disease and other copper toxic disorders? *Mol Cell*. 2006;21:775–785.

Schilsky ML. Treatment of Wilson's disease: What are the roles of penicillamine, trientine, and zinc supplementation? *Curr Gastroenterol Rep*. 2001;3:54.

Sternlieb I. Wilson's disease and pregnancy. *Hepatology*. 2000;31:304.

Taly AB, et al. Wilson's disease: description of 282 patients evaluated over 3 decades. *Medicine (Baltimore)*. 2007;86:112–121.

Hemochromatosis

Brunt EM, et al. Histologic evaluation of iron in liver biopsies: Relationship of HFE mutations. *Am J Gastroenterol*. 2000;95:1788.

Harrison-Findik DD, et al. Alcohol metabolism mediated oxidative stress down porter expression. *J Biol Chem*. 2006;281:22974–22982.

Papanikolanon G, et al. Mutations in HFE2 cause iron overload in chromosome 1g-linked juvenile hemochromatosis. *Nat Genet*. 2004;36:77–82.

Pietrangelo A. Hereditary hemochromasis—a new look at an old disease. *N Eng J Med*. 2004;350:2382–2397.

Pietrangelo A. Hereditary hemochromatosis: Biochemia and biophysician. *Acta*. 2006; 1763:700–710.

α_1-Antitrypsin Deficiency

Arroyo M, et al. Hepatic inherited Metabolic disorders. *Semin Diag Pathol*. 2006; 23:182–189.

Perlmutter DH. The cellular basis of liver injury in alpha-1-antitrypsin deficiency. *Hepatology*. 1990;13:172.

Perlmutter DH, et al. Molecular pathogenesis of alpha-1-antitrypsin deficiency associated liver disease. A meeting review. *Hepatology*. 2007;45:1313–1323.

Pietrangelo A. The ferroportin disease. *Blood Cells Mol D13*. 2004;32:131–138.

Pietrangelo A, et al. Genetics in liver diseases. *J Hepot*. 2007;46:1143–1146.

Powell PF, et al. Steatosis is a cofactor in liver injury in hemochromatosis. *Gastroenterol*. 2005;129:1932–1943.

Sveger T, et al. The liver in adolescents with a1-antitrypsin deficiency. *Hepatology*. 1995;22:514.

Whiting PF. Fetal and infantile hemochromatosis. *Hepatology*. 2006;43:654–660.

Wong K, et al. The diversity of liver disease associated with an elevated ferratin. *Con J Gastro*. 2007;20:467–470.

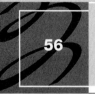

I. Cirrhosis is a disease state that is the consequence of a wide variety of chronic, progressive liver diseases. These result in diffuse destruction of hepatic parenchyma and its replacement with collagenous scar tissue and regenerating nodules with disruption of the normal hepatic lobular and vascular architecture. Regardless of etiology, the triad of parenchymal necrosis, regeneration, and scarring is present in all cirrhotic patients.

  A. Classification

   1. Morphologic. The pattern of scarring and gross appearance of the liver can be used to classify cirrhosis into three groups:

   a. Micronodular (Laënnec's)

   b. Macronodular

   c. Mixed

   Morphologic classification seldom permits the determination of the specific etiology. However, micronodular cirrhosis is most commonly seen as the consequence of alcoholic liver disease, and macronodular and mixed cirrhosis are the result of most other inflammatory or infiltrative diseases of the liver.

   2. Etiologic

   a. Alcohol

   b. Viral hepatitis B, C, and D—most common causes of cirrhosis in the United States

   c. Drug- or toxin-induced

   d. Hemochromatosis

   e. Wilson's disease

   f. α_1-Antitrypsin deficiency

   g. Autoimmune hepatitis

   h. Nonalcoholic steatohepatitis (NASH)

   i. Biliary obstruction

     i. Primary biliary cirrhosis (without extrahepatic bile duct obstruction)

     ii. Secondary biliary cirrhosis (with extrahepatic bile duct obstruction)

   j. Venous outflow obstruction

     i. Budd-Chiari syndrome

     ii. Venoocclusive disease

   k. Cardiac failure

     i. Chronic right-sided failure

     ii. Tricuspid insufficiency

   l. Malnutrition

     i. Jejunoileal bypass surgery

     ii. Gastroplasty

   m. Miscellaneous

     i. Schistosomiasis

     ii. Congenital syphilis

     iii. Cystic fibrosis

     iv. Glycogen storage disease (type IV)

   n. Idiopathic

  B. Diagnosis. A specific diagnosis generally requires a combination of history, physical findings, laboratory tests, and the identification of characteristic histologic features.

1. **History.** Most symptoms found in patients with cirrhosis are nonspecific. Fatigue, malaise, and loss of vigor are common. There may be other symptoms caused by a complication of the disease leading to cirrhosis or of cirrhosis itself. These are discussed in the corresponding chapters or sections.
2. **Physical examination.** No physical abnormality establishes the diagnosis of cirrhosis.
    a. **Characteristic findings** include palmar erythema, spider angiomata, gynecomastia, testicular atrophy, Dupuytren's contractures, and findings due to portal hypertension such as splenomegaly, ascites, esophageal varices, and prominent superficial veins of the abdominal wall (caput medusae).
    b. **The liver** in most patients with cirrhosis is enlarged and palpable below the costal margin. The left lobe often extends to the left upper quadrant below the xiphoid process. A small, hard, shrunken liver is a sign of very advanced cirrhosis. The liver edge in most patients with cirrhosis feels firm. Occasionally, regenerating nodules may be palpable in macronodular cirrhosis. Micronodules are not palpable.

C. **Pathophysiologic consequences of cirrhosis**
   1. Alteration of hepatic blood flow: portal hypertension
   2. Reduction in functional cell mass
       a. Decreased synthesis: albumin, coagulation proteins, other proteins
       b. Decreased detoxification: bilirubin, ammonia, drugs

II. PORTAL HYPERTENSION

A. **Pathogenesis.** The normal adult liver is perfused by about 1,500 mL of blood per minute. Two thirds of this blood flow and one half of the oxygen supply are provided by the portal vein, the rest by the hepatic artery. Normally, the pressure in the portal vein is low because the vascular resistance in the hepatic sinusoids is also low. A sustained elevation of portal venous pressure above the normal of 6 to 10 mmHg is called portal hypertension. There are many causes of portal hypertension, but cirrhosis is the most common cause in the United States. Portal venous pressure is primarily a function of volume of and resistance to the blood flow. Factors contributing to distortion of the portal venous bed resulting in increased resistance to blood flow in cirrhosis include the following:
   1. Deposition of collagen in the space of Disse with consequent narrowing of the sinusoids.
   2. Distortion of sinusoids and the hepatic venous system by regenerating nodules.
   3. The distortion of the hepatic parenchyma results in not only the development of portal hypertension but also intrahepatic intravascular shunts between portal venules through sinusoids to hepatic venules. Up to one third of the hepatic blood flow may bypass the functioning liver tissue because of these shunts.

B. **Classification.** The current classification (Table 56-1) of portal hypertension is based on the major location of increased vascular resistance. Anatomically, the obstruction to portal blood flow can occur at three levels:
   1. Portal vein (prehepatic)
   2. Intrahepatic (presinusoidal, sinusoidal, postsinusoidal)
   3. Hepatic veins (posthepatic)

C. **Complications resulting from portal hypertension and cirrhosis**
   1. Collateral circulation and varices
   2. Ascites
   3. Congestive splenomegaly
   4. Encephalopathy

III. COLLATERAL CIRCULATION (VARICES).
Extensive portosystemic venous collaterals develop as a direct consequence of portal hypertension. These vessels form through the dilatation of preexisting venous channels to decompress the high-pressure portal venous system. Maintenance of portal hypertension, once collaterals are formed, is attributed to a resultant increase in splanchnic blood flow.

TABLE 56-1	Classification of Portal Hypertension (A Partial Listing)

	Intrahepatic			
Prehepatic	**Presinusoidal**	**Sinusoidal**	**Postsinusoidal**	**Posthepatic**
Portal vein thrombosis	Schistosomiasis	Cirrhosis	Alcoholic hepatitis	Inferior vena cava web
Splenic arteriovenous fistula	Sarcoidosis	Primary biliary cirrhosis	Venoocclusive disease	Tricuspid insufficiency
Constrictive	Metastatic carcinoma	Cryptogenic; alcohol-induced cirrhosis	Hepatic vein thrombosis	Pericarditis

Major sites of collateral flow include the following:

A. The left gastric vein and short gastric veins join with intercostal, diaphragm esophageal, and azygos veins of the caval system. This results in the formation of **esophageal** and **gastric varices.**

B. The hemorrhoidal vein of the portal system joins hemorrhoidal veins of the caval system. This results in the formation of **large hemorrhoidal veins.**

C. Remnants of the umbilical circulation of the fetus present in the falciform ligament may form **a large paraumbilical vein (caput medusae).**

D. Others. **Retroperitoneal veins, lumbar veins, omental veins.**

IV. VARICES. The thin-walled varices in the lower esophagus and upper stomach may bleed extensively and constitute the major complication of portal hypertension. Variceal bleeding occurs without an obvious precipitating cause and presents usually as a painless massive hematemesis or melena.

Variceal bleeding primarily reflects portal hypertension. The role of acid reflux and its contribution to initiation of variceal bleeding is not clear. Even though there is no clear agreement as to whether bleeding correlates with the severity of portal hypertension, it is generally accepted that hemorrhage usually is seen with a portal pressure above 12 mm Hg and is more likely in patients with large varices.

A. Diagnosis. The presence of varices may be detected by barium swallow and upper gastrointestinal (GI) series (40% sensitivity), angiography, and endoscopy. Upper GI endoscopy is preferred; it not only shows the presence and size of the varices but also reveals whether they are the sites of bleeding. Forty percent of the bleeding in patients with cirrhosis with known varices has a nonvariceal source. Congestive or portal hypertensive gastropathy is a major source of bleeding in these patients.

B. Prognosis. Once esophageal varices are diagnosed, the risk of bleeding ranges from 25% to 35% within 1 year of diagnosis of large varices. Risk factors for variceal bleeding include size of varices, severity of liver disease, and presence of active alcohol consumption. The overall mortality of variceal bleeding is 70% to 80% in patients with cirrhosis. The prognosis is dependent on the patient's nutritional status, presence or absence of ascites; encephalopathy, bilirubin level, albumin level, and prothrombin time (see modified Child's criteria in Table 56-2).

C. Treatment. Prompt care of the patient with massive hematemesis or melena from bleeding esophageal or gastric varices requires coordinated medical and surgical efforts.

1. Transfusion. The first step is to ensure adequate circulation with transfusion of blood, fresh-frozen plasma, and, if necessary, platelets. Because patients with

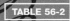

TABLE 56-2 Modified Child's Classification

Variable	Score[a]		
	1	**2**	**3**
Encephalopathy (degree)	Nil	Slight–moderate	Moderate–severe
Ascites (degree)	Nil	Slight	Moderate–severe
Bilirubin[b] (mg/dL)	<2	2–3	>3
Albumin (g/dL)	≥3.5	2.8–3.4	<2.8
Prothrombin index (%)	>70	40–70	<40
Prothrombin time(s) (our modification)	≤14	15–17	≥18

[a]Scores are summed to determine Child's class: class A, 5–7; class B, >7–10; class C, >10–15.
[b]For primary biliary cirrhosis, the bilirubin score is adjusted: 1 = <4; 2 = 4–10; 3 = >10 mg/dL.
From DiMagno EP, et al. Influence of hepatic reserve and cause of esophageal varices on survival and rebleeding before and after the introduction of sclerotherapy: A retrospective analysis. *Mayo Clin Proc.* 1985;60:149. Reprinted with permission.

liver disease often have deficiency of clotting factors, the infusion of fresh blood or fresh-frozen plasma is important.

2. **Endoscopy or angiography.** After the vital signs are stabilized, the site and cause of the bleeding should be established by endoscopy. If bleeding is too brisk and endoscopic diagnosis is not possible, angiography may be performed to determine the site of bleeding and the vascular anatomy of the portal circulation.

3. **Choice of therapeutic method.** Once the diagnosis of active variceal bleeding is made, there are several therapeutic options. The treatment of choice is endoscopic sclerotherapy or endoscopic variceal banding.

   If these methods are not immediately available, medical drug therapy, balloon tamponade, or transhepatic variceal obliteration may be used. Surgical therapy with a portosystemic shunt (PSS) carries a very high mortality but may be lifesaving. Transjugular introduction of an expandable stent (transjugular intrahepatic portosystemic shunt [TIPS]) into the liver may create a PSS with much less morbidity or mortality.

4. **Endoscopic sclerotherapy,** the direct injection of a sclerosing agent into the esophageal varices, is effective in the immediate control of variceal bleeding. This technique is preferentially used as an initial therapy before the infusion of vasopressin or balloon tamponade. The sclerosants most commonly used are tetradecyl, sodium morrhuate, and ethanolamine oleate. The sclerosing agent is injected directly into the variceal wall or into the mucosa between the varices. It causes clotting of the varices and a severe necrotizing inflammation of the esophageal wall followed by a marked fibrotic reaction.

   After control of the bleeding, the endoscopic sclerotherapy is repeated at weekly or monthly intervals until the varices are totally obliterated, leaving a scarred esophagus. Sclerotherapy of gastric varices has not been shown conclusively to be effective and may result in gastric ulceration. The complications of endoscopic sclerotherapy of esophageal varices include ulceration, hemorrhage, perforation, stricture, and pleural effusion. Sclerotherapy controls acute variceal hemorrhage in 80% to 90% of patients. Chronic sclerotherapy that obliterates the esophagus and varices decreases the risk of rebleeding.

5. **Endoscopic banding of esophageal varices** has been shown to be as effective as or slightly more effective than injection sclerotherapy in the initial treatment of bleeding esophageal varices. The technique requires expertise and a

cooperative patient. Tracheal intubation and sedation of the patient may be necessary.

6. **Drug therapy.** Although endoscopic banding or sclerotherapy is widely accepted as the treatment of choice for acutely bleeding esophageal varices, drug therapy may be a useful adjunctive treatment, particularly in severe hemorrhage and when bleeding is present from sites inaccessible to sclerotherapy (e.g., portal hypertensive gastropathy, gastric fundal varices, and varices in the more distal gastrointestinal tract). Several agents have been evaluated in the setting of acute portal hypertensive bleeding: **vasopressin** and its analogs with or without short-acting **nitrates** and **somatostatin** and its analog **octreotide.**

   a. **Vasopressin (Pitressin).** Parenteral vasopressin results in constriction of the splanchnic blood flow and subsequent decrease in portal venous pressure. There is no clear evidence that direct infusion of vasopressin into the superior mesenteric artery is more effective or less toxic than intravenous (IV) administration of the drug. The IV route is preferred initially.

      A continuous infusion of 0.4 unit per minute (or up to 0.9 U/min if necessary) is given for 4 to 12 hours with subsequent gradual decrease in the dose for duration up to 36 to 48 hours. The complications of vasopressin therapy are generalized vasoconstriction leading to myocardial and peripheral ischemia, lactic acidosis, cardiac arrhythmias, and hyponatremia (antidiuretic hormone effect).

   b. **Short-acting nitrates.** The addition of **nitroglycerin** administered via transdermal, sublingual, or IV routes reduces the peripheral vasospastic effects of vasopressin and lowers the portal pressure further via direct vasodilation of portosystemic collaterals. The **dosages** are as follows: transdermal: 10 mg applied to skin q12h; sublingual: 0.6 mg every 30 minutes; IV: 40 μg/min increasing to 400 μg/min, adjusting doses to keep systolic blood pressure greater than 90 mmHg.

   c. **Somatostatin.** Somatostatin appears to be highly selective in its ability to reduce splanchnic blood flow and hence reduce portal pressure. It has been shown to be as effective as vasopressin with considerably fewer hemodynamic effects. It can be administered for prolonged periods. The possible side effects are nausea, abdominal pain, and minor disturbances in glucose tolerance with prolonged use. **Octreotide,** the synthetic somatostatin analog, appears to be as effective as somatostatin. The **dosages** are as follows: **somatostatin:** 250-μg IV bolus followed by 250 μg per hour IV continuous infusion up to 5 days; **octreotide:** 50-mg IV bolus followed by 50 mg per hour IV. In cases of severe bleeding, the bolus dose may be repeated and the dose of somatostatin or octreotide in the continuous infusion may be doubled.

      Octreotide has replaced vasopressin in the treatment of bleeding esophageal varices.

7. **Balloon tamponade. The Sengstaken-Blakemore (SB)** and **the Minnesota tube** consist of two balloons, an elongated esophageal and a round gastric balloon, with orifices in the tube to suction the stomach and upper esophagus of collecting secretions. Variceal tamponade with the SB tube stops the bleeding, at least temporarily, in more than 90% of patients. Many difficulties that have been associated with the procedure can be avoided if the patient is monitored in an intensive care unit. The proper procedure requires inserting the tube through either the mouth or the nose, inflating the gastric balloon with 250 to 300 mL of air, and positioning the balloon tightly against the gastroesophageal junction. In most patients, this procedure alone stops the bleeding. If the bleeding persists, the esophageal balloon must be inflated to a pressure of 30 to 40 mmHg. The main complications of the SB tube are esophageal or gastric ischemia, rupture, and aspiration. Because the chance for complications from the SB tube increases with the length of time the balloon is kept inflated, the balloon should be deflated after 24 hours. If bleeding has stopped, the SB tube may be removed in another 24 hours.

8. **Percutaneous transhepatic obliteration** of the varices with either a sclerosant or embolization controls active variceal bleeding 70% of the time. However, bleeding usually recurs. It should be used only as a secondary approach after other therapy has failed or for bleeding gastric varices in patients who are poor surgical risks.

9. **Portosystemic shunts (PSSs).** Recurrent or continued bleeding may indicate a need for a PSS with surgical decompression of the portal venous pressure. This major surgery, when performed on an emergency basis, carries a mortality of 40%. If the surgery can be performed electively, mortality declines substantially. PSS procedures do not appear to prolong survival, but they do prevent subsequent bleeding. Because PSS diverts much of the blood away from the liver into the vena cava, the underperfusion of the liver results in liver failure and intractable hepatic encephalopathy in most of the patients. A variation of the PSS, the distal splenorenal shunt with concomitant gastroesophageal devascularization, selectively decompresses esophageal varices while maintaining mesenteric blood flow to the liver. In many studies, the use of the distal splenorenal shunt has been shown to reduce the incidence of severe encephalopathy as a late complication following surgery compared to other PSSs. This procedure is technically difficult, however, and is not advised in the presence of significant nonresponsive ascites, which it tends to worsen.

   Emergency PSSs have been compared with endoscopic sclerotherapy in the treatment of patients with severely decompensated alcoholic liver disease and active variceal bleeding. Subsequent recurrence of bleeding may be less frequent in the shunted patients, but liver failure and encephalopathy were greater in this group. The survival was comparable in the two groups.

   Insertion of a prophylactic PSS prior to bleeding is not recommended for patients with cirrhosis and varices. The resultant overall survival is not improved. There is evidence to suggest that prophylactic endoscopic sclerotherapy and obliteration of large esophageal varices prevents bleeding.

10. **Transjugular intrahepatic portosystemic shunts.** Partial portal decompression may be achieved by creating a channel between the hepatic vein and the portal vein via a percutaneous transjugular approach.

    Elastic recoil of the liver parenchyma occluding the shunt lumen is prevented by the use of an expandable metallic endoprosthesis. With use of TIPS, portal pressure has been reduced from 34 to 22 mmHg, with effective control of variceal bleeding. Shunt patency is 90% up to 6 months afterward and may be restored by shunt dilatation or restenting. Late complications of TIPS are encephalopathy and ascites in about 10% to 20% of the patients.

11. **Other surgical therapy.** Surgical transection of the esophagus, devascularization of the distal esophagus and proximal stomach, and splenectomy has been used in patients with acute refractory variceal bleeding. These operations carry a very high mortality and are not routinely recommended.

12. **Liver transplantation** is curative for portal hypertension, but it is impractical in the acute setting of variceal bleeding. It is not necessary in patients with only moderate liver disease and should be reserved for patients with irreversible advanced liver disease.

13. **Prevention of first variceal bleeding and rebleeding** in cirrhosis. Nonselective beta-adrenergic receptor blockers (e.g., **propranolol** 20–180 mg b.i.d.—a dose that reduces the resting heart rate by 25%) have been shown to reduce portal hypertension and prevent the first variceal bleeding in patients with large varices or gastropathic hemorrhage and to decrease rebleeding; these drugs probably improve survival in patients with cirrhosis. Long-acting nitrates (e.g., **isosorbide-5-mononitrate**) have been shown to be at least as effective as propranolol in the prevention of first bleeding in cirrhosis. It has fewer side effects than propranolol and may be used as an alternative.

    Beta-blockers are minimally effective in patients with decompensated cirrhosis. Propranolol also has been shown to prevent bleeding from portal hypertensive gastropathy. Beta-blocker therapy should not replace sclerotherapy or variceal band ligation in the early management of variceal bleeding. It should be considered as adjunctive therapy in the long-term management of portal hypertension.

V. Ascites refers to the accumulation of excessive volumes of fluid within the peritoneal cavity. Cirrhosis is the most common cause of ascites. The other main causes are infection (acute and chronic, including tuberculosis), malignancy, pancreatitis, heart failure, hepatic venous obstruction, nephrotic syndrome, and myxedema.

  A. Pathogenesis. Ascites forms because of an imbalance between the formation and resorption of peritoneal fluid. Distribution of fluid between vascular and tissue spaces is determined by the equilibrium of hydrostatic and oncotic pressures in the two compartments. The accumulation of fluid in the peritoneal cavity of patients with cirrhosis results from an interaction of a number of factors:

   1. Portal hypertension with increased total splanchnic plasma volume.

   2. Renal changes favoring increased sodium and water resorption and retention include the following:

       a. Stimulation of the renin-aldosterone system

       b. Increased antidiuretic hormone release

       c. Decreased release of "natriuretic" hormone or third factor

   3. Imbalance in the formation and removal of hepatic and gut lymph. Lymphatic drainage (removal) fails to compensate for the increased lymph leakage, mainly due to elevated hepatic sinusoidal pressure, leading to formation of ascites.

   4. Hypoalbuminemia from decreased hepatic synthesis, which results in decreased intravascular oncotic pressure. The leakage of albumin through lymph into the peritoneal cavity increases the intraperitoneal oncotic pressure, favoring ascites formation.

   5. Elevated plasma vasopressin and epinephrine levels. These hormonal responses to a volume-depleted state further accentuate renal and vascular factors.

  B. Diagnosis

   1. Clinical presentation. The physical findings of ascites include the puddle sign, bulging flanks, flank and shifting dullness, and fluid wave. Abdominal or umbilical herniation, penile or scrotal edema, or right-sided pleural effusion may be present.

       Detection of more than 2 L of ascites is not difficult, but less than this amount is not always ascertained by physical examination. The percussion maneuvers require the presence of at least 500 mL of fluid. The diagnostic accuracy of all the maneuvers described is only about 50%. The maneuver to determine flank and shifting dullness is probably the most reliable.

   2. Radiologic studies

       a. Plain abdominal x-ray films may reveal general haziness of the abdomen with loss of the psoas shadow. Usually, there is centralization and separation of bowel loops.

       b. Ultrasonography can detect as little as 30 mL of ascitic fluid with the patient in the right lateral decubitus position. Free and loculated collections can be identified.

       c. Computed tomography (CT) scans of the abdomen may detect small amounts of ascites and at the same time evaluate intraabdominal anatomy, giving important information on the size and state of the liver and spleen and on the presence or absence of varices and tumors.

   3. Characterization of ascitic fluid

       a. Paracentesis. A diagnostic paracentesis should be performed for new onset ascites or when a complication is suspected. The procedure is performed under sterile conditions using a 20- to 23-gauge angiocatheter. The most frequent site of puncture is on the linea alba slightly below the umbilicus. The iliac fossa also may be used. Paracentesis rarely leads to serious complications (<1%), which include bowel perforation, hemorrhage, and persistent ascitic fluid leakage. It is much safer to perform the paracentesis under ultrasound guidance with proper localization of ascitic fluid away from bowel loops.

b. Laboratory studies

i. Approximately 50 mL of ascitic fluid is withdrawn for diagnostic purposes. The ascitic fluid is analyzed for appearance, color, red and white blood cell counts, and percentage of neutrophils, total protein, albumin, glucose, triglycerides, and amylase determination. The fluid should be inoculated into blood culture bottles at the bedside for aerobic and anaerobic organisms. Samples should be sent for Gram's and acid-fast bacillus (AFB) stains, tuberculin and fungal cultures, and cytologic study to look for malignant cells. Gram's stain is helpful only in the setting of gut perforation. A concomitant serum sample is also analyzed for the preceding chemical parameters.

ii. A serum ascites albumin gradient equal to or greater than 1.1 g/dL is consistent with ascites secondary to portal hypertension and cirrhosis. The cell count in cirrhotic ascites is usually less than 500 white cells/μL with less than 25% neutrophils (polymorphonuclear [PMN] cells). PMN counts greater than 250/μl/L strongly suggest bacterial infection either from spontaneous bacterial peritonitis or from perforation of a viscus. Patients with bloody ascites should have a corrected PMN count calculated, as one PMN is subtracted from the total absolute PMN count for every 250 red blood cells. Ascitic fluid, lactate, and pH values are not helpful in diagnosing infection.

iii. The presence of blood in the ascitic fluid suggests infection with tuberculosis, fungi, or, more commonly, malignancy. **Pancreatic ascites** has a high protein concentration, increased number of neutrophils, and elevated amylase levels. Increased triglycerides in the ascitic fluid indicate **chylous ascites** and suggest the presence of lymphatic obstruction and disruption by trauma, lymphoma, tumor, or infection.

C. Spontaneous bacterial peritonitis

1. Spontaneous bacterial peritonitis (SBP) seems to occur in 8% to 10% of patients with alcoholic cirrhosis. The patient may be totally asymptomatic or present with signs and symptoms of peritonitis or increased liver failure and encephalopathy or both. When SBP is suspected, ascitic fluid and blood cultures should be obtained, and the patient should be treated promptly with broad-spectrum antibiotics (e.g., a third-generation cephalosporin). Because untreated SBP results in high mortality, overtreatment rather than delayed treatment is recommended. The antibiotic coverage may be altered following culture results. Five days of IV antibiotic therapy is sufficient even for patients with bacteremia.

2. The organisms most commonly found in the infected ascitic fluid belong to the gut flora such as *Escherichia coli*, pneumococcus, and *Klebsiella* organisms. Anaerobic infection is rare. In 70% of patients, the blood cultures are also positive for bacteria. The pathogenesis of SBP is multifactorial. The decreased hepatic reticuloendothelial filtration of gut bacteria and the decreased antimicrobial activity of ascitic fluid with low opsonic activity due to low complement and antibody levels and neutrophil dysfunction are thought to play a large role. Possible routes of entry for the bacteria are transmurally from the gastrointestinal tract, from the lymphatics, or, in women, from the genital tract and fallopian tubes. Recurrent SBP may be seen in a high percentage of patients. An ascitic fluid protein concentration less than 1.0 g/dL is the best predictor of recurrence. Oral quinolone therapy (e.g., norfloxacin) has been shown to be effective in decreasing the rate of recurrence of infection. Diuresis also may help in SBP by increasing ascitic fluid opsonic and total protein concentrations.

3. SBP is sometimes difficult to distinguish from secondary peritonitis resulting from rupture of an abscess or bowel perforation. The number and type of infecting organisms may be helpful in distinguishing spontaneous from secondary peritonitis. Unlike secondary peritonitis, in which there are always multiple organisms, a single organism is cultured in 78% to 88% of SBP cases.

If present, pneumoperitoneum strongly suggests secondary bacterial peritonitis. The treatment of secondary peritonitis is surgical. However, all patients require proper broad-spectrum antibiotic coverage.

D. Complications of ascites. Most of the complications of ascites result from increased intraabdominal pressure and are proportional to the volume and rate of fluid accumulation. The most common complications are dyspnea, decreased cardiac input, anorexia, reflux esophagitis, vomiting, ventral hernia, and escape of the ascitic fluid along tissue planes to the chest (hydrothorax) and the scrotum. By increasing the portal hypertension, the risk of upper gastrointestinal bleeding may also be increased.

E. Treatment of ascites. The treatment of uncomplicated ascites should start with attempts to improve the hepatic function. Patients should abstain from alcohol and other hepatotoxic drugs and should receive good nutrition to promote hepatic regeneration. When drug therapy may be helpful in decreasing hepatic inflammation, patients should be treated appropriately. Hepatic healing and regeneration have resulted in decrease of ascites.

Most patients, especially those with urine sodium concentrations less than 10 mEq/L, respond to moderate periods of bed rest and restriction of dietary sodium to 0.5 to 1.0 g per day and fluid intake to less than 1 L per day with spontaneous diuresis.

1. Diuretics. If the preceding measures do not induce spontaneous diuresis, diuretics may be used. Optimally, diuresis should result in loss of 1 L or 1 to 2 lb (0.4–0.9 kg) per day. Peripheral edema is more easily mobilized by diuretics than ascites and serves as a safety valve for fluid loss. Excessive diuresis may result in azotemia, hyponatremia, hepatorenal syndrome, and encephalopathy.

a. Spironolactone (Aldactone) is usually the diuretic of choice at 100 to 200 mg per day given in a single dose. If the urinary sodium concentration remains less than 10 mEq/L and the diuresis is suboptimal, doses up to 600 mg per day may be used. The effect of the drug (inhibition of the effect of aldosterone at the distal tube) is slow, and initial diuresis begins after 2 to 3 days. The possible side effects are gynecomastia, lactation, and hyperkalemia.

b. Furosemide. In patients in whom diuresis is not successful with spironolactone, furosemide (Lasix) may be added, starting at 40 mg per day. The dosage may be increased to 240 mg per day, especially in patients with peripheral edema.

c. Combination therapy. Although single-agent spironolactone has been shown to be superior to single-agent furosemide, it is usually preferable to start spironolactone and furosemide together, beginning with 100 mg and 40 mg, respectively, given as a single dose.

Single daily doses of medications are most appropriate and enhance compliance. **Amiloride hydrochloride** 10 mg per day can be substituted for spironolactone; amiloride hydrochloride is less available and more expensive than spironolactone, but it is more rapidly effective and does not cause gynecomastia. If the combination of 100 mg per day of spironolactone (or 10 mg of amiloride hydrochloride) and 40 mg per day of furosemide is ineffective in increasing urinary sodium or decreasing body weight, the dosages of both drugs should be simultaneously increased as needed (e.g., 200 plus 80, then 300 plus 120, and finally 400 mg per day of spironolactone [or 40 mg per day of amiloride hydrochloride] plus 160 mg per day of furosemide). Doses higher than 400 mg per day plus 160 mg per day can be given, but additional increments in urine sodium are marginal. Addition of a third diuretic such as **hydrochlorothiazide** can lead to a natriuresis in such a patient but may result in hyponatremia. Although the preceding ratios of spironolactone and furosemide usually maintain normokalemia, the doses of these two drugs can be adjusted to correct serum potassium imbalance.

F. Treatment of refractory ascites. In 10% to 20% of patients with ascites, the standard medical therapy is ineffective or causes serious side effects. Ascites that is resistant to mobilization with the usual therapy is not always the result of refractory hepatorenal failure. The conditions that may contribute to refractory ascites include worsening of the primary liver disease, such as active inflammation, portal or hepatic vein thrombosis, gastrointestinal bleeding, infection, SBP, malnutrition, hepatocellular carcinoma, superimposed cardiac or renal disease, and hepatotoxic (e.g., alcohol and acetaminophen) and nephrotoxic substances. Nonsteroidal antiinflammatory drugs (NSAIDs) reduce renal blood flow by reducing renal vasodilating prostaglandins, glomerular filtration rate, and response to diuretics. Angiotensin-converting enzyme (ACE) inhibitors and some calcium channel blockers decrease peripheral vascular resistance, effective vascular volume, and renal perfusion. Aminoglycoside nephrotoxicity is more prevalent in patients with cirrhosis and may result in renal failure.

Current options for the 10% of patients whose condition is refractory to routine medical therapy include **therapeutic paracentesis, PV shunt,** and **liver transplantation**. Side-to-side portacaval shunts have been used in the treatment of refractory ascites, but operative hemorrhagic complications and portosystemic encephalopathy have led to the abandonment of this approach. Whether TIPS will be of value in the treatment of patients with diuretic resistant ascites remains to be seen.

1. **Therapeutic paracentesis.** The safety and efficacy of large-volume paracentesis have been confirmed. The procedure involves the daily removal of 4 to 6 L of ascitic fluid until the abdomen is completely evacuated. After paracentesis, adjunctive therapy with diuretics and dietary sodium restriction should be continued to prevent rapid reaccumulation of ascitic fluid. The procedure may be repeated at intervals of 2 to 4 weeks.

   In view of the ease and efficacy of diuretic therapy in more than 90% of patients, therapeutic paracentesis should be reserved for treatment of tense ascites and ascites that is refractory to diuretic therapy. In addition to being time-consuming for both the physician and the patient, the procedure leads to protein and opsonin depletion; diuresis, on the other hand, conserves proteins and opsonins. Depletion of opsonins could predispose to spontaneous bacterial peritonitis.

   Colloid replacement after large-volume paracentesis remains controversial. The cost of albumin infusion ranges from $120 to $1,250 per tap. The changes noted in plasma renin and serum electrolytes and creatinine in patients who receive no colloid replacement do not seem to be clinically significant and have not resulted in increases in morbidity or mortality.

2. **Shunts.** In about 5% of patients, ascites does not respond to the usual dosages of diuretics, and increases in diuretic dosages result in the deterioration of renal function. In these patients, a shunting procedure may be considered. A side-to-side portosystemic shunt has been used in some patients, but the procedure is associated with high mortality.

3. **Peritoneovenous shunts.** The reinfusion of ascitic fluid by a peritoneovenous (PV) shunt (e.g., LeVeen or Denver shunt) may be therapeutic in selected patients. The PV shunt routes the ascitic fluid subcutaneously from the peritoneal cavity into the internal jugular vein through a pressure activated one-way valve. Most patients still require diuretics but at reduced doses. There is also a concomitant improvement in renal blood flow. Serious complications of the PV shunt occur in more than 10% of the patients and may lead to death. The complications include peritoneal infection and sepsis, disseminated intravascular coagulation (DIC), congestive heart failure, and ruptured esophageal varices. The shunt may clot in about 30% of the recipients and require replacement. The procedure is contraindicated in patients with sepsis, heart failure, malignancy, and history of variceal bleeding. The morbidity and survival rates of patients with cirrhosis treated with PV shunts correlate with the degree of impairment of liver and renal functions. The best results are obtained in the few patients with diuretic-resistant ascites and relatively preserved hepatic function.

   At the present time, PV shunting is reserved for a very small group of patients who fail to improve with both diuretic and paracentesis therapy or patients in whom diuretic therapy has failed, or who live too far from medical care to receive large-volume paracentesis every other week.

4. Liver transplantation. Orthotopic liver transplantation should be considered among the treatment options of a patient with refractory ascites who is otherwise a transplant candidate. The 12-month survival of patients with ascites refractory to medical therapy is only 25%. With liver transplantation, however, the 12-month survival is 70% to 75%.

VI. Hepatorenal syndrome is a progressive, functional renal failure that occurs in patients with severe liver disease. Most of these patients have decompensated cirrhosis and tense ascites. Similar syndromes may be seen in metastatic liver disease and fulminant hepatitis from viral, alcoholic, or toxic causes.

The kidneys are anatomically and histologically normal and capable of normal function. The functional integrity of the renal tubules is maintained during the renal failure, as manifested by relatively normal capacity for both sodium resorption and urine concentration. When transplanted into patients without liver disease, these kidneys have been shown to function normally. Conversely, normal function has returned when liver transplantation is carried out successfully.

A. Pathogenesis. The exact pathogenesis of hepatorenal syndrome is unclear. Most evidence suggests that the primary abnormality in the kidneys is altered blood flow. Hepatorenal syndrome is presently viewed as a perturbation of renal hemodynamics characterized by vasoconstriction of arterioles of the outer renal cortex with shunting of blood to the renal medulla, which results in decreased glomerular filtration rate and urine flow.

The renal hemodynamic alterations in hepatorenal syndrome are thought to be a consequence of decreased "effective" blood volume and increased sympathetic tone, increased intraabdominal and renal venous pressure, and alteration of the normal balance of vasoactive humoral agents such as renin-angiotensin, prostaglandins, thromboxanes, kinins, endotoxins, and renal kallikrein. Newer studies suggest the involvement of endothelin-1 and endothelin-3 in hepatorenal syndrome. Other studies focus on the florid systemic hemodynamic disturbances that accompany this syndrome. These include a hyperdynamic circulation, increased heart rate and cardiac output, and decreased blood pressure and systemic vascular resistance. The identity of the "excess" vasodilator has not been elucidated. Nitric oxide, a vasodilator synthesized from L-arginine and released from vascular endothelium, has been proposed as the mediator for both the hyperdynamic circulation and renal failure. Nitric oxide synthetase can be induced by bacterial lipopolysaccharide endotoxin and leads to peripheral vasodilatation, tachycardia, and a decline in blood pressure.

B. Diagnosis. Hepatorenal syndrome is characterized by progressive azotemia (serum creatinine >2.5 mg/dL) oliguria (urine volume <500 mL per day), a concentrated urine with a urine-plasma osmolality ratio greater than 1.0, urinary sodium concentration less than 10 mEq/L, and normal urine analysis. The urine may contain small amounts of protein, hyaline, and granular casts. The oliguria may occur spontaneously but usually follows diuretic-therapy diarrhea, paracentesis, gastrointestinal hemorrhage, or sepsis. Hyponatremia, hyperkalemia, hepatic encephalopathy, and coma may precede or accompany the renal functional deterioration. A modest decrease in systemic blood pressure is present, but profound hypotension is not part of the syndrome.

C. Differential diagnosis. Hepatorenal syndrome must be differentiated from other types of renal failure that can occur in patients with liver disease. These include renal failure from exposure to toxins such as acetaminophen, NSAIDs, and carbon tetrachloride; infections; acute tubular necrosis due to hypotension or exposure to aminoglycoside or angiographic dyes; and obstructive uropathy.

D. The prognosis of hepatorenal syndrome is very poor with an associated mortality greater than 90%.

E. Treatment

1. Factors precipitating renal failure. The management of these patients should include the identification, removal, and treatment of any factors known to precipitate renal failure. Diuretics should be stopped, blood volume lost due to hemorrhage or dehydration should be replaced, serum electrolyte abnormalities (hyponatremia and hypokalemia) corrected, and infections promptly treated. Drugs that inhibit prostaglandin synthesis such as aspirin and NSAIDs should not be given to patients with severe liver disease, because these drugs may precipitate renal failure.

2. **Fluid challenge.** All patients should undergo a trial of fluid challenge to increase the "effective" plasma volume, using saline with salt-poor albumin or plasma. Administration of fluid should be closely monitored, preferably with measurement of the central venous pressure to document adequacy of the fluid replacement as well as to prevent congestive heart failure. If diuresis does not occur, the fluid challenge should be stopped.

3. **Drugs.** There is no effective treatment for hepatorenal syndrome. Numerous agents have been tried in a limited number of patients to reverse the renal vasoconstriction, including phentolamine, papaverine, aminophylline, metaraminol, dopamine, phenoxybenzamine hydrochloride, and prostaglandin E_1. No consistent benefit has been observed with any of these agents. The current treatment of hepatorenal syndrome remains conservative with supportive measures.

4. **Dialysis.** It is advisable to use dialysis for patients with potentially reversible liver disease, such as fulminant hepatitis, to allow the liver to heal with the hope that renal function will benefit. Spontaneous reversion of the syndrome, although infrequent, occurs when the liver disease begins to improve.

5. **Surgery.** There are a few reports of recovery from hepatorenal syndrome following portacaval shunt or liver transplantation. However, these major surgical interventions are inapplicable to most patients with this disorder. Reversal of the hepatorenal syndrome after insertion of a PV shunt has been reported.

6. **Liver transplantation** is a frequently successful therapy for the hepatorenal syndrome. It is currently the only definitive treatment; the improvement in liver function that follows liver transplantation is associated with complete recovery from the hepatorenal syndrome.

VII. HYPERSPLENISM. Portal hypertension and obstruction to portal flow may cause enlargement and engorgement of the spleen. The resulting hypersplenism causes sequestration and destruction of all or some of the blood cells, leading to decreased red cell survival, neutropenia, and thrombocytopenia. These hematologic abnormalities are usually not severe and do not require specific therapy.

In patients with thrombocytopenia who require a surgical procedure, a normal bleeding time is a good index of adequacy of hemostasis. If it is abnormal, cryoprecipitate and platelet transfusions should be administered prior to surgery. Splenectomy is not routinely recommended for patients with hypersplenism. The effect of surgical portal decompression on hypersplenism is unpredictable.

VIII. Hepatic encephalopathy is a neuropsychiatric syndrome occurring in patients with acute or chronic liver failure. The acute disorder seen in fulminant hepatic failure is discussed in Chapter 17. Patients with chronic liver disease develop a more indolent encephalopathy, called **portosystemic encephalopathy (PSE).** It accompanies the development of portal systemic collaterals that arise from portal hypertension, most often due to cirrhosis. PSE involves the alteration of mental state and behavior. PSE may be subclinical, recurrent with overt episodes, or chronic, and may lead to hepatocerebral degeneration. In most instances, PSE is precipitated by a specific cause such as gastrointestinal bleeding, acid-base disorders, electrolyte abnormalities, hypoxia, carbon dioxide retention, azotemia, infection, or use of sedatives or other medications.

A. **The pathogenesis** of hepatic encephalopathy is incompletely understood. Using sensitive CT scan and magnetic resonance imaging (MRI), significant frontoparietal atrophy of the cortical brain has been found in patients with PSE including those with subclinical PSE. The findings were dramatic in alcoholic cirrhotics. Histopathologic evaluation of brain tissue from patients with PSE reveals astrocytic changes (Alzheimer type II astrocytosis). The degree of astrocytic damage was directly related to the severity and duration of PSE. It is thought to be a metabolic disorder, and in most patients the cerebral dysfunction is reversible. However, in patients with hepatocerebral degeneration and spastic paraparesis, it may be progressive. Reduced neuronal activity and brain energy metabolism and decreased brain glucose utilization in PSE is due to neurotransmission failure, rather than primary energy failure.

The shunting of blood from the gut directly to the systemic circulation, bypassing the liver, due to portal hypertension and the poor function of the diseased liver, allows the accumulation of various "toxins," leading to deranged cerebral function. The various toxins and states implicated in the pathogenesis of hepatic encephalopathy include ammonia, γ-aminobutyric acid (GABA), mercaptan, short-chain fatty acids, false neurotransmitters, an imbalance of excitatory and inhibitory neurotransmitters, and the reversed ratio of serum aromatic amino acids to branched-chain amino acids.

Several pathogenetic mechanisms involving neurotransmitter systems have been proposed to explain hepatic encephalopathy, including the following:

1. Ammonia neurotoxicity (most commonly accepted theory)
   a. Direct effects of ammonia on inhibitory and excitatory synaptic transmission
   b. Glutamate synaptic dysregulation due to astrocytic changes
   c. Increased serotonin turnover (especially in preclinical PSE)
2. The GABA-benzodiazepine system
   a. Increased brain GABA uptake
   b. Increased GABA-ergic tone
   c. Presence of "endogenous" benzodiazepines
3. Other neurotransmitter systems (acetylcholine, histamine, taurine, opioid system, other peptides).

   Moreover, in these patients, other metabolic disturbances such as azotemia, electrolyte abnormalities, acid-base disorders, such as hypokalemic alkalosis, and infections may also contribute to the cerebral dysfunction. In addition, in patients with cirrhosis and PSE, the central nervous system (CNS) appears to be very sensitive to the sedative effects of drugs. Decreased hepatic drug metabolism with subsequent accumulation of the drug, decreased binding of the drug to decreased plasma proteins (making more free drug available to penetrate the altered, "more porous" blood-brain barrier), and enhanced cerebral receptor sensitivity to sedative drugs such as benzodiazepines and barbiturates probably combine to increase susceptibility of the patient to development of encephalopathy and coma.

B. Diagnosis
   1. Clinical presentation. The diagnosis of hepatic encephalopathy is clinical and depends on documentation of the presence of mental status changes, fetor hepaticus, and asterixis in a patient with parenchymal liver disease. Fetor hepaticus refers to the feculent-fruity odor of the breath in these patients. Asterixis is a flapping motion of the hands caused by intermittent loss of extensor tone. It is best elicited by asking the patient to outstretch his or her arms, with hands extended at the wrist and fingers separated. The flap is maximal with sustained posture. The motor disturbance can also be detected in tightly closed eyelids, pursed lips, and protruded tongue. Asterixis is not specific for hepatic encephalopathy. It can also occur in patients with uremia, severe pulmonary disease, and sedative overdose.
      a. Stages. Hepatic encephalopathy can be subclinical or overt; the overt form can be classified roughly into four stages of increasing severity as follows:
         i. Stage I. Patients exhibit inappropriate behavior, altered sleep pattern, loss of affect, depression, or euphoria. There is usually asterixis and difficulty with writing and other fine motor skills.
         ii. Stage II. Patients are moderately obtunded, confused, and disoriented. There is accompanying fetor hepaticus and asterixis.
         iii. Stage III. Patients are stuporous with marked confusion. They are barely responsive to painful stimuli. If it can be elicited, asterixis should

be present. There is usually hyperreflexia, clonus, and rigidity of limbs, extensor response, grasping, and sucking responses.

    iv. Stage IV. Patients are in deep coma, usually with no response to stimuli. Muscle tone may be totally absent, limbs flaccid, and reflexes depressed.

  b. The **neurologic signs** in hepatic encephalopathy are caused by metabolic abnormalities and in most instances are transient, changing, and potentially reversible.

2. Diagnostic studies

  a. Laboratory abnormalities found in patients with hepatic encephalopathy may include abnormal liver chemistry tests, which reflect the state of the underlying parenchymal liver disease. Respiratory alkalosis with central hyperventilation is usually present. In 90% of the patients with hepatic encephalopathy, the arterial ammonia concentration is increased. The arterial ammonia level does not correlate linearly with the depth of the coma. However, serial measurements are helpful in following the course of the hepatic encephalopathy in individual patients. Since the brain does not have a urea cycle, the removal of ammonia depends on glutamine synthesis. Thus the spinal fluid glutamine is a more sensitive test than arterial ammonia and correlates closely with the depth of the coma.

    In patients with PSE, blood levels of free fatty acids are elevated. There is also an increase in the aromatic amino acids and methionine in the blood, whereas branched-chain amino acid levels are decreased.

  b. The electroencephalogram (EEG) and evoked potentials (visual, auditory, somatosensory) offer little additional useful information to the clinician except in atypical cases. The EEG shows characteristic slowing or flattening of the waves with 3:1 high-voltage waves. Similar EEG changes may be seen in patients with other metabolic encephalopathies.

    Focal abnormalities should not be present. Some investigators believe visual **evoked potential recording** is a useful tool in the diagnosis of hepatic encephalopathy. It has been demonstrated that latency of the N_3 component of the flash visual evoked response (VER) is useful for the diagnosis of preclinical PSE and the assessment of patients with clinically overt PSE. VER may replace the tedious psychometric testing of patients suspected to have preclinical PSE.

C. The treatment of PSE includes the following:

  1. Improvement of the hepatic function, if possible, by treatment of the underlying parenchymal liver disease.

  2. Identification and removal or correction of the precipitating causes.

  3. Removal of any sedative drugs.

  4. Reduction of the "influx" of the putative cerebral "toxins." Most of the putative toxins implicated in PSE such as ammonia, GABA, and mercaptans are protein breakdown products from the gut. Due to portal hypertension and PSS, these toxins are more available to the "sensitive" CNS in these patients. The reduction of the formation and influx of these toxins into the CNS is accomplished by the following:

    a. Supportive care is crucial in these patients. Catabolism of patients' own endogenous protein should be prevented by providing adequate calories (1,800–2,400 per day) in the form of glucose or carbohydrates. Vitamins and minerals such as magnesium, calcium, phosphorus, and zinc may be deficient and should be replenished. Electrolytes, acid-base imbalances, and prerenal azotemia should be corrected. Gastrointestinal bleeding and infections should be meticulously searched for and treated.

    b. Restriction of dietary protein. The degree of restriction of dietary protein depends on the severity of the mental status changes. Dairy and vegetable proteins are much better tolerated than animal protein. In most patients who can eat, the dietary protein is initially restricted to 40 g per day. Since these patients require protein for hepatic regeneration and protein synthesis (anabolism), complete withdrawal of protein should be brief. As the mental status improves, protein should be reintroduced, preferably in the form of vegetable protein, and advanced to 60 to 110 g as tolerated. Amino acid mixtures, rich in branched-chain amino acids and low in aromatic amino acids and methionine, such as HepatAmine or Hepatic-Aid may be used as protein source or supplement.

c. **Intestinal cleansing**, especially if there is gastrointestinal bleeding. Bowel cleansing is initially accomplished by enemas or intestinal lavage solutions such as GoLYTELY or Colyte. However, these patients require prolonged bowel cleansing to eliminate the contents as well as the organisms that break down proteins and "convert" them to the putative toxins. This is accomplished by the use of antibiotics or nonabsorbable sugars.

d. **Antibiotics**
   i. **Neomycin** is a nonabsorbable aminoglycoside given orally in doses of 2 to 6 g per day or as a 1% enema if the patient has ileus. Its effect is thought to be by the inactivation of gut bacteria. About 1% to 3% of the drug is absorbed and excreted by the kidneys. Prolonged use of the drug may lead to renal failure as well as eighth cranial nerve damage.
   ii. **Vancomycin** has been shown to be effective in the management of resistant hepatic encephalopathy, but its high cost is prohibitive.
   iii. **Metronidazole** has become the oral antibiotic of choice for acute management of hepatic encephalopathy when lactulose alone does not achieve adequate results. It must be used with caution in this setting because the drug is cleared by the liver and thus is likely to accumulate in patients with chronic liver disease. The recommended dosage is 250 mg by mouth three or four times daily. Use of metronidazole beyond 7 to 10 days is not advisable.
   iv. **Rifaximin (Xifaxan)** has recently shown to be effective in the treatment of PSE in the dose range of 400 mg 2–3 times daily. It is a nonabsorbable, gut-specific antibiotic that alters the intestinal flora with any systemic side effects.

e. **Nonabsorbable sugars**
   i. **Lactulose** is a nonabsorbable disaccharide (galactoside fructose). It is given orally in dosages of 60 to 120 mg of syrup per day. The goal is initially to achieve diarrhea, then to produce two to three soft bowel movements per day. The mechanism of action of lactulose is multifactorial:
      a) It causes an osmotic diarrhea, providing for a rapid evacuation of nitrogenous toxins from the bowel.
      b) It is broken down in the colon by gut bacteria to short-chain fatty acids, which lower the pH of stool. The low pH promotes ammonia (NH_3) to ammonium (NH_4^+) well as the $-NH_2$ group of other amines, thus making them less lipid soluble and less apt to cross cell membranes of enterocytes to be absorbed into the circulation. Also, the low pH promotes the growth of low-ammonia producing gut bacteria.
      c) It serves as a substrate for bacteria in utilizing ammonia.
   ii. **Lactitol** is similar to lactulose but has a less sweet taste (hence is less likely to cause aversion and noncompliance). It is as effective as lactulose but is not yet available in the United States.

f. **Lactulose and neomycin or metronidazole.** Since lactulose has no toxicity, it is usually preferred over neomycin or metronidazole. In some patients, the two types of drugs may be used concomitantly for further therapeutic benefit. As long as the stool pH remains less than 5, the antibiotic is not interfering with the action of lactulose. Thus the stool pH should be checked periodically to ensure that the addition of neomycin does not prevent bacterial action required to reduce lactulose to the active organic acids.

g. **Branched-chain amino acid (BCAA)**-enriched formulas. No consensus has been reached on whether the use of IV BCAA-enriched formulas leads to more rapid resolution of hepatic encephalopathy. The results of oral BCAA regimens have strongly suggested that this dietary strategy may be useful.

Since the cost of these formulations is very high, they may be reserved for patients in whom other measures have failed.

h. Zinc. Zinc deficiency has been suggested to play a role in hepatic encephalopathy, but few data are available to support this hypothesis. Zinc sulfate and zinc acetate supplementation have been studied in limited trials. Zinc histidine holds promise as a superior oral preparation to use in future trials.

i. Benzodiazepine receptor antagonists such as **flumazenil** (Romazicon) have been used in several trials. Sixty to seventy percent of patients improved after IV flumazenil administration. Larger trials are under way at this time.

j. Surgical considerations

i. Portosystemic shunts. Distal splenorenal shunts, portacaval H-graft shunts, mesocaval calibrated shunts, and TIPS have been successful in decompressing portal hypertension and ameliorating PSE. All of these special shunt procedures do not completely decompress the **preexisting portal hypertension and allow hepatic perfusion.**

ii. Liver transplantation. Intractable hepatic encephalopathy unmanageable by medical treatment is a clear indication for liver transplantation. Nontransplant surgical procedures, with the exception of TIPS, should be considered only for patients who are not transplant candidates.

iii. Other procedures. Patients with demonstrated large, spontaneous, or surgically created PSSs and intractable hepatic encephalopathy sometimes benefit from the **closure of the shunt**. This operation should be accompanied by additional procedures to prevent variceal bleeding. Shunt occlusion by radiologic techniques has been described. Duplex ultrasound may be used instead of angiography to identify patients with large spontaneous PSSs. Portosystemic shunts, especially end-to-side shunts and sometimes side-to-side shunts, can induce hepatic encephalopathy. **Colonic exclusion** has been used in selected patients for the management of severe post–PSS hepatic encephalopathy.

Selected Readings

Cirrhosis

Fellowfield JA, et al. Reversal of fibrosis: no longer a pipedream? *Clin Liver Dis.* 2006;10:481–497.

Friedman SL. Reversibility of hepatic fibrosis and cirrhosis. Is it all hype? *Nat Clin Pract Gastroenterol Hepatol.* 2007;4:236–237.

Groszman R, et al. Measurement of portal pressure: when, how, and why to do it. *Clin Liver Dis.* 2006;10:499–512.

Tripodi A, et al. Abnormalities of hemostasitis in chronic liver disease. Reappraisal of their clinical significance and need for clinical and laboratory research. *J Hepatol.* 2007;46:727–733.

Variceal Bleeding

Bosch J, et al. Prevention of variceal rebleeding. *Lancet.* 2003;361:952–954.

Corley DA, et al. Octreotide for acute esophageal variceal bleeding: A meta-analysis. *Gastroenterology.* 2001;120:946.

Fernandez J, et al. Norfloxactlin versus ceftriaxone in the prophylasix of infections in patients with advanced cirrhosis and hemorrhage. *Gastroenterology.* 2006;131:1049–1056.

Hegab AM, et al. Bleeding esophageal varices. *Postgrad Med.* 2001;109:75.

Lower C, et al. Pharmacologic therapy of portal hypertension. *Curr Gastroenterol Rep.* 2001;24.

Luketic VA, et al. Esophageal Varices I. Clinical presentation, medical therapy and endoscopic therapy. *Gastroenterol Clin North Am.* 2000;29:337.

Luketic VA, et al. Esophageal Varices II: Transjugular intrahepatic portosystemic shunt and surgical therapy. *Gastroenterol Clin North Am.* 2000;29:387.

Sarin SK, et al. Comparison of endoscopic ligation and propranolol for the primary prevention of variceal bleeding. *N Engl J Med.* 1999;340:988.

Hepatorenal Syndrome

Arroyo V, et al. Advances in the pathogenesis and treatment of type-1 and type-2 hepatorenal syndrome. *J Hepatol.* 2007;46(5):935–946.
Moreau R, et al. The use of vasoconstrictors in patients with cirrhosis: type 1 HRS. *Hepatology.* 2006;43(3):385–394.
Salerno F, et al. Diagnosis prevention and treatment of hepatorenal syndrome in cirrhosis. A consensus workshop of the international ascites club. *Gut.* 2007;56(9):1310–1318.
Wong F, et al. Midodrive, octreodde, albumin and TIPs in selected patients with cirrhosis and type 2 hepatorenal syndrome. *Hepatology.* 2004;40(1):55–64.

Hepatic Encephalopathy

Abon-Assi S, et al. Hepatic encephalopathy. *Postgrad Med.* 2001;109:52.
Ahboacha S, et al. Increased brain concentrations of endogenous (nonbenzodiazepine) GABA-A receptor lizards in human hepatic encephalopathy. *Metab Brain Dis.* 2004;19:241–251.
Feeney ER, et al. Hepatic encephalopathy. *Pract Gastroenterol.* 2001;25:45.
Huassinger D. Low grade hepatic encephalopathy in cirrhosis. *Hepatology.* 2006;43: 1187–1190.

Ascites and Spontaneous Bacterial Peritonitis

Fernandez J, et al. Primary prophylaxis of spontaneous bacterial peritonitis delays hepatorenal syndrome and improves survival in cirrhosis. *Gastroenterology.* 2007;133:818–824.
Gives P, et al. Transjular intrahepatic protosystemic shunting versus paracentesis plus albumin for refractory ascites in cirrhosis. *Gastroenterology.* 2002;123:1839–1847.
Moore KP, et al. The management of ascites in cirrhosis: report on the consensus conference of the international ascites club. *Hepatology.* 2003;38(1):258–266.
Zucker SD. Management of refractory ascites: Are TIPs or TAPs tops? *Gastroenterology.* 2001;120:311.

Nutrition

Als-Nielsen B, et al. Branched-chain aminoacids for hepatic encephalopathy Cochrane Database. *Syst Rev.* 2003;(2)CD 001939.
Als-Nielsen B, et al. Non-absorbable disaceharides for hepatic encephalopathy: systematic review of randomized trials. *Brit Med J.* 2004;324:1046.

Hepatocellular Carcinoma

Bruix J, et al. Management of hepatocellular carcinoma. *Hepatology.* 2005;42:1208–1236.
Bruix J, et al. Diagnosis of small HCC. *Gastroenterology.* 2005;129:1364.
Colli A, et al. Accuracy of ultrasonography, spiral CT, magnetic resonance and alphatoprotein in diagnosing a systematic review. *Am J Gastroenterol.* 2006;101(3):513–523.
Ioannou GN, et al. Incidence and predictors of hepatocellular carcinoma in patients with cirrhosis. *Clin Gastroenterol Hepatol.* 2007;5(8):938–945.
Llover JM, et al. Resection and liver transplantation for hepatocellular carcinoma. *Semin Liver Dis.* 2005;25:181–200.
Lopez PM, et al. Systematic review: evidence based management of hepatocellular carcinoma—an updated analysis of randomized controlled trials. *Aliment Parmacol Ther.* 2006;23:1537–1547.

I. LIVER TUMORS. The liver filters both arterial and portal venous blood and thus is a major site for the spread of metastatic cancers, particularly those that originate in the abdomen. Metastatic liver tumors can develop after the primary tumor has been identified, or patients can present initially with the signs and symptoms of metastatic liver disease. Common primary tumors that metastasize to the liver are colon, pancreas, stomach, breast, lung, gallbladder, and bile duct tumors, and lymphoma.

The most common primary liver cancer is hepatoma, or hepatocellular carcinoma (HCC). HCC often is a consequence of cirrhosis. Worldwide, chronic hepatitis B and C are major causes of HCC. Other primary liver malignancies are fibrolamellar carcinoma and cholangiohepatocellular carcinoma and sarcoma, including angiosarcoma, leiomyosarcoma, fibrosarcoma, and mesenchymal sarcoma.

Benign tumors of the liver include hepatic hemangioma, adenoma, focal nodular hyperplasia, and focal regenerative hyperplasia.

A. Clinical presentation

    1. History. Primary hepatoma often occurs in the setting of established cirrhosis of any cause. In fact, abrupt deterioration of a patient with known cirrhosis is a signal to consider the possibility of HCC. Other pathogenic antecedents of HCC include hepatitis C virus, chronic hepatitis B virus infection (HBV) with or without cirrhosis, exposure to aflatoxins in food (implicated in parts of Africa and Asia), and exposure in the distant past to thorium dioxide, a radiologic contrast material, nonalcoholic steatohepatitis (NASH) associated with obesity and diabetes mellitus. Uncommon consequences of HCC include fever of unknown origin, portal vein thrombosis, hypoglycemia, polycythemia, hypercalcemia, porphyria, and dysglobulinemia.

        The incidence of HCC has doubled in the United States for the past 20 years and continues to increase due to HCV- and HBV-related complications and NASH-related cirrhosis.

        The mean age at the time of diagnosis of HCC in the United States is 65 years. Seventy-four percent of cases occur in men. In patients younger than 40 years of age who present with liver cancer, only a third are HCC; others include fibrolamellar carcinoma, which has a much better prognosis, and metastatic cancer.

        In patients with metastatic liver cancer, the primary lesion may not be known. Thus the initial presentation may be due to the metastatic disease to the liver. About half of the patients who die from malignant disease have metastases in the liver at postmortem examination.

        Abdominal pain is a common complaint of patients with primary HCC or metastatic liver disease. Some patients have nonspecific complaints, such as anorexia, weight loss, and malaise.

    2. Physical examination. The liver typically is enlarged and nodular and may be tender. Ascites often has developed. A friction rub heard over the liver with respiration indicates involvement of the liver capsule. Rarely, a bruit is heard, reflecting the vascular nature of most HCC and some metastatic tumors. Jaundice usually develops later in the course of both HCC and metastatic liver disease. If jaundice is present initially, it means that preexisting liver disease is present, the tumor involves much of the liver parenchyma, or a large bile duct is obstructed.

455

B. Diagnostic studies

1. **Laboratory studies.** Anemia is common in patients with liver cancer. It may be the nonspecific anemia of chronic disease or the macrocytic anemia associated with a chronic liver disorder. Bilirubin is elevated for the same reasons that the patient may be jaundiced (see section I.A.2). Elevation of alkaline phosphatase is common simply because obstruction of even the small biliary radicals causes generation and release of this enzyme. If the source of an elevated alkaline phosphatase level is in question, a 59-nucleotidase elevation will confirm its origin in the liver. Often mild elevations of aspartate aminotransferase (AST) and alanine aminotransferase (ALT) occur.

   The serum alpha-fetoprotein concentration is elevated in about half of the patients with hepatoma in the United States; thus, the measurement is useful in helping make the diagnosis. However, some patients with gonadal malignancies and metastatic disease to the liver also have elevated serum alpha-fetoprotein.

2. **Radiologic studies** include ultrasound, computed tomography (CT), magnetic resonance imaging (MRI), dimethylphenylcarbamylmethyliminiodiacetic acid (HIDA) scan, and sulfur colloid liver scan.

   Many physicians proceed immediately to CT in the evaluation of liver tumors after the initial blood chemistry studies have been done. The CT scan has the advantage of not only providing accurate information about the liver but also identifying enlarged lymph nodes and other abnormalities of the abdominal organs. Furthermore, a CT-guided needle biopsy of a liver lesion or other abdominal mass may provide important diagnostic information.

3. **Liver biopsy.** Percutaneous liver biopsy is diagnostic of liver cancer in about 80% of patients in whom alkaline phosphatase is elevated due to intrahepatic cancer. Biopsy of the liver under direct laparoscopic vision is an alternative to percutaneous liver biopsy. Laparoscopy also can assess the spread of tumor to the peritoneum, lymph nodes, and other abdominal organs.

4. **Angiography.** Celiac axis angiography can determine operability in a patient with a HCC or with a solitary metastatic lesion to the liver. If the CT scan suggests tumor in both lobes of the liver, arteriography is not indicated. An arteriogram is helpful in differentiating a benign hemangioma from a malignant tumor when the CT scan suggests a vascular lesion.

C. Natural history and treatment. Survival of patients diagnosed with HCC remains very poor. Survival is related to tumor size, liver function, and the receipt of effective and potentially curative treatment (resection or orthotopic liver transplantation [OLT]). In recent years, living-donor partial liver transplantation (LT) has made transplantation more available for this indication. Five-year survival rates after OLT may be as high as 70% for a Child class A patient with one tumor less than 2 to 5 cm in diameter. Patients with intermediate to advanced HCC tend to have uniformly poor prognosis.

1. **Surgical resection** is possible only for a small number of patients. Tumor spread, poor liver function, and the presence of portal hypertension preclude patients for surgery. Even with resectable tumors, there is a high recurrence rate. This increases with large tumors, those with vascular invasion, and those with poor differentiation. Well-differentiated and encapsulated HCC especially less than 3 cm in size has been associated with lower recurrence rates after resection.

2. **Liver transplantation (OLT or living-donor partial LF)** may be offered to patients with HCC. The eligibility criteria include solitary tumors less than 5 cm or up to three tumors each less than 3 cm. Recurrence is much lower than that of resection if these criteria are used.

3. **Local ablation** using US- or CT-guided percutaneous ethanol injection (PEI) or radiofrequency ablation have become established modes of therapy for patients with HCC with no significant coagulopathy or ascites. For patients with a single tumor less than 3 cm, HCC recurrence-free survival is similar to that surgical resection.

4. **Palliative therapy** is used for patients not suitable for potentially curative therapy. Unfortunately, several studies have confirmed no survival benefit with

treatments of 5-fluorouracil, tamoxifen, or PEI. Transarterial chemoembolization (TACE) was found to have a small, but significant benefit in prolonging survival.

II. BILIARY TUMORS.
Biliary tumors include those that arise in the gallbladder and in the intra- and extrahepatic biliary system. Benign tumors are rare and include papilloma, leiomyoma, lipoma, myxoma, and fibroma. On the other hand, adenocarcinomas of the **gallbladder** and **bile ducts (cholangiocarcinomas)** are not rare, accounting for about 5% of all malignancies.

A. Carcinoma of the gallbladder (CG)

1. **Epidemiology.** CG is extremely rare in the United States. However, CG is the most common gastrointestinal malignancy in the Native Americans living in the Southwest and in Mexican Americans. The incidence is highest in Chile and Bolivia. The risk is higher in women and in the elderly. If it is diagnosed early or incidentally on routine cholecystectomy for gallstone disease, the prognosis is very good. Incidental CG is noted in 1% to 3% of cholecystectomy specimens.

2. **Risk factors** for CG include gallstones, chronic cholecystitis, and porcelain gallbladder. Adenomatous polyps of the gallbladder may progress to cancer. Polyps smaller than 1 cm seldom undergo malignant change. Other risk factors for CG include congenital biliary cysts, anomalous drainage of the pancreatic duct to the common bile duct (CBD), and chronic infection of the gallbladder with *Salmonella*.

   CG associated with gallstones are most commonly seen with large gallstones (>2.5 cm) and in patients with long duration of gallstone disease. Use of certain drugs (i.e. isoniazid, methyldopa, and oral contraceptive) may also be associated with CG.

3. **Clinical picture.** Most patients with CG may present with symptoms of gallstone disease (i.e., right upper quadrant pain, malaise, anorexia, nausea, vomiting, weight loss, and jaundice). Unfortunately, most patients at the time of diagnosis have tumors that have invaded adjacent organs and lymph nodes and may even have distant metastases. The 5-year survival for such patients is usually less than 5%.

4. **Diagnosis** is usually obtained by imaging techniques including abdominal US, CT, MRI (magnetic resonance imaging), and MRCP (magnetic resonance cholangiopancreatography). Tumor markers such as CEA and CA-19-9 are not helpful.

5. **Prognosis and treatment.** Prognosis depends on the stage of CG. If the CG is thought to be a T_1 lesion, surgical resection (i.e., simple cholecystectomy) may be sufficient. Advanced cases may require radical resection. Postoperative radiation and chemotherapy may reduce rates of recurrence.

B. Cholangiocarcinoma (CGC)

1. **Epidemiology.** CGC arises from the epithelium of the intra- or extrahepatic biliary ductular system. It is less common than HCC and tends to occur at an older age than HCC. The incidence is similar in both men and women.

2. **Risk factors** of CGC include primary sclerosing cholangitis (PSC), ulcerative colitis, inflammatory bowel disease (IBD), choledochal cysts, biliary ductal ectasia (Caroli's disease), intrahepatic gallstones, biliary duct infections (chronic cholangitis), infections with *Clonorchis sinensis* and *Opisthorchis viverrini*, multiple biliary papillomatosis, bile duct adenoma, and exposure to thorotrast (contrast agent used in the past for radiologic imaging).

3. **Clinical features** depend on whether CGC is central or peripheral.
   a. **Central CGC** arises in major bile ducts and is often associated with chronic inflammation of the bile ducts (i.e., with PSC). **Klatskin tumor** arises in the bifurcation of the CBC. Central CGC is often present with obstructive jaundice.
   b. **Peripheral CGC** is rarely associated with PSC or cirrhosis. It often presents with weight loss and abdominal pain.
   c. **Mixed HCC and CGC** may be found in association with cirrhosis.

4. **Diagnosis.** Abnormal laboratory tests include elevated levels of alkaline phosphatase, bilirubin, 5′nucleotidase, γ-glutamyltransferase, and serum CA19-9 above 100 mm/mL.

Central tumors may be more difficult to diagnose. Cytologic and histologic examination of tissue obtained from endoscopic brushing and biopsy during ERCP as well as direct cholangioscopy may help make the diagnosis.

Peripheral tumors may be amenable to needle biopsy during CT or MRCP.

5. Treatment. Peripheral and central CGC may be resectable when the tumor is small; however, the recurrence rate after surgical resection is high and survival is poor. Liver transplantation is not a viable alternative for treatment of HCC due to high posttransplant recurrence rates. Radiation and chemotherapy may provide symptomatic relief. Placement of stents in the obstructive ducts during ERCP may be palliative.

Selected Readings

Bruix J, et al. Management of hepatocellular carcinoma. *Hepatology*. 2006;42:1202–1236.

Case Records of the Massachusetts General Hospital (Case 13-2006). A man with bone mass and lesions in the liver. *N Engl J Med*. 2006;354:1828–1837.

Colli A, et al. Accuracy of ultrasonography, spiral CT, magnetic resonance and alfa-etoprotein diagnosing hepatocellular carcinoma. A systematic review. *Am J Gastroenterol*. 2006; 101:513–523.

deGroen PC. Cholangiocarcinoma: Making the diagnosis. *Clin Perspect Gastroenterol*. 2001;4:77–89.

DeVreede T, et al. Prolonged disease five-year survival after orthotopic liver transplantation plus adjuvant chemo-irradiation for cholangiocarcinoma. *Liver Transplant*. 2000;6:399.

DiBisceylia AM. Liver tumors. *Clin Liver Dis*. 2001;5:1–286.

Geahigan TA. Primary hepatic lymphoma: A case report and discussion. *Pract Gastroenterol*. 2001;25:58.

Heimbach JK, et al. Liver transplantation for perihilar cholangiocarcinoma after aggressive neoadjuvant therapy: a new paradigm for liver and biliary malignancies? *Surgery*. 2006;140:331–334.

Koslin DB. Hepatocellular carcinoma. *Rev Gastroenterol Disord*. 2001;1:58.

Larsson SC. Coffee consumption and risk of liver cancer: A metaanalysis. *Gastroenterology*. 2007 May;132:1740–1745.

Llover JM, et al. Resection and liver transplantation for hepatocellular carcinoma. *Seminar Liver Dis*. 2005;25:181–200.

Llovert JM, et al. Hepatocellular carcinoma. *Lancet*. 2003;362:1907–1917.

Lopez PM, et al. Systematic review: evidence based management of hepatocelluar carcinoma—an updated analysis of randomized controlled trials. *Ailment Pharmacol Ther*. 2006;23:1537–1547.

Rea DJ, et al. Liver transplantation with neoadjuvant chemoradiation is more effective than resection for hilar cholangiocarcinoma. *Ann Surg*. 2005;242:451–461.

Sheth S, et al. Primary gallbladder cancer: Recognition of risk factors and the role of prophylactic cholecystectomy. *Am J Gastroenterol*. 2000;95(6):1402–1409.

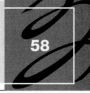
*L*iver transplantation is an effective and accepted therapy for a variety of chronic, irreversible liver diseases for which no other therapy has proved to be satisfactory. The liver can be transplanted as an extra (auxiliary) organ at another site (Fig. 58-1) or in the orthotopic location after the removal of the host liver (Figs. 58-2 and 58-3). The discussions of this chapter mainly concern the orthotopic liver transplantation (OLT).

Split liver and living-donor liver transplantation has become available and successful. Although the number of patients requiring OLT continues to grow steadily, the number of available donors remains unchanged. Fifteen percent to 20% of patients awaiting liver transplantation die prior to receiving an organ. Currently the majority of patients wait 6 to 24 months for OLT. Although the number of patients requiring OLT continues to grow steadily the number of available organ donors remains unchanged. The referring physician faces three important questions regarding liver transplantation: first, candidacy (patient selection); second, appropriate timing for referral; and third, follow-up care of patients returning from a successful operation.

I. **GENERAL INFORMATION. The American Liver Foundation** estimates that in the United States at any one time as many as 5,000 people with end-stage liver disease could benefit from liver transplantation. The two major factors limiting the number of liver transplantations performed are the **availability of suitable donor organs** and the fact that donor livers are recovered from only about 25% of potential donors.

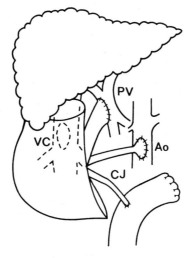

Figure 58-1. Anastomoses in auxiliary partial liver transplantation. VC, inferior vena cava; PV, portal vein; AO, aorta; CJ, choledochojejunostomy. (From Terpstra OT, et al. Auxiliary partial liver transplantation for end-stage chronic liver disease. *N Engl J Med.* 1988;319:1507. Reprinted with permission. Copyright © 1988 Massachusetts Medical Society. All rights reserved.)

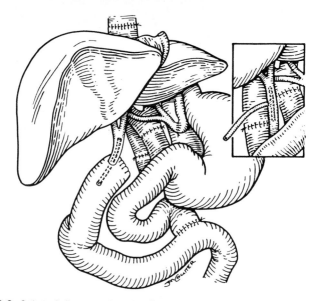

Figure 58-2. Orthotopic liver transplantation. Biliary reconstruction can be accomplished through choledochojejunostomy or duct-to-duct anastomosis (*inset*). (From Starzl TE. Liver transplantation, II. *N Engl J Med.* 1989;321:1092. Reprinted with permission. Copyright © 1989 Massachusetts Medical Society. All rights reserved.)

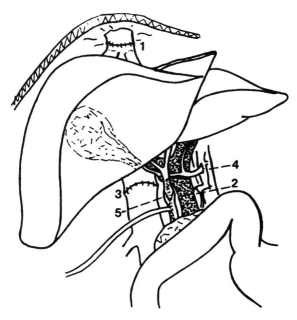

Figure 58-3. Diagram of appearance after orthotopic liver transplantation. Sequence of anastomoses is as follows: upper vena caval anastomosis above the liver (1), lower vena caval anastomosis beneath the liver (3), end-to-side hepatic artery anastomosis (4), portal vein anastomosis (2), and common bile duct anastomosis over a T tube (5). (From Krom RAF. Liver transplantation at the Mayo Clinic. *Mayo Clin Proc.* 1986;61:278–282. Reprinted with permission.)

The second factor is due partly to inadequate **identification** of potential organ donors by physicians. Members of the medical community, especially physicians dealing with patients who may require transplantation (internists, nephrologists, gastroenterologists, cardiologists), must begin to increase their own and their patients' awareness of the need for donor organs.

In an attempt to increase the number of organ donors, 27 states have passed legislation for required request. This legislation obligates hospitals to have policies in place to offer organ donation as an option to families of patients dying in that hospital. These laws are designed to relieve the attending physician of the burden of requesting organ donation from grieving families by making the request for organ donation part of the routine hospital policy.

Many patients do not receive a liver transplant because they are never referred to a transplantation center. Other patients are referred only after their liver disease has reached its terminal stage, and they often die before a suitable donor organ can be found. To allow all appropriate patients the opportunity to undergo liver transplantation and survive the procedure, physicians must be aware of the criteria for candidacy and for timing of the referral.

There are more than 30 active centers in which liver transplant operations are performed in the United States. For the success of this procedure, centers must maintain high standards and achieve and maintain acceptable 1- and 5-year survival rates. Centers performing fewer than 10 liver transplantations each year are unlikely to maintain the necessary expertise for optimal management of patients with this extremely complex disease. Currently 1-year survival rates range from 80% to 95% and 5-year survival rates are 80% to 85%. The dramatic increase in the survival rates results from the following factors:

A. Advances in standardization and refinement of the transplantation procedure.

B. Expertise of anesthesiologists in the prevention and treatment of the metabolic abnormalities that occur in patients with end-stage liver disease during the transplantation procedure.

C. Use of the venovenous bypass system, which ensures venous return to the heart from both the portal and systemic venous systems during the hepatic phase of the transplantation procedure, reduces blood loss, decreases the incidence of postoperative renal failure, and generally results in less hemodynamic instability during the procedure.

D. Improved techniques for the identification and support of potential organ donors.

E. Refinement of operative techniques for the recovery and preservation of the donor livers.

F. Use of more effective and less toxic immunosuppressive regimens. It is important to remember that successful liver transplantation does not return a patient to normal. Rather, a new disease, a "transplanted liver," replaces the former disease. However, this new state allows patients a chance for both long-term survival and a more normal lifestyle than were possible during the late stages of their liver disease. After liver transplantation, patients must take immunosuppressive medications for the remainder of their lives. Discontinuation of the prescribed medications may lead to rejection and rapid deterioration in the patient's condition.

II. CANDIDACY (PATIENT SELECTION). In the past, patients were referred for liver transplantation only after their disease had reached its end stage. For best results, however, earlier referral to a transplantation center is desirable for all appropriate patients. Because of the variable course of many liver diseases, the determination of the most appropriate time for referral of any patient for transplantation is difficult.

A. Criteria. There are three general criteria used in most transplantation centers. These are as follows:

   1. The unavailability of other surgical or medical therapies that offer the patient an opportunity for long-term survival.

   2. Absence of complications of chronic liver disease that may significantly increase the patient's operative risk or lead to the development of absolute or relative contraindications to transplantation.

3. Understanding by the patient and family of the physical and psychological consequences of the transplantation procedure including the risks, potential benefits, and costs.
B. Indications. The indications for liver transplantation have been expanding. Currently the indications can best be grouped into four major categories of liver disease:
    1. Chronic irreversible advanced liver disease of any cause
    2. Nonmetastatic hepatic malignancies
    3. Fulminant hepatic failure
    4. Inborn errors of metabolism
        Table 58-1 summarizes the indications for liver transplantation used in most transplant centers. More than 60 distinct diseases have been treated with liver transplantation. In adults, the most common diagnoses have been fulminant hepatic failure, chronic active hepatitis, cryptogenic cirrhosis, primary biliary cirrhosis, alcoholic cirrhosis, and inborn errors of metabolism. In pediatric patients, biliary atresia and inborn errors of metabolism are the most common indications (Table 58-2).
C. OLT for specific disease indications
    1. Hepatitis C virus (HCV)-induced cirrhosis is the most common indication for OLT in adults, accounting for 40% to 60% of OLTs in some centers. The overall 3- to 5-year survival rate after OLT for HCV cirrhosis is 80% to 85%.

 TABLE 58-1   **Indications for Liver Transplantation**

Adults	Children
Primary biliary cirrhosis	Biliary atresia
Sclerosing cholangitis	Inborn errors of metabolism (see Table 58-2)
Fulminant liver failure	Acute liver failure (viral, toxic, metabolic)
Hepatitis (viral, drug, or toxin induced)	Reye's syndrome
Metabolic liver diseases	Neonatal hepatitis
Alcoholic liver disease	Chronic hepatitis
Postnecrotic cirrhosis	Cryptogenic cirrhosis
Secondary biliary cirrhosis	Familial cholestasis
Autoimmune liver disease	Arterial thrombosis
Hepatic traumas	Benign or malignant hepatic tumors
Polycystic liver	Rejection
Budd-Chiari syndrome	
Venoocclusive disease	
Liver tumors (benign, malignant, metastatic)	
Primary nonfunction	
Rejection	

 TABLE 58-2   **Inborn Errors of Metabolism Treated with Liver Transplantation**

Cystic fibrosis	Erythropoietic protoporphyria
Alpha-1 antitrypsin deficiency	Crigler-Najjar syndrome type I
Wilson's disease	Urea-cycle enzyme deficiencies
Type I and type IV glycogen storage disease	Type I hyperoxaluria
	Hemophilia A and B
Niemann-Pick disease	Homozygous type II hyperlipoproteinemia
Tyrosinemia	Protein C deficiency

Prognosis after OLT may be affected by comorbid conditions including renal insufficiency, cryoglobulinemia, and hepatocellular carcinoma (HCC).

There is no effective antiviral regimen to prevent recurrence of HCV in allograft. Fortunately, reinfection rarely (5%–10% of patients) leads to graft failure within the first 3 to 5 years after OLT, but survival rates are lower than in patients with OLT for other causes of cirrhosis in seven or more years after OLT. Cirrhosis occurs in 10% to 30% of patients post-OLT. HCV recurrence in the allograft may be treated by reduction of immunosuppression antiviral therapy or both. Retransplantation for patients with graft failure due to HCV recurrence is controversial and is associated with poor survival (40% 1-year survival).

2. **Hepatitis B virus (HBV)-induced cirrhosis** is also a common indication for OLT; however, HBV also recurs in the allograft.

3. **Alcoholic cirrhosis/liver disease.** Strict selection of criteria is necessary to identify appropriate patients for OLT. A period of >6 months of sobriety is usually required, but this factor alone is not sufficient for post-OLT recidivism. Many of these patients present with multiple organ systems' dysfunction and severe malnutrition that requires aggressive preoperative management. Also, other coexistent liver diseases need to be identified (i.e., hemochromatosis, alpha-1-antitrypsin deficiency, viral hepatitis [B, D, C], and ACC). The 5-year survival of patients with alcoholic cirrhosis post-OLT is similar to other patients who undergo OLT for other indications.

4. **Liver tumors.** OLT may be indicated for patients with liver tumors who are unable to undergo surgical resection either due to the anatomic location of the tumor or due to the severity of the underlying liver disease (cirrhosis).

Tumors of the liver for which OLT should be considered are HCC, fibrolamellar HCC, epithelioid hemangioendothelioma, hepatoblastoma, and metastatic neuroendocrine tumors.

For HCC, OLT may be offered if the tumor is confined to the liver, documented by imaging (CT or MRI); if the tumor is single (<5 cm) and/or there are fewer than three tumors, each <3 cm in diameter; there is no invasion or thrombosis of the portal vein; and there is no lymph node involvement. For patients fulfilling these criteria, the 5-year survival may approach that of patients who undergo OLT for other causes.

5. **Cholestatic liver diseases.** In children, OLT is performed for patients with biliary atresia and Alagille syndrome. In adults, OLT is performed for primary biliary cirrhosis (PBC) and primary sclerotic cholangitis (PSC). A risk score for PBC has been formulated based on patients' serum bilirubin, albumin, prothrombintre, presence of edema, and variceal bleeding. Patients should be referred for OLT when the lirubin is >10 mg/dL. Posttransplant recurrence of PBC is rare. Patients' 5-year survival is 80% to 85%.

For PSC, a similar criteria as for PBC has been formulated for OLT and provides more accurate prognostic information. Patients with PSC should be referred for OLT when serum bilirubin is >10 mg/dL. In a small number of patients, PSC may recur in the allograft.

6. **Fulminant hepatic failure (FHF).** OLT may be lifesaving in patients with FHF (see Chapter 17). Early referral to a transplant center is necessary to ensure a good outcome. Death of patients with FHF is usually due to late referral and/or inability to find an appropriate donor within the necessary timeframe. Five-year survival of patients with FHF is in the range of 70% to 80%.

D. **Contraindications.** Absolute and relative contraindications to liver transplantation include the conditions listed in Table 58-3. The absolute contraindications are conditions that would result in a prohibitively high mortality risk after transplant surgery.

A number of diseases for which transplantation might have been precluded 5 or 10 years ago are no longer absolute contraindications to the procedure. An upper age limit has been eliminated because recipients over 50 years of age have a 5-year survival after transplantation similar to that of younger adults. Also, liver transplantation in very young infants and even newborns has become common, although the results are better with older children.

TABLE 58-3	Contraindications to Liver Transplantation

Absolute contraindications
  Extrahepatic malignancy
  Advanced cardiopulmonary disease
  Acquired immunodeficiency syndrome (AIDS)
  Active substance abuse
  Other organ system failure not curable with hepatic transplantation
Relative contraindications
  Active sepsis outside the hepatobiliary tract
  Renal insufficiency/failure
  Advanced protein-calorie malnutrition
  Portal vein thrombosis
  Operative procedures, such as end-to-side portacaval shunt or complex hepatobiliary surgery
  Previous extrahepatic malignancies

Preoperative diagnosis by advanced imaging techniques and intrasurgical use of vein grafts have made it possible for patients with extensive thromboses of the portal, mesenteric, or splenic veins to be candidates for liver transplantation. The routine use of imaging techniques to measure the size of the liver and determine the state of the host vessels helps identify these patients in advance so that appropriate plans can be made.

Previous upper abdominal surgery, especially splenectomy and portosystemic shunts, that may affect the portal vein reconstruction during transplantation previously were considered absolute contraindications. With the advanced surgical techniques used today, however, many of these patients, especially those with mesocaval and distal splenorenal shunts, have had successful transplantations.

Primary liver malignancy is still a relative contraindication for liver transplantation. Hepatocellular carcinoma other than fibrolamellar hepatoma has a recurrence rate of approximately 80% at 1 year after transplantation. Because of this high recurrence rate, most centers do not recommend liver transplantation for patients with large or advanced hepatocellular malignancy.

Transplantation in patients with fulminant hepatic failure secondary to drugs or viral hepatitis provides good results if the patient receives the transplant before the onset of major systemic complications. Stage IV hepatic coma in adult patients is a relative contraindication to transplantation. Referral before development of this level of coma and other complications (see Chapter 56) is the key to successful transplantation in this group of critically ill patients. Most patients with fulminant hepatic failure should be transferred to a transplantation center once the diagnosis is established. With worsening of the patient's condition (increasing coagulopathy and encephalopathy), the patient should be placed on the center's active transplantation list at the highest possible status.

Before the availability of HIV antibody testing, a group of patients who received liver transplants were subsequently found to be HIV positive. The AIDS-related mortality in this group was 37% in a 6-year follow-up period. The most commonly accepted policy in the United States is to screen all recipients for HIV, but not to exclude transplantation because of a positive test.

III. EVALUATION

A. Goals. Once the attending physician identifies a patient as a potential candidate for liver transplantation, he or she refers the patient to a transplant center where the patient undergoes a thorough evaluation to satisfy four specific goals:

1. The establishment of a specific diagnosis

2. Documentation of the severity of the disease

3. Identification of all complications of the disease or concomitant diseases that might adversely affect the patient's survival
4. Estimation of the long-term prognosis of the disease with or without orthotopic liver transplantation

B. Criteria for organ donation include confirmation of
1. Consent signed by family
2. Brain death of the donor
3. Absence of systemic diseases, including HIV, HBV, HCV, bacterial and fungal infection, and neoplasia
4. Presence of normal or near-normal liver tests
5. Absence of incorrectable coagulopathy and disseminated intravascular coagulopathy (DIC)
6. Liver size and blood-type compatibility
   The donor factors associated with poor graft function include steatosis (>30% fat), prolonged cold preservation time (>12 hours), and initial poor function of graft after transplantation.

C. Criteria for OLT recipient. The following criteria (score) are used to determine a patient's candidacy for OLT: **Model for end-stage liver disease (MELD)** and **pediatric end-stage liver disease (PELD).**
   MELD uses readily available tests to predict mortality risk: 3.8 log (bilirubin) + 11.2 log (INR) + 9.6 log (Creative) + 6.4. MELD scores range from 6 to 40. MELD has been validated as a predictor of mortality in adult patients with end-stage liver disease.

D. Testing. The routine evaluation process involves a number of laboratory tests and imaging studies. Additional studies are tailored to the individual patient after a thorough review of the patient's records from the referring physician. All patients undergo Doppler ultrasonography of the portal venous system to measure portal vein flow and to confirm its patency. Adult patients also undergo pulmonary function testing and electrocardiography. In patients suspected of having coronary artery or valvular disease, a stress test or coronary angiography may be required. In addition, patients with significant nutritional deficiencies are identified and treated with an intensive program of nutritional support while they are awaiting a donor liver.

   Patients are also evaluated by a psychiatrist, a social worker, and a hospital finance officer. The social worker ensures that all appropriate arrangements have been made to allow the patient to return to the transplantation center when a suitable donor liver is located.

   After completion of the evaluation process, each patient's situation is discussed by a transplantation committee, and he or she is placed into one of four categories:
1. Active candidate
2. Active candidate pending additional evaluation
3. Inactive candidate (liver disease not far enough advanced for transplantation)
4. Unacceptable candidate for transplantation. In addition, a decision is made regarding the urgency of the need for transplantation.
   Once accepted as an active candidate for liver transplantation, the patient is placed on the active transplantation list. The waiting period varies widely among transplantation centers. When a potential liver donor is identified and located, all suitable candidates on the active list are reviewed by the transplantation committee and priority is given to the patient with the most urgent need. The chosen recipient is admitted to the transplant hospital on an emergency basis and is surgically prepared to receive the donor organ. The recipient operation is precisely timed with the donor liver procurement procedure, and the donor and recipient operating teams maintain close communication regarding the progress of the two operative procedures. If the two procedures are performed at different sites, the donor liver is preserved and transported to the recipient team under cold ischemia conditions within 6 to 20 hours of procurement.

IV. OPERATIVE PROCEDURE

A. Technical (procedure-related) complications. The abdominal wall incision used by most transplant surgeons is a bilateral subcostal incision that is extended in the upper midline. The xiphoid process is excised. Complications of these incisions include infections, hernias, and granulomas of the fascial sutures, which may occur as late as several years after transplantation. In addition to the abdominal incisions, adult patients also have cutdowns performed in the groin and axilla to accommodate the venovenous bypass system (placed in the axillary and saphenous veins) (Fig. 58-4). In addition to wound infections, **lymphoceles** are a frequent complication in these sites. Lymphoceles may require repeated aspirations or the placement of drains to allow complete resolution.

The four vascular anastomoses established in the transplantation procedure involve the suprahepatic inferior vena cava, infrahepatic inferior vena cava, portal vein, and hepatic artery. Complications related to these anastomoses usually present in the early postoperative period but may occur as late as several months to years after transplantation. These complications include **bleeding, thrombosis, stenosis, infection,** and **pseudoaneurysm formation.** Postoperative anastomotic bleeding requires reoperation in the immediately postoperative period and has been associated with a higher early mortality. Arterial thrombosis is the most frequent vascular complication in the early postoperative period and usually requires immediate retransplantation. Thrombosis of the portal vein or inferior vena cava is rare.

The biliary system of the recipient is reconstructed in one of two ways (see Fig. 58-4). If the patient has no intrinsic disease of the bile duct, a duct-to-duct

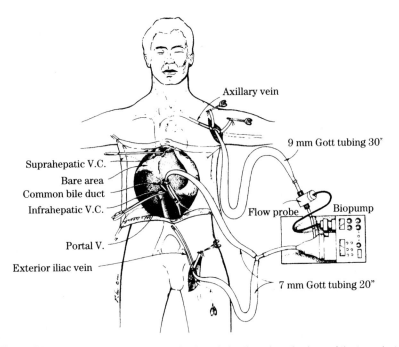

Figure 58-4. Venovenous bypass system in place during the anhepatic phase of the transplant procedure. Venous blood from the femoral and portal veins is returned to the heart via the axillary vein. (From Griffith BP, et al. Venovenous bypass without systemic anticoagulation for transplantation of the human liver. *Surg Gynecol Obstet.* 1985;160:270. Reprinted with permission.)

anastomosis (choledochocholedochostomy) is performed over a T tube usually brought out through the recipient's native bile duct. The T tube is left on dependent drainage until the patient's total bilirubin level falls below 4 mg/dL. The tube is then clamped; it is usually removed as an outpatient procedure approximately 3 months later. Even after this prolonged period of clamping, T-tube removal may result in either bile peritonitis or a localized bile collection.

In the recent years, T tubes are not being used in OLT. Primary areas to miosis are being constructed to avoid possible bile ductular complications.

In patients in whom the native bile duct is diseased or judged too small to accommodate a T tube, the donor bile duct is anastomosed end-to-side to a Roux-en-Y limb of jejunum (choledochojejunostomy). The Roux-en-Y reconstruction drains all bile internally. A localized bile collection is usually amenable to percutaneous drainage, but bile peritonitis requires operative repair of the leaking common bile duct.

The **biliary reconstruction** is a frequent cause of early and late postoperative complications. Complications related to either type of biliary reconstruction are **leak, stricture, infection,** and **formation of gallstones or sludge.** Any patient who is noted to have laboratory evidence of liver dysfunction unrelated to a rejection episode or who has episodes of cholangitis during the first several months to years after liver transplantation should be evaluated radiologically or endoscopically (e.g., ERCP) to ascertain biliary patency and function. If the problem cannot be resolved percutaneously or endoscopically, operative reconstruction of the biliary tract may be required, often including the conversion of a choledochocholedochostomy to a Roux-en-Y choledochojejunostomy.

B. Perioperative graft failure. If a transplanted liver fails to function, the only recourse is retransplantation to prevent complications of fulminant hepatic failure before cerebral edema and brainstem herniation occur. Graft injury can allow short-term survival, but retransplantation or death remains the end point. Currently, the rate of retransplantation in the first 3 postoperative months is 10% to 20%. There are four general reasons for graft failure:

1. A technically imperfect operation
2. Unrecognized liver disease in the donor liver
3. An ischemic injury to the graft
4. Accelerated rejection

Obvious technical complications account for less than 10% of the primary graft failures in adults but 30% of those in infants and children. The risk in infants is inversely related to the patient's size, and complications are mainly attributable to vascular thromboses.

Portal vein thrombosis is rare and usually occurs only when the recipient's splanchnic venous bed has been altered by a portosystemic shunt, a splenectomy, or another operation. Early portal vein thrombosis usually requires retransplantation, but a few patients have been saved by immediate or delayed secondary reconstruction of the portal vein.

Thrombosis of the hepatic artery may be asymptomatic in 20% to 30% of instances, and the diagnosis can be made only with the routine use of Doppler ultrasonography. The complications that can result are serious; they include failure of the primary graft to function, hepatic infarction, bacteremia, abscess, rupture of the dearterialized ducts resulting in bile peritonitis orbile leakage and the formation of biloma within the graft parenchyma.

Later, these biliary duct lesions may form multiple intrahepatic biliary strictures that resemble sclerosing cholangitis. Although secondary rearterialization has been attempted, retransplantation is usually the only alternative.

The most common cause of postoperative graft dysfunction is **ischemic injury** to the donor liver, which may occur during the death of the donor, the procurement operation, or the period of refrigeration. The preservation solution, which is infused through the portal vein or hepatic artery, allows the safe cold storage of donor livers for at least 24 hours. The restoration of clotting function and the absence of lactic acidosis are also important predictors of success of the transplanted liver. Measurements of blood amino acid clearance and other products of intermediary metabolism have been used to distinguish between patients in whom the new liver is expected to recover and those in whom it is not.

Host immune factors and hyperacute rejection may result in primary failure of the liver graft. Compared to other transplanted organs such as kidney and heart, the human liver seems to be more resistant to antibody-mediated injury. Because of this resistance, liver transplantation is often performed in spite of major blood-group incompatibilities. However, a progressive and severe coagulopathy that develops shortly after hepatic revascularization should arouse suspicion of an accelerated rejection.

C. Nontechnical complications

1. **Hypertension** is almost universally present in a transplant recipient, especially in the early postoperative period, and requires aggressive treatment. The cause of the hypertension is probably multifactorial and includes the use of cyclosporine. Blood pressure control often requires at least two antihypertensive medications, usually a vasodilator and a beta-blocker. In addition, patients need diuretics both for blood pressure control and to relieve the ascites that usually develops after transplantation. Hypertension is usually less severe after the first 6 months after transplantation, and many patients require no antihypertensive medications by 1 year after the procedure.

2. **Infection.** Serious bacterial, viral, and fungal infections may occur in "routine" liver transplantation patients up to several years after the transplant operation. However, infectious complications are much more common in patients who require multiple reoperations or who have poor initial function of the transplanted liver. Therefore, **fever** in any posttransplant patient requires a thorough investigation to rule out infection. The initial workup of fever should begin with a detailed history and physical examination and appropriate cultures of blood, urine, and sputum. Suspected **bacterial infections** should be treated aggressively with broad-spectrum antibiotics, which are modified when culture results become available.

Fever may be one of the earliest signs of rejection of the transplanted liver, and patients experiencing an acute rejection episode may complain of flulike symptoms. Therefore, the workup of any fever must include a close examination of the patient's most recent liver function tests.

Liver transplantation patients do not appear to be more susceptible to common viral illnesses than other people. However, if the physical examination reveals oral or cutaneous lesions compatible with either **herpes simplex** or **herpes zoster,** the lesions should be cultured and acyclovir therapy instituted for at least 2 weeks. When the cause of the fever cannot be identified or the patient fails to respond to initial treatment, repeat cultures and serum titers for **cytomegalovirus** and **Epstein-Barr virus** should be obtained and compared to those obtained before transplantation to identify patients with acute viral infections. Biopsy specimens, especially of liver, skin, and lung, should be cultured and histologically examined for evidence of virus. Any patient with evidence of a severe viral infection should return to the transplantation center for treatment. Appropriate management includes careful reduction in the patient's immunosuppression and treatment with antiviral agents.

Opportunistic infections may occur in the posttransplant patient and require prompt diagnosis and treatment. *Pneumocystis carinii* **pneumonitis,** rare in the early posttransplantation period, most commonly presents between 3 and 6 months after surgery. In most patients, the presenting symptom is tachypnea. Physical examination and chest x-ray are usually normal initially, but arterial blood gases reveal moderate-to-severe hypoxemia. All patients with suspected pneumocystic pneumonia should be started on intravenous trimethoprim/sulfamethoxazole and undergo immediate bronchoscopy with bronchoalveolar lavage to confirm the diagnosis. A dramatic worsening of the pulmonary status commonly occurs after treatment is initiated, and the patient may require intubation and mechanical ventilation. Early diagnosis and treatment usually result in a relatively brief, limited illness, whereas failure to make the diagnosis expediently may prove fatal.

Other opportunistic infections include **Cryptococcal meningitis, coccidiomycosis, *Listeria* meningitis, and tuberculosis.**

Because a reduction in the dosage of immunosuppressive medications is essential, a transplant patient with a serious infection should return to the transplantation center for treatment of the infection. Too rapid or aggressive a reduction in the immunosuppressive regimen may put the patient at risk for acute rejection. Full immunosuppressive therapy should be reinstituted as soon as possible. If full immunosuppression is reinstituted before complete recovery, however, the infection may recur; on the other hand, failure to resume full immunosuppressive therapy at the appropriate time may lead to an acute rejection episode, which could result in loss of the transplanted liver.

3. **Rejection.** Despite advances in immunosuppression, rejection of the grafted liver is one of the most common indications for retransplantation. Acute rejection episodes may occur at any time after transplantation but become less frequent with time. Severe rejection episodes should be treated at the liver transplant center, but mild rejection episodes usually can be handled by the patient's physician in consultation with the transplant surgeons.

After transplantation, the follow-up of the patient may continue at the transplantation center or may be done by the patient's physician. Initially, routine blood work is performed three times per week, including a complete blood count with platelet count, electrolytes, blood urea nitrogen, creatinine, aspartate aminotransferase (AST), alanine aminotransferase (ALT), gamma-glutamyl transpeptidase (GGTP), alkaline phosphatase, total and direct bilirubin, and a cyclosporine trough level. If the patient remains stable, the frequency of routine blood work may be decreased to once or twice a month by 6 months after transplantation.

Most acute rejection episodes that occur in the late postoperative period are due to either too rapid a reduction in immunosuppressive drugs or a decreased cyclosporine level. The cyclosporine level depends on absorption from the small intestine and is affected by vomiting, diarrhea, and interaction with other drugs taken by the patient (e.g., phenytoin [Dilantin], ketoconazole, and rifampin). Gastroenteritis and diarrheal illnesses may be associated with a rapid fall in the patient's cyclosporine level and may result in a severe rejection episode. Therefore, these patients may require hospitalization for the administration of intravenous cyclosporine and corticosteroids until the gastrointestinal function returns to normal. Drug interactions that may affect cyclosporine levels also should be closely monitored. Patients with mild rejection episodes may be entirely asymptomatic or may have flulike symptoms. Such episodes are generally diagnosed by a slight elevation in any of the liver chemistry tests; after consultation with the transplant surgeons, they are usually treated with a single 500- to 1,000-mg bolus of methylprednisolone or with a short course (usually 5 days) of an increased dosage of oral prednisone. If the liver chemistry tests improve, nothing else may be required except a temporary increase in the frequency of laboratory tests.

Patients who fail to respond to steroid therapy or respond only temporarily should be returned to the transplant center for additional investigation and treatment of the suspected rejection episode. The workup includes a liver biopsy and an ultrasound study of the biliary tract to rule out obstruction, and Doppler ultrasound to ascertain the patency of the hepatic artery and portal vein. The liver biopsy may differentiate rejection from cholangitis, hepatitis, and ischemic injury, all of which may clinically mimic rejection. Because therapy for most of these disorders is vastly different from treatment of acute rejection, making an accurate and prompt diagnosis is essential.

Treatment of biopsy-confirmed rejection is initiated with a short course of high-dose steroids. Patients who fail to respond to this therapy are usually given a 10- to 14-day course of either antilymphocyte globulin or the monoclonal antibody OKT3. Repeat liver biopsy to confirm continued rejection and to rule out the other diagnoses should be performed if liver chemistry tests do not improve after a course of either of these drugs. Patients in whom rejection is confirmed should be treated with whichever therapy they have not yet received. Cytomegalovirus hepatitis may develop during the antirejection therapy. A liver biopsy is necessary to make this diagnosis so that appropriate antiviral therapy may be initiated.

If repeat biopsy reveals a severely damaged liver secondary to rejection, additional antirejection therapy is not administered, and the patient is considered at high priority for retransplantation. Retransplantation should be considered for any patient who continues to demonstrate severe liver dysfunction despite adequate therapy for rejection.

Chronic rejection, in contrast to acute rejection, often fails to respond to any form of antirejection therapy. It is a more indolent process, characterized by a gradual, progressive, and unrelenting rise in the patient's liver chemistry tests. This form of rejection may occur at any time after transplantation, and most of these patients eventually require retransplantation. Approximately 20% of all liver transplantation patients require retransplantation. The 1-year survival rate after retransplantation is approximately 50%.

D. Immunosuppression. Most transplant centers use similar immunosuppression protocols. The primary immunosuppressive agents currently used are cyclosporine and corticosteroids.

1. **Corticosteroids.** Adults receive 1,000 mg of methylprednisolone intravenously after revascularization of the donor liver. The dosage of methylprednisolone is tapered rapidly over the first 6 days by 40 mg/day until a baseline of 20 mg/day is reached. By day 6, most patients are able to tolerate oral medications, and prednisone 20 mg/day is begun. Most adult patients are discharged with this dosage of prednisone; depending on the frequency and severity of rejection episodes, the dosage is reduced in 2.5 mg increments in the first year until a baseline of 5 to 10 mg is reached in adult patients.

2. **Cyclosporine and tacrolimus** are the two agents used in combination with prednisone.

    a. **Cyclosporine** is given as a single dose (2 mg/kg IV) before the start of the transplantation procedure, and the next dose is given immediately postoperatively when the patient is in the intensive care unit. If urinary output is adequate, a dose of 2 mg/kg is administered q8h. The frequency of the cyclosporine dose of 2 mg/kg may be reduced to twice daily in patients with marginal urinary output or with prior evidence of renal dysfunction. Oral cyclosporine is initiated at a dosage of 10 mg/kg twice daily as soon as adequate gastrointestinal function has returned. When oral cyclosporine therapy is begun, the intravenous dose of cyclosporine is gradually reduced and eventually eliminated. All additional adjustments in dosage are based on daily cyclosporine trough levels. A cyclosporine level of 1,000 ng/dL by radioimmunoassay (RIA) is accepted as ideal. The intestinal absorption of cyclosporine tends to be erratic, and the maintenance of stable blood levels is sometimes difficult. The cyclosporine level is maintained at a level that is proportionately lower than 1,000 ng/dL if toxicity develops.

    In patients in whom cyclosporine is not well tolerated, it may be necessary to add azathioprine 1.5 to 2.5 mg/kg daily to ensure adequate immunosuppression. After a stable course of several months, the dosage of cyclosporine may be reduced gradually to obtain a blood level of 500 to 800 ng/dL by 1 year after transplantation. During the late postoperative period, it is difficult to predict how much the dosages of immunosuppressive medications can be lowered without causing an acute rejection episode. However, doses should be maintained at as low a level as possible because most side effects of immunosuppressive drugs are dose related. Except for the immunosuppressive regimen, which is usually managed indefinitely by the transplant surgeon, care is resumed by the referring physician when the patient returns home.

b. Side effects. The most common side effects directly related to cyclosporine are hypertension, nephrotoxicity, hepatotoxicity, hirsutism, gum hyperplasia, and a fine motor tremor.

 i. Hypertension. The hypertension may be quite severe initially but becomes less severe during the first year after transplantation. Often the referring physician is left with the task of gradually reducing the patient's antihypertensive medications during the first year after transplantation.

 ii. Nephrotoxicity. Some degree of nephrotoxicity is experienced by most patients taking cyclosporine, but in most cases it is not clinically significant. During the early postoperative period, some degree of nephrotoxicity is tolerated because the patient is most vulnerable to severe rejection episodes during this time. This nephrotoxicity is usually reversible when the dosage of cyclosporine is reduced. However, patients who require continued high dosages of cyclosporine because of repeated rejection episodes might have a significant deterioration in renal function after an otherwise successful liver transplantation. Azathioprine may be added as a third immunosuppressive drug in patients in whom severe nephrotoxicity develops so that the dosage of cyclosporine may be reduced. In most liver transplant patients, however, close monitoring of the patient's renal function and cyclosporine trough levels allows the cyclosporine dosage to be adjusted appropriately both to prevent rejection and to avoid significant toxicity without the addition of a third drug.

 iii. Hepatotoxicity is common when the patient's cyclosporine level is greater than 1,200 ng/dL; therefore, it is rarely seen in patients who take a lower dosage of cyclosporine.

 iv. Hirsutism, tremor, and gum hyperplasia. These side effects are less serious but may be indicative of overimmunosuppression. If clinically possible, the transplant surgeon may reduce the dose of the immunosuppressants. To prevent serious gum disease, all liver transplant patients should receive frequent dental examinations. Excessive hair growth may require the use of a depilatory, especially in young female patients with body and facial hair.

 Tacrolimus has similar pharmacologic properties as cyclosporine and gives similar patient and graft survival rates. It is available as 0.5 mg, 1 mg, and 5 mg capsules for oral use and as a solution 5 mg/mL for parenteral use. The principal side effects include nephrotoxicity and neurotoxicity, hypertension, hyperbulemia, hyperglycemia, and nausea, vomiting, and diarrhea.

 Patients receiving cyclosporine and tacrolimus may develop lymphoprolerative disorders.

3. Carcinogenesis. The incidence of cancer is significantly increased in immunosuppressed patients. The most common cancers are carcinoma of the cervix, vulva, perineum, shin, and lip; Kaposi's sarcoma; and non-Hodgkin's lymphoma. Most lymphomas appear to be related to infection with or reactivation of the Epstein-Barr virus. In most patients, the presenting problem is fever, lymphadenopathy, gastrointestinal perforation, obstruction, or hemorrhage. The treatment of these lymphomas is controversial. Some authorities believe that reduction of immunosuppression is sufficient, and others recommend chemotherapy or radiation therapy or both. All physicians involved in the long-term care of transplantation patients must be aware that these patients are at increased risk of the development of some cancers (especially lymphomas). Any patient suspected of having a lymphoma should be evaluated promptly and referred back to the transplant center.

E. Long-term management of the liver transplant patient. Adult patients' hospital stay for OLT is 7 to 14 days and children's 10 to 20 days. After discharge, patients are asked to remain near the transplant center for 2 to 6 weeks for intensive monitoring of liver function and immunosuppression. They are also monitored for the need for nutritional support, antibiotics, and/or antiviral therapy. Initially, outpatient visits occur twice weekly, then weekly for the first month, then less frequently. Laboratory tests are initially performed weekly, then monthly indefinitely. In the outpatient setting, patient's primary caregivers need to follow patient's symptoms, assess and encourage strict compliance with medications, perform physical exams and appropriate laboratory testing, including a chemistry panel, complete blood count, trough levels for cyclosporine, and tacrolimus at the indicated intervals. Patients should be referred to the transplant center if at any time rejection is suspected.

V. QUALITY OF LIFE. Even though a successful liver transplantation does not return a patient to "normal" but to a life of indefinite immunosuppression, the operation allows patients a chance for long-term survival and a much more productive lifestyle than they experienced during the late stages of their liver disease. Most patients are able to return to work in 3 to 6 months after OLT. Active physical fitness programs and psychotherapeutic support facilitate patients' return to normal daily activities.

Selected Readings
Alexander JW, et al. The influence of immunomodulatory diets on transplant success and complications. *Transplantation.* 2005;79:460–465.
Clavien PA, et al. Strategies for safer liver surgery and partial liver transplantation. *N Eng J Med.* 2007;356:1545–1550.
Di Bisceglie A. Pretransplant treatments for hepatocellular carcinoma: Do they improve outcomes? *Liver Transplantation.* 2005;11:510–513.
Fausto N, et al. Liver regeneration. *Hepatology.* 2006;43(suppl 1):S45–S53.
Lee J, et al. Transplantation trends in primary biliary cirrhosis. *Clin Gastroenterol Hepatol.* 2007;5(11):1313–1315.
Levy M, et al. The elderly liver transplant recipient: A call for caution. *Ann Surg.* 2001; 233:107.
Mantel HT, Heimbach JK, et al. Vascular complications after orthotopic liver transplantation following neoadjuvant therapy for hilar cholangiocarcinoma. *Liver Transpl.* 2006;82.
Middleton PF, et al. Living donor liver transplantation—adjust donor outcomes: a systematic review. *Liver Transpl.* 2006;12:24–30.
Pomfret EA, et al. Liver and intestine transplantation in the United States. *Am J Transpl.* 2007;7:1376–1389. ′
Tan HP, et al. Adult living donor liver transplantation: Who are the ideal donor and recipient: *J Hepatol.* 2005;43:13–17.
Tillman HL. Successful orthotopic liver transplantation. *Gastroenterology.* 2001;120:1561.
VanThiel D, et al. Liver transplantation: What the non-hepatologist should know. *Pract Gastroenterol.* 2001;25(4):46.

ANOREXIA NERVOSA AND BULIMIA NERVOSA

59

*A*norexia nervosa and bulimia nervosa are eating disorders that are distinct but related syndromes that have in common an intense preoccupation with food. Patients with anorexia nervosa are characterized by a fear of becoming obese, disturbance in body image, anorexia, extreme weight loss, and amenorrhea. On the other hand, bulimia is characterized by periods of binge eating, alternating with fasting; self-induced vomiting; and the use of diuretics and cathartics. Bulimic behavior is seen in some patients with anorexia.

I. **EPIDEMIOLOGY.** Eating disorders affect an estimated 5 million Americans every year. It is estimated that about 6% to 10% of all young women have an eating disorder. Eating disorders typically run in adolescent girls or young women; however, 5% to 15% of cases of anorexia and bulimia nervosa occur in young boys and men. The age of onset most commonly is the teenage years, but these diseases also occur in young children and in older adults (e.g., after age 40).

II. **ETIOLOGY.** The cause of these disorders has been attributed in part to the great emphasis our society places on thinness. However, the disorders are caused by a combination of genetic, neurochemical, psychological, and sociocultural factors.

Despite profound weight loss, patients with anorexia usually regard themselves as being too fat. They may be reluctant to admit this and, in fact, often agree to increase their food intake when prompted by relatives and friends. However, they typically continue to avoid food, indulge in excessive physical exercise, and consume medications to inhibit appetite and promote diuresis and catharsis. Emotionally, the anorectic patient tends to be isolated and shuns relationships, whereas the bulimic patient is likely to be outgoing and sociable. Weight may fluctuate in bulimics because of the alternate food binging and purging, but the low points in weight usually do not reach the point of dangerous weight loss that sometimes occurs in anorectics.

III. **COMPLICATIONS AND CONSEQUENCES.** Starvation is the most serious complication of anorexia nervosa. Mortality in excess of 5% has been estimated, but this figure may reflect the experience in large referral centers that deal with the most severe cases. Amenorrhea is common, and other organ system abnormalities may develop (Table 59-1). Particularly worrisome are the cardiac arrhythmias, diuretic-induced changes in electrolytes, and complications of vomiting, such as gastric and esophageal rupture and aspiration pneumonia.

IV. **CLINICAL PRESENTATION.** The diagnosis of anorexia nervosa or bulimia should be considered when a young woman has had severe weight loss but denies that anything is wrong. A preoccupation with weight and food, distortion of body image, or any of the characteristics mentioned previously strengthens the suspicion.

The physical examination often is normal, unless a serious complication, such as cardiac arrhythmia or aspiration pneumonia, has developed. Patients with anorexia nervosa characteristically are thin or even emaciated, whereas bulimics range from underweight to overweight.

473

| TABLE 59-1 | Medical Complications of Anorexia Nervosa and Bulimia Nervosa |

Organ system	Complication
General	Dry skin and hair, hair loss, altered temperature regulations
Cardiovascular	Hypotension, abnormal electrocardiogram: bradycardia, low voltage, prolonged Q interval, arrhythmias, mitral valve prolapse, cardiomyopathy
Renal	Edema, decreased glomerular filtration rate, increased blood urea nitrogen level, renal calculi
Endocrine/Metabolic	Electrolyte abnormalities, hypoglycemia, hypomagnesemia, hyperphosphatemia, euthyroid sick syndrome, delay in puberty, menorrhea, infertility, decreased estradiol and testosterone, lipid abnormalities, osteoporosis
Gastrointestinal	Constipation, rectal prolapse, decreased intestinal motility, esophagitis, Mallory-Weiss tear, gastric dilatation, delayed emptying, elevated liver enzymes, elevated amylase level
Hematologic	Anemia, leukopenia, thrombocytopenia, elevated prothrombin time
Pulmonary	Aspiration pneumonia
Neurologic	Peripheral neuropathy

V. DIFFERENTIAL DIAGNOSIS. Clearly, other disorders that cause anorexia, weight loss, or vomiting must be considered. Crohn's disease, which typically begins in adolescence or young adulthood, can present with many of the signs and symptoms of anorexia nervosa. Malabsorption syndromes (see Chapter 31) also can cause profound weight loss and diarrhea (steatorrhea). Neoplasia, unusual in the age group under consideration, may also be considered. Finally, metabolic, endocrinologic, cardiovascular, renal, pulmonary, and hematologic disorders must be considered when appropriate. The complications of anorexia nervosa or bulimia may mimic those conditions.

VI. Diagnostic studies are performed in patients suspected of having anorexia nervosa or bulimia for two reasons: to document the severity and complications of the disease and to exclude other disorders. Thus a complete blood count, serum electrolytes, serum proteins, liver tests, and renal function tests should be obtained. Examination of the entire gastrointestinal tract by sigmoidoscopy, barium enema or colonoscopy, and barium swallow–upper gastrointestinal– small-bowel x-ray series may be done. If vomiting persists, upper gastrointestinal endoscopy and esophageal motility testing are appropriate in most patients because of the high frequency of Crohn's disease, gastrointestinal motility disorders, and other conditions in patients originally thought to have anorexia nervosa. Studies for the evaluation of diarrhea or malabsorption may be indicated in some patients.

VII. TREATMENT. Typically, anorectic patients deny the severity of their illness and evade adequate psychiatric and medical care or fail to comply with the treatment regimen. Bulimic patients are more motivated to seek treatment but do not tolerate therapeutic regimens that fail to give immediate relief of symptoms.

Treatment includes improvement of medical and nutritional status, reestablishment of healthful patterns of eating, and identification and resolution of psychosocial precipitants of the disorder. Most patients are treated on an outpatient basis; however, some patients may require inpatient medical and psychiatric care. Rapid weight loss, intractable purging, severe electrolyte imbalances, cardiac disturbances, and a high suicide risk are some of the indications for inpatient care.

A. Restoring adequate nutrition is essential to effective treatment. This may be accomplished on an outpatient basis in some instances, but hospitalization may be necessary. Some patients respond to a system of goals and rewards, that is, setting goals in terms of food intake each day and rewarding success with privileges. Malnutrition and protein deficiency may be associated with impairment of pancreatic exocrine function and mucosal lactase deficiency. Thus, initial oral feedings may result in diarrhea and failure to respond unless lactose is omitted and food is administered in small amounts. Severely malnourished patients may require enteral or parenteral nutrition, with special attention to correction of electrolyte and metabolic disorders. Vitamin supplementation should be provided as well as calcium 1,000 to 1,500 mg and vitamin D 400 IU per day to prevent osteopenia and osteoporosis.

B. Psychiatric therapy and pharmacotherapy. Several psychiatric methods have been used, including individual psychotherapy, group therapy, and family therapy. Psychodynamic psychotherapy with concomitant use of behavioral strategies to control symptoms has been found to be effective. Education of the patient's family and enlisting their support in the treatment increases the chances of success. Psychopharmacologic therapy is moderately effective in treating bulimia nervosa, less so anorexia nervosa. The most effective and studied drugs are the serotonin reuptake inhibitors (SSRIs), such as fluoxetine hydrochloride (Prozac) 20 to 80 mg per day, and sertraline hydrochloride (Zoloft) 20 to 80 mg per day. Desipramine hydrochloride 50 to 300 mg per day has also been beneficial; however, it is contraindicated for patients with Q-T interval prolongation and for those taking other tricyclic antidepressants.

Selected Readings

Becker AE, et al. Eating disorders. *N Engl J Med.* 1999;340:1092.

Gard ME, et al. The dismantling of a myth: A review of eating disorder and socioeconomic status. *Int J Eat Disord.* 1996;20:1.

Kohn MR, et al. Cardiac arrest and delirium: Presentations of the refeeding syndrome in severely malnourished adolescents with anorexia nervosa. *J Adolesc Health.* 1998;22:239.

Pike KM, et al. Ethnicity and eating disorders. *Psychopharmacol Bull.* 1996;32:265.

Vitiello B, et al. Research on eating disorders: Current status and future of prospects. *Biol Psychiatry.* 2000;47:777.

Walsh BT, et al. Medication and psychotherapy in the treatment of bulimia nervosa. *Am J Psychiatry.* 1997;154:523.

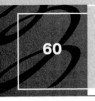

60 OBESITY

I. EPIDEMIOLOGY. Obesity has become an epidemic throughout the world, even in the Third World countries. In the United States it is estimated that three of five American adults are overweight or obese and the cost of obesity is in excess of $100 billion annually. In the last 35 years, the prevalence of obesity has more than doubled in the United States. The prevalence of obesity is particularly high in many ethnic minority women (e.g., African American, Mexican American, Native American, Pacific Islander American, Puerto Rican, and Cuban American). Obesity, in fact, is equal to tobacco use as a public health hazard, contributing to more than 500,000 premature deaths annually and is associated with a twofold increase in mortality. Obesity is a major health problem in young adults and children. In minority populations, up to 30% to 40% of the children and adolescents are overweight.

II. DEFINITION. *Obesity* is defined as a complex multifactorial chronic disease that develops from an interaction of genotype and environment. The type of fat accumulated and the site where the fat is deposited has different health implications and require different approaches to management. The precise amount of body fat mass that causes medical complications depends on patient's gender, body fat distribution, and weight (fat) gain since early adulthood, level of fitness and genetic factors.

  A. Body mass index. Table 60-1 represents the relationship between weight and height. Body mass index (BMI) is calculated as weight in kilograms divided by height in square meters or as weight in pounds multiplied by 704.5 and divided by height in square inches. The National Institutes of Health has issued guidelines for the classification of weight status by BMI that separates patients by risk: Those with a BMI of 25.0 to 29.9 kg/m^2 are considered **overweight;** those with a BMI more than 30 kg/m^2 are considered **obese.** Extreme obesity is defined as a BMI more than 40 kg/m^2 and carries a much higher risk for morbidity and mortality. The optimal BMI to minimize the consequences of obesity-related diseases is probably in the range of 19 to 21 kg/m^2 for women and 20 to 22 kg/m^2 for men. It is reported that American adults, especially women, who weigh 15% less than their age-matched, normal-weight peers have a significant reduction in projected mortality. Additional factors such as fat distribution and recent weight gain also modify the risk within each BMI category. Persons with increased abdominal fat have increased risk for hypertension, ischemic heart disease, dyslipidemia, diabetes mellitus, and insulin resistance syndrome over those with increased gluteal and femoral fat.

  Weight gain during adulthood is an additional risk factor for medical complications. Weight gain of 75 kg in body weight since the age of 12 to 20 years increases the relative risk for cholelithiasis, diabetes mellitus, hypertension, and ischemic heart disease.

  B. Waist circumference correlates adequately with abdominal fat distribution. Deposition of fat in the abdomen, particularly if it is out of proportion to fat distribution elsewhere in the body, represents a health risk for morbidity and mortality that is independent of being overweight or obese. Measuring waist circumference, best taken at the level of the umbilicus with the patient in the supine position, is a reasonable method for assessing a patient's health risk and monitoring weight-reduction interventions (Table 60-2).

TABLE 60-1 Body Mass Index

BMI =	19	20	21	22	23	24	25	26	27	28	29	30	31	32	33	34	35
Height (in.)								Body Weight (lb)									
58	91	96	100	105	110	115	119	124	129	134	138	143	148	153	158	162	167
59	94	99	104	109	114	119	124	128	133	138	143	148	153	158	163	168	173
60	97	102	107	112	118	123	128	133	138	143	148	153	158	163	168	174	179
61	100	106	111	116	122	127	132	137	143	148	153	158	164	169	174	180	185
62	104	109	115	120	126	131	136	142	147	153	158	164	169	175	180	186	191
63	107	113	118	124	130	135	141	146	152	158	163	169	175	180	186	191	197
64	110	116	122	128	134	140	145	151	157	163	169	174	180	186	192	197	204
65	114	120	126	132	138	144	150	156	162	168	174	180	186	192	198	204	210
66	118	124	130	136	142	148	155	161	167	173	179	186	192	198	204	210	216
67	121	127	134	140	146	153	159	166	172	178	185	191	198	204	211	217	223
68	125	131	138	144	151	158	164	170	177	184	190	197	203	210	216	223	230
69	128	135	142	149	155	162	169	176	182	189	196	203	209	216	223	230	236
70	132	139	146	153	160	167	174	181	188	195	202	209	216	222	229	236	243
71	136	143	150	157	165	172	179	186	193	200	208	215	222	229	236	243	250
72	140	147	154	162	169	177	184	191	199	206	213	221	228	235	242	250	258
73	144	151	159	166	174	182	189	197	204	212	219	227	235	242	250	257	265
74	148	155	163	171	179	184	194	202	210	218	225	233	241	249	256	264	272
75	152	160	168	176	184	189	200	208	216	224	232	240	248	256	264	272	279
76	156	164	172	180	189	193	205	213	221	230	238	246	254	263	271	279	287
77	160	168	177	185	193	202	210	219	227	235	244	252	261	269	278	286	294
78	164	173	181	190	198	207	216	224	233	232	250	259	268	276	285	293	302

To obtain the BMI, locate height on the left, then move across the line to the weight; the BMI will be on the top. BMI, body mass index.

TABLE 60-2	Weight-Associated Disease Risk	

Weight class	Body mass index (kg/m²)	Waist circumference women >88 cm or 35 in. Men >102 cm or 40 in.
Extreme obesity	>40	Extremely high risk
Obesity II	>35.0–39.9	Very high risk
Obesity I	>30.0–34.9	High risk
Overweight	>25.0–29.9	Increased risk
Normal	18.0–24.9	Increased risk
Underweight	<18.5	Increased risk

    C. Waist-to-hip ratio (WHR) is another measurement that may be helpful in assessing the risk of morbidity and mortality in relation to excess weight. The waist circumference is measured at the level of the umbilicus with the patient in the supine position and the hip circumference should be measured at the maximal girth around the buttocks. The WHR is calculated as:

WHR = waist circumference (cm or in)/hip circumference (cm or in)

    A WHR of more than 0.95 for males and more than 0.80 for females is associated with an increased risk of morbidity and mortality.

III. PATHOGENESIS. Both genetic and environmental factors contribute to body size. Genetic background can explain up to 40% of the variance in body mass in humans. However, the marked increase in the prevalence of obesity in the last 20 years cannot be attributed to genetic change and may be caused by alterations in the environment, such as sleep deprivation, increased stress at work and home, lack of regular meal times, and choices of foods, i.e., fast food versus mediterranian-type diet.

    Simplistically, obesity originates from ingesting more energy and calories than is expended over a long period of time. The excess ingested calories are stored as fat. Even small, but persistent differences between energy intake and energy expenditure can lead to large increases in body fat. For example, ingestion of only 5% more calories than expended could result in the accumulation of about 5 kg of adipose tissue in one year. Ingestion of 7 kcal/day more than expended over 30 years can lead to an increase of 10 kg body weight, which is the average amount of weight gained by American adults from 25 to 55 years of age.

    Technological advances have led to changes in lifestyle that favor a positive energy balance due to an increased availability and palatability of inexpensive energy-dense foods, decreased daily physical activity because of labor-saving devices, changes in job-work patterns, and accessibility to mechanical transportation. Persons with certain genetic backgrounds are particularly predisposed to weight gain when they are exposed to this "modern" lifestyle. For example, Pima Indians living in reservations in Arizona have a much greater prevalence of obesity and diabetes mellitus than their genetic counterparts who live in rural areas of Mexico.

    The modern American diet of fast food and beverages are high in fat and calories and low in nutritional value. An estimated 60% to 90% of Americans are undernourished meaning that despite excessive caloric intake, they do not meet their daily recommended dietary allowances (RDAs) in one or more food groups. In addition to increased caloric intake, only about 9% of men and 3% of women exercise vigorously on a regular basis as part of their leisure time activities.

IV. MEDICAL COMPLICATIONS ASSOCIATED WITH OBESITY. Obesity is a significant risk factor for many medical diseases, impaired quality of life, and premature

TABLE 60-3	Obesity-Associated Medical Complications
Cardiovascular	Hypertension, congestive heart failure, pulmonary hypertension, coronary artery disease, arrhythmia, ischemic stroke, venous stasis, deep vein thrombosis, pulmonary embolism
Pulmonary	Pulmonary hypertension, sleep apnea, obesity-hypoventilation syndrome
Gastrointestinal	Ventral hernia, gastroesophageal reflux, gallstone, steatohepatitis
Musculoskeletal	Osteoarthritis, lower-back problem, gout
Endocrine-metabolic	Diabetes mellitus, insulin resistance, dyslipoproteinemia (hypertriglyceridemia, hypercholesterolemia)
Genitourinary	Menstrual dysfunction, infertility, complication of pregnancy, urinary stress incontinence
Postoperative risk	Deep vein thrombosis, pulmonary embolism, atelectasis, and pneumonia
Cancer	Breast, uterus, prostate, colon, gallbladder, cervix
Psychiatric	Social stigmatization, psychoemotional disorder

death (Table 60-3). In addition, obese individuals experience depression, frustration, insecurity, and other negative feelings because of the way society reacts to them and the way they feel about themselves.

V. THERAPY

A. General principles. Table 60-4 lists the key principles involved in the therapy of obesity. Americans spend in excess of $70 billion a year on commercial weight-loss products. Most persons lose weight on these diets, but unfortunately within 1 to 5 years the weight is gained back with extra pounds.

Obesity is a chronic illness and requires long-term management for long-term success. Behavior modification is necessary for long-term lifestyle changes. Dietary and nutritional education is also very important. Patients should be encouraged to lose weight in a systemic and modest way through increased insulin sensitivity, decreased blood pressure and blood lipid levels, and reduction of fatty infiltration of the liver.

Caloric reduction needs to be individualized based on the individual's age and comorbid risk factors. A useful formula for losing about a pound a week is as follows:

Current weight in pounds × 13 kcal − 500 kcal = daily caloric requirement

Reduction of fat intake is essential in a successful weight-reduction program. Many patients will do well by reducing their total dietary fat intake to 10% to 20% of their total caloric intake (about 20–30 g of total dietary fat daily). Most commercial weight loss programs limit caloric intake to 800 to 1,200 calories a day. When followed carefully, these programs will induce a weight loss of 0.5 to 2.0 lbs a week for up to 30 weeks.

TABLE 60-4	Principles of Weight Reduction and Maintenance

1. Long-term weight loss and management	4. Behavior modification
2. Gradual and modest weight loss in increments	5. Physical activity
	6. Pharmacotherapy
3. Nutrition education	7. Surgery

Many **"fad diets"** have little merit. Some of these diets may be actually harmful. For example, avoiding carbohydrates will induce ketosis; excessively high protein intake may adversely affect the kidneys and accelerate calcium loss from bones, thereby promoting or enhancing osteoporosis. In addition, reduced caloric intake may lead to micronutrient deficiencies that impair metabolic fitness.

The assistance of a **dietitian** is very important. The National Registry of Dietitians may be contacted for recommendations of a dietitian in patients' living areas (telephone: 1-800-366-1655). Diet advice should include encouraging patients to eat three meals a day, avoid snacking between meals, avoid energy-dense and high-fat foods, and increase the intake of fruits and vegetables.

Physical activity is important for long-term weight management and improved health. Physical activity should be increased slowly over time. Studies suggest that about 80 minutes per day of moderate-intensity exercise (e.g., brisk walking or 35 minutes per day of vigorous activity such as fast bicycling or aerobic exercise) is needed for long-term weight maintenance after initial weight loss has been achieved. Physical activity does not necessarily have to be part of a structured exercise program. Increasing daily lifestyle activities is just as effective in maintaining weight loss as participating in an aerobic program exercise.

Recent data indicate that weight-resistance training appears to be the most beneficial form of exercise for successful weight management. By improving the integrity of existing muscle or by developing muscle mass, this type of exercise increases overall metabolism and enhances the oxidation of fat as fuel. These effects make long-term weight control far more likely.

B. **Very-low-calorie diets (VLCDs) or protein-sparing diets** are proven, safe alternatives to starvation for significant sustained and progressive weight loss. These diets deliver a total daily caloric intake of 400 to 800 calories. Successful and safe programs include a daily intake of 0.8 to 1.0 g of protein per kilogram of desirable body weight or about 70 to 100 g of protein and at least 45 to 50 g of carbohydrate to minimize nitrogen losses and ketosis, respectively. All VLCDs require careful physician supervision and close patient monitoring. Generally, weight loss is rapid and progressive for several weeks to months. After about 6 months, weight loss slows and plateaus and further weight loss becomes difficult to achieve. Unfortunately, once the VLCD is discontinued, initial weight-loss maintenance is also difficult to sustain. Incorporation of regular exercise and lifestyle changes improve the likelihood of sustaining the weight loss. Intermittent use of VLCD products or meal substitutions along with restrained eating patterns offers considerable promise.

C. **Pharmacotherapy.** It is extremely difficult to achieve and sustain significant reductions in weight and body fat in obese patients without pharmacotherapy or VLCDs. Pharmacotherapy can help selected patients maintain long-term weight loss, but it should not be considered a short-term treatment approach. Obesity is a chronic disease and patients who respond to drug therapy usually regain weight when the drug therapy is stopped. Also, the effectiveness of pharmacotherapy may diminish with time. It is of paramount importance that pharmacotherapy be coupled with dietary, lifestyle, and behavioral changes.

1. **Sibutramine hydrochloride maleate (Meridia)** is a relatively new drug that was approved by the U.S. Food and Drug Administration (FDA) for long-term use in 1997. It is a monoamine reuptake inhibitor that was initially developed as an antidepressant to prevent the reuptake of serotonin, dopamine, and norepinephrine; thus, it synergistically promotes enhanced satiety and a reduction in food intake. In most patients, it induces a dose-dependent reduction in weight. The drug is available in capsule form in once-daily doses of 5, 10, and 15 mg. In one study, at 1 year, 39% of patients randomized to sibutramine hydrochloride maleate (15 mg per day) lost 70% of their initial body weight compared to 9% of those randomized to receive placebo. Based on clinical trials, it appears to be safe. With long-term use, parallel to the weight loss, successful reduction in obesity associated comorbid conditions has also been observed.

The most common side effects associated with sibutramine hydrochloride maleate therapy are dry mouth, headache, constipation, and insomnia. These were usually mild and transient. Small increases in systolic rate (1–3 mmHg) and heart rate (4–5 beats per minute) occur in some patients. However, in a very small percentage of patients, greater increases in blood pressure and pulse may occur and reduction of dose or discontinuation of the drug may be necessary.

2. **Orlistat (Xenical)** was approved by the FDA in 1999 for control of obesity. Orlistat inhibits gastric and pancreatic lipases and impedes the hydrolysis of dietary triglycerides into fatty acids; consequently, a significant portion of dietary fat is not absorbed and passes undigested through the small intestine to the colon for elimination in stool. In clinical trials of Orlistat given in dosages of 120 mg t.i.d. with meals, at 1 year, 40% of the patients had lost more than 10% of their initial body weight compared with 20% of patients receiving placebo. Thus, Orlistat was noted to be effective in inducing weight loss and reducing abdominal adiposity regardless of meal composition. The drug does not ameliorate hunger or enhance satiety. The side effects include abdominal cramping, loose stools, and flatulence; however, with a high dietary fat intake, reducing fat intake to less than 60 g a day eliminates most of these gastrointestinal (GI) side effects. A slight decrease in plasma concentration of fat-soluble vitamins A and D and B-carotene was observed, but their levels remained in the normal range. Orlistat is contraindicated in patients with chronic malabsorption or cholestasis. Orlistat is currently available as an over-the-counter medicine **(Alli)** as 60 mg tablets to be taken per 2 tablets t.i.d.

3. **Olestra** is a fat substitute that consists of six to eight fatty acids esterified to a sucrose molecule. Olestra resembles fat (butter) in texture and taste, but it is not hydrolyzed by the lipolytic enzymes of the GI tract and is excreted unchanged with stool. It is commercially used in the production of potato chips and is also marketed as a butter substitute; thus, the drug may help patients reduce their fat intake by satisfying the taste for butter or fat.

D. **Surgery (bariatric surgery)** is the most effective approach for achieving weight loss in extremely obese patients (BMI >40 kg/m^2) or patients with a BMI of 35 to 40 kg/m^2 and obesity-related diseases who are unlikely to lose weight with nonsurgical therapy. Patients need to be well enough to have acceptable surgical risks and are able to comply with long-term follow-up treatment.

The **goal of bariatric surgery** is to either reduce the size or bypass the stomach and part of the small intestine (SI) to enhance satiety and create malabsorption.

1. **Surgical procedures.** There are three main categories of bariatric surgery:

   a. **Restrictive surgery** involves changing the GI anatomy to limit food intake with no interference to the absorptive process (i.e., **gastric stapling, vertical banded gastroplasty (VBG), Silastic ring gastroplasty, horizontal gastroplasty, gastric banding,** and **adjustable silicone gastric band).**

   b. **Malabsorptive surgery** involves changes in GI anatomy to impair the absorption of calories and nutrients (i.e., **biliopancreatic diversion with** or **without duodenal switch (BPC) and jejunoileal bypass** [no longer performed due to causing cirrhosis of the liver]).

   c. **Combined restrictive and malabsorptive surgery** involves changes in GI anatomy to limit food intake as well as impair absorption of calories and nutrients (i.e., **Roux-en-Y gastric bypass, transected vertical gastric bypass, distal Roux-en-Y gastric bypass,** and **intestinal bypass).**

   The most commonly used bariatric surgery types are **gastric banding** and **gastric bypass operation.** Laparoscopic approach has become the preferred method.

2. **Surgery types**

   a. **Gastric bypass** involves the stapling of the upper stomach into a vertical or horizontal 15- to 25-mL pouch and creating an outlet to the SI. Surgery is reversible and can be performed laparoscopically or with the open approach. The gastric outlet joins with the limb of the SI containing bile and pancreatic juice. The standard SI Roux limb is 75 cm long, the SI limb is 150 cm, and distal gastric bypass is >150 cm. Weight loss occurs due to early satiety from the small gastric size and induction of mild malabsorption. If weight loss is not satisfactory the standard Roux gastric bypass can be revised to a very long limb Roux-en-Y procedure.

b. Laparoscopic mini-gastric bypass (LMGB) is a modification of gastric bypass with a longer lesser curvature tube.

c. Gastric banding or laparoscopic adjustable gastric banding (LABG) is usually performed laparoscopically. It involves placement of a "band" high on the stomach creating a pouch of 15-mL capacity without cutting the stomach. Adjustments are made up to six times per year to limit gastric capacity.

LABG is reversible by the removal of the band, tubing and port or it can be revised by removal of the device and performance of a restrictive-malabsorptive or malabsorptive procedure.

d. Vertical banded gastroplasty (VBG) is usually performed using an open surgical approach and involves the creation of a small 15-to 25-mL linear gastric pouch along the lesser curve of the stomach with an outlet of 0.75 to 1.25 cm in diameter. This procedure may be revised by the removal of the ring or the band allowing the outlet to dilate. In patients with inadequate weight loss, VGB may be revised by conversion to gastric bypass or duodenal switch.

3. Results

a. Benefits. Weight loss is greater with gastric bypass (about 70 kg vs. 30 kg in 12 months) than with gastroplasty or gastric banding procedures. Postoperatively, patients experience prolonged satiety and have improved well-being, attractiveness, self-regard, and social or physical activity. There is a significant reduction in the incidence of diabetes, hyperlipidemia, hyperuricemia, sleep apnea, hypertension, and mortality rate. In addition, there are significant risk reductions for developing cardiovascular, malignant, endocrine, infectious, psychiatric, and mental disorders.

b. Complications. Short-term complications are those expected as in any postoperative period.

Long-term complications may include anastomotic ulceration, bleeding, stenosis, and possible increase in certain GI symptoms such as diarrhea. Deficiencies in certain vitamins and nutrients and neurologic and psychiatric complications may occur. Patients should be monitored for vitamin and nutrient deficiencies and should be placed on replacement therapies as needed.

Selected Readings

Balasekasan R, et al. Positive results in tests for steatorrhea in person consuming olestra potato chips. *Am Intern Med.* 2000;132:279.

Bardia A, et al. Diagnosis of obesity by primary care physicians and impact on obesity management. *Mayo Clin Prac.* 2007;82(8):927–932.

Bloomberg RD, et al. Nutritional deficiencies following bariatric surgery: What have we learned? *Obes Surg.* 2005;15(2):145–154.

Buchwald H, et al. Bariatric surgery: A systematic review and meta-analysis. *JAMA.* 2004; 292(14):1724–1737.

Choban PS, Dickerson RN. Morbid obesity and nutrition support: is bigger different? *Nutr Clin Pract.* 2005;20:480–487.

Christou NV, et al. Surgery decreases long-term mortality, morbidity and health care use in morbidly obese patients. *Ann Surg.* 2004;240(3):416–423.

DeMaria EJ. Bariatric surgery for morbid obesity. *N Eng J Med.* 2007;356:2176–2183.

Dixon AF, et al. Laparoscopic adjustable gastric banding induces prolonged satiety: A randomized blind crossover study. *J Clin Endocrinol Metab.* 2005;90(2):813–819.

Flum DR, et al. Impact of gastric bypass on survival: A population-based analysis. *J Am Coll Surg.* 2004;199(4):543–551.

Inabnet WB, et al. Laparoscopic Roux-en-Y gastric bypass in patients with BMI <50: A prospective randomized trial comparing short and long limb lengths. *Obes Surg.* 2005;15(1):51–57.

Koffman BM, et al. Neurologic complications after surgery for obesity. *Muscle Nerve.* June 22, 2005 (Epub ahead of print).

Kruger J, et al. Attempting to lose weight: specific practices among adults. *Am J Prev Med.* 2004;26:402–406.

Lee WJ, et al. Laparoscopic vertical banded gastroplasty and laparoscopic gastric bypass: A comparison. *Obes Surg.* 2004;14(5):626–634.

Lujan JA, et al. Laparoscopic versus open gastric bypass in the treatment of morbid obesity: A randomized study. *Ann Surg.* 2004;239(4):433–437.

Madan A. Laparoscopic bariatric surgery. *US Gastroneterol Rev.* 2007;1:29–331.

Maggard MA, et al. Meta-analysis: Surgical treatment of obesity. *Ann Intern Med.* 2005;142(7):547–559.

Malone AM. Permissive underfeeding: Its appropriateness in patients with obesity, patients on parenateral nutrition, and non-obese patients receiving enteral nutrition. *Curr Gastroenterol Rep.* 2007;9(4):317–322.

Padwal RS, et al. Drug treatments for obesity: orlistat, sibutramine, and rimonabant. *Lancet.* 2007:369:71–77.

Perrin EM. Preventing and treating obesity: pediatricians' self-efficacy, barriers, resources, and advocacy. *Ambul Pediatr.* 2005;5:150–156.

Redinges RN. The pathophysiology of obesity and its clinical manifestations. *Gastroenteric Hepatol.* 2007;3(11):856–874.

Sjostrom L, et al. Lifestyle, diabetes, and cardiovascular risk factors 10 years after bariatric surgery. *N Engl J Med.* 2004;351(26):2683–2693.

Slater GH, et al. Serum fat-soluble vitamin deficiency and abnormal calcium metabolism after malabsorptive bariatric surgery. *J Gastrointest Surg.* 2004;8(1):48–55.

Wang W, et al. Short-term results of laparoscopic mini-gastric bypass. *Obes Surg.* 2005; 15(5):648–654.

Yan LL, et al. Midlife body mass index and hospitalization and mortality in older age. *JAMA.* 2006;295:190–1989.

INDEX

Page numbers followed by "f" indicate figures; those followed by "t" indicate tables.